CARDIOLOGY RESEARCH AND CLINICAL DEVELOPMENTS

PERSPECTIVES IN AORTIC VALVE DISEASE

CLINICAL AND MORPHOLOGICAL CHARACTERISTICS, DIAGNOSIS AND TREATMENTS

CARDIOLOGY RESEARCH AND CLINICAL DEVELOPMENTS

Additional books and e-books in this series can be found on Nova's website under the Series tab.

CARDIOLOGY RESEARCH AND CLINICAL DEVELOPMENTS

PERSPECTIVES IN AORTIC VALVE DISEASE

CLINICAL AND MORPHOLOGICAL CHARACTERISTICS, DIAGNOSIS AND TREATMENTS

GIOVANNI CONCISTRÈ
EDITOR

nova
Medicine & Health
New York

Library of Congress Cataloging-in-Publication Data

ISBN: 978-1-53618-769-4

Published by Nova Science Publishers, Inc. † New York

to my father

CONTENTS

FOREWORD

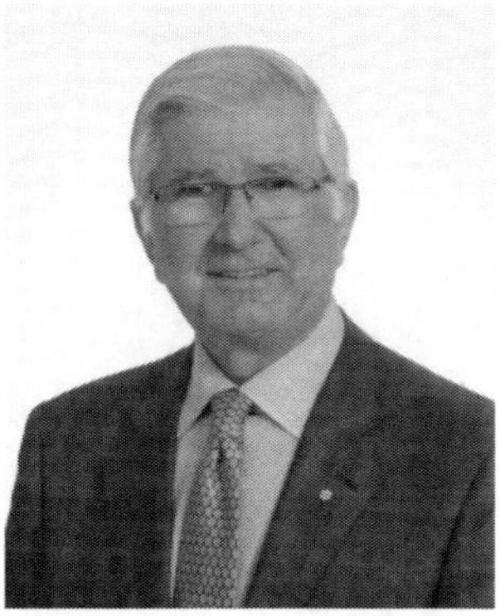

I enjoyed reading this monograph on aortic valve diseases. Giovanni Concistrè and colleagues from Italy put a lot of thought in producing *Perspectives in Aortic Valve Disease*, hundreds of pages of detailed description of practically all aortic valve themes from basic sciences to the latest modalities of treatment, all well documented with pertinent and current references. It is often difficult to compile a multi-author textbook and maintain the standard in breadth and depth in its various sections, but our Italian colleagues delivered excellence in each of the 21 chapters. Medical students, cardiac surgical trainees and practicing cardiac surgeons and cardiologists will enrich their knowledge in aortic valve disorders by spending the hours required to read the entire monograph. By the end, they will feel that the time was well spent and they know more about this topic than ever before. I read it during the Covid-19 pandemic and I encourage you to read too. It is not a Shakespearean piece but it is a very good didactic book.

Aortic valve diseases have become an important subject for cardiologists and surgeons. This is due to a multitude of factors such as an increase in the median age of the population in Western countries with a consequent increase in the incidence of calcific aortic stenosis, older people who want to remain physically active, better diagnostic and operative techniques to treat congenital and acquired disorders sporadic or associated with genetic syndromes, and the development of transcatheter therapies to treat aortic valve disease. The book describes how aortic valve disorders are dealt at the present but undoubtedly it will continue to evolve. Reading Concistrè's work will bring you up to speed and will prepare you to understand what is yet to come in managing patients with aortic valve diseases.

Tirone David, MD

PREFACE

The aortic valve is located at the center of the heart and is the core of the cardiac anatomy. The disease of this valve is an important cause of morbidity worldwide. Rheumatic heart disease is the most common cause of both aortic stenosis (AS) and aortic regurgitation (AR) in developing countries, while fibro-calcific degeneration and conditions causing aortic root dilation are the leading causes of AS and AR, respectively, in industrialized countries. A careful search for signs and symptoms may provide the first clues to the presence of aortic valve disease, which can then be verified and characterized by imaging techniques, starting from transthoracic echocardiography. In patients with known aortic valve disease, identification of disease grade and prompt detection of symptom onset are crucial to refer them to pharmacological therapy or aortic valve surgery or transcatether technology. Furthermore, a correct interpretation of the signs and symptoms of acute AR can result in a rapid diagnostic workup and prompt patient referral to surgery. In the history of cardiac surgery, the aortic valve prosthesis was the first target of the cardiac surgery, which was performed by Dr. Hufnagel at Georgetown University, Washington DC, in 1952. Since then, aortic valve surgery has led the field of cardiac surgery. Many prosthetic heart valves have been developed to replace defective valves, and numerous surgical procedures have been created to deal with the complexities of aortic valve surgery. Aortic valve surgery has developed from a single valve replacement to more complex procedures, such as the Ross procedure or valve sparing surgery. Recently, a transcatheter aortic valve replacement has evolved as well. All aspects regarding of the aortic valve are addressed in this book, including anatomy, physiology, preoperative examination by techniques such as echocardiography, as well as various surgical procedures, operative risk analysis especially in the senile population, and newly emerging technologies. The authors are italian cardiologists, radiologists, pathologists and cardiac surgeons who work in Italy and in Europe. This work is aimed at cardiology fellows in training, while also helpful to surgeons, cardiologists, imagers, interventionalists, as well as other clinicians and students involved in the diagnosis and treatment of aortic valve. I believe this book will help clarify daily questions regarding the clinical and surgical practice in aortic valve disease, as well as induce inspiration and new insights into this field. I would like to thank all the chapter authors who sent us splendid manuscripts albeit their tight schedules and current terrible pandemic situation. I thank Professor Tirone David who honored the work with his Foreword. I could not have accomplished editing this book without the help and tremendous support of the staff at Nova

Science Publishers. Finally, I thank my family and my friends for encouraging me to proceed with this project.

Giovanni Concistrè, MD

In: Perspectives in Aortic Valve Disease
Editor: Giovanni Concistrè

ISBN: 978-1-53618-769-4

Chapter 1

SURGICAL ANATOMY AND PATHOLOGY OF AORTIC VALVE: MORPHOGENESIS, NORMAL AND PATHOLOGICAL ANATOMY

Giacomo Bianchi*, MD, PhD
Adult Cardiac Surgery, Ospedale del Cuore, Massa, Italy

ABSTRACT

The systematic study of the aortic valve in the surgical perspective should include an integrated approach. The embryology of semilunar valves and cono-truncal division are the cornerstone of the entire surgical anatomy. Like other cardiac valve structures, the aortic valve cannot be analyzed separately but must be framed within the aortic root, both morphologically and functionally. These aspects not only guide the clinician in the diagnosis but also the surgeon and the interventionalist in the treatment of aortic structural heart disease.

Keywords: surgical anatomy, morphogenesis, pathology, aortic valve

INTRODUCTION

The study of aortic valve pathology for the clinician, surgeon and researcher cannot ignore the knowledge of the mechanisms of formation, its normal and pathological anatomy. Embryology applied to the surgical anatomy is the basis for the exact knowledge of the pathological pictures and methods of intervention today. In this chapter, importance is given both to the molecular processes that determine the development of semilunar valves, with particular reference to the aortic valve, and to the anatomical pictures and their pathological variants.

* Corresponding Author's Email: gbianchi@ftgm.it.

Aortic Valve Morphogenesis

Structural Components

In the 4-chambered heart of the vertebrates, the presence of atrioventricular valves (tricuspid and mitral) that separate the atria from the ventricles and semilunar (aorta and pulmonic) to the arterial poles, ensure the unidirectional flow of blood [1]. The leaflets of the semilunar (SL) valves are composed of superimposed layers of extra-cellular matrix (ECM), each characterized by a prevalent component: *pars ventricularis* (elastin), *spongiosa* (proteoglycans) and *fibrosa* (collagen).

The SL valves do not require a supporting apparatus. Instead, the aortic valve (AoV) cusps are self-supporting and attach to crown-shaped arterial roots via the annulus fibrosus. Supporting connective tissue is present in the aortic and pulmonic roots and hinge regions of the SL valves [2].

The first evidence of valvulogenesis during embryonic development is the formation of endocardial cushions in the AV canal (AVC) and outflow tract (OFT) of the primitive looped heart tube [3].

The SL valves arise from the complex arrangement of proximal and distal cushions that form in the OFT. The valve progenitor cells of the endocardial cushions are highly proliferative, whereas little or no cell cycling is apparent later in remodeling and mature valves [4].

At E10.5, the OFT cushions are populated by mesenchyme originating from two distinct lineages. The contribution of endocardially derived cells is restricted to the proximal portion of the conal cushions and distal part of the truncal ridges [5, 6]. The cranial neural crest cells (CNCCs) are found mostly in the distal portion wherein they form two prongs of mesenchymal cells [7]. By E11.5, the interface of endocardium and neural crest-derived mesenchyme at the conotruncal junction delineates a boundary corresponding to the site of SL valve development in humans [8].

The fate of CNCCs is controversial: initial studies had shown that these cells were selectively eliminated during embryonic development, while more recent studies have found their persistence even in the final stage of development and in the adult [4, 7].

In particular, evidence emerges about the concentration of these cells in the leaflets adjacent to the aortic-pulmonary septum, i.e., the R-L cusp of the aortic valve and the pulmonary valve, respectively [7]. This discovery is interesting in the light of hypothesis about the origin of the bicuspid aortic valve from the neural crest, with the fusion of the R-L cusp [9].

The secondary heart field (SHF) might constitute a third source of OFT mesenchyme. These cells cells are added to the myocardial wall as the OFT elongates before septation and contribute to endocardial lineages within the OFT [10].

Postnatally, bone marrow (BM) – derived cells can contribute to the valve leaflets. Those cells might be important for valve homeostasis, for example, by providing a population of valve-interstitial cells (VICs) responsive to injury.

From E11.5 onward, the ECs expand by mesenchyme proliferation driven by Bmp/TGF-b, Egf, Nf1/ras, and Wnt signaling. Septation of the OFT and AV junctions into separate R–L ventricular inlets is mediated by fusion of the EC structures. In the OFT, the fusion of the larger cushions at midline yields separate outlet lumens, connecting the left and right ventricles to the AoV and PV, respectively. The primary ECs in the AVC form a partition between atria and ventricles and determine the alignment of the R–L AV valves and proper relationship of the great arteries to the ventricular chambers.

In humans, R – L fusion is the most common, followed by R-NC [11]. A comparative study of inbred Syrian hamsters with R–L morphology and Nos3-knockout mice with R-NC morphology suggests that the etiologies of these phenotypes are different [9]. R – L fusion may be the result of defective OFT septation, implicating the neural crest, whereas R-NC fusion may be caused by defec- tive lateral cushion formation, suggesting in- adequate EMT. The BAV is usually detected in isolation, but can also coexist with other cardio- vascular malformations, suggesting a multigenic etiology [11].

The later phases of valve development are char- acterized by the gradual transition from undifferentiated mesenchyme to specialized VICs. This process is strongly influenced by hemodynamic stimuli.

Cell proliferation, density, and turnover, substantial in early valvulogenesis, become less pronounced at this stage; in the OFT cushions the apoptosis process predominates. While in AV valves a differential and spatial expression of the genes in the leaflets and in the chordal apparatus is noted, in SL valves the genes are expressed at the same time and space, since they must give rise to a cellular structure with internal support apparatus [12].

The final process is the complex and continuous extracellular matrix (ECM) stratification and remodeling driven by the hemodynamic forces.

Dysregulation of the ECM appears to be a general feature of valve disease regardless of etiology; for example, BAVs from pediatric patients have increased collagen and proteoglycan content, whereas myxomatous MVs have loose collagen, increased proteoglycan, and reduced elastin content with altered fiber orientation in all layers.

THE AORTIC ROOT

Anatomical Landmarks and Uniform Terminology

The definitive outflow tracts in the postnatal hearts possess three components. These are the intrapericardial arterial trunks, the arterial roots, and the subvalvar ventricular outflow tracts. The distal boundary of the aortic root with the intrapericardial component of the ascending aorta is clearly marked by the sinutubular junction. The proximal boundary, in contrast, has no direct anatomic substrate.

The aortic root forms the centerpiece of the cardiac base. It is at the junction of the left ventricular outflow tract and the intrapericardial component of the ascending aorta. In surgical view, all cardiac structures normally referred to as “right” and “left” are instead “anterior” and “posterior,” respectively.

Definition of the Aortic Root

The aortic root is a complex and functional unit situated between the left ventricular outflow tract (LVOT) and the ascending aorta (Figure 1). It supports the leaflets of the aortic valve and gives the origin to the coronary arteries. Delineated superiorly by the sinotubular junction (STJ) and inferiorly by the ventriculoaortic junction (or "aortic annulus"), consists of:

- Sinotubular ridge/junction
- The Valsalva sinuses
- The leaflets
- The commisures
- The interleaflets triangles
- The ventriculoaortic junction.

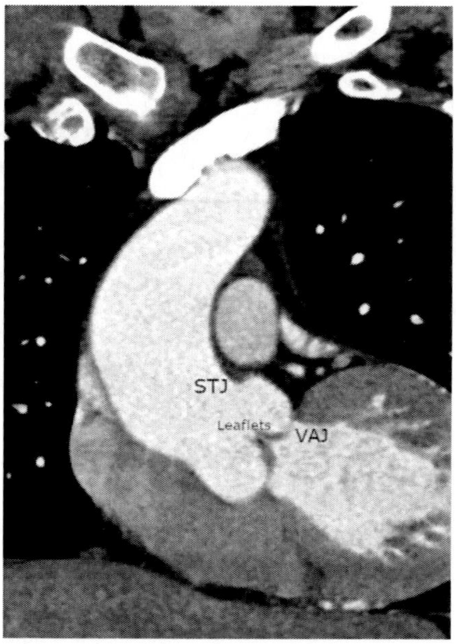

Figure 1. CT scan of the thoracic aorta. STJ: sino-tubular junction; VAJ: ventriculo-aortic junction. Leaflets: thickened aortic valve leaflets.

The Sinotubular Junction

The sino-tubular junction joins upwards the tubular portion of the aorta and downwards the sinuses of Valsalva and the aortic commissure with which is in direct continuity. On the aortic lumen the STJ usually presents a slightly raised ridge of thickened aortic wall, while on the outside it is smooth and. The sino-tubular junction takes on the contour of the three sinuses, thus it is not perfectly circular and evidences a mildly trefoil or scalloped outline.

STJ play a fundamental role in the structure of the aortic root and in the function of the aortic valve being a component of the functional aortic annulus [13]. It has specific geometrical relationship with the other components of the root. In fact, despite the area of the STJ increased with age and with hypertensive cardiomyopathy [14], in normal healthy hearts echocardiographic diameter of the STJ is about 75% of the maximal sinus diameter [15], while is larger than aortic annulus at the level of the VBR with a ratio of 1.3.

At the level of the aortic commissures forms a circular ring [16]; its diameter is 10-15% smaller than that of the ventriculo-aortic junction (VAJ). It provides most of the support for the valve cusps at their commissures and its integrity is essential fo the correct function of the valve.

The Valsalva Sinuses

The three-dimensional space of the aortic root surrounding the aortic leaflets are known as the sinuses of Valsalva. The sinuses of Valsalva represent the most proximal portion of the arterial system above the aortic valve. In a cross-sectional view the three bulges have a clover shape, and due to its physiological morphology, characterized by a dilatation, the root is much wider at the midpoint of the sinuses than at either the STJ or at the basal attachment of the leaflets.

Although the three sinuses af the root and their leaflets play an identical function, they anatomy differ [16, 17]. Two of them give rise to the coronary arteries and are named the right and the left coronary sinuses. A crescent of ventricular musculature, relative to the VAJ, is incorporated all along the base of the right coronary sinus and in the part of the left coronary sinuses close to the right sinus. The third sinus, called the non-coronary aortic sinus, consists exclusively of fibrous wall; its base is part of the mitro-aortic continuity, thus at this level the VAJ and the VBR coincide.

The base od the left coronary leaflet partially attaches to the septal muscle and partly to the fibrous skeleton of the heart, as well as to the base of the anterior mitral leaflet. The right coronary cusp is attached to both the septal muscle and the membranous septum. The non-coronary leaflet attaches to the membranous septum and then along the fibrous skeleton in continuity with the anterior leaflet of the mitral valve. The fibrous tissue constitutes approximatively 55% of the posterior aspect of the aortic root, ranging from the membranous septum to the left trigone.

The Aortic Valve Structure (Semilunar Leaflets and Commissures)

The normal aortic valve is composed of three leaflets that represent the moving parts of the valve. Each leaflet has a base that contributes to the definition of the ventriculoaortic junction, a "body," and a free margin. The superior aspect ends at the level of the sinotubular junction.

Normal aortic leaflets are soft and pliable. Each leaflet is composed of a free margin that is slightly thicker than the basal portion and is responsible of the closure of the valve during the diastole.

The apposition zone, the "lunule," is on the ventricular surface of the free margin and represents the place where each leaflet meets the adjacent leaflets during valvar closure. At the mid-portion of the "lunule," there is a further thickening called the "nodule of Arantius." Leaflets fenestrations above the closure line are common. The valve competence depends on the coaptation of the three leaflets; at the midline level of each cusp, the coaptation depth is 8-10 mm.

The basal margin of the leaflets is attached in a semilunar fashion to the aortic root. This basal attachment has the nadir below the VAJ and the zenith at the level of the STJ, where each leaflet, joining the adjacent leaflet, form the three commissures respectively. Beneath the apex of the commissures, a thin layer of fibrous tissue go down, between the respective leaflets, towards the VAJ and forms the final part.

Histologically, aortic leaflets show dense collagen bundles at the level of their semilunar hinge on the arterial wall and of their free margin. The insertion of the apices of the semilunar hinges on the aortic wall corresponds to the apices of the interleaflets triangles. These regions are strongly reinforced with connective fibers and elastic aortic lamellae, thus holding the semilunar leaflets and distributing the tension forces that would otherwise break and distort the leaflets [18].

Each cusp consists of three layers: the *fibrosa*, on the aortic side, the *spongiosa* in the middle, and the *ventricularis*. The *fibrosa* is mostly constituted of collagen fibers, which are primarily arranged in a circumferential direction, from one commissure to the other. The *spongiosa* consists of collagen and elastic fibers, proteoglycans, and mucopolysaccharides that give it a soft consistency. The *ventricularis* mainly consists of elastic fibers, structured in thin sheets, randomly oriented as compared with the highly organized structure of the fibrosa; it provides the tensile recoil to retain the folded and corrugated shape of the *fibrosa* and also prevents diastolic overdistension.

The Interleaflet Triangles

The interleaflets triangles are bordered by insertion of the leaflets and of the leaflet attachments of the aortic sinuses at their base. They are triangular extensions of the LVOT. The triangle between the left and the right coronary cusps is partly constituted of myocardial tissue, the triangle between the right and the noncoronary cusps consists of fibrous tissue and contains the atrio-ventricular (AV) bundle of the conduction axis, and the triangle between the noncoronary and the left cusps is only composed of fibrous tissue. The border of the triangles are delimited on the cusps' side by a dense collagen fibers layer, forming also the fibrous layer of the VAJ. The area delimited is the "body" of the triangle. A thin layer of elastic fibers is also present and in continuity with the elastic layer beneath the endocardium.

The Ventriculo-Aortic Junction

Unlike the 'annulus,' the anatomic ventriculo-arterial junction is more reminiscent of a circle. It is where ventricular myocardium terminates and gives way to the wall of the aortic sleeve. But, on account of the region of aortic-mitral valvar continuity and the central fibrous body forming the remaining 60% or so of the ventriculo-arterial junction, the slightly larger portion of the junction is fibrous. Here, precise location of the junction is not possible and we can only extrapolate by completing the circle around the outflow tract, and making the assumption that there is a sharp line between myocardium and sleeve. Nevertheless, the semilunar hingelines of the valvar leaflets create an intricate arrangement at this junction. The nadirs of the hingelines are locates below the ventriculo-arterial junction. Thus, where the hingelines cross muscle, myocar- dial segments are included into the aortic sinuses.

In human, myocardium is present in the non-coronary and posterior half of the left-coronary sinus only when there is persistence of the left ventriculo-infundibular fold (inner heart curvature) but this seldom happens. The area of valvar continuity is thickened at both ends to form the right and left fibrous trigones; the right trigone contributing to the central fibrous body of the heart.

The anatomic ventriculo-arterial junction, however, does not coincide with the functional junction, again owing to the configuration of the semilunar hingelines. First, the ventricular parts within the aortic sinuses become incorporated, functionally, into the aorta. Second, the parts of the wall of the aortic sleeve that are in between adjacent leaflets, lie above the anatomic ventriculo-arterial junction but become, haemodynamically, a part of the ventricle when the valve is closed.

Functional Anatomy

Considering the aortic root as one functional unit, it is a three-dimensional structure adjoining distally to the aorta and proximally to the ventricle, and all parts have to work in harmony. When there is dysfunction it is unlikely to involve only a single element, apart from, for example, isolated perforation of the leaflet.

In a series of fixed preparations of human aortic roots, the mean circumference was found to be 65.8 mm at the sinutubular junction and 69.2 mm at the base of the root [19]; in another series of cadaveric studies, the sinutubular junction was found to be narrower than the basal part and the middle of the sinusal part was the widest [20].

The diameter at the sinutubular junction and at the nadirs of the leaflets change continuously during the cardiac cycle in experimental studies [21]. During systole the sinutubular junction increases initially as aortic pressure increases and decreases later as aortic pressure drops, and the base decreases so the root adopts a cylindrical shape [22]. During diastole the sinutubular junction moves inwards and the base moves outwards commissures, changing the cylindrical shape to a more conical shape.

The sinuses of Valsalva play an important role in the local hydrodynamic forces that exert their effects on both cup motion and coronary flow; they generate a space behind the open aortic leaflets, preventing closure of the coronary artery orifices. This space favors the generation of "eddy currents" (first described by Leonardo da Vinci) behind the leaflets when these are open. The "eddy currents" prevent the contact of the valve leaflets with the aortic wall and promote smooth valve closure. The peripheral laminae of the flow in systole encounter the "bottle neck" of the sinotubular junction that forces these laminae back down, along the borders of the sinuses, distend the cusp borders at the end of systole, and finally close the cusps during diastole.

The aortic root undergoes complex deformations during the cardiac cycle, which consists in the strain of the aorto-ventricular base (putative annulus) and sinotubular junction, aortic root elongation and compression, and shear and torsion deformities. During the first third of systole, the aortic root gains its maximal expansion, approaching a cylindrical shape. Then its volume decreases in mid-diastole, then it reapproaches a truncated cone shape in end-diastole. The 39% increase of the ventriculoaortic junction ring area and the 63% expansion of the apexes of the interleaflets triangles during systole reduce the opposition to ejection, facilitating left ventricular unload.

The elastic properties of the root are crucial for the omeostatis of this complex structure. The maximal stress on the leaflets is concentrated on their insertion at the sinotubular junction and progressively decreases along the border of cusp insertion. During diastole, the stress on the leaflets is almost four times higher than that on the sinuses. If the three sinuses do not uniformly share the stress, the sinus wall would draw inward in diastole. Vice versa, the sinus walls move outward, thus decreasing the stress and wear and tear on the aortic leaflets.

Aortic Stenosis

Valve calcification is classified according to the extent and localization of the calcium deposits [23]. In all imaging evaluations of the aortic root (echocardiography, CT scan, and nuclear magnetic imaging), aortic valve calcification should be graded/classified as follows:

- Grade 1: absence of calcification,
- Grade 2: isolated small calcification spots,
- Grade 3: bigger calcification spots interfering with cuspsmotion, and
- Grade 4: extensive calcification of all cusps with restricted cusp motion.

For calcifications of ≤ grade 3, the localization of the calcium deposits should be specified.

The early stages of aortic stenosis are in many ways similar to atherosclerosis. Indeed, the 2 conditions share many common risk factors, with large longitudinal studies consistently demonstrating that the incidence of aortic stenosis is linked to factors such as smoking, age, and hypertension [24]. As in atherosclerosis, endothelial damage due to increased mechanical stress and reduced shear stress is believed to be the initiating injury, perhaps best illustrated by bicuspid valve disease. In this congenital valve malformation, the characteristic 2-leaflet structure of these valves results in less efficient dissipation of mechanical stress and accelerated endothelial damage, so that patients almost universally develop aortic stenosis and display more rapid disease progression [25].

Following endothelial damage, the same lipids implicated in atherosclerosis infiltrate the valve, in particular, lipoprotein(a) and oxidized low-density lipoprotein (LDL) cholesterol. Consequently, observational studies have identified cholesterol and its related lipoproteins as independent risk factors for the development of aortic stenosis [26]. Progressive endothelial injury and lipid oxidization then establishes an inflammatory response within the valve that is characterized predominantly by infiltration of macrophages, but also involves T lymphocytes and mast cells [27]. Features of fibrosis, calcification and activation of genes for osteoblastic differentitation within the valve along with angiogenesis, lead to valve ossification in an active, highly regulated pathological process [28].

Aortic Regurgitation

Aortic valve regurgitation may depend either on the valve or on the dysfunction of each of the nonvalvular components of the aortic root. In a schematic way, the pathophysiology of the aortic valve incompetence may result from failure of each of the six components of the root, either variably combined or as isolated abnormali- ties of the sinotubular junction or sinuses of Valsalva, or semilunar leaflets or three-coronet shaped ventriculoaor-tic junction.

Aortic regurgitation may be caused by age-related atherosclerosis and hypertension; infective aortic disease (endocarditis); chronic inflammatory aortic valve disease such as rheumatic disease; heritable connective tissue disease; congenital diseases such as true or false bicuspid aortic valve (BAV); or acquired valve disease (aged aortic valve calcific degeneration leading to mixed steno-insufficient valve). Whatever is the cause of valve insufficiency, once established, all aortic root components enter a vicious circle with corresponding damage and dysfunction, all contributing to worsening the regurgitation.

Morphofunctional Classification of Aortic Regurgitation

Based on above considerations, the mechanisms that may cause aortic regurgitation in the presence of normal mor- phology of the aortic cusps are:

1. Dilatation of the aortic annulus, generally associated with dilation of the sinuses of Valsalva (known as "annuloaortic ectasia")
2. Isolated single sinus of Valsalva aneurysm affecting the function of a single leaflet
3. Loss of the sinotubular junction shape which assumes a rectilinear and enlarged morphology
4. Isolated ascending aortic aneurysm (not involving the aortic root) that can stretch the sinotubular junction, valve commissures, and interleaflets triangles.

El Khoury and co-workers [29] proposed a simplified functional anatomy classification of the aortic root considering the two main components:

- The functional aortic annulus (FAA) that includes the ventriculoaortic junction, the sinuses of Valsalva, and the sinotubular junction
- The three semilunar leaflets.

The two basic mechanisms of aortic regurgitation, i.e., FAA dilatation and pathology of the leaflets are classified as follows:

Table 1. Functional classification of aortic regurgitation. STJ: Sino-Tubular Junction; FAA: Functional Aortic Annulus

TYPE I	TYPE II	TYPE III
Ia: ascending aorta dilatation	Cusp Prolapse	Cusp retraction and thickening
Ib: Valsalva sinuses and STJ dilatation		
Ic: FAA dilatation		
Id: cusp perforation		

THE BICUSPID VALVE

Bicuspid aortic valve (BAV) disease has the characteristic of heredity with variable genetic penetrance. And 0.5–2% of the population worldwide have the possibility to be attacked by this disease, which 75% of them are male [30]. BAVs are known to prematurely calcify leading to calcific aortic valve disease (CAVD), the second most common cause of aortic valve stenosis. In addition, BAV predisposes affected individuals to aortic aneurysms and infective endocarditis [31]. BAV has strong genetic components, as evidenced by reports of familial clustering and calculated heritability [32].

Morphology of BAV

The typical structure of the aortic valve had three semilunar leaflets in shape. Due to the fusion of two cusps out of three, BAV usually included two unequal cusps and a central raphe. From a surgical point of view, Sievers classification system was used widely [33]. Based on number of raphes, three categories of BAV are presented in patients including type 0 (no raphe in the valve), type 1 (only one raphe in the valve) and type 2 (two raphes in the valve). And the most common type is type 1, which accounting for about 90% of the patients [34]. On the basis of the raphe position with coronary sinuses, types 1 and 2 were classified as left (L), right (R) and none (N) type. The right and left coronary leaflet (RL) were most common accounted for about 80%, the right and non-coronary leaflet (RN) was about 17% and left and non-coronary leaflet (LN) was 2%. Compared to Asians, type 0 BAV was more frequently among Europeans, whereas the incidence of RN-BAV with a raphe was higher in Asian [35].

Aortic stiffness was measured by pulse wave velocity (PWV) using velocity-encoded magnetic resonance imaging (VENC-MRI) and patients with R-NC fusion were manifested as greater PWV than patients with R-L fusion phenotype.

In order to show the relationship between BAV morphology type and valvulopathy or aortopathy, the dichotomous classification method was introduced. The right and left coronary leaflet cusp fusion was defined as the coronary cusp fusion (CCF) and all other types were defined as the mixed cusp fusion (MCF). The MCF type of BAV was considered as one of risk factors for the occurrence of aortic stenosis and associated aortopathy, which resulted in significant hemodynamic changes [36]. Calcification of a bicuspid valve begins first along the raphe and also on the aortic surface of the other leaflet.

Genetics of BAV

Although the initial potential genetic link for human BAV was mutations in the gene KCNJ2 in the setting of Anderson syndrome, no mutations in this gene had been reported in nonsyndromic BAV. The first genetic etiology of nonsyndromic BAV was identified through the use of genome-wide linkage analysis by studying families with autosomal-dominant disease. NOTCH1 is a transmembrane receptor known to function in highly conserved signaling pathways that play important roles in cell fate and cardiovascular developmental processes [37]. Since then, several mutations in NOTCH1 have been found to be associated with aortic valve disease [38]. GATA5 belongs to the family of GATA transcription factors, and several of these factors have been implicated in human disease. It was recently shown that targeted deletion of GaTa5 in mice leads to a partially penetrant BAV phenotypes [39]. Mutations in SMAD6, a member of the Bmp signaling pathway, display functional deficits in vitro and have been found in humans with BAV [40]. Consistent with this, cardiac cushion abnormalities have also been observed in Smad6-null mice [41].

Aortic Stenosis in BAV

In adults, the development of aortic stenosis is often due to leaflet calcification, which occurs in a similar fashion to that seen in patients with trileaflet leaflet calcification. This process is felt to be an active process, perhaps initiated by endothelial dysfunction and involving inflammation, lipoprotein deposition, calcification, and ossification of the aortic side of the valve leaflets [42]. The folding and creasing of the valves and the turbulent flow are felt to contribute to development of fibrosis and calcification [43]. The combination of these processes results in an accelerated disease progression. Calcification is often present by 40 years of age. Although in some series a peculiar arrangement of valve morphology (raphe location) was found to be associated with increased risk of valve calcification [44, 45], two large studies in adults have not identified leaflet orientation as a risk factor for late adverse events [46, 47]. This finding that valve orientation was not predictive of outcomes in adults may reflect the modifying role of atherosclerosis risk factors and/or more advanced degenerative process encountered in adults. A composite index of valve degeneration, which incorporated valve thickening, calcification, and mobility, that was an independent predictor of long-term cardiac events in a population of adults with no baseline valve dysfunction. The predictive role of both morphology and function in adults with BAV parallels that observed in series examining older adults with aortic stenosis mostly of acquired basis.

Aortic Regurgitation in BAV

Aortic incompetence can develop in the setting of redundant or prolapsing cusps, endocarditis, or after balloon valvuloplasty. With age, aortic incom- petence may also develop secondary to dilation of the ascending aorta. Although adults with BAV often have some degree of aortic regurgitation, the actual prevalence of pure aortic incompetence has varied, with some suggesting it is rare and others suggesting that it is common. In the Olmstead county echocardio- graphic study of asymptomatic adults [46], 47% had some degree of aortic incompetence at baseline; however, interventions for severe aortic incompetence were relatively uncommon, occurring in only 3% of the cohort during follow-up. In the Toronto study [47], 21% of the population had moderate or severe aortic incompetence at baseline; however, only 6% had an intervention for symptomatic aortic incompetence or progressive left ventricular dysfunc- tion. Despite variations in prevalence, moderate or severe aortic incompetence is clinically important and is an independent predictor for late adverse cardiac events.

Aortopathy and Aortic Dissection in BAV

In BAV disease, the aortic annulus, sinus, and proximal ascending aorta are larger than those found in adults with trileaflet valves [48, 49]. These differences persist even after adjusting for blood pressure (systolic and diastolic), peak aortic velocities, and left ventricular ejection time. Aortic root size is shown to be related to valve morphology and the presence of significant valve disease (82, 84). Specifically, the increased stroke volume from aortic incompetence is felt to result in stress on the diseased aorta and subsequent aortic dilation. The most feared complication is aortic dissection, pri- marily due to the high associated mortality rate; however, the actual incidence of this complication is debated. In the Toronto series (7), the prevalence of dissection was 0.1% per patient-year of follow-up, and in the Olmsted County study (6), there were no cases of dissection. Despite the low rates of dissection, the increased prevalence of BAV disease relative to Marfan syndrome make dissections due to BAV equal to or more common than dissections due to Marfan syndrome [50]. Dissection in BAV, when it occurs, typically involves the ascending aorta, but involvement of the descending aorta has been reported in older patients. Risk factors for dissection have included aortic size, aortic stiffness, male sex, family history, and the presence of other lesions such as coarc- tation of the aorta or Turner syndrome.

REFERENCES

[1] Schoen FJ. Evolving concepts of cardiac valve dynamics: the continuum of development, functional structure, pathobiology, and tissue engineering. *Circulation* 2008;118:1864–80. https://doi.org/10.1161/CIRCULATIONAHA.108.805911.

[2] Hinton RB, Lincoln J, Deutsch GH, Osinska H, Manning PB, Benson DW, et al. Extracellular matrix remodeling and organization in developing and diseased aortic valves. *Circ Res* 2006;98:1431–8. https://doi.org/10.1161/01.RES.0000224114.65109.4e.

[3] Person AD, Klewer SE, Runyan RB. Cell biology of cardiac cushion development. *Int Rev Cytol* 2005;243:287–335. https://doi.org/10.1016/S0074-7696(05)43005-3.

[4] de Lange FJ, Moorman AFM, Anderson RH, Männer J, Soufan AT, de Gier-de Vries C, et al. Lineage and morphogenetic analysis of the cardiac valves. *Circ Res* 2004;95:645–54. https://doi.org/10.1161/01.RES.0000141429.13560.cb.

[5] Snarr BS, Kern CB, Wessels A. Origin and fate of cardiac mesenchyme. *Dev Dyn Off Publ Am Assoc Anat* 2008;237:2804–19. https://doi.org/10.1002/dvdy.21725.

[6] Wu B, Wang Y, Lui W, Langworthy M, Tompkins KL, Hatzopoulos AK, et al. Nfatc1 coordinates valve endocardial cell lineage development required for heart valve formation. *Circ Res* 2011;109:183–92. https://doi.org/10.1161/CIRCRESAHA.111.245035.

[7] Nakamura T, Colbert MC, Robbins J. Neural crest cells retain multipotential characteristics in the developing valves and label the cardiac conduction system. *Circ Res* 2006;98:1547–54. https://doi.org/10.1161/01.RES.0000227505.19472.69.

[8] Anderson RH. Development of the heart: (2) Septation of the atriums and ventricles. *Heart* 2003;89:949–958. https://doi.org/10.1136/heart.89.8.949.

[9] Fernández B, Durán AC, Fernández-Gallego T, Fernández MC, Such M, Arqué JM, et al. Bicuspid aortic valves with different spatial orientations of the leaflets are distinct etiological entities. *J Am Coll Cardiol* 2009;54:2312–8. https://doi.org/10.1016/j.jacc.2009.07.044.

[10] Yang L, Cai C-L, Lin L, Qyang Y, Chung C, Monteiro RM, et al. Isl1Cre reveals a common Bmp pathway in heart and limb development. *Dev Camb Engl* 2006;133:1575–85. https://doi.org/10.1242/dev.02322.

[11] Siu SC, Silversides CK. Bicuspid aortic valve disease. *J Am Coll Cardiol* 2010; 55:2789–800. https://doi.org/10.1016/j.jacc.2009.12.068.

[12] Zhao B, Etter L, Hinton RB, Benson DW. BMP and FGF regulatory pathways in semilunar valve precursor cells. *Dev Dyn Off Publ Am Assoc Anat* 2007;236:971–80. https://doi.org/10.1002/dvdy.21097.

[13] El Khoury G, Glineur D, Rubay J, Verhelst R, d'Acoz Y d'Udekem, Poncelet A, et al. Functional classification of aortic root/valve abnormalities and their correlation with etiologies and surgical procedures. *Curr Opin Cardiol* 2005;20:115–21. https://doi.org/10.1097/01.hco.0000153951.31887.a6.

[14] Silver MA, Roberts WC. Detailed anatomy of the normally functioning aortic valve in hearts of normal and increased weight. *Am J Cardiol* 1985;55:454–61. https://doi.org/10.1016/0002-9149(85)90393-5.

[15] Tamás E, Nylander E. Echocardiographic description of the anatomic relations within the normal aortic root. *J Heart Valve Dis* 2007;16:240–6.

[16] Underwood MJ, El Khoury G, Deronck D, Glineur D, Dion R. The aortic root: structure, function, and surgical reconstruction. *Heart Br Card Soc* 2000;83:376–80. https://doi.org/10.1136/heart.83.4.376.

[17] Loukas M, Bilinsky E, Bilinsky S, Blaak C, Tubbs RS, Anderson RH. The anatomy of the aortic root. *Clin Anat N Y N* 2014;27:748–56. https://doi.org/10.1002/ca.22295.

[18] Sutton III JP, Ho SY, Anderson RH. The forgotten interleaflet triangles: a review of the surgical anatomy of the aortic valve. *Ann Thorac Surg* 1995;59:419–427.

[19] Berdajs D, Lajos P, Turina M. The anatomy of the aortic root. *Cardiovasc Surg* 2002;10:320–7.

[20] Kunzelman KS, Grande KJ, David TE, Cochran RP, Verrier ED. Aortic root and valve relationships. Impact on surgical repair. *J Thorac Cardiovasc Surg* 1994;107:162–70.

[21] Thubrikar M, Nolan SP, Bosher LP, Deck JD. The cyclic changes and structure of the base of the aortic valve. *Am Heart J* 1980;99:217–24. https://doi.org/10.1016/0002-8703(80)90768-1.

[22] Thubrikar M, Piepgrass WC, Shaner TW, Nolan SP. The design of the normal aortic valve. *Am J Physiol* 1981;241:H795-801. https://doi.org/10.1152/ajpheart.1981.241.6.H795.

[23] le Polain de Waroux J-B, Pouleur A-C, Goffinet C, Vancraeynest D, Van Dyck M, Robert A, et al. Functional anatomy of aortic regurgitation: accuracy, prediction of surgical repairability, and outcome implications of transesophageal echocardiography. *Circulation* 2007;116:I264-269. https://doi.org/10.1161/CIRCULATIONAHA.106.680074.

[24] Stewart BF, Siscovick D, Lind BK, Gardin JM, Gottdiener JS, Smith VE, et al. Clinical factors associated with calcific aortic valve disease. Cardiovascular Health Study. *J Am Coll Cardiol* 1997;29:630–4. https://doi.org/10.1016/s0735-1097(96)00563-3.

[25] Pachulski RT, Chan KL. Progression of aortic valve dysfunction in 51 adult patients with congenital bicuspid aortic valve: assessment and follow up by Doppler echocardiography. *Br Heart J* 1993;69:237–40. https://doi.org/10.1136/hrt.69.3.237.

[26] Smith JG, Luk K, Schulz C-A, Engert JC, Do R, Hindy G, et al. Association of low-density lipoprotein cholesterol-related genetic variants with aortic valve calcium and incident aortic stenosis. *JAMA* 2014;312:1764–71. https://doi.org/10.1001/jama.2014.13959.

[27] Otto CM, Kuusisto J, Reichenbach DD, Gown AM, O'Brien KD. Characterization of the early lesion of "degenerative" valvular aortic stenosis. Histological and immunohistochemical studies. *Circulation* 1994;90:844–53. https://doi.org/10.1161/01.cir.90.2.844.

[28] Mohler ER, Gannon F, Reynolds C, Zimmerman R, Keane MG, Kaplan FS. Bone formation and inflammation in cardiac valves. *Circulation* 2001;103:1522–8. https://doi.org/10.1161/01.cir.103.11.1522.

[29] Jeanmart H, de Kerchove L, Glineur D, Goffinet J-M, Rougui I, Van Dyck M, et al. Aortic valve repair: the functional approach to leaflet prolapse and valve-sparing surgery. *Ann Thorac Surg* 2007;83:S746-751; discussion S785-790. https://doi.org/10.1016/j.athoracsur.2006.10.089.

[30] Dargis N, Lamontagne M, Gaudreault N, Sbarra L, Henry C, Pibarot P, et al. Identification of Gender-Specific Genetic Variants in Patients With Bicuspid Aortic Valve. *Am J Cardiol* 2016;117:420–6. https://doi.org/10.1016/j.amjcard.2015.10.058.

[31] Fedak PWM, Verma S, David TE, Leask RL, Weisel RD, Butany J. Clinical and pathophysiological implications of a bicuspid aortic valve. *Circulation* 2002;106:900–4. https://doi.org/10.1161/01.cir.0000027905.26586.e8.

[32] McBride KL, Garg V. Heredity of bicuspid aortic valve: is family screening indicated? *Heart Br Card Soc* 2011;97:1193–5. https://doi.org/10.1136/hrt.2011.222489.

[33] Sievers H-H, Schmidtke C. A classification system for the bicuspid aortic valve from 304 surgical specimens. *J Thorac Cardiovasc Surg* 2007;133:1226–33. https://doi.org/10.1016/j.jtcvs.2007.01.039.

[34] Sievers H-H, Stierle U, Mohamed SA, Hanke T, Richardt D, Schmidtke C, et al. Toward individualized management of the ascending aorta in bicuspid aortic valve surgery: the role of valve phenotype in 1362 patients. *J Thorac Cardiovasc Surg* 2014;148:2072–80. https://doi.org/10.1016/j.jtcvs.2014.04.007.

[35] Kong WKF, Regeer MV, Poh KK, Yip JW, van Rosendael PJ, Yeo TC, et al. Inter-ethnic differences in valve morphology, valvular dysfunction, and aortopathy between Asian and European patients with bicuspid aortic valve. *Eur Heart J* 2018;39:1308–13. https://doi.org/10.1093/eurheartj/ehx562.

[36] Sun BJ, Lee S, Jang JY, Kwon O, Bae JS, Lee JH, et al. Performance of a Simplified Dichotomous Phenotypic Classification of Bicuspid Aortic Valve to Predict Type of Valvulopathy and Combined Aortopathy. *J Am Soc Echocardiogr Off Publ Am Soc Echocardiogr* 2017;30:1152–61. https://doi.org/10.1016/j.echo.2017.08.002.

[37] de la Pompa JL, Epstein JA. Coordinating tissue interactions: Notch signaling in cardiac development and disease. *Dev Cell* 2012;22:244–54. https://doi.org/10.1016/j.devcel.2012.01.014.

[38] Foffa I, Ait Alì L, Panesi P, Mariani M, Festa P, Botto N, et al. Sequencing of NOTCH1, GATA5, TGFBR1 and TGFBR2 genes in familial cases of bicuspid aortic valve. *BMC Med Genet* 2013;14:44. https://doi.org/10.1186/1471-2350-14-44.

[39] Laforest B, Andelfinger G, Nemer M. Loss of Gata5 in mice leads to bicuspid aortic valve. *J Clin Invest* 2011;121:2876–87. https://doi.org/10.1172/JCI44555.

[40] Tan HL, Glen E, Töpf A, Hall D, O'Sullivan JJ, Sneddon L, et al. Nonsynonymous variants in the SMAD6 gene predispose to congenital cardiovascular malformation. *Hum Mutat* 2012;33:720–7. https://doi.org/10.1002/humu.22030.

[41] Galvin KM, Donovan MJ, Lynch CA, Meyer RI, Paul RJ, Lorenz JN, et al. A role for smad6 in development and homeostasis of the cardiovascular system. *Nat Genet* 2000;24:171–4. https://doi.org/10.1038/72835.

[42] Wallby L, Janerot-Sjöberg B, Steffensen T, Broqvist M. T lymphocyte infiltration in non-rheumatic aortic stenosis: a comparative descriptive study between tricuspid and

bicuspid aortic valves. *Heart Br Card Soc* 2002;88:348–51. https://doi.org/10.1136/heart.88.4.348.

[43] Robicsek F, Thubrikar MJ, Cook JW, Fowler B. The congenitally bicuspid aortic valve: how does it function? Why does it fail? *Ann Thorac Surg* 2004;77:177–85. https://doi.org/10.1016/s0003-4975(03)01249-9.

[44] Beppu S, Suzuki S, Matsuda H, Ohmori F, Nagata S, Miyatake K. Rapidity of progression of aortic stenosis in patients with congenital bicuspid aortic valves. *Am J Cardiol* 1993;71:322–7. https://doi.org/10.1016/0002-9149(93)90799-i.

[45] Fernandes SM, Khairy P, Sanders SP, Colan SD. Bicuspid aortic valve morphology and interventions in the young. *J Am Coll Cardiol* 2007;49:2211–4. https://doi.org/10.1016/j.jacc.2007.01.090.

[46] Michelena HI, Desjardins VA, Avierinos J-F, Russo A, Nkomo VT, Sundt TM, et al. Natural history of asymptomatic patients with normally functioning or minimally dysfunctional bicuspid aortic valve in the community. *Circulation* 2008;117:2776–84. https://doi.org/10.1161/CIRCULATIONAHA.107.740878.

[47] Tzemos N, Therrien J, Yip J, Thanassoulis G, Tremblay S, Jamorski MT, et al. Outcomes in adults with bicuspid aortic valves. *JAMA* 2008;300:1317–25. https://doi.org/10.1001/jama.300.11.1317.

[48] Nkomo VT, Enriquez-Sarano M, Ammash NM, Melton LJ, Bailey KR, Desjardins V, et al. Bicuspid aortic valve associated with aortic dilatation: a community-based study. *Arterioscler Thromb Vasc Biol* 2003;23:351–6. https://doi.org/10.1161/01.atv.0000055441.28842.0a.

[49] Cecconi M, Manfrin M, Moraca A, Zanoli R, Colonna PL, Bettuzzi MG, et al. Aortic dimensions in patients with bicuspid aortic valve without significant valve dysfunction. *Am J Cardiol* 2005;95:292–4. https://doi.org/10.1016/j.amjcard.2004.08.098.

[50] Pape LA, Tsai TT, Isselbacher EM, Oh JK, O'gara PT, Evangelista A, et al. Aortic diameter > or = 5.5 cm is not a good predictor of type A aortic dissection: observations from the International Registry of Acute Aortic Dissection (IRAD). *Circulation* 2007;116:1120–7. https://doi.org/10.1161/CIRCULATIONAHA.107.702720.

In: Perspectives in Aortic Valve Disease
Editor: Giovanni Concistrè
ISBN: 978-1-53618-769-4

Chapter 2

EPIDEMIOLOGY AND CLINICAL APPROACH TO AORTIC VALVE DISEASE

Claudio Passino[1,2,*], Valentina Galfo[1], Simone Gasparini[1], Filippo Quattrone[1], Octavian Vatavu[1] and Alberto Aimo[1]
[1]Institute of Life Sciences, Scuola Superiore Sant'Anna, Pisa, Italy
[2]Fondazione G. Monasterio, Pisa, Italy

ABSTRACT

Aortic valve disease is an important cause of morbidity worldwide. Rheumatic heart disease is the most common cause of both aortic stenosis (AS) and aortic regurgitation (AR) in developing countries, while fibro-calcific degeneration and conditions causing aortic root dilation are the leading causes of AS and AR, respectively, in industrialized countries. A careful search for signs and symptoms may provide the first clues to the presence of aortic valve disease, which can then be verified and characterized by imaging techniques, starting from transthoracic echocardiography. In patients with known severe aortic valve disease, prompt detection of symptom onset is crucial to refer them to aortic valve replacement (AVR) or transcatether aortic valve implantation (in AS) or AVR (in AR). Furthermore, a correct interpretation of the signs and symptoms of acute AR can result in a rapid diagnostic workup and prompt patient referral to surgery

Keywords: epidemiology, aortic valve disease, aortic valve replacement, transcatheter aortic valve

ABBREVIATIONS

A2	aortic component of the second heart sound
AF	atrial fibrillation
AR	aortic regurgitation

* Corresponding Author's Email: passino@ftgm.it.

AS	aortic stenosis
AVR	aortic valve replacement
BNP	B-type natriuretic peptide
CAD	coronary artery disease
CMR	cardiovascular magnetic resonance
CT	computed tomography
ECG	electrocardiogram
HF	heart failure
HR	hazard ratio
LV	left ventricle
LVEF	LV ejection fraction
MDCT	multidetector computed tomography
NT-proBNP	N-terminal fraction of pro-BNP
P2	pulmonic component of the second heart sound
PET	positron emission tomography
S1	first heart sound
S2	second heart sound
S3	third heart sound
S4	fourth heart sound
SCD	sudden cardiac death
TAVI	transcatheter aortic valve implantation
TEE	transesophageal echocardiogram
TTE	transthoracic echocardiogram

INTRODUCTION

Stenosis of the aortic valve is the most common cause of left ventricular (LV) outflow obstruction in children and adults. The three main manifestations of severe aortic stenosis (AS) are angina, syncope or heart failure (HF). Symptomatic AS has a poor prognosis and requires surgical or percutaneous treatment. The acute onset of severe aortic regurgitation (AR) is usually a medical emergency due to the inability of the LV to quickly adapt to the abrupt increase in end-diastolic volume caused by the regurgitant flow. If not surgically corrected, acute severe AR commonly results in cardiogenic shock. By contrast, clinical symptoms are a relatively late feature of chronic AR, since the gradually dilating LV and the chronically increased diastolic volume dampens many of the hemodynamic effects of AR.

EPIDEMIOLOGY AND ETIOLOGIES

There are 3 main causes of valvular aortic stenosis (AS):

- a congenitally abnormal valve, often with superimposed calcification (unicuspid or bicuspid);
- calcific disease of a trileaflet valve (degenerative aortic valve disease);

- rheumatic valve disease, which is characterized by fusion of commissures between the leaflets, leaving a small central orifice. The rheumatic process typically involves the mitral valve as well; as a result, most patients with rheumatic AS also have mitral stenosis and/or mitral regurgitation.

Rare causes of AS include metabolic disorders (e.g., Fabry's disease), systemic lupus erythematosus and alkaptonuria. In patients with Paget disease or end-stage kidney disease, calcific AS presents at a younger age and progresses more rapidly [1, 2]. Different causes of AS have different relative frequencies according to geographical regions. Worldwide, rheumatic valve disease is the most common cause of aortic valve disease and mitral valve involvement is almost always present. In North America and Europe, aortic valve disease is primarily due to calcific disease of a native trileaflet valve or a congenitally bicuspid valve [1, 2]. The prevalence of AS increases with age, as demonstrated by a prospective population-based study of 3,273 participants including 164 subjects with AS. The prevalence of AS varied from 0.2% at ages 50 to 59 years, to 1.3% at ages 60 to 69, 3.9% at ages 70 to 79 years, and 9.8% at ages 80 to 89 years [3]. Compared with the general population, mortality was not significantly increased in the group with asymptomatic AS (hazard ratio [HR] 1.28), nor in those who received aortic valve replacement (AVR) (HR 0.93) [3]. The relative prevalence of trileaflet versus congenitally abnormal valves varies according to age, as illustrated by a series of 932 adults who underwent surgery for isolated AS [4]. Patients undergoing mitral valve replacement or with mitral stenosis were excluded to ensure exclusion of rheumatic valve disease. An anatomically abnormal valve was present in 54%: 49% had a bicuspid valve and 4% had a unicuspid valve, but the frequency displayed a significant variation with age:

- approximately two-thirds of 7% of patients who underwent surgery at ≤50 years of age had a bicuspid valve and one-third had a unicuspid valve;
- approximately two-thirds of 40% of patients who underwent surgery between 50 and 70 years had a bicuspid valve and one-third a tricuspid valve; only few patients had a unicuspid valve;
- approximately 60% of patients over 70 years had a tricuspid valve and 40% had a bicuspid valve [4].

The possible causes of acute AR with a native aortic valve include:

- infective endocarditis, because of valve destruction and leaflet perforation, or the rupture of a perivalvular abscess into the LV [5, 6];
- aortic dissection, which can lead to AR by four mechanisms: dilation of the sinuses with incomplete coaptation of the leaflets at the center of the valve; involvement of a valve commissure resulting in inadequate leaflet support; direct extension of the dissection into the base of a leaflet, resulting in a flail valve leaflet; and prolapse of the dissection flap across the aortic valve into the LV outflow tract in diastole impeding leaflet closure [5, 6];
- rupture of a congenitally fenestrated cusp [7-9];

- traumatic rupture of valve leaflets after a chest trauma [10, 11];
- complications of percutaneous procedures on the aortic valve [12, 13].

In a single-center series of 268 adults referred for AVR for isolated AR, 18% had acute AR. All of the cases were due to active infective endocarditis (56%) or acute aortic dissection (44%) [14]. Acute AR may also develop in patients with prosthetic aortic valves. AR may occur with structural valve deterioration or leaflet destruction due to infective endocarditis. Acute mechanical valve regurgitation can be caused by valve thrombosis or pannus formation with incomplete leaflet closure. Paravalvular AR is caused by prosthetic valve dehiscence occurring as a complication of infective endocarditis or inadequate valve attachment, as in the case of aortopathy associated with Marfan syndrome [15]. As for chronic AR, a study from the Framingham Heart Study found that AR of at least trace severity on color Doppler echocardiography was present in 13% of men and 9% of women. The prevalence of AR varied with age and disease severity. More than trace AR was unusual before 50 years and then increased progressively. For mild AR, the prevalence was 3.7, 12.1, and 12.2% in men at ages 50 to 59, 60 to 69, and 70 to 83, respectively. The corresponding values in women were 1.9, 6.0, and 14.6%. For moderate to severe AR, the prevalence was 0.5, 0.6, and 2.2% in men at ages 50 to 59, 60 to 69, and 70 to 83, respectively, and 0.2, 0.8, and 2.3% in women [16]. Chronic AR is caused by diseased valve leaflets or enlargement of the aortic root. In the developing world, the most common cause of AR is rheumatic heart disease. However, in developed countries, AR is most often due to aortic root dilation, congenital bicuspid aortic valve, and degenerative aortic valve disease (Table 1).

Table 1. Causes of chronic aortic regurgitation

Valve disease	Aortic root dilatation
Degenerative aortic valve disease	Hypertension
Myxomatous degeneration	
Congenital heart disease Bicuspid aortic valve Ventricular septal defect (infundibular or membranous)	Congenital heart disease Bicuspid aortic valve Sinus of Valsalva aneurysm
Genetic syndromes Pseudoxanthoma elasticum	Genetic syndromes Marfan syndrome Familial thoracic aneurysm Ehlers-Danlos syndrome Osteogenesis imperfecta
Systemic rheumatic disorders Ankylosing spondylitis Rheumatoid arthritis Systemic lupus erythematosus Antiphospholipid syndrome	Systemic rheumatic disorders Giant cell arteritis Takayasu arteritis Ankylosing spondylitis
Infective endocarditis	Infectious aortitis (e.g., syphilis)
Aortic dissection	Aortic dissection
Trauma	Trauma
Rheumatic heart disease	

Clinical Approach to Aortic Valve Disease

Aortic Stenosis

Symptoms

The “classic” manifestations of AS are angina pectoris, syncope, and HF, but the following symptoms are currently those most frequently encountered thanks to an earlier diagnosis:

- exertional dyspnea or decreased exercise tolerance,
- presyncope or syncope during exercise,
- angina pectoris [1, 17].

Patients with AS are typically asymptomatic for a long period despite the increased pressure load on the LV [3, 46]. A wide variability exists in the degree of outflow obstruction that causes symptoms, depending in part on patient size and level of physical activity. However, in most patients with AS and normal LV systolic function, symptoms uncommonly occur until stenosis is severe (defined as a valve area ≤1.0 cm2, an aortic velocity of 4.0 m/s or higher, and/or a mean transvalvular gradient ≥40 mmHg) [18]. Notably, many patients who meet the criteria for severe AS are still asymptomatic. The most common symptom of AS is dyspnea during exercise, usually due to the diastolic dysfunction with a backward increase in pulmonary pressures with exercise and an inability of the LV to increase the cardiac output during exercise. Systolic LV dysfunction develops in a later stage. Once overt HF occurs, the patient may complain of shortness of breath, fatigue, debilitation, and other signs and symptoms of a low cardiac output state [17]. Presyncope or syncope is the presenting symptom in around 10% of patients with symptomatic severe AS [19]. Several mechanisms may lead to syncope: exercise-induced vasodilation in the presence of an obstruction with fixed cardiac output can result in hypotension, a transient bradyarrhythmia during or immediately after exercise, abnormalities in the baroreceptor response with a resulting failure to appropriately increase the blood pressure, or arrhythmias such as atrial fibrillation (AF) [17]. Approximately 50% of patients with angina pectoris have concomitant coronary artery disease (CAD) [20-22]. AS without significant CAD can cause myocardial ischemia by several mechanisms: increased total LV oxygen demand as a result of increased LV mass; reduced coronary flow reserve related to myocardial and vascular factors; elevated LV diastolic pressure contributes to a reduction in the perfusion pressure gradient, especially in the subendocardial myocardium; reduced diastolic coronary perfusion time during tachycardia [23].

Signs

The physical examination may provide the first clue to the presence of AS [24]. The three findings most useful to diagnose severe AS are: a low volume and slow-rising carotid pulse; a loud mid- or late-peaking systolic murmur in the right intercostal space; a single second heart sound [24]. On the other hand, these findings can be absent due to concurrent vascular disease [24-26]. The most useful signs to rule out significant AS are the absence of any systolic murmur and normal physiologic splitting of the second heart sound (S2). A transthoracic echocardiogram (TTE) is recommended when AS cannot be excluded on physical examination in a patient with symptoms possibly due to AS [17]. The typical arterial pulse in severe AS has been described as "parvus and tardus" (i.e., with a low volume and slowly rising). It can be appreciated in the carotid artery, and the delay can be detected by simultaneous palpation of the apex (point of maximum impulse) and the carotid artery. The amplitude of the carotid upstroke may be preserved in older patients with AS due to vascular changes. An associated carotid artery thrill or coarse vibration due to the turbulence of blood flow across the stenotic valve can be sometimes remarked [27]. Stenosis of the aortic leaflets is associated with reduced mobility and delayed closure [46]. S2 is soft and single since the aortic component of the second heart sound (A2), which is due to aortic valve closure, is delayed and tends to occur simultaneously with the pulmonic component of the second heart sound (P2), due to pulmonary valve closure. S2 may be paradoxically split when the stenosis is severe and associated with LV dysfunction. With increasingly severe, fixed AS, the A2 closing sound may disappear. The first heart sound (S1) is usually normal. However, an aortic ejection click, which is more common in patients with a bicuspid aortic valve, may be heard after S1 when the leaflets are still compliant and mobile. Vigorous left atrial contraction against a stiff, noncompliant ventricle can produce a fourth heart sound (S4) [17, 27]. The murmur associated with AS is described as a systolic "ejection" murmur, typically heard best at the base of the heart in the right intercostal space. The murmur generally begins after S1 and ends before S2. The intensity of the murmur reflects the amount and velocity of blood flow across the valve and the turbulence produced by the stenosis. A loud murmur has a high specificity for severe AS. However, most patients with severe stenosis have a grade 3 murmur, and many have only a grade 1 or 2 murmur. In patients with concomitant AS and LV dysfunction resulting in low-flow low-gradient, the murmur may be soft and almost inaudible. The timing of the murmur also correlates with AS severity. An early-peaking murmur is typical of mild to moderate AS, while a late-peaking murmur is consistent with severe AS. The murmur is well transmitted to carotid arteries and may also radiate to the apex (Gallavardin phenomenon); the murmur at the apex can be louder when there is an associated mitral regurgitation [27]. AS is often associated with a small degree of AR since the stiff, calcified, and rigid aortic valve leaflets may not coapt normally. In this case, a soft diastolic murmur may be heard [27].

Diagnosis and Evaluation

A TTE is the primary test for the diagnosis and characterization of AS. The exam includes evaluation of valve anatomy and structure, hemodynamic consequences, concomitant AR or other valve disorders. In patients with AS, the aortic leaflets are generally thickened and calcified with reduced systolic motion and a small orifice during systole. Thin aortic leaflets with normal systolic excursion, a normal aortic root, and normal LV wall thickness and systolic function suggest absence of significant AS. Patients with LV systolic dysfunction may have reduced leaflet excursion, even when AS is not severe. When a bicuspid aortic valve is present, systolic images show the two leaflets (and two commissures) of the open valve. A bicuspid valve may appear trileaflet when a raphe is present. In patients with a bicuspid aortic valve, the risk of associated aortic root involvement may be related to the specific bicuspid valve phenotype (congenital fusion of the right and left versus the right and noncoronary cusps) [28]. Doppler echocardiography allows measurement of transaortic velocity and calculation of the LV-aorta gradient and the valve area, which are the standard parameters used to evaluate stenosis severity. Over 80% of patients with AS display also AR, which is usually mild. The LV has usually normal size and systolic function, but the LV wall is concentrically hypertrophied, and LV longitudinal strain is reduced. Mitral regurgitation is common and may be exacerbated by the high systolic LV pressure due to LV outflow obstruction. The most reliable measure of AS severity is aortic velocity (or gradient) alone when LV ejection fraction (LVEF) is normal [27]. Valve area measurements are generally important only in patients with a low forward stroke volume due to a low LVEF or a small LV size. Body size should be considered in assessing aortic valve area (AVA) in smaller patients because a small aortic valve area may be normal for body size in smaller individuals [28]. A transesophageal echocardiogram (TEE) may be helpful in selected cases as it provides better images of aortic valve anatomy, and is more accurate for the diagnosis of a sub- or supra-aortic membrane. An electrocardiogram (ECG) is not needed for AS diagnosis, but is generally performed as part of the initial evaluation. A chest radiograph is not generally required when evaluating AS, but can aid in the differential diagnosis of dyspnea [27]. Exercise testing is suggested in patients with asymptomatic severe AS (maximum aortic valve velocity of ≥4.0 m/s or mean aortic valve pressure gradient ≥40 mmHg) who are sedentary to confirm asymptomatic status. Such evaluation is particularly helpful when the level of physical activity is unclear or low. Patients with severe AS who develop typical symptoms of AS during exercise testing should be considered symptomatic even if the clinical history is uncertain [18]. Exercise testing should not be performed in patients with symptomatic severe AS [27]. For patients with equivocal symptoms and severe AS, measurement of B-type natriuretic peptide (BNP) or N-terminal fraction of pro-BNP (NT-proBNP) levels may be helpful, as their elevation suggests that symptoms may be due to AS or other causes of high cardiac filling pressures [27]. Among patients with severe AS, BNP and NT-proBNP are higher in symptomatic than in asymptomatic patients [29, 30] and fall after AVR [31]. Higher BNP values are independent predictors of reduced symptom-free survival [32] and overall survival [33]. Among patients with low gradient AS, low-dose dobutamine stress TTE allows to differentiate true severe AS (with a fixed small valve area) from pseudo-severe AS (with a functionally small valve area due to reduced driving forces). Low-dose dobutamine stress test may also be helpful in symptomatic patients with findings consistent with paradoxical low-flow low-gradient AS. In addition, the test provides information on LV contractile reserve, which is helpful for prognostic purposes in contemplating possible surgical AVR or transcatheter aortic valve implantation (TAVI) [17, 27]. Cardiac computed tomography (CT) implements the evaluation in patients with low-gradient AS, particularly patients with classical low-flow low-gradient AS with inconclusive low-dose dobutamine stress TTE, with symptomatic paradoxical low-flow low-gradient AS who have inconclusive low-dose dobutamine stress TTE, or symptomatic patients with normal flow, low gradient AS. The degree of aortic valve calcification correlates with both echocardiographic determination of stenosis severity and clinical outcomes. Different cutoff values of aortic valve calcium score should be used in women compared with men to identify severe AS (≥1200 vs. 2000) [34]. Multidetector CT (MDCT) also allows measurement of aortic valve calcium density (the ratio of calcium load to cross-sectional area of the aortic annulus), which might be useful in the identification of patients at risk of rapid progression and adverse clinical outcomes [35, 36]. Cardiovascular magnetic resonance (CMR) is not performed routinely for clinical evaluation of AS, but it provides accurate measurements of the size and shape of the aortic sinuses and ascending aorta [37, 38], as well as antegrade velocity through the stenotic valve without angle dependence [39], and 4D flow patterns. Cardiac catheterization is not routinely required to assess the aortic valve gradient but is indicated for patients with suspected significant AS when noninvasive data are nondiagnostic or if there is a discrepancy between the clinical evaluation and noninvasive testing [18]. Coronary angiography is recommended in patients with apparently mild to moderate AS who have one or more of the general indications for coronary angiography such as progressive angina, objective evidence of ischemia, or either asymptomatic or symptomatic LV dysfunction. Coronary angiography is also mandatory in patients referred to AVR or transcatheter aortic valve implantation. Noninvasive stress imaging tests have low sensitivity and specificity for ischemia in patients with AS [17, 27].

Table 2. Stages of aortic stenosis (AS) and aortic regurgitation (AR)

Stage	AS	AR
A	Asymptomatic. V_{max} < 2 m/s; bicuspid aortic valve or other congenital anomalies, aortic sclerosis.	Asymptomatic At risk of AR, bicuspid aortic valve or other congenital valve anomaly, aortic valve sclerosis, diseases of the aortic sinuses or ascending aorta, history of RHD or IE.
B	Asymptomatic Mild: V_{max} 2.0 to 2.9 m/s or mean transvalvular pressure gradient < 20 mmHg; Moderate: V_{max} 3.0-3.9 m/s or mean transvalvular pressure gradient 20-39 mmHg	Asymptomatic Progressive AR; mild or moderate AR with normal LV systolic function and normal or mildly dilated LV volumes.
C	Asymptomatic. Severe leaflet calcification/thickening, reduced leaflet motion and Vmax ≥ 4 m/s; AVA ≤ 1.0 cm^2 (or AVA indexed ≤ 0.6 cm^2/m^2).	Asymptomatic. Alterations identified by Doppler echocardiography, CMR or cardiac catheterization.
C1	LVEF > 50%	LVEF ≥ 50%, LVESD ≤ 50 mm. Compensated phase of chronic AR.
C2	LVEF < 50%.	Precedes HF. LVEF < 50% and/or LVESD > 50mm or indexed LVESD > 25 mm/m^2.
D		Symptomatic LVEF 40-50% or < 40%.
D1	Symptomatic Vmax ≥ 4 m/s or mean transvalvular pressure gradient is ≥ 40 mmHg. AVA ≤ 1.0 cm^2 (or AVA indexed to body surface area is ≤ 0.6 cm^2/m^2) but may be larger with mixed AS/AR.	
D2	Symptomatic LFLG AS with LVEF < 50%. AVA ≤ 1.0 cm^2 and Vmax < 4 m/s or mean pressure gradient < 40 mmHg. AVA ≤ 1.0 cm^2 and Vmax ≥ 4 m/s at low-dose dobutamine stress echocardiography.	
D3	Symptomatic Severe low-gradient AS with LVEF ≥ 50% (paradoxical low-gradient severe AS). AVA ≤ 1.0 cm^2 (or AVA indexed ≤ 0.6 cm^2/m^2) and Vmax < 4 m/s or mean transvalvular pressure gradient < 40 mmHg; SVi < 35 mL/m^2.	

AR, aortic regurgitation; AVA, aortic valve area; AVD, aortic valve degeneration; CMR, cardiovascular magnetic resonance; HF, heart failure; IE, infective endocarditis; LFLG, low flow, low gradient; LV, left ventricle; LVEF, LV ejection fraction; LVESD, LV end-systolic dimension; RHD, rheumatic heart disease; SVi, stroke volume index; Vmax, maximum transvalvular velocity. Adapted from American Heart Association/American College of Cardiology Guidelines [18].

AS is a progressive disease and 4 stages have been identified based on TTE findings and symptoms (Table 2). Asymptomatic patients with AS with normal LVEF should be evaluated serially by history, physical examination and TTE to search for evidence of progression. Exercise testing is recommended if exercise tolerance is uncertain. The frequency of recommended evaluation varies with the severity of disease:

- for patients with mild AS and no significant calcification, evaluation is recommended every 2 to 3 years;
- for patients with moderate AS, evaluation should be performed every 1 to 2 years;
- for patients with asymptomatic severe AS, clinical evaluation should be performed every 6 to 12 months or sooner if symptoms develop or if there is a change in physical exam suggestive of worsening AS [18, 34].

Clinical Features of Advanced AS

Diastolic dysfunction, secondary to hypertrophy and fibrosis, is common and often persists after AVR. These patients may present with HF with preserved ejection fraction. A subset of patients presents with LV systolic dysfunction due to the high afterload imposed by the stenotic valve resulting in a low LVEF and symptoms of HF with reduced ejection fraction. LV dysfunction due to valve obstruction improves rapidly after AVR. The pulmonary artery pressure may be increased in AS because of the chronic elevation in LV diastolic filling pressure. A severe elevation in pulmonary artery pressure (systolic pressure >50 mmHg) occurs in approximately 15% of patients [40]. In some cases, pulmonary hypertension is due to coexisting lung disease rather than to the effects of aortic valve obstruction. Symptomatic severe AS is associated with a high risk of sudden cardiac death (SCD). The incidence of SCD is around 1% per year in patients with asymptomatic severe AS, and 8 to 34% in symptomatic patients [41]. The mechanism of SCD has not been established. A potential cause is activation of ventricular baro-chemoreceptors resulting in paradoxical bradycardia, decreased contractility, and hypotension (Bezold-Jarisch reflex). Ventricular tachyarrhythmias are another possible cause. The risk of SCD is reduced by AVR or TAVI [17, 27]. Intraventricular or atrioventricular conduction abnormalities are uncommon and, when present, may be due to severe hypertrophy, extension of calcium from valve structures into the interventricular septum, or concomitant heart disease [17]. Ventricular and supraventricular arrhythmias usually occur in patients with LV dysfunction. Risk factors for AF include older age, more severe AS, LV hypertrophy and systolic dysfunction [42, 43]. Among adults with mild to moderate AS, AF occurs in 5-6%, with an incidence of 1.2% new cases per year, and highest when LV systolic dysfunction is present [43]. AF is common in adults with severe AS (for example, in 34% in a series of patients referred to TAVI) [44]. New-onset AF can precipitate symptom onset in adults with severe AS because the loss of atrial contraction and the rapid heart rate both limit diastolic filling of a small, stiff LV. AF increases the risk of HF and non-hemorrhagic stroke [27, 45]. Infective endocarditis can occur in patients with AS, particularly those with a bicuspid AV. In a series of 2,401 patients with congenital heart lesions who were followed prospectively, those with AS developed infective endocarditis at a rate of 0.27 percent per year [46]. A higher peak gradient across the AV was associated with a greater risk of infective endocarditis. Although definite evidence is lacking, it has been proposed that the risk of infective endocarditis is lower in older patients with heavily calcified valves than in younger patients with less severe abnormalities.

Antibiotic prophylaxis is no longer recommended when patients with AS undergo dental or other invasive procedures that produce significant bacteremia with organisms associated with infective endocarditis. Antibiotic prophylaxis is recommended in certain high-risk groups (e.g., patients with prior infective endocarditis) [18, 34]. Patients with AS have an increased risk of bleeding, particularly in the gastrointestinal tract and at skin and mucosal sites [47]. The association between chronic gastrointestinal bleeding due to angiodysplasia and degenerative aortic valve disease has been named Heyde syndrome [48]. In a series of 42 patients with severe AS undergoing AVR, 9 had a history of skin or mucosal bleeding, and 4 had a history of gastrointestinal bleeding. The increased risk of bleeding is attributed to an acquired von Willebrand syndrome, which has been described in 67 to 92% of patients with severe AS. This abnormality is thought to result from mechanical disruption of von Willebrand multimers during turbulent passage through the narrowed valve and an interaction between the von Willebrand factor and platelets that promotes platelet clearance [47, 49]. The severity of the von Willebrand factor abnormality is directly related to the mean transvalvular gradient [47, 50, 51]. The hemostatic abnormality is corrected after surgery but recurs within 6 months of AVR in two-thirds of patients, especially when there is a mismatch between patient and prosthesis (an effective orifice area $<0.8\ cm^2/m^2$). The association between AS and angiodysplasia seems apparent, since patients with AS have an increased bleeding tendency, leading to the identification of angiodysplasia [17, 27].

Aortic Regurgitation

Acute Aortic Regurgitation

Symptoms and Signs

Severe acute AR commonly presents with acute HF or cardiogenic shock, with profound hypotension, pallor, diaphoresis, signs of peripheral vasoconstriction, and pulmonary edema. The pulse pressure may be normal or reduced, but the arterial pulsation is rapid and usually with low amplitude [5]. The cardiac apex is generally not displaced and not hyperdynamic [5]. In cases of aortic dissection, pulses and blood pressure values in the left and right arms may be inequal [52]. The peripheral manifestations of chronic AR, associated with an increased pulse pressure (listed below) may be absent in patients with acute AR, since LV stroke volume and pulse pressure are not significantly increased [5].

Acute AR is often characterized by a low-pitched early diastolic murmur beginning after S2. The murmur is sometimes not audible and its location may be variable. A systolic murmur resulting from the increased volume of blood crossing the aortic valve may be heard, but is usually not loud. Furthermore, acute AR alters the quality of heart sounds: the early closure of the mitral valve generally produces a soft or absent S1, which can occasionally be heard in mid-diastole; the aortic component of S2 is often soft, while P2 is usually increased, reflecting pulmonary hypertension; an S3 is often heard, but an S4 is absent [5].

Other possible symptoms are related to the cause of acute AR, such as infective endocarditis or aortic dissection. In some cases, acute AR is the first diagnostic clue to these conditions. Aortic dissection should always be suspected in patients with AR and chest or back pain [52].

Diagnosis and Evaluation

Echocardiography allows to diagnose acute AR, assess its severity, and in some cases to identify the underlying cause (such as infective endocarditis or aortic dissection). Color Doppler echocardiography demonstrates the backflow of blood across the aortic valve in diastole. The regurgitant jet is either central or eccentric, and the vena contracta width might be >6 mm. Holodiastolic flow reversal can be observed in the descending thoracic and proximal abdominal aorta [5]. In very severe cases, the late diastolic velocity approaches zero, indicating that aortic diastolic pressure and LV diastolic pressure are virtually identical [53, 54]. Signs of rapid pressure equalization of diastolic aortic and LV pressures include a dense continuous wave Doppler signal with a steep diastolic slope (pressure half-time <200 ms), and a short mitral deceleration time (<150 ms) and premature closure of the mitral valve. Importantly, the criteria for severe chronic AR may underestimate the severity of acute AR [55]. Echocardiography also enables evaluation of LV size and systolic function (which are often normal), and may provide information on the cause of valve dysfunction, by showing for example aortic dilatation and dissection or the presence of valvular vegetations. TEE is useful for identifying the mechanism of acute AR in the setting of aortic dissection, which may affect decision-making about the surgical procedure [56]. ECG changes are nonspecific. ST and T wave abnormalities are common, and patients may develop a myocardial infarction because of coronary occlusion in the setting of aortic dissection. Chest radiograph may show evidence of pulmonary edema, an enlarged cardiac silhouette because of pericardial effusion, or aortic root dilation [5]. When aortic dissection is suspected, TEE or CT can be performed, with high and similar values of sensitivity and specificity. CT imaging may help identify the intimal flap, the site and extent of dissection and the possible involvement of major branch arteries. Emergency valve surgery should not be delayed for coronary angiography if there is severe acute AR with hemodynamic instability. If the patient is reasonably stable, coronary angiography is generally performed in patients with CAD [18]. Aortography is indicated only when the diagnosis cannot be established by noninvasive imaging [5].

Chronic Aortic Regurgitation

Symptoms

Patients with chronic AR may remain asymptomatic for decades, even if there is progressive LV dilation. Symptoms that develop in some patients with severe AR include exertional dyspnea, angina, and other symptoms of HF. Dyspnea on effort and other HF symptoms (such as orthopnea or paroxysmal nocturnal dyspnea) are usually associated with LV systolic dysfunction. Angina during exercise can occur in the absence of significant CAD and is caused by reduced coronary flow reserve, as epicardial coronary flow shifts from predominantly diastolic to predominantly systolic. Angina can also occur at night when the heart rate slows, arterial diastolic pressure falls, and regurgitant volume increases, thus reducing coronary diastolic perfusion pressure. Some patients with severe AR may complain of symptoms related to the increased LV size and stroke volume. These include an uncomfortable awareness of the heartbeat, and atypical chest pain. These symptoms are especially pronounced when lying down or lying on the left side, which brings the LV apex closer to the chest wall.

Signs

The physical examination in patients with chronic severe AR provides many clues to the diagnosis, though findings are frequently more subtle in patients with milder disease. A variety of signs are caused by the wide pulse pressure in patients with chronic AR (Table 3). Among the four signs with sufficient literature for review (Corrigan pulse, Duroziez sign, Hill sign, and Austin Flint murmur), the Hill sign had a 75-100% sensitivity and a 71-100% specificity [57]. On precordial inspection and palpation, the apical impulse is displaced laterally and inferiorly and becomes diffuse and hyperdynamic. A prominent pulsation (and occasionally a thrill) may be felt at the sternal notch due to concurrent dilation of the ascending aorta. A diastolic murmur is a key sign favoring the diagnosis of AR, although the absence of a diastolic murmur does not exclude the diagnosis. The presence of an early diastolic murmur, as heard by a cardiologist, was the most useful finding for establishing the presence of AR (positive likelihood ratio 8.8) and its absence the most useful finding for reducing the likelihood of AR (negative likelihood ratio 0.2-0.3) [58]. On the other hand, widely different frequencies of a diastolic murmur among patients with chronic AR have been reported (14 to 73%) [59]. The diastolic murmur of AR begins immediately after A2. It has a high pitch, often blowing quality, and may be sustained or having a decreasing intensity. It may be soft and barely audible, often appreciated only when the patient is sitting up, leaning forward, and holding his or her breath in end-expiration. The intensity of the diastolic murmur does not correlate well with the severity of AR. The timing and duration of the murmur may be helpful in assessing the severity of AR:

- In mild AR, the murmur occurs only in early diastole and is blowing.
- As the regurgitation becomes more severe, the murmur extends through more of diastole, may become holodiastolic, and is often rougher in quality. Patients with a longer diastolic murmur, a displaced LV impulse, a wide pulse pressure, and the peripheral findings of a wide pulse pressure cited in the previous section are considered to have severe AR.
- In very severe regurgitation with ventricular decompensation, the murmur may become soft or even absent. This change in character reflects the near equalization of aortic diastolic and LV diastolic pressures, which diminish regurgitant flow. A similar situation can occur when AR is acute and the LV diastolic pressure is very high. The intensity of the murmur can also be affected by certain maneuvers. For example, the intensity of the murmur increases with squatting and decreases with the Valsalva maneuver. The site at which the murmur is best heard varies with the cause. The murmur is heard best along the left sternal border, at the third and fourth intercostal space, when AR is due to valvular disease. In contrast, abnormalities of the aortic root produce murmurs that are best heard at the right sternal border and apex. A mid-systolic murmur is heard in many patients with AR [59, 60]. The systolic murmur typically resembles the ejection type of murmur heard in aortic stenosis, i.e., a crescendo-decrescendo harsh murmur beginning after S1. This murmur is caused by a large ejection volume and thus does not necessarily reflect concurrent AS. A second type of diastolic murmur (the Austin Flint murmur) may also be appreciated. This murmur is a low-pitched, mid-to-late diastolic rumble, best heard at the apex. The murmur has been attributed to the effects of competing antegrade turbulent diastolic blood flow from the left atrium and the retrograde

regurgitant flow from the aorta. The sensitivity and specificity of the Austin Flint murmur is uncertain. A review found a higher sensitivity (57 to 100%) among patients with severe AR compared with patients with mild to moderate disease (0 to 50%) [57]. The heart sounds typically have the following characteristics: S1 may be soft, often reflecting a long PR interval; S2 is variable; it may be soft, absent, or single; A2 is often soft or absent while P2 may be normal, but obscured by the diastolic murmur; a systolic ejection sound may be due to abrupt aortic distension caused by the large stroke volume; a third heart sound (S3 gallop) is heard when LV function is severely depressed.

Table 3. Signs of aortic regurgitation

Sign	Manifestations
Corrigan pulse	"Water hammer" or "collapsing" pulse (rapidly rising and falling arterial pulse with a wide pulse pressure). Best appreciated in correspondence of radial, brachial, and carotid arteries.
de Musset's sign	Head bob in correspondence of each heartbeat.
Traube's sign	"Pistol shot" pulse (systolic and diastolic sounds) in correspondence of femoral arteries.
Duroziez's sign	Systolic and diastolic bruit heard when the femoral artery is partially compressed.
Quincke's pulses	Capillary pulsations in the fingertips or lips.
Mueller's sign	Systolic pulsations of the uvula.
Becker's sign	Visible pulsation of the retinal arteries.
Landolfi's sign	Constriction and dilation of the pupils with each heartbeat.
Hill's sign	Popliteal cuff systolic pressure exceeding brachial cuff pressure by more than 20 mmHg with patient in the recumbent position.
Mayne's sign	>15 mmHg decrease in diastolic blood pressure with arm elevation from the value obtained with the arm in the standard position.
Rosenbach's sign	Systolic pulsations of the liver.
Gerhard's sign	Systolic pulsations of the spleen.

Adapted from: Babu et al., 2003 [57].

Diagnosis and Evaluation

Chronic AR should be suspected in patients with physical examination findings consistent with AR, as symptoms develop only in a late disease stage. In addition, AR should be suspected in patients with dilated aortic sinuses or ascending aorta and in patients with bicuspid aortic valve, even if no murmur is apparent [18]. A TTE examination confirms the diagnosis of AR, establishes its severity, provides an assessment of aortic root and ascending aorta dilation, and evaluates LV size and function. Characteristic echocardiographic findings include the following:

- valve leaflets may be abnormal or may be normal but stretched due to aortic dilation, depending on the etiology of the AR. Abnormalities that may be seen include thickening, vegetations, calcification, a bicuspid valve, and prolapsed or flail leaflets;
- the aortic sinuses are often dilated with or without dilation of the ascending aorta. A thoracic aortic aneurysm is defined as an aortic diameter is ≥50% greater than the expected normal diameter but many patients have valve dysfunction due to aortic enlargement with a smaller degree of dilation;

- there is often restriction of opening of the anterior mitral leaflet and M-mode showing high frequency diastolic fluttering, which are due to the diastolic regurgitant jet of blood from the aorta;
- Doppler echocardiography (transthoracic or transesophageal) is the most sensitive noninvasive technique for detecting the regurgitant AR jet;
- the LV end-systolic and end-diastolic dimensions and volumes are increased in chronic AR. Wall motion is increased in parallel with the large stroke volume, but the ejection fraction does not increase. When LV decompensation occurs, the ejection fraction declines and end-systolic dimension and volume increases. Together with clinical evaluation of patient symptoms, echocardiography helps define the disease stage according to valve anatomy, severity of AR, and LV size and function, which in turn determines the need for AVR. The European Society of Cardiology guidelines have proposed qualitative, semiquantitative and quantitative criteria to define chronic AR as severe (Table 4). An ECG is not indicated for diagnosis of AR but is commonly included in the evaluation of patients with AR. ECG findings may reflect the adaptive changes that occur in the LV as a result of the volume overload, and typically shows evidence of LV eccentric hypertrophy. Conduction abnormalities are usually not seen, but can occur late in the course of AR when significant LV dysfunction occurs. Isolated atrial and ventricular premature beats are common, but sustained supraventricular or ventricular tachyarrhythmias are unusual in the absence of significant LV dysfunction. A chest radiograph may be obtained in selected patients with AR such as those in whom the cause of dyspnea is uncertain. In patients with severe AR, chest radiograph shows cardiac enlargement in an inferior and leftward direction. The ascending aorta (and often the aortic arch or knob) are often dilated. Left atrial enlargement does not occur unless there is significant LV dysfunction. In patients with a suboptimal or inconclusive TTE, CMR imaging is indicated to quantify AR severity, measure LV diastolic and systolic volumes, and assess LV systolic function [18]. Aortic regurgitant volume and regurgitant orifice area can be quantified. Aortic root angiography and cardiac catheterization with measurement of LV pressures are indicated when noninvasive tests are inconclusive or provide discrepant results from clinical findings [18].

Table 4. Features of severe aortic regurgitation

Qualitative	**Semiquantitative**	**Quantitative**
Valve morphology: abnormal/flail/large coaptation defect	***Vena contracta width:*** >6 mm	***EROA:*** $\geq$30 mm^2
Color flow regurgitant jet: large in central jets, variable in eccentric jets	***Pressure half-time:*** <200 ms	***Regurgitant volume:*** $\geq$60 mL/beat
CW signal of regurgitant jet: dense		***Increased LV volume***
Holodiatolic flow reversal in descending aorta: EDV >20 cm/s		

CW, Continuous-wave; EROA, effective regurgitant orifice area; EDV, end-diastolic volume; LV, left ventricle.

Staging and Serial Monitoring

A staging system considering valve anatomy and hemodynamics as well as symptoms has been proposed (Table 2) [18]. The frequency of serial clinical and echocardiographic monitoring in patients with asymptomatic aortic regurgitation varies with the severity of the disease, LV dimensions and LVEF, and the rate of disease progression on previous examinations.

CONCLUSION

Aortic valve disease is an important cause of morbidity in both industrialized and developing countries, although the etiology is profoundly different in the two settings. A careful search for signs and symptoms may provide the first clues to the presence of aortic valve disease, which can then be verified and characterized by imaging techniques, starting from TTE. In patients with known severe aortic valve disease, prompt detection of symptom onset is crucial to refer them to AVR or TAVI (in the case of AS), or AVR (in AR). Furthermore, a correct interpretation of the signs and symptoms of acute AR can result in a rapid diagnostic workup and prompt patient referral to surgery.

REFERENCES

[1] Braunwald, E. Aortic Stenosis: Then and Now. *Circulation.*, 2018, 137(20), 2099-100.

[2] Joseph, J; Naqvi, SY; Giri, J; Goldberg, S. Aortic Stenosis: Pathophysiology, Diagnosis, and Therapy. *The American journal of medicine.*, 2017, 130(3), 253-63.

[3] Eveborn, GW; Schirmer, H; Heggelund, G; Lunde, P; Rasmussen, K. The evolving epidemiology of valvular aortic stenosis. the Tromso study. *Heart (British Cardiac Society).*, 2013, 99(6), 396-400.

[4] Roberts, WC; Ko, JM. Frequency by decades of unicuspid, bicuspid, and tricuspid aortic valves in adults having isolated aortic valve replacement for aortic stenosis, with or without associated aortic regurgitation. *Circulation.*, 2005, 111(7), 920-5.

[5] Flint, N; Wunderlich, NC; Shmueli, H; Ben-Zekry, S; Siegel, RJ; Beigel, R. Aortic Regurgitation. *Current cardiology reports.*, 2019, 21(7), 65.

[6] Akinseye, OA; Pathak, A; Ibebuogu, UN. Aortic Valve Regurgitation: A Comprehensive Review. *Current problems in cardiology.*, 2018, 43(8), 315-34.

[7] Blaszyk, H; Witkiewicz, AJ; Edwards, WD. Acute aortic regurgitation due to spontaneous rupture of a fenestrated cusp: report in a 65-year-old man and review of seven additional cases. *Cardiovascular pathology: the official journal of the Society for Cardiovascular Pathology.*, 1999, 8(4), 213-6.

[8] Yang, LT; Liu, PY; Lee, CH; Kan, CD; Li, YH; Tsai, LM; et al. Acute aortic regurgitation caused by spontaneous aortic valve rupture. *The Annals of thoracic surgery.*, 2013, 96(6), e147-9.

[9] Mahara, K; Ota, M; Kishiki, K; Takanashi, S. Acute Aortic Valve Regurgitation Due to Spontaneous Rupture of Fenestrated Cusp Treated With Aortic Valve Repair. *Circulation journal: official journal of the Japanese Circulation Society.*, 2017, 81(2), 241-2.

[10] Pretre, R; Faidutti, B. Surgical management of aortic valve injury after nonpenetrating trauma. *The Annals of thoracic surgery.*, 1993, 56(6), 1426-31.

[11] Onorati, F; De Santo, LS; Carozza, A; De Feo, M; Renzulli, A; Cotrufo, M. Marfan syndrome as a predisposing factor for traumatic aortic insufficiency. *The Annals of thoracic surgery.*, 2004, 77(6), 2192-4.

[12] Isner, JM. Acute catastrophic complications of balloon aortic valvuloplasty. The Mansfield Scientific Aortic Valvuloplasty Registry Investigators. *Journal of the American College of Cardiology.*, 1991, 17(6), 1436-44.

[13] Dall'Ara, G; Saia, F; Moretti, C; Marrozzini, C; Taglieri, N; Bordoni, B; et al. Incidence, treatment, and outcome of acute aortic valve regurgitation complicating percutaneous balloon aortic valvuloplasty. *Catheterization and cardiovascular interventions: official journal of the Society for Cardiac Angiography & Interventions.*, 2017, 89(4), E145-e52.

[14] Roberts, WC; Ko, JM; Moore, TR; Jones, WH. 3rd. Causes of pure aortic regurgitation in patients having isolated aortic valve replacement at a single US tertiary hospital (1993 to 2005). *Circulation.*, 2006, 114(5), 422-9.

[15] Stout, KK; Verrier, ED. Acute valvular regurgitation. *Circulation.*, 2009, 119(25), 3232-41.

[16] Singh, JP; Evans, JC; Levy, D; Larson, MG; Freed, LA; Fuller, DL; et al. Prevalence and clinical determinants of mitral, tricuspid, and aortic regurgitation (the Framingham Heart Study). *The American journal of cardiology.*, 1999, 83(6), 897-902.

[17] Otto, CM; Prendergast B. Aortic-valve stenosis--from patients at risk to severe valve obstruction. *The New England journal of medicine.*, 2014, 371(8), 744-56.

[18] Nishimura, RA; Otto, CM; Bonow, RO; Carabello, BA; Erwin, JP; 3rd. Guyton, RA; et al. 2014 AHA/ACC guideline for the management of patients with valvular heart disease: executive summary: a report of the American College of Cardiology/American Heart Association Task Force on Practice Guidelines. *Journal of the American College of Cardiology.*, 2014, 63(22), 2438-88.

[19] Park, SJ; Enriquez-Sarano, M; Chang, SA; Choi, JO; Lee, SC; Park, SW; et al. Hemodynamic patterns for symptomatic presentations of severe aortic stenosis. *JACC Cardiovascular imaging.*, 2013, 6(2), 137-46.

[20] Silaruks, S; Clark, D; Thinkhamrop, B; Sia, B; Buxton, B; Tonkin, A. Angina pectoris and coronary artery disease in severe isolated valvular aortic stenosis. *Heart, lung & circulation.*, 2001, 10(1), 14-23.

[21] Tansuphaswadikul, S; Silaruks, S; Lehmongkol, R; Chakorn, T. Frequency of angina pectoris and coronary artery disease in severe isolated valvular aortic stenosis. *Journal of the Medical Association of Thailand = Chotmaihet thangphaet.*, 1999, 82(2), 140-9.

[22] Green, SJ; Pizzarello, RA; Padmanabhan, VT; Ong, LY; Hall, MH; Tortolani, AJ. Relation of angina pectoris to coronary artery disease in aortic valve stenosis. *The American journal of cardiology.*, 1985, 55(8), 1063-5.

[23] Julius, BK; Spillmann, M; Vassalli, G; Villari, B; Eberli, FR; Hess, OM. Angina pectoris in patients with aortic stenosis and normal coronary arteries. Mechanisms and pathophysiological concepts. *Circulation.*, 1997, 95(4), 892-8.

[24] Munt, B; Legget, ME; Kraft, CD; Miyake-Hull, CY; Fujioka, M; Otto, CM. Physical examination in valvular aortic stenosis: correlation with stenosis severity and prediction of clinical outcome. *American heart journal.*, 1999, 137(2), 298-306.

[25] Etchells, E; Bell, C; Robb, K. Does this patient have an abnormal systolic murmur? *Jama.*, 1997, 277(7), 564-71.

[26] Etchells, E; Glenns, V; Shadowitz, S; Bell, C; Siu, S. A bedside clinical prediction rule for detecting moderate or severe aortic stenosis. *Journal of general internal medicine.*, 1998, 13(10), 699-704.

[27] Otto, CM. Aortic stenosis. Clinical evaluation and optimal timing of surgery. *Cardiology clinics.*, 1998, 16(3), 353-73, vii.

[28] Baumgartner, HC; Hung, JCC; Bermejo, J; Chambers, JB; Edvardsen, T; Goldstein, S; et al. Recommendations on the echocardiographic assessment of aortic valve stenosis: a focused update from the European Association of Cardiovascular Imaging and the American Society of Echocardiography. *European heart journal cardiovascular Imaging.*, 2017, 18(3), 254-75.

[29] Gerber, IL; Stewart, RA; Legget, ME; West, TM; French, RL; Sutton, TM; et al. Increased plasma natriuretic peptide levels reflect symptom onset in aortic stenosis. *Circulation.*, 2003, 107(14), 1884-90.

[30] Lim, P; Monin, JL; Monchi, M; Garot, J; Pasquet, A; Hittinger, L; et al. Predictors of outcome in patients with severe aortic stenosis and normal LV function: role of B-type natriuretic peptide. *European heart journal.*, 2004, 25(22), 2048-53.

[31] Weber, M; Arnold, R; Rau, M; Elsaesser, A; Brandt, R; Mitrovic, V; et al. Relation of N-terminal pro B-type natriuretic peptide to progression of aortic valve disease. *European heart journal.*, 2005, 26(10), 1023-30.

[32] Bergler-Klein, J; Klaar, U; Heger, M; Rosenhek, R; Mundigler, G; Gabriel, H; et al. Natriuretic peptides predict symptom-free survival and postoperative outcome in severe aortic stenosis. *Circulation.*, 2004, 109(19), 2302-8.

[33] Clavel, MA; Malouf, J; Michelena, HI; Suri, RM; Jaffe, AS; Mahoney, DW; et al. B-type natriuretic peptide clinical activation in aortic stenosis: impact on long-term survival. *Journal of the American College of Cardiology.*, 2014, 63(19), 2016-25.

[34] Baumgartner, H; Falk, V; Bax, JJ; De Bonis, M; Hamm, C; Holm, PJ; et al. 2017 ESC/EACTS Guidelines for the management of valvular heart disease. *European heart journal.*, 2017, 38(36), 2739-91.

[35] Clavel, MA; Messika-Zeitoun, D; Pibarot, P; Aggarwal, SR; Malouf, J; Araoz, PA; et al. The complex nature of discordant severe calcified aortic valve disease grading: new insights from combined Doppler echocardiographic and computed tomographic study. *Journal of the American College of Cardiology.*, 2013, 62(24), 2329-38.

[36] Clavel, MA; Pibarot, P; Messika-Zeitoun, D; Capoulade, R; Malouf, J; Aggarval, S; et al. Impact of aortic valve calcification, as measured by MDCT, on survival in patients with aortic stenosis: results of an international registry study. *Journal of the American College of Cardiology.*, 2014, 64(12), 1202-13.

[37] John, AS; Dill, T; Brandt, RR; Rau, M; Ricken, W; Bachmann, G; et al. Magnetic resonance to assess the aortic valve area in aortic stenosis: how does it compare to current diagnostic standards? *Journal of the American College of Cardiology.*, 2003, 42(3), 519-26.

[38] Friedrich, MG; Schulz-Menger, J; Poetsch, T; Pilz, B; Uhlich, F; Dietz, R. Quantification of valvular aortic stenosis by magnetic resonance imaging. *American heart journal.*, 2002, 144(2), 329-34.

[39] Kilner, PJ; Manzara, CC; Mohiaddin, RH; Pennell, DJ; Sutton, MG; Firmin, DN; et al. Magnetic resonance jet velocity mapping in mitral and aortic valve stenosis. *Circulation.*, 1993, 87(4), 1239-48.

[40] Faggiano, P; Antonini-Canterin, F; Ribichini, F; D'Aloia A; Ferrero, V; Cervesato, E; et al. Pulmonary artery hypertension in adult patients with symptomatic valvular aortic stenosis. *The American journal of cardiology.*, 2000, 85(2), 204-8.

[41] Sorgato, A; Faggiano, P; Aurigemma, GP; Rusconi, C; Gaasch, WH. Ventricular arrhythmias in adult aortic stenosis: prevalence, mechanisms, and clinical relevance. *Chest.*, 1998, 113(2), 482-91.

[42] Bang, CN; Greve, AM; Boman, K; Egstrup, K; Gohlke-Baerwolf, C; Kober, L; et al. Effect of lipid lowering on new-onset atrial fibrillation in patients with asymptomatic aortic stenosis: the Simvastatin and Ezetimibe in Aortic Stenosis (SEAS) study. *American heart journal.*, 2012, 163(4), 690-6.

[43] Greve, AM; Gerdts, E; Boman, K; Gohlke-Baerwolf, C; Rossebo, AB; Nienaber, CA; et al. Prognostic importance of atrial fibrillation in asymptomatic aortic stenosis: the Simvastatin and Ezetimibe in Aortic Stenosis study. *International journal of cardiology.*, 2013, 166(1), 72-6.

[44] Stortecky, S; Buellesfeld, L; Wenaweser, P; Heg, D; Pilgrim, T; Khattab, AA; et al. Atrial fibrillation and aortic stenosis: impact on clinical outcomes among patients undergoing transcatheter aortic valve implantation. *Circulation Cardiovascular interventions.*, 2013, 6(1), 77-84.

[45] Tarantini, G; Mojoli, M; Urena, M; Vahanian, A. Atrial fibrillation in patients undergoing transcatheter aortic valve implantation: epidemiology, timing, predictors, and outcome. *European heart journal.*, 2017, 38(17), 1285-93.

[46] Gersony, WM; Hayes, CJ; Driscoll, DJ; Keane, JF; Kidd, L; O'Fallon, WM; et al. Bacterial endocarditis in patients with aortic stenosis, pulmonary stenosis, or ventricular septal defect. *Circulation.*, 1993, 87(2 Suppl), I121-6.

[47] Vincentelli, A; Susen, S; Le Tourneau, T; Six, I; Fabre, O; Juthier, F; et al. Acquired von Willebrand syndrome in aortic stenosis. *The New England journal of medicine.*, 2003, 349(4), 343-9.

[48] Hudzik, B; Wilczek, K; Gasior, M. Heyde syndrome: gastrointestinal bleeding and aortic stenosis. *CMAJ: Canadian Medical Association journal = journal de l'Association medicale canadienne.*, 2016, 188(2), 135-8.

[49] Pareti, FI; Lattuada, A; Bressi, C; Zanobini, M; Sala, A; Steffan, A; et al. Proteolysis of von Willebrand factor and shear stress-induced platelet aggregation in patients with aortic valve stenosis. *Circulation.*, 2000, 102(11), 1290-5.

[50] Natorska, J; Bykowska, K; Hlawaty, M; Marek, G; Sadowski, J; Undas, A. Increased thrombin generation and platelet activation are associated with deficiency in high molecular weight multimers of von Willebrand factor in patients with moderate-to-severe aortic stenosis. *Heart (British Cardiac Society).*, 2011, 97(24), 2023-8.

[51] Blackshear, JL; Wysokinska, EM; Safford, RE; Thomas, CS; Stark, ME; Shapiro, BP; et al. Indexes of von Willebrand factor as biomarkers of aortic stenosis severity (from the Biomarkers of Aortic Stenosis Severity [BASS] study). *The American journal of cardiology.*, 2013, 111(3), 374-81.

[52] Pretre, R; Von Segesser, LK. Aortic dissection. *Lancet* (London, England)., 1997, 349(9063), 1461-4.

[53] Grande, RD; Katz, WE. Acute aortic regurgitation secondary to disk embolization of a Bjork-Shiley prosthetic aortic valve. *Journal of the American Society of*

Echocardiography: official publication of the American Society of Echocardiography., 2011, 24(3), 350.e5-6.

[54] Saranteas, T; Christodoulaki, K; Rinaki, D; Kostopanagiotou, G. Transthoracic echocardiography for the identification of acute aortic regurgitation in the intensive care unit. *Journal of cardiothoracic and vascular anesthesia.*, 2011, 25(1), 204-5.

[55] Zoghbi, WA; Enriquez-Sarano, M; Foster, E; Grayburn, PA; Kraft, CD; Levine, RA; et al. Recommendations for evaluation of the severity of native valvular regurgitation with two-dimensional and Doppler echocardiography. *Journal of the American Society of Echocardiography: official publication of the American Society of Echocardiography.*, 2003, 16(7), 777-802.

[56] Patel, PA; Bavaria, JE; Ghadimi, K; Gutsche, JT; Vallabhajosyula, P; Ko, HA; et al. Aortic Regurgitation in Acute Type-A Aortic Dissection: A Clinical Classification for the Perioperative Echocardiographer in the Era of the Functional Aortic Annulus. *Journal of cardiothoracic and vascular anesthesia.*, 2018, 32(1), 586-97.

[57] Babu, AN; Kymes, SM; Carpenter Fryer, SM. Eponyms and the diagnosis of aortic regurgitation, what says the evidence? *Annals of internal medicine.*, 2003, 138(9), 736-42.

[58] Choudhry, NK; Etchells, EE. The rational clinical examination. Does this patient have aortic regurgitation? *Jama.*, 1999, 281(23), 2231-8.

[59] Heidenreich, PA; Schnittger, I; Hancock, SL; Atwood, JE. A systolic murmur is a common presentation of aortic regurgitation detected by echocardiography. *Clinical cardiology.*, 2004, 27(9), 502-6.

[60] Attenhofer Jost, CH; Turina, J; Mayer, K; Seifert, B; Amann, FW; Buechi, M; et al. Echocardiography in the evaluation of systolic murmurs of unknown cause. *The American journal of medicine.*, 2000, 108(8), 614-20.

In: Perspectives in Aortic Valve Disease
Editor: Giovanni Concistrè

ISBN: 978-1-53618-769-4

Chapter 3

NON-INVASIVE IMAGING OF AORTIC VALVE – ULTRASOUNDS: TRANS-THORACIC, TRANS-ESOPHAGEAL AND STRESS ECHOCARDIOGRAPHY

Alberto Giannoni[1,2,*], MD, PhD, Chiara Borrelli[1,3], MD, Giulia Elena Mandoli[4], MD and Francesco Gentile[5], MD

[1]Institute of Life Sciences, Scuola Superiore Sant'Anna, Pisa, Italy
[2]Division of Cardiology and Cardiovascular Medicine, Fondazione Toscana G. Monasterio, Pisa, Italy
[3]Division of Emergency Medicine, University of Pisa, Pisa, Italy
[4]Department of Medical Biotechnologies, Division of Cardiology, University of Siena, Siena, Italy.
[5]Division of Cardiology and Cardiovascular Medicine University of Pisa, Pisa, Italy

ABSTRACT

Echocardiography is the main imaging modality for the characterization of the aortic valve (AV) anatomy and function and the test of choice for following-up patients with AV disease. The combination of two dimensional trans-thoracic echocardiography, transesophageal echocardiography and stress echocardiography togheter with other imaging modalities and biomarkers help to refine the perfect timing and choice of treatment (surgical/percutaneus).

Keywords: trans-thoracic, trans-esophageal and stress echocardiography, aortic valve disease

* Corresponding Author's Email: alberto.giannoni@ftgm.it.

INTRODUCTION

Echocardiography still remains the most important imaging modality for the characterization of the aortic valve (AV) anatomy and function. Due to its widespread availability, superior assessment of flow haemodynamics, and the possibility to acquire in a single examination several prognostic parameters, echocardiography is routinely the test of choice for the assessment and follow-up of patients with AV disease and for the determination of the timing for surgical referral.

Two dimensional (2D) trans-thoracic echocardiography (TTE) is a key technique to confirm the diagnosis of AV disease and to assess its severity and prognosis. An integrated approach taking into accpunt several haemodynamic parameters rather than relying on a single measurement is usually recommended, together with a thorough clinical evaluation of patient's symptoms and potential confounders.

Transesophageal echocardiography (TEE) should be considered when TTE is of suboptimal quality, when further details on AV anatomy or pathophysiology are needed, or when thrombosis, prosthetic valve dysfunction or endocarditis is suspected. Three-dimensional (3D) echocardiography may warrant unlimited perspective and better outline complex anatomy of the AV and aortic root, in spite of potentially inaccurate geometric assumptions.

Finally, stress echocardiography (SE) may implement the assessment of the physical, haemodynamic, and echocardiographic consequences of exercise, unmasking symptoms in patients with poorly active lifestyles. Likewise, SE may help stratifying patients showing discrepancies between the AV area and the transvalvular gradients at rest, in the suspicion of the so called low-flow/low-gradient aortic stenosis.

TRANS-THORACIC ECHOCARDIOGRAPHY

Anatomic Assessment of the Aortic Valve in Physiology and Pathology

TTE, for its non-invasiveness, feasibility and availability, is the first and most used approach for the assessment of AV anatomy and disease (aortic stenosis - AS and aortic regurgitation - AR). The AV apparatus consists of three semilunar leaflets, three interleaflet triangles, three commissures, the annulus and the aortic wall. The aortic cusps are classified according to the emergency of the coronary arteries as left, right and non-coronary cusp (LCC, RCC and NCC, respectively); the latter is adjacent to the interatrial septum and in direct fibrous continuity with the anterior mitral leaflet [1]. The highest point of attachment of the cusps to the aortic wall is the sinotubular junction, while the nadir defines the annular plane [1].

There are different projections for TTE assessment of AV anatomy.

In the parasternal long axis (PLAX) view, the NCC and RCC are visualized, alongside the aortic root (Figure 1, panel a). This view allows the evaluation of left ventricular outflow tract (LVOT) and ascending aorta, thus enabling the assessment of left ventricular (LV) hypertrophy/dilation, aortic coartation or dilation (of the sinotubular junction or the annular plane), proximal aortic dissection and the presence of membranes, which is essential to determine the etiology of AS and AR [1].

By rotating the probe clockwise of 90° from the PLAX view, the parasternal short axis (PSAX) view is obtained. This is the best view for the evaluation of the whole aortic apparatus, as well as structural and functional anatomy of the three cusps (Figure 1, panel b).

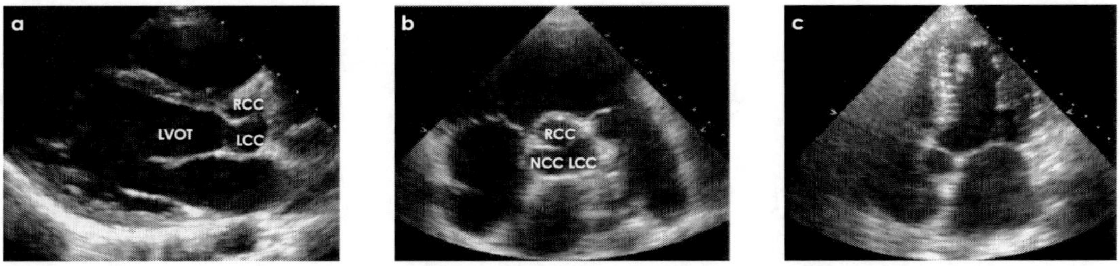

Figure 1. Transthoracic projections for the evaluation of the aortic valve (AV). The parasternal long axis view allows the evaluation of the right and non-coronary cusps (RCC and NCC, respectively), the aortic root, the left ventricular outflow tract (LVOT) and left ventricular dimensions (panel a). The parasternal short axis view allows the evaluation of the whole AV apparatus (from the lower left going clockwise: NCC, RCC and LCC, left cornary cusp) (panel b). The apical 5 chambers view allows the evaluation of the LVOT and aorta and it is used for continous wave Doppler evaluation of the aortic flow.

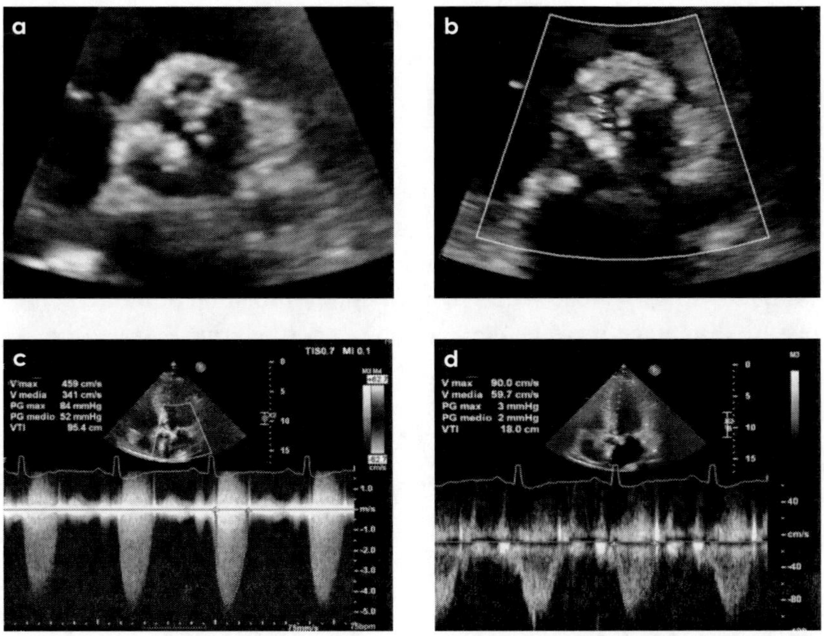

Figure 2. Echocardiographic evaluation of aortic stenosis (AS). Anatomic parasternal short axis view of a bicuspid aortic valve with Color Doppler evaluation of valve opening (panels a and b). Velocity time integral (VTI) of the aortic valve with continuous wave Doppler in apical 5 chambers view (A5Ch) showing severe AS: Vmax 4.6 m/s, mean pressure gradient 52 mmHg (panel c). VTI of the left ventricular outflow tract (LVOT) in A5Ch (panel d). Both aortic and LVOT VTI are necessary for the estimation of the aortic valve area.

When evaluating AS, the number and mobility of the cusps must be assessed to detect anatomical or functional (leaflet fusion, presence of raphe) bicuspid valve (see further on); cusps thickness and presence and severity of calcifications (bright, hyperechoic spots seen on leaflet edges with commissural fusion in rheumatic valve disease; central and annular calcifications in degenerative valve disease) must also be described (Figure 2, panel a and b) [2].

When assessing AR, leaflet motion, prolapse, perforation or the presence of calcifications or vegetations should be evaluated in both PLAX and PSAX views. In PLAX, measurements of the sinotubular junction and aortic annulus should also be acquired for AR classification [2].

Another important projection is the apical 5-chambers (A5Ch) view, which is obtained from the standard apical 4-chamber view, tilting the probe downwards (Figure 1, panel c). This view is fundamental for accurate Doppler measurements is AS and AR (see below). Additional views for the AV and aorta are the apical 3-chamber, the subcostal and the sovraclavear views.

Doppler-Based Assessment of Aortic Stenosis

When assessing AS, integration of 2D and Doppler data with patient's symptoms is crucial. The anatomical 2D alterations in AS have been discussed in the previous paragraph.

Simultaneous assessment of flow dependent (peak jet velocity and mean pressure gradient) and flow independent (AV area – AVA) measures, together with LV systolic function are required, as summarized in Table 1.

Transaortic jet velocities are measured by recording the maximal transaortic flow signal using continuous wave (CW) Doppler in different projections, the best one being A5Ch [3]. Peak velocity is measured at the outer edge of the dense spectrum, while velocity time integral (VTI) is calculated by tracing the entire spectral Doppler (Figure 2, panel c). Precise alignment with blood flow is required to prevent underestimation of the velocities [3].

The pressure difference between the LV and the aorta during systole (transvalvular aortic gradient, ΔP) are measured from CW velocity (v) with the simplified Bernoulli equation, as follows:

$$\Delta P = 4v^2$$

Table 1. Quantification of aortic stenosis (AS) severity with 2D echocardiography

Quantification of AS severity				
Parameters	**Sclerosis**	**Mild**	**Moderate**	**Severe**
Peak velocity (m/s)	≤2.5	2.5-2.9	3.0-3.9	≥4.0
Mean Gradient (mmHg)	-	<20	20-39	≥40
AVA (cm^2)	-	≥ 1.5	1.0-1.5	≤1.0

AVA: aortic valve area.

While maximum ΔP is estimated from peak velocity, mean ΔP is calculated averaging the instantaneous gradients over the whole ejection period [4].

Finally, AVA is calculated with the continuity equation, which is based on the principle that stroke volume (SV) ejected through the LVOT must be equal to SV at valve orifice level:

$$SV_{LVOT}=SV_{AV}$$

Because SV equals cross sectional area (CSA) times velocity over a set period (hence, VTI), the above equation can be rewritten as follows:

$$AVA = CSA_{LVOT} * VTI_{LVOT}/VTI_{AV}$$

The VTI_{AV} can be traced with CW over the entire Doppler spectrum, as previously mentioned; while the VTI_{LVOT} is estimated with pulsed wave (PW) at LVOT level in the A5Ch (Figure 2, panel d) or A3Ch [2].

The standard approach for CSA_{LVOT} calculation is the estimation of the diameter of the LVOT (D_{LVOT}), which is assumed to be circular. This measure is obtained in the PLAX view, measuring from septal endocardial border to the anterior mitral leaflet in mid-systole [2].

When interpreting the results, attention should be paid to discrepancies from velocity/gradient measures and AVA. In case of high flow states (i.e., AR, shunts, hyperdynamic states), markers of severe hemodynamic impairment can be registered in presence of an AVA ≥ 1 cm^2.

On the other hand, AVA $\leq 1 cm^2$ with non-severe gradients can be seen in case of LVEF <50% and/or SVi <35 mL/m^2, a condition known as low-flow low-gradient AS [3].

In this setting, dobutamine SE might help differentiating true from pseudosevere AS, as described below. Finally, the entity of low-flow low-gradient

AS with preserved EF has been introduced in the recent Guidelines in patients with small, hypertrophied LV despite normal LVEF [3]. However, this is a rare condition and should be diagnosed with extreme care.

Doppler-Based Assessment of Aortic Regurgitation

Anatomical 2D evaluation is mandatory to identify the mechanisms of AR (as explained above), while Color-Doppler (CD), CW and PW measurements are required for severity assessment (Table 2) [4, 5].

PSAX and A5Ch are the best views to assess AR severity (Figure 3, panel a and b), although multiple evaluations from different projections should be warranted, especially for eccentric jets. A comprehensive evaluation of LV function and dimension should also be performed, especially for chronic severe AR [4].

CD is the most immediate and intuitive way to assess AR severity from the degree of its extension in the LVOT. However, CD also allows the quantitative evaluation of the three components of the regurgitant jet: jet width, vena contracta (VC) and flow convergence.

Table 2. Quantification of aortic regurgitation (AR) severity with 2D echocardiography.

Quantification of AR severity			
	Mild	**Moderate**	**Severe**
Qualitative			
CD jet in LVOT	small	intermediate	large
CW jet density	faint	inermediate	dense
PHT (msec)	>500	200-500	<200
Semiquantitative			
Jet width/D_{LVOT} (%)	<25	25-64	≥65
VC (cm)	<0.3	0.3-0.6	>0.6
Quantitative			
EROA (cm^2)	<0.10	0.10-0.29	≥0.30
R_F (%)	<30	30-49	≥50
R_{VOL} (mL/beat)	<30	30-59	≥60

CD: Color Doppler; CW: continuous flow Doppler; D_{LVOT}: diameter of the LVOT; EROA: effective regurgitant orifice area; LVOT: left ventricular outflow tract; PHT: pressure half-time; R_F: regurgitant fraction; R_{VOL}: regurgitant volume; VC: vena contracta.

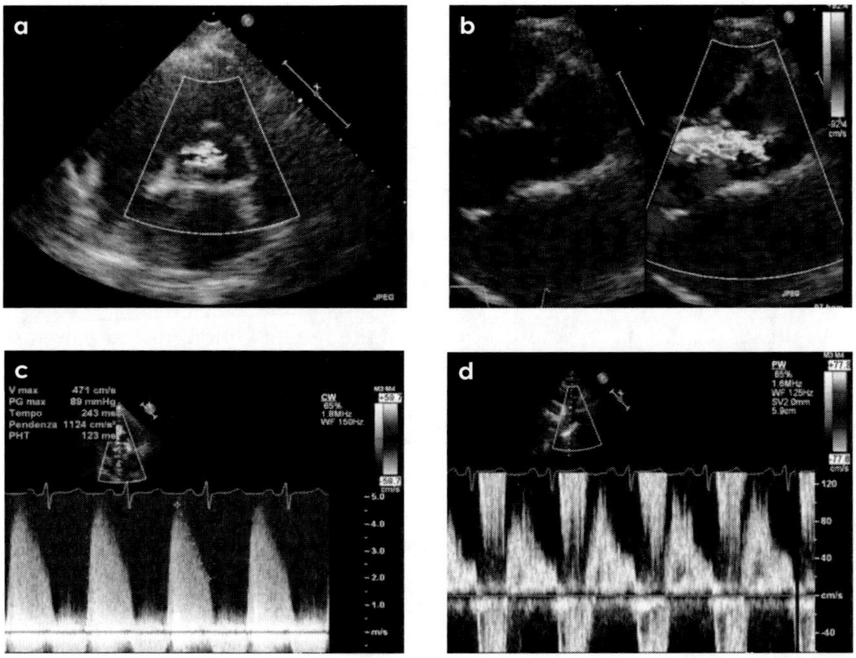

Figure 3. Echocardiographic evaluation of aortic regurgitation (AR). Anatomic parasternal short axis view of aortic valve regurgitation (panel a). Parasternal long axis view of left ventricular outflow tract (LVOT), with and without color Doppler. In this projection the diameter of the LVOT (dLVOT) and the jet width are calculated, allowing for the estimation of jet width/dLVOT ratio (panel b). The vena contracta can also be calculated in this projection. Pressure half time of AR in apical 5 chambers view with continuous wave Doppler (panel c). Diastolic flow reversal in the aortic arch with pulsed wave Doppler (panel d).

Jet width to D_{LVOT} ratio can be assessed for central jets only; it is measured in PLAX, just below the AV. VC is defined as the smallest neck of the regurgitant jet at the level of the AV, immediately below the flow convergence region, and is preferably measured in PLAX. Flow convergence (with proximal isovelocity surface area - PISA method) allows the quantification of the effective regurgitant orifice area (EROA), regurgitant volume (R_{vol}) and regurgitant fraction (R_F). This method is based on the principle that blood flow converges to the regurgitant orifice in hemispheric shells of increasing velocity and decreasing area. At this level, lowering the Nyquist limit in the direction of the flow to 30-40 cm/s, the velocity is known as the aliasing velocity (V_a) at the brusk red-blue interface. The PISA radius (rPISA) can also be measured from the aliasing interface to the regurgitant orifice. Finally, knowing the VTI of the regurgitant jet (VTI_{AR}) with CW, R_F, EROA and R_{VOL} can be calculated:

$$R_F = 2\pi rPISA^2 * V_a$$

$$EROA = R_F/VTI_{AR}$$

$$R_{VOL} = EROA * VTI_{AR}$$

The isovelocity surface area is not always optimally visualized. In such cases, an alternative option is the comparison of SV at both mitral annulus (MA) and LVOT with PW as follows:

$$R_{VOL} = SV_{LVOT}-SV_{MA}$$

$$R_F = R_{VOL}/SV_{LVOT} * 100$$

$$EROA = R_{VOL} * VTI_{AR}$$

CW is used for the calculation of VTI_{AR} (as explained above) and of pressure half-time (PHT) (Figure 3, panel c). PHT is derived from the regurgitant velocity spectrum and it is defined as the time required for the difference in pressure across the aorta to be halved; the fastest the equilibration, the steepest the PHT. Nevertheless, PHT is highly dependent on LV compliance and therefore loses its accuracy in cases of abnormal relaxation or acute AR [5]. Lastly, the density of the regurgitant spectrum is also considered as a marker of AR severity [4].

Finally, the combined use of PW and CD allows the detection of backflow in thoracic or abdominal aorta, which is present if AR is at least moderate (Figure 3, panel d).

TRANS-ESOPHAGEAL ECHOCARDIOGRAPHY

TEE allows a complete assessment of the AV apparatus. Anatomy is easily examined using standard views, mostly from mid-esophagus. The use of CD is essential to assess valvular function and can be applied to each view while the correct alignment for spectral Doppler is only obtained in deep transgastric (TG) view.

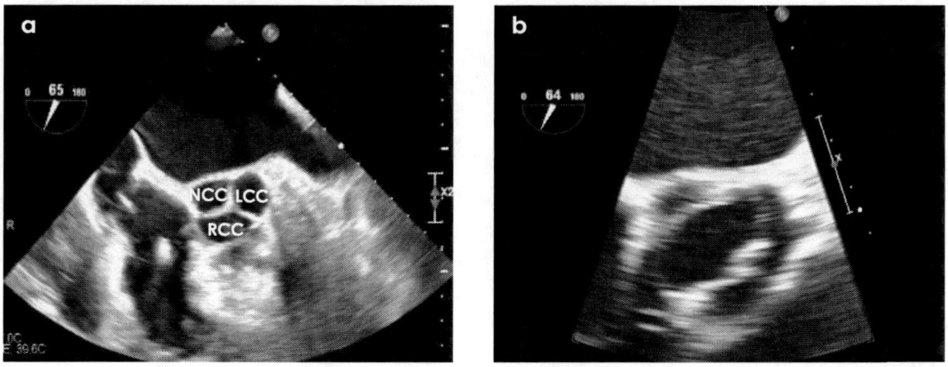

Figure 4. Transesophageal mid-esophageal (ME) AV short axis view (SAX). ME AV SAX is displayed starting from a standard ME 4 chamber view, with a slight probe withdrawal and rotation, up to 30-45°. In case of a tricuspid valve, the typical Mercedes Benz sign in diastole is displayed (the non coronary cusp - NCC on the left, close to interatrial septum, the left coronary cusp - LCC on the right and posterior, the right coronary cusp - RCC on the right and anterior). SAX is the key view for the diagnosis of bicuspid AV (BAV). In panel b the most common phenotype or type I BAV is shown with LCC-RCC fusion.

The mid-esophageal (ME) AV short axis view (SAX) is displayed starting from a standard ME 4 chamber view, with a slight probe withdrawal and rotation, up to 30-45°. Its position is then varied, with clockwise or counterclockwise small movements, to put the valve in the middle of the screen, ensuring the identification of all AV cusps and commissures. In a tricuspid AV a triangular orifice during systole and the typical Mercedes Benz sign in diastole are observed; the NCC is on the left, close to interatrial septum, the LCC is on the right and posterior, the RCC is the anterior leaflet (at the bottom of the screen) (Figure 4, panel a).

A minimal further withdrawal of the probe shows the origin of the coronary arteries from the left and right cusps (helping in the detection of abnormal origin and proximal course). SAX is the key view for the diagnosis of bicuspid AV (BAV), showing the 2 unequal-sized leaflets with the typical systolic fish mouth sign (Figure 4, panel b). Congenital type I BAV is characterized by an LCC-RCC fusion and represents the most common phenotype followed by RCC-NCC fusion (type II). Usually, a raphe replaces the corresponding commissure. Starting from the paramount assumption that BAV is not only an AV disease but also an aortic vessel disease, aortic root and ascending aorta must be carefully evaluated in all patients. Interestingly, the rheologic differences, consequent to the fusion pattern, lead to variable changes in aortic shear stress. The blood flow passing through a type I BAV usually promotes aortic root and ascending aorta dilatation while RCC-NCC fusion is most commonly associated with dilatation of the tubular portion of the ascending aorta and the aortic arch (the root is preserved) [6]. BAV can also be associated with other congenital defects, the most common of which being aortic coartation [7]. Thus, TEE examination must evaluate all accessible aortic portions. TEE report should describe the degree of atrioventricular sclero-calcific remodeling up to acquired form of BAV (consequent to extensive calcifications, previous endocarditis – rare – or rheumatic disease). Quadricuspid or unicuspid AV are other extremely rare congenital abnormalities.

From standard ME long-axis view, with a slight withdrawal or rotation of the probe up to 120-140° from an AV short axis-view, the ME AV long-axis view (LAX) is obtained. The anterior (inferior) aortic leaflet is the RCC while the closest cusp to the probe is either NCC or LCC (accordingly to rotation) (Figure 5, panel a). A magnified visualization of the aorta (by applying zoom mode or by reducing depth) is recommended to reduce errors in the measurement of aortic sections (annulus, sinuses of Valsalva, sino-tubular-junction). Normal cut-off values are listed in Table 3. Systolic valve doming, asymmetrical diastolic coaptation (both typical of BAV) and diastolic prolapse can be easily seen in this view. LVOT can also be measured.

The assessment of the LVOT and the AV can be completed at mid-esophagus with a five-chambers view, opened by slightly withdrawing or ante-flexing the probe from a standard ME four-chambers view. The anterior cusp is the RCC while the closest to the left atrium is the NCC.

Advancing the probe into the stomach and increasing the angle up to 120-140°, both the LVOT and the AV are included in the image (TG long axis view). Cusps motion and structure can be further evaluated here. Finally, going back to 0°, with an additional advance and anteflexion of the probe (in contact with gastric wall), we display a deep TG view, in which the LVOT anatomy and dimension can be studied and the perfect alignment with the AV allows spectral Doppler interrogation.

Table 3. Aortic root dimensions: reference values

	Absolute values (cm)		**Indexed values (cm/m^2)**	
	Men	**Women**	**Men**	**Women**
Mid-systolic*				
Annulus	2.6 ± 0.3	2.3 ± 0.2	1.3 ± 0.1	1.3 ± 0.1
End-diastolic**				
Sinuses of Valsalva	3.4 ± 0.3	3.0 ± 0.3	1.7 ± 0.2	1.8 ± 0.2
STJ	2.9 ± 0.3	2.6 ± 0.3	1.5 ± 0.2	1.5 ± 0.2
Proximal ascending aorta	3.0 ± 0.4	20.7 ± 0.4	1.5 ± 0.2	1.6 ± 0.3

*inner edge to inner edge ** leading edge to leading edge.
Adapted from Lang et al. [8] STJ = Sinotubular junction.

Aortic Stenosis

TEE examination helps to discriminate between the valvular stenosis and the much rarer sub- and supra-valvular defects. In ME AV short axis view, planimetry of the valve (anatomical area) can be obtained in systole even if it is more complicated in case of very severe calcifications. CD imaging can reveal a typical mosaic pattern in the LVOT due to the turbulent blood flow. CW and LVOT PW interrogation in deep TG view allow the calculations of jet velocity and gradients across AV and the estimation of AVA by continuity equation. However, TTE remains the best method for this purpose.

Aortic Regurgitation

The assessment of AR starts from the investigation of its etiology. In each view, the AV anatomy should be accurately evaluated to verify if AR is related to acquired or congenital diseases. The surgical classification of AR recognizes 3 different patterns: enlargement of aortic root with normal cusps (type 1); cusps prolapse or fenestration with excessive motion (type 2); poor cusp tissue quality or quantity with restricted motion (type 3) [9]. If the clinical suspect is endocarditis, vegetations must be carefully investigated (Figure 5, panel a and b).

The use of CD must complete every TEE exam. In ME AV SAX, AR is seen as a continuous flow during diastole and the origin of the jet can be described as central or commissural. In all other views, the direction of the flow can be central or eccentric (typical of BAV, fenestrated or prolapsed cusps, with an opposite-directed jet). In ME AV LAX, quantitative parameters for the estimation of AR can be calculated, including jet width/LVOT width, jet area/LVOT area, VC width, PISA radius (Figure 6, panel b).

A good alignment of the ultrasound beam in the deep TG view is useful to obtain the CW Doppler spectral trace for the evaluation of other AR indexes such as PHT, EROA, R_{VOL} and R_F. Methods and cut-off values are described in TTE section. The demonstration of reversal flow in descending aorta by PW is associated with a higher AR severity.

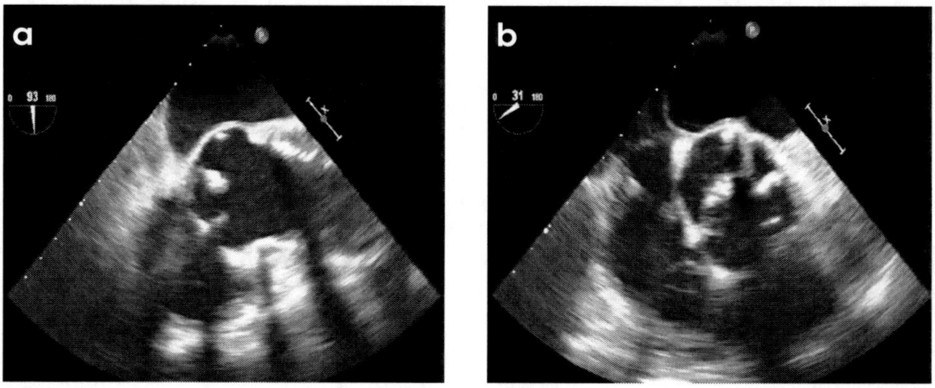

Figure 5. Transesophageal evaluation of aortic valve (AV) endocarditis. Mid-esophageal long axis (panel a) and short axis (panel b) views of AV showing an endocarditis mass on the non coronary cusp.

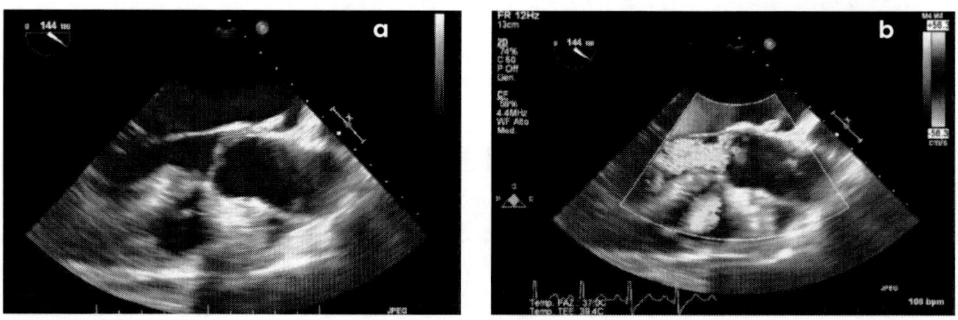

Figure 6. Transesophageal mid-esophageal (ME) aortic valve (AV) long-axis view (LAX). From a ME AV short axis-view (SAX) with a slight withdrawal or rotation of the probe up to 120-140°, we obtain a ME AV LAX (panel a). The anterior (inferior) aortic leaflet is the RCC while the closest cusp to the probe is either NCC or LCC (accordingly to rotation). From this view it is possible to obtain measurements of different aortic sections (annulus, sinuses of Valsalva, sino-tubular-junction) and left ventricular outflow tract (LVOT). By applying color-Doppler (panel b) the regurgitant jet may be visualized (central/eccentric) and quantitative parameters for the estimation of aortic regurgitation AR can be calculated, including jet width/LVOT width, jet area/LVOT area, vena contracta width and PISA radius.

Thoracic Aorta and Aortic Arch

Beyond the measurement of the aortic root and the ascending aorta, every TEE should be completed by the evaluation of thoracic aorta and aortic arch. Starting from a TG or ME at 0°, the probe must be rotated counterclockwise (to the left of the patient) to display the posterior descending aorta short axis view (Figure 7).

An image optimization by reducing image depth, setting the focus in the near field and increasing the gain is recommended. A slow continuous withdrawal of the probe allows to follow and evaluate the whole wall structure and lumen.

Long axis view is obtainable when increasing the angle up to 90-110°; however, thanks to the widely available probes with biplane mode, simultaneous short and long axis views are displayed (Figure 7). At the level of left subclavian artery, the aorta will appear elongated: this is the cut plane at which aortic arch begins. Usually a slight clockwise rotation of the probe is needed to show a correct long axis view. Aortic arch short axis view is detected at 70-90°.

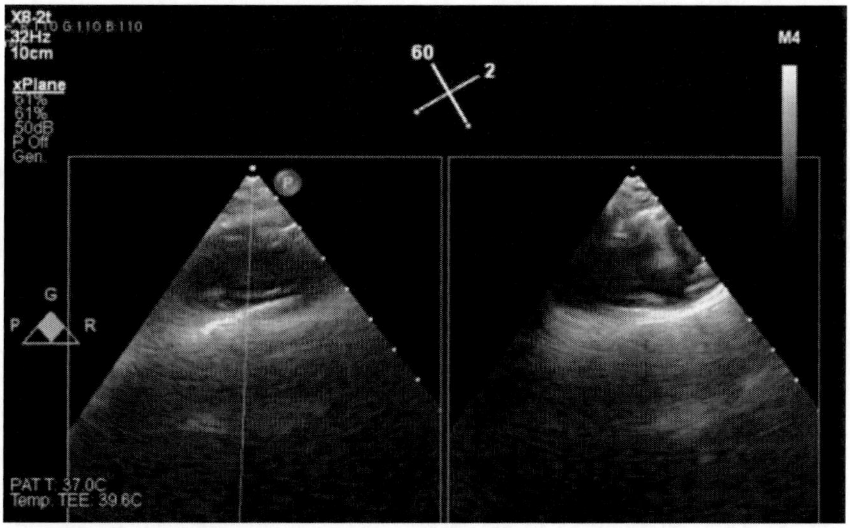

Figure 7. Transesophageal evaluation of the thoracic aorta with the X-plane view. The thoracic aorta is displaced along its long axis (left) and shor axis (right).

3D-Transesophageal Assessment

The use of 3D TEE aims to integrate the AV and LVOT visualization and planimetry, mostly when 2D images are sub-optimal or partially defined (Figure 8).

Full volume 3D dataset is usually built from the ME AV short and long axis views or from a ME 60° view, simultaneously optimizing the two 2D images [10]. The size of 3D box will determine spatial and temporal resolution. Once the 3D image is modeled, the surgical view of the AV is usually firstly displayed. Moving the crop planes, the AV and LVOT areas can be traced and calculated with a good accuracy compared to multislice computed tomography [11]. Experience in 3D echocardiography is needed for the correct interpretation of images (i.e., discrimination between drop out artifacts and cusps abnormalities). Applying

CD, 3D VC has been used to estimate AR severity, showing significant correlation with 2D VC [12].

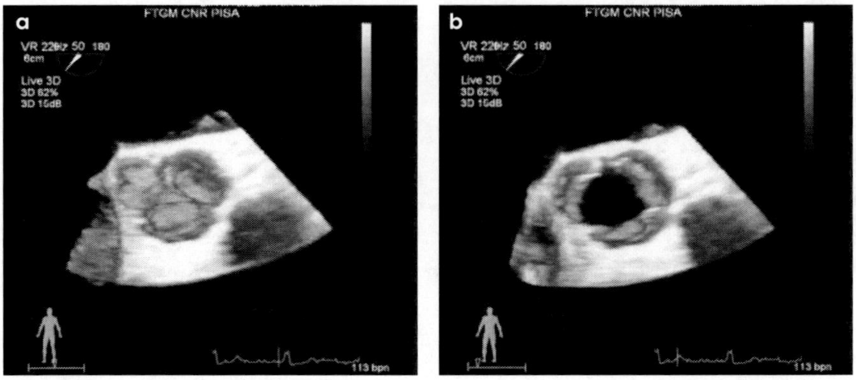

Figure 8. 3D-transesophageal mid-esophageal (ME) AV short axis view (SAX). The use of 3D transesophageal echochardiography aims to integrate the AV visualization and planimetry. Full volume 3D dataset is here built from the ME AV SAX simultaneously optimizing 2D images. Once the 3D image is modeled, the surgical view of the AV is usually displayed. Moving the crop planes, the AV area can be traced and calculated.

TEE as a Key Tool before and after Percutaneous and Surgical Procedures

The role of TEE is relevant in the decision making of AV functional defects. A complete report should include: AS/AR etiology, AV anatomic features (BAV or other defects), dimensions of the whole AV apparatus (crucial for prosthesis sizing), LVOT dimension, AVA, origin of coronary ostia, degree of calcification of ascending aorta (in case of aortic clamp). The functional and anatomical data from TEE are integrated with computed tomography data. During follow up, aortic prostheses are periodically evaluated by TTE.

However, TEE can help in searching perivalvular leaks (due to technical issues during implant or suture dehiscence) or prosthesis degeneration causing relevant regurgitation, if TTE images are of poor quality. In addition, a TEE can be requested for the differential diagnosis between pannus and thrombosis in mechanical prosthesis, even if technically difficult. Usually, clinical history and the aspect of thrombus (more commonly hyperechoic and large, with greater interference with disks motion) are key features. Finally, TEE is an integral diagnostic technique when suspecting prosthesis endocarditis: vegetations, abnormal valve function, peri-annular abscesses are usually found and quite easily detected [13].

Stress Echocardiography

Stress echocardiography (SE), meant as either exercise stress-testing or pharmacological stress with dobutamine, is widely accepted as a key exam in the diagnostic workup and risk stratification of patients with AV disease.

Indeed, when appropriate, SE may yield straightforward information about the severity of valvular dysfunction along with the potential hemodynamic consequences, such as pressure and volume overload and impaired contractile reserve (CR) [14]. Moreover, the relatively low-cost, safety, and wide diffusion, make SE an ideal choice in patients with a slow-progressive valve disease and with a poorly active lifestyle, combing information derived from the exercise-challenge and potentially useful imaging markers [15].

Therefore, during last decades, the clinical setting of AS has seen an increasing demand of SE, along with the growing number of potential candidates to valve replacement, due to the ageing population and to the widespread diffusion of percutaneous approaches. In particular, the main applications of SE in the patient with AS are:

1. The assessment of the physical, hemodynamic, and echocardiographic consequences of exercise in patients with a known severe AS but with poor active lifestyles, potentially masking symptoms occurrence.
2. The further stratification of patients showing discrepancies between the AVA and the transvalvular gradients at rest, in the suspicion of low-flow/low-gradient AS [16].

Conversely, only a marginal role is attributed to SE in patients with chronic AR, probably due to the lack of large studies in this context [14].

Stress Echocardiography in Aortic Stenosis

Nowadays, due to ageing population, ever more patients receiving a diagnosis of severe AS complain few symptoms, probably because of sedentary lifestyles. Therefore, it may be tricky to attribute physical limitations and symptoms to the valvular disease. Moreover, while AV replacement is clearly indicated in case of reduced LVEF, only symptomatic patients with severe AS and preserved LVEF should undergo surgery, unless meeting criteria of very severe AS.

Exercise-testing may then unmask symptoms, significant blood pressure drops and/or changes in ST-segment, and thus be useful to identify the subgroup of patients that would benefit more from surgical intervention [17, 18, 19].

In this respect, stress-related increase in mean transvalvular gradient >20 mmHg and a pulmonary systolic artery pressure >60 mmHg during exercise have been related with a 3.8-fold and 2-fold greater risk of cardiac event at follow-up, respectively, also in absence of other SE criteria [20, 21]. Notwithstanding, the utility of SE in asymptomatic AS has been challenged in a recent study, in which, among the 112 patients with an otherwise negative exercise-test, neither the increase in mean transvalvular gradient nor in pulmonary systolic artery pressure were predictive of outcome [22]. Discrepancies in methodology and study populations or endpoints have been advocated to explain those contrasting results.

Other parameters have been also proposed in asymptomatic patients with severe AS : an increase in average E/e' > 14; a worsening in left ventricular wall motion; a reduced CR (meant either as LVEF fall/increase <5% or left ventricular global longitudinal strain fall/increase <-1.4%); an S'-wave velocity increase <5 cm/s [23].

Whether SE may help to properly select the subset of “truly” asymptomatic patients in which AV surgery may be beneficial is yet to be clarified by large and multicenter prospective studies.

Low-Flow Low-Gradient Aortic Stenosis

Dobutamine SE (DSE) represents a key test in the diagnostic algorithm of patients with a suspected low-flow/low-gradient AS, both in the classical (i.e., in case of reduced LVEF) and in the paradoxical subtype (i.e., in case of preserved LVEF) [16]. Due to the frailty of such subgroup of patients, a low-dose dobutamine protocol is usually indicated, with a starting dose of 2.5 or 5 mg/kg/min and a progressive increment up to 10–20 mg/kg/min, until study targets have been achieved [3].

The first aim of DSE is to evaluate whether CR is present or absent. In particular, a recovery of the SV >35 mL/m^2, a rise >20% from baseline, and/or a transvalvular flow rate >200-250 mL/s (as calculated from the ratio between SV and systolic ejection time) are commonly used as signs of preserved CR. In this case, re-evaluating the AVA in optimized flow condition may allow to distinguish between a truly severe AS or a pseudo-severe AS. An increase in the AVA up to value >1 cm^2 at any stage of DSE indicates a pseudo-severe AS and it is often accompanied by no change or only a slight rise of transvalvular gradients.

On the contrary, truly severe AS is suggested by an AS jet velocity ≥4.0 m/s or a mean gradient ≥40 mmHg, while the AVA remains <1 cm^2 [24] (Figure 9).

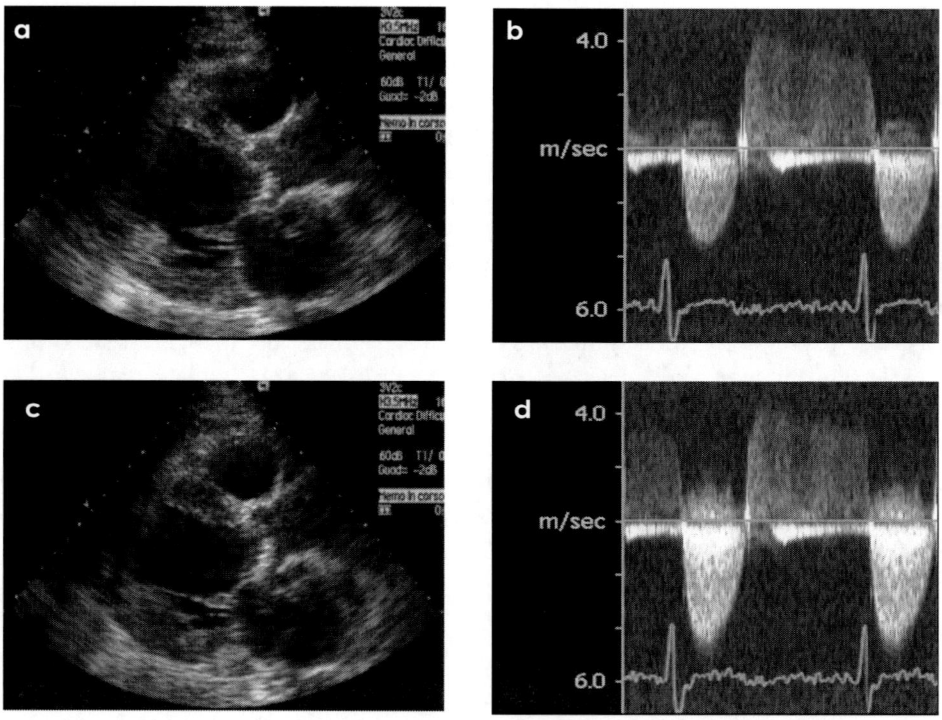

Figure 9. Dobutamine stress echocardiography for the evaluation of low-flow low-gradient aortic valve (AV). Parasternal long axis view of the AV showing aortic stenosis (AS) with aortic valve area (AVA) = 0.7 cm^2 in presence of an ejection fraction <50% (panel a). Doppler evaluation of the AV shows a peak velocity of 3.5 m/s and a mean gradient of 27 mmHg (panel b). To assess the severity of AS in presence of discordant anatomical and Doppler data, dobutamine stress echo is performed, confirming an AVA = 0.7 cm^2 (panel c). Doppler based data show a peak velocity of 4.3 m/s and a mean gradient of 43 mmHg, confirming the severity of the stenosis (panel d).

Whether diagnostic uncertainty still persists after the test, calculating the projected AVA (i.e., AVA at a normalized flow rate of 250 mL/s) may be considered, by means of a mathematical formula, firstly proposed by Blais et al.:

$$\text{Projected AVA} = \text{AVArest} + (\Delta\text{AVA}/\Delta\text{Q}) * (250 - \text{Qrest})$$

where Q indicates the flow rate and ΔAVA and ΔQ are the differences between the values obtained during DSE and at rest. A projected AVA <1 cm^2 indicates a truly severe AS [25].

The clinical relevance of distinguishing between a truly severe and a pseudo-severe AS lays in the assumption that AV replacement is indicated only in the former situation, while clinical follow-up is indicated in the latter [17, 18]. Furthermore, the absence of CR at DSE helps to identify a subset of patients at very high operative risk, to be consequently candidate to less invasive approaches [16].

Finally, similar criteria may be applied to patients with a suspected paradoxical low-flow/low-gradient AS. Nevertheless, the small cardiac volumes and the restrictive filling pattern that often characterize these patients, may affect DSE interpretation and require the use of other diagnostic tools, such as computed tomography, to obtain definitive conclusions [26].

Stress Echocardiography in Aortic Regurgitation

Exercise-SE may help to unmask symptoms in poorly active patients also in the setting of AR. Nevertheless, whether exercise-testing may provide a better risk stratification in otherwise asymptomatic patients with AR is still to be elucidated [27]. Therefore, while the use of SE is considered reasonable in this setting according to American guidelines [17], it is not even mentioned in the latest European guidelines [18].

A few and relatively small studies have shown that a preserved pre-operative CR could be a predictor of survival and ventricular decompensation better than other parameters obtained at resting conditions [28, 29]. Moreover, in the study of Park et al. one-third of patients with a preserved CR had a LV end-systolic diameter >50 mm, that would have indicated AV replacement according to current guidelines (class IIa) [17, 18]. The evaluation of CR may then improve the current ability to allocate asymptomatic patients as potential candidates to AV replacement [29]. Finally, the possible role of other markers, such as stress-related changes in longitudinal LV function assessed with tissue Doppler [30, 31] and tricuspid annular plane systolic excursion measured during exercise [32] seem also to improve risk stratification of asymptomatic patients with severe AR and preserved LVEF, encouraging future research in this field.

CONCLUSION

Echocardiography is the first imaging technique of choice to diagnose and grade AS and AR. The use of multiple views and several qualitative, semiquantitative and quantitative parameters derived from transthoracic, transesophageal and stress echocardiography may help to understand the clinical relevance of AV diseases, to stratify patients' prognosis and to understand both the need of an intervention and the timing and choice of the best treatment modality. With expanding technologies and increasing availability of treatment options such as transcatheter aortic valve interventions, in addition to conventional surgical approaches, accurate and precise assessment of AV conformation and disease severity is critical to guide clinical decisions.

A multiparametric echocardiographic approach, along with the incorporation in certain scenarios of multimodality imaging (cardiac computed tomography or magnetic resonance imaging), is now mandatory to avoid incorrect misclassification of AS/AR and to ensure appropriate selection of patients who would most benefit from AV interventions.

REFERENCES

[1] Basso C, Thiene G, and Ho SV. "Heart valve disease (aortic valve disease): anatomy and pathology of the aortic valve." In *The EACVI textbook of echocardigraphy, 2nd edition*, edited by Lancellotti PP, Zamorano JL, Habib G, Badano L. 231-233. Oxford: Oxford University Press (2017).

[2] Baumgartner H, Orwat S, Sade E, and Bermejo J. "Heart valve disease (aortic valve disease): aortic stenosis. In "*The EACVI textbook of echocardigraphy, 2nd edition*," edited by Lancellotti PP, Zamorano JL, Habib G, Badano L. 234-250. Oxford: Oxford University Press, (2017).

[3] Baumgartner H, Hung J, Bermejo J, Chambers JB, Edvardsen T, Goldstein S, Lancellotti P, LeFevre M, Miller F, and Otto CM. "Recommendations on the echocardiographic assessment of aortic valve stenosis: a focused update from the European Association of Cardiovascular Imaging and the American Society of Echocardiography." *J Am Soc Echocardiogr* (2017): 373-392.

[4] Zoghbi WA, Adams D, Bonow RO, Enriquez-Sarano M, Foster E, Grayburn, PA Hahn RT, Han Y, Hung J, Lang RM, Little SH, Shah DJ, Shernan S, Thavendiranathan P, Thomas JD, and Weissman NJ. "Recommendations for noninvasive evaluation of native valvular regurgitation. A Report from the American Society of Echocardiography Developed in Collaboration with the Society for Cardiovascular Magnetic Resonance." *J Am Soc Echocardiogr* (2017): 303-371.

[5] Otto CM. "Valvular regurgitation." In "*Textbook of clinical echocardiography, 6th edition*" edited by Otto CM. 364-345. Philadelphia, Elsevier, (2018).

[6] Verma S, Siu SC. "Aortic Dilatation in Patients with Bicuspid Aortic Valve." *N Engl J Med* (2014): 1920-1929.

[7] Roos-Hesselink JW, Schölzel BE, Heijdra RJ, Spitaels SE, Meijboom FJ, Boersma E, Bogers AJ, Simoons ML. "Aortic valve and aortic arch pathology after coarctation repair." *Heart* (2003): 1074-1077.

[8] Lang RM, Badano LP, Mor-Avi V, Afilalo J, Armstrong A, Ernande L, Flachskampf FA, Foster E, Goldstein SA, Kuznetsova T, Lancellotti P, Muraru D, Picard MH, Rietzschel ER, Rudski L, Spencer KT, Tsang W, Voigt JU. "Recommendations for cardiac chamber quantification by echocardiography in adults: an update from the

American Society of Echocardiography and the European Association of Cardiovascular Imaging." *J Am Soc Echocardiogr* (2015): 1-39.e14.

[9] El Khoury G, Glineur D, Rubay J, Verhelst R, d'Acoz Yd, Poncelet A, Astarci P, Noirhomme P, van Dyck M. "Functional classification of aortic root/valve abnormalities and their correlation with etiologies and surgical procedures." *Curr Opin Cardiol* (2005): 115-121.

[10] Hahn RT, Abraham T, Adams MS, Bruce CJ, Glas KE, Lang RM, Reeves ST, Shanewise JS, Siu SC, Stewart W, Picard MH. "Guidelines for performing a comprehensive transesophageal echocardiographic examination: recommendations from the American Society of Echocardiography and the Society of Cardiovascular Anesthesiologists." *J Am Soc Echocardiogr* (2013): 921-964.

[11] Khalique OK, Kodali SK, Paradis JM, Nazif TM, Williams MR, Einstein AJ, Pearson GD, Harjai K, Grubb K, George I, Leon MB, Hahn RT. "Aortic annular sizing using a novel 3-dimensional echocardiographic method: use and comparison with cardiac computed tomography." *Circ Cardiovasc Imaging* (2014): 155–163.

[12] Sato H, Ohta T, Hiroe K, Okada S, Shimizu K, Murakami R, Tanabe K. "Severity of aortic regurgitation assessed by area of vena contracta: a clinical two-dimensional and three-dimensional color Doppler imaging study." *Cardiovasc Ultrasound* (2015): 24.

[13] Flachskampf FA, Wouters PF, Edvardsen T, Evangelista A, Habib G, Hoffman P, Hoffmann R, Lancellotti P, Pepi M. "Recommendations for transoesophageal echocardiography: EACVI update 2014." *Eur Heart J Cardiovasc Imaging* (2014): 353-365.

[14] Gentry Iii JL, Phelan D, Desai MY, Griffin BP. "The Role of Stress Echocardiography in Valvular Heart Disease: A Current Appraisal." *Cardiology* (2017): 137-150.

[15] Pierard LA, Lancellotti P. "Stress testing in valve disease." *Heart* (2007): 766–772.

[16] Lancellotti P, Pellikka PA, Budts W, Chaudhry FA, Donal E, Dulgheru R, Edvardsen T, Garbi M, Ha JW, Kane GC, Kreeger J, Mertens L, Pibarot P, Picano E, Ryan T, Tsutsui JM, Varga A. "The Clinical Use of Stress Echocardiography in Non-Ischaemic Heart Disease: Recommendations from the European Association of Cardiovascular Imaging and the American Society of Echocardiography." *J Am Soc Echocardiogr* (2017): 101-138.

[17] Nishimura RA, Otto CM, Bonow RO, Carabello BA, Erwin JP 3rd, Guyton RA, O'Gara PT, Ruiz CE, Skubas NJ, Sorajja P, Sundt TM 3rd, Thomas JD; ACC/AHA Task Force Members. "2014 AHA/ACC Guideline for the Management of Patients With Valvular Heart Disease: a report of the American College of Cardiology/American Heart Association Task Force on Practice Guidelines." *Circulation* (2014): e521-643.

[18] Baumgartner H, Falk V, Bax JJ, De Bonis M, Hamm C, Holm PJ, Iung B, Lancellotti P, Lansac E, Rodriguez Muñoz D, Rosenhek R, Sjögren J, Tornos Mas P, Vahanian A, Walther T, Wendler O, Windecker S, Zamorano JL; ESC Scientific Document Group. "2017 ESC/EACTS Guidelines for the management of valvular heart disease." *Eur Heart J* (2017): 2739-2791.

[19] Magne J, Lancellotti P, Piérard LA. "Exercise testing in asymptomatic severe aortic stenosis." *JACC Cardiovasc Imaging* (2014): 188-199.

[20] Lancellotti P, Lebois F, Simon M, Tombeux C, Chauvel C, Pierard LA. “Prognostic importance of quantitative exercise Doppler echocardiography in asymptomatic valvular aortic stenosis.” *Circulation* (2005): 1377–1382.

[21] Lancellotti P, Magne J, Donal E, O’Connor K, Dulgheru R, Rosca M, Pierard LA. “Determinants and prognostic significance of exercise pulmonary hypertension in asymptomatic severe aortic stenosis.” *Circulation* (2012): 851–859.

[22] Goublaire C, Melissopoulou M, Lobo D, Kubota N, Verdonk C, Cimadevilla C, Codogno I, Brochet E, Vahanian A, Messika-Zeitoun D. “Prognostic value of exercise-stress echocardiography in asymptomatic patients with aortic valve stenosis.” *JACC Cardiovasc Imaging* (2018): 787-795.

[23] Burkule N. “Stress echocardiography in aortic stenosis.” *J Clin Prev Cardiol* (2019): 64-70.

[24] deFilippi CR, Willett DL, Brickner ME, Appleton CP, Yancy CW, Eichhorn EJ, Grayburn PA. “Usefulness of dobutamine echocardiography in distinguishing severe from nonsevere valvular aortic stenosis in patients with depressed left ventricular function and low transvalvular gradients.” *Am J Cardiol* (1995): 191-194.

[25] Blais C, Burwash IG, Mundigler G, Dumesnil JG, Loho N, Rader F, Baumgartner H, Beanlands RS, Chayer B, Kadem L, Garcia D, Durand LG, Pibarot P. “Projected valve area at normal flow rate improves the assessment of stenosis severity in patients with low-flow, low-gradient aortic stenosis: the multicenter TOPAS (Truly or Pseudo-Severe Aortic Stenosis) study.” *Circulation* (2006): 711-721.

[26] Clavel MA, Ennezat PV, Maréchaux S, Dumesnil JG, Capoulade R, Hachicha Z, Mathieu P, Bellouin A, Bergeron S, Meimoun P, Arsenault M, Le Tourneau T, Pasquet A, Couture C, Pibarot P. “Stress echocardiography to assess stenosis severity and predict outcome in patients with paradoxical low-flow, low-gradient aortic stenosis and preserved LVEF.” *JACC Cardiovasc Imaging* (2013): 175-183.

[27] Lancellotti P and Magne J. “Stress Echocardiography in Regurgitant Valve Disease.” *Circ Cardiovasc Imaging* (2013): 840-849.

[28] Wahi S, Haluska B, Pasquet A, Case C, Rimmerman CM and Marwick TH. “Exercise echocardiography predicts development of left ventricular dysfunction in medically and surgically treated patients with asymptomatic severe aortic regurgitation.” *Heart* (2000): 606-614.

[29] Park SJ, Enriquez-Sarano M, Song JE, Lee YJ, Ha MR, Chang SA, Choi JO, Lee SC, Park SW, Oh JK. “Contractile reserve determined on exercise echocardiography in patients with severe aortic regurgitation.” *Circ J* (2013): 2390-2398.

[30] Helin LM1, Tamás E, Nylander E. “Preoperative longitudinal left ventricular function by tissue Doppler echocardiography at rest and during exercise is valuable in timing of aortic valve surgery in male aortic regurgitation patients.” *J Am Soc Echocardiogr* (2010): 387-395.

[31] Forsberg LM, Nylander E, Tamás É. “Exercise echocardiography predicts postoperative left ventricular remodeling in aortic regurgitation.” *Scand Cardiovasc J* (2014): 4-12.

[32] Kusunose K, Agarwal S, Marwick TH, Griffin BP, Popović ZB. “Decision making in asymptomatic aortic regurgitation in the era of guidelines: incremental values of resting and exercise cardiac dysfunction.” *Circ Cardiovasc Imaging* (2014): 352-362.

In: Perspectives in Aortic Valve Disease
Editor: Giovanni Concistrè

ISBN: 978-1-53618-769-4

Chapter 4

ADVANCED IMAGING AND FUNCTIONAL TOOLS FOR AORTIC VALVE ASSESSMENT: CARDIOVASCULAR MAGNETIC RESONANCE AND CARDIAC COMPUTED TOMOGRAPHY ANGIOGRAPHY

Andrea Barison and Alberto Clemente*
Fondazione Toscana Gabriele Moonasterio, Pisa-Massa, Italy

ABSTRACT

Cardiovascular Magnetic Resonance (CMR) and Cardiac Computed Tomography Angiography (CCTA) provide three-dimensional, high resolution view of the thoracic aorta, aortic root, aortic valve and the underlying myocardium. In particular, CCTA represents the reference standard for anatomic assessment of the aortic valve, the coronary tree and for calcium detection in relation to its submillimetric spatial resolution with enough temporal resolution to clearly plan interventions.

CMR represents the reference standard for biventricular volume and function calculation, for flow measurements and for tissue characterization. Both CMR and CCTA allow a three-dimensional and multiplanar reconstruction of the thoracic aorta and great vessels. This review encompasses the existing literature regarding the role of CMR and CCTA in aortic valve disease, including diagnosis, prognosis and follow-up.

Keywords: aortic stenosis, aortic regurgitation, aortic valve, magnetic resonance, computed tomography

INTRODUCTION

Aortic valve disease shows a relatively high prevalence in the general population, particularly in the elderly [1]. Crucial to patient management is the early diagnosis and

* Corresponding Author's Email: clemente@ftgm.it.

correct grading of disease severity, which depends on multiple factors such as the anatomy of the leaflets, valve hemodynamics and left ventricular (LV) function, in addition to patient symptoms [2]. Cardiac imaging is necessary not only for early diagnosis, but also for prognosis, therapeutic management and follow-up. Besides surgical aortic valve replacement (SAVR), minimally invasive percutaneous interventional techniques, like transcatheter aortic valve implantation (TAVI), have been recently established as a valid alternative option: a crucial task of cardiac imaging is to guide clinicians to plan the appropriate time and techniques of aortic valve treatment.

In this complex clinical scenario, although echocardiography remains the primary imaging modality for both initial assessment and longitudinal evaluation of aortic valve disease, cardiovascular magnetic resonance (CMR) and computed tomography (CT) are being increasingly used in daily clinical practice due to their versatility, which allows a comprehensive evaluation of the different aspects of valvular disease. CMR is a robust alternative for aortic valve assessment in patients with a poor acoustic window, and represents the reference stardard for biventricular volume and function calculation, for flow measurements and for tissue characterization. Both CMR and CT allow a three-dimensional and multiplanar reconstruction of the thoracic aorta and great vessels. CT represents the reference standard for anatomic assessment of the aortic valve, the coronary tree and for calcium detection (Table 1).

This review encompasses the existing literature regarding the role of CMR and CT in morphological and functional assessment of aortic valve stenosis and regurgitation, from disease staging, to surgical/percutaneous interventional planning, to post-operative follow-up. Moreover, the prognostic implications related to the concomitant presence of myocardial ischaemia, systolic/diastolic dysfunction or fibrosis will be analysed, with CMR providing a unique tissue characterization and CT a unique anatomical definition.

Table 1. Technical characteristics of different imaging modalities

	Spatial resolution	Dimensionality	Temporal resolution	Contrast resolution
Catheter angiography	0.15 mm	2D	1-10 ms	Moderate
CCTA	0.23-0.5 mm	2D/3D	29-175 ms	Moderate/High*
Echocardiography	0.5-2 mm	2D/3D	<10 ms	Low
CMR	1-2 mm	2D/3D	20-50 ms	High
PET	4-8 mm	3D	100-300 ms	High
SPECT	5-15 mm	3D	100-300 ms	High

CCTA, Cardiac Computed Tomography Angiography, CMR, Cardiac Magnetic Resonance; SPECT, Single-Photon Emission Computed Tomography; PET, Positron Emission Tomography.

*: High contrast resolution for vascular structures and moderate contrast resolution for myocardial characterization.

Aortic Valve Morphology

Normal Anatomy

The aortic valve is a trifoliate structure supported by a fibrous skeleton, linked with the anterior leaflet of the mitral valve. The three valve cusps (left, right and non-coronary) are thin and symmetric leaflets of fibrous tissue that open uniformly, pushing into their respective sinuses of Valsalva during systole. The free edge of cusps is suspended within the aortic lumen in systole, whereas it is pushed back by retrograde aortic flow in diastole. The joining points between the valve cusp attachments and the root are called commissures The aortic root comprises the aortic valve leaflets, their attachments, the sinuses of Valsalva and inter leaflet trigones. It is a complex structure, schematically outlined with three parallel virtual rings (sino-tubular junction, ventricular-aortic junction and basal attachment of AV leaflets) and one crown-shaped line (representing the attachment of each cusp to the respective Valsalva sinus, sometimes called "surgical annulus") [3]. The sinotubular junction represents the ring connecting the aortic root with the ascending aorta; the ventriculo-aortic junction (VAJ) is a circle positioned slightly above the basal ring, between the aortic wall and left ventricular myocardium; the basal ring is the ring defined by the three anchors at the bottom of each aortic cusp attachments, usually inhomogeneous because of calcifications.

The normal tricuspid morphology is easily recognized by the so-called "Mercedes sign" (three-pointed star) on cine-CMR images obtained on axial planes passing through the aortic bulb. Echocardiography is generally sufficient to assess AV morphology; however in the case of poor acoustic window or unclear morphology, CMR is indicated to provide a detailed assessment of valve and root anatomy [2, 4].

Aortic Valve Variants

The most common anatomical abnormalities of the aortic valve are represented by the numeric variants of the leaflets and the fusion of the commissures.

The unicuspid variant is rare (0.02% of general population) and is frequently associated with early severe aortic stenosis occurring in infancy or childhood and with ascending aortic dilatation [5]. Unicuspid aortic valve may be classified into a unicommissural form, which has an eccentric loophole-shaped orifice (Figure 1A, B), and an acommissural form with a central orifice similar to a diaphragm [6].

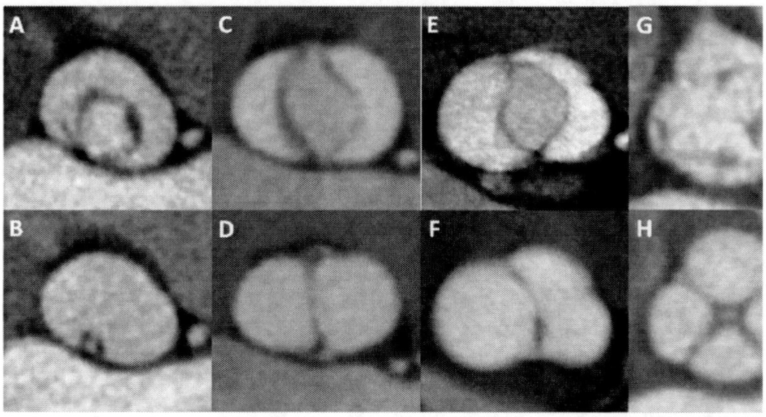

Figure 1. CCTA images depicting the aortic valve variants. Unicommissural unicuspid valve with an eccentric loophole-shaped orifice in systole (A) and diastole (B); bicuspid valve without raphe having two cusps and commissures, in systole (C) and diastole (D); bicuspid valve with raphe between two fused cusps, in systole (E) and diastole (F); quadricuspid aortic valve in systole (G) and diastole (H).

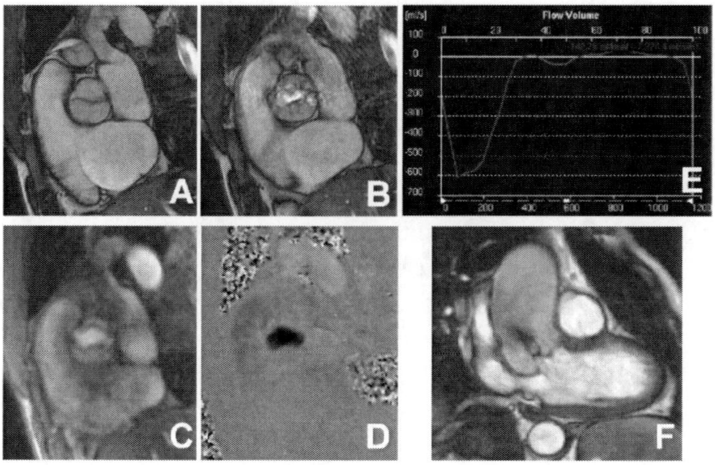

Figure 2. CMR short axis cine images of a mildly stenotic bicuspid aortic valve, showing a complete closure in diastole (A) but a reduced opening with flow turbolence in systole (B). Phase contrast short-axis images in sytole (C, magnitude; D flow) show an oval-shaped opening, corresponding to a steep systolic flow in the flow/time diagram with no significant diastolic regurgitant flow (E). Three-chamber left ventricular cine image in systole, confirming the transvalvular stenotic turbulence (F).

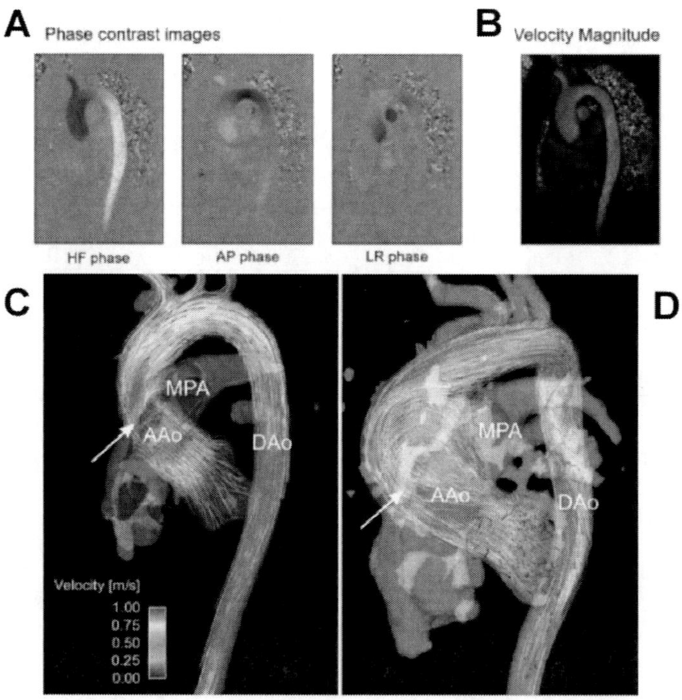

Figure 3. Four-D flow sequences allows to detect blood flows across the three orthogonal planes at the same time (A) and to depict velocity magnitude (B). In two different patients with bicuspid aortic valve (C, D), a posteriorly directed high velocity flow jet (white arrow) is present in the ascending aorta suggesting aortic stenosis, either with minimal ascending aortic dilation (C) or with an enlarged ascending aorta aneurysm (D). AAo, ascending aorta; MPA, main pulmonary artery; DAo, descending aorta. Modified from Stankovic et al.

Biscuspid aortic valve (BAV) is the most common congenital heart disease (1-2% of the population, familial in 9% of cases), often associated with other congenital cardiovascular abnormalities (coartaction, supra- o subvalvar aortic stenosis, ventricular septal defect) or genetics disorders, such as Marfan's syndrome and Turner syndrome [7]. The "purely" BAV is composed of two cusps, morphologically and functionally (Figure 1C, D), even though the most frequent form of BAV consists of three developmental remnants of cusps with variable fusion (raphe) (Figure 1E, F).

Several classifications of BAV exist, based on the presence/absence of raphes, on cusp fusion, size and position, and on the number of sinuses [8]. The most common type is the fusion between the right and left coronary cusps (RL-BAV, 85% of cases), followed by the fusion between the non-coronary and right coronary cusps (RN-BAV, 12% of cases) and by the fusion between the left and non-coronary cusps (LN-BAV, 3% of cases). BAV is commonly complicated by valvular stenosis (51% of cases), aortic regurgitation (17%) or mixed lesions (9%) [9] (Figure 2).

The impaired valve opening confers the typical "fish mouth" appearance in systole and modifies aortic hemodynamics, by distorting the LV outflow, with an eccentric jet directed towards the mid ascending aortic wall, resulting in an increased localized wall shear stress: there has been growing interest in exploring the relationships between specific anatomy, downstream flow pattern and pathophysiology of aortic dilatation by using the novel 4D flow CMR imaging [10, 11] (Figure 3).

Dilatation of Valsalva sinuses or ascending aorta is frequently reported in patients with BAV, independent of valve function, with a prevalence ranging from 20% to 84% [12]. Serial evaluation of the size and morphology of the aortic sinuses and ascending aorta is recommended in patients with a bicuspid aortic valve: while an aortic diameter greater than 55 mm is a general surgical indication, this cut-off is lower for partients with BAV or Marfan disease with specific risk factors [2]. Nowadays, the only considered quantitative criterion predicting aortic dissection in BAV is the diameter, while it is still controversial whether specific BAV phenotypes entail an increased risk of aneurysmal dilatation and aortic dissection.

Quadricuspid aortic valves are extremely rare variants (0.01% at autopsy), generally associated with abnormal valve function (84% of cases, 75% of which have aortic regurgitation) [13, 14] (Figure 1 G, H).

AORTIC VALVE STENOSIS

Aortic stenosis (AS) is defined as an impaired valve opening, leading to left ventricular outflow obstruction. The prevalence of AS in the general population is 0.3-0.5%, rising to 3% in people >75 years old[1]. The survival rate, without repair, is 50% at 10 years. Clinical grading of AS is currently performed noninvasively by Doppler transthoracic echocardiography through measurement of the aortic peak velocity, mean transaortic pressure gradient, and the effective aortic valve area (AVA). Severe AS is defined as peak velocity >4.0 m/s, corresponding to a mean aortic valve gradient >40 mmHg and an AVA <1.0 cm2[2].

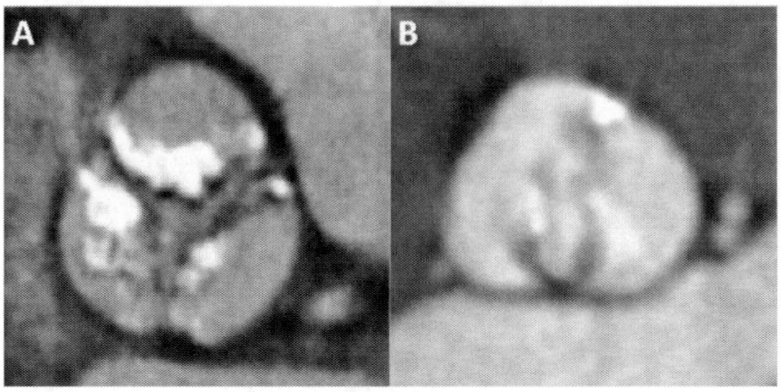

Figure 4. CCTA axial image of a fibro-calcific degenerated and stenotic tricuspid (A) and bicuspi (B) aortic valve during systole.

Fibrocalcific degeneration of the aortic cusps is related to valve stenosis. Calcification mainly occurs in regions characterized by an altered shear stress flow (e.g., oscillatory shear stress on the non-coronary leaflet of the aortic valve during diastole and non-uniform, irregular, and disturbed blood flow at vessel bifurcations): endothelial dysfunction and nitric oxide reduction are common events in valvular diseases[15] (Figure 4).

Coronary as well as extra coronary calcium, can be qualitatively and quantitatively evaluated by CT with and/or without ECG-synchronization (by analyzing the calcium volume such as the calcium score provided by Agatston) [16, 17]. Retrospective ECG-gated cardiac computed tomography angiography (CCTA) acquisition permits nowadays a fast scan with both systolic and diastolic cardiac phases clearly showing the presence, severity and extension of aortic valvular fibrocalcific degeneration together with cusps movements; in addition the calcific involvement of the left anterior mitral leaflet can be identified and the residual area of a stenotic aortic valve can be evaluated during systole. Characterizing the extent of calcium can help predict the risk of annular rupture and the likelihood of post valve implantation perivalvular leak [18].

CMR evaluation is indicated mainly in cases of inappropriate acoustic windows, which occurs in up to 30% of cases, or complex valve anatomy. Cine CMR imaging allows also to visualize the aortic valve, the aortic root, the systo/diastolic movement of aortic cusps and to take 2D measurements. Cine CMR allows also to visualize the stenotic jet (as a flow void artefact) and to determine its geometry, direction and location, for example to differentiate between valvular, subvalvular and post-valvular stenosis. On the other hand, phase-constrast (PC)-CMR enables to encoding the blood flow as velocity maps and to quantify functional parameters (e.g., flow, velocity, pressure gradient) (Figure 2). Flow analysis performed by 2D PC-CMR typically utilizes a monodirectional 2D ECG-triggered acquisition, able to quantify velocities in a single direction perpendicular to the acquired plane ("through-plane" velocity encoding orientation) [19]. This sequence requires proper slice orientation that should be exactly perpendicular to the AS jet direction and located at the level of the opening of the valve orifice, which is commonly the point of maximum flow acceleration, otherwise Vpeak is underestimated. A precise flow velocity measurement is particularly challenging in valvular abnormalities associated with multiple or eccentric jets. Compared to Doppler echocardiography, PC-CMR has a lower temporal resolution (about 30-40 ms vs. <10 ms), and the acquisition is segmented over several heart beats, which increases acquisition length and makes PC-CMR more susceptible to arrhythmias or patient movements. For these reasons, flow velocities measured through PC-CMR are tightly correlated with echo Doppler measurements, but are systematically lower. Some of these limitations can be overcome by the novel 3-dimensional (3D) and 4-dimensional (4D) flow sequences, which allow multidirectional, time-resolved simultaneous visualization and quantification of all cardiac and extracardiac flows, through a dedicated postprocessing with 3D or multiplanar reconstruction. In particular, 4D flow not only allows to orientate the three-dimensional geometric position of the sampling plan during post-processing, but also to adapt the plan orientation in each timeframe, as the jet direction may vary throughout the cardiac cycle (Figure 3).

Two methods have been described for AVA measurement with CMR: direct planimetry from short axis cine images at the valvular level, by manually tracing the opening area in systole, and the continuity equation from corresponding phase contrast (AVA=stroke volume/velocity-time integral at the aortic flow velocity peak). These two techniques present good agreement (correlation: R2 = 0.86, $p < 0.0001$) [20], even if they are prone to measurement errors because of the signal loss due to calcifications and turbulence. Multimodality comparisons showed no major differences between AVA measurements obtained by cine CMR versus transthoracic echocardiography (TTE), transoesophageal echocardiography (TOE) and cardiac catheterization, even if the sensitivity and specificity of CMR to detect AVA $\leqslant$ 0.80 cm2 were higher (78% and 89%, respectively) than TOE (70% and 70%) and TTE (74% and 67%) [21]. Moreover, annular measurement at CMR and TOE present a better accuracy compared to transthoracic echocardiography and angiography [22]. 4D flow measurements (mean and peak velocity and gradient, AVA) show an even higher correlation (Pearson's correlation coefficient from 0.61 to 0.81) with TTE than with traditional 2D-PC CMR [23].

Regarding AVA measurement with CT, aortic valve area at CT is larger than that measured by TTE and does not improve the correlation with transvalvular gradient, the concordance between gradient and AVA, or the mortality prediction compared with TTE [24].

AORTIC VALVE REGURGITATION

Aortic regurgitation (AR) is defined as the diastolic reflux of blood from the aorta to the LV, caused by primary impairment of valve leaflets, by an alteration of aortic root morphology, or both(Maurer, 2006). Similar to AS, correct clinical grading is pivotal to prevent and predict morbidity and mortality, with prognosis ranging from excellent, in asymptomatic patients with normal LV function, to poor in subjects with moderate to severe disease.

The CCTA use in aortic valve regurgitation allows a very fast anatomical evaluation of the aortic root morphology, it shows the incomplete coaptation of the cusps related to the degree of aortic regurgitation and quantifies morphological and functional data of both ventricles (Figure 5).

CMR may offer both qualitative and quantitative analysis of AR and LV response to volume overload. AR severity can be approximately assessed on cine CMR images using long axis LV outflow tract views, where it is represented by the typical signal void of the regurgitation jet, backflowing into the ventricular lumen during diastole, which in some cases may impact on the anterior leaflet of the mitral valve, preventing its correct opening. Even though the wider is the jet, the more severe is AR, a simplistic visual assessment is prone to many potential errors because the jet size is determined by flow acceleration and turbolence, rather than by regurgitant volume (Figure 6).

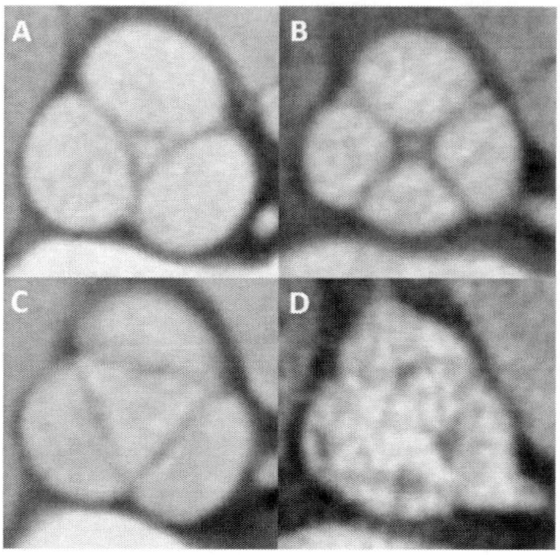

Figure 5. CCTA of a dilated tricuspid aortic valve in diastole (A) and systole (C) and of a quadricuspid aortic valve in diastole (B) and systole (D); please note the incomplete coaptation of the cusps (A, B) in both cases, causing aortic regurgitation.

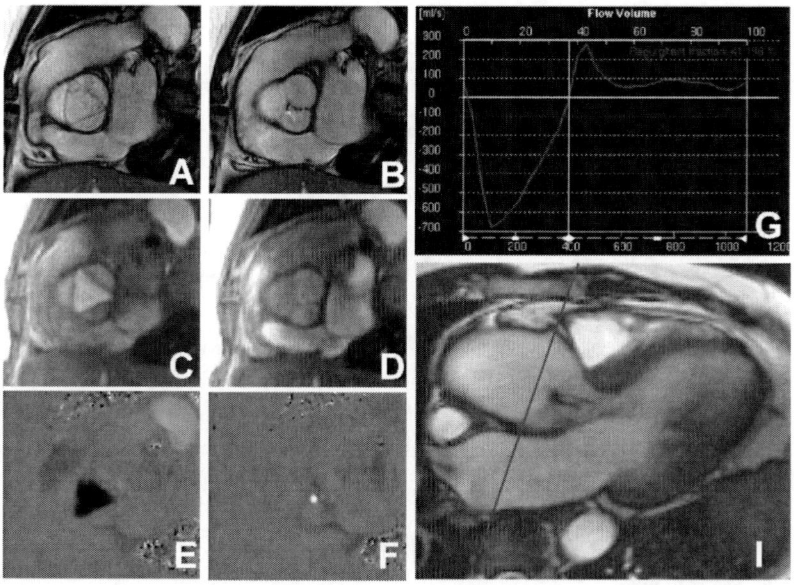

Figure 6. CMR short axis cine images of a regurgitant tricuspid aortic valve, showing a normal, wide opening in systole (A) and incomplete closure in diastole (B). Phase contrast short-axis images in systole (C, magnitude; E flow) show an triangular-shaped opening, while in diastole (D, magnitude; F flow) they show a backward flow (white spot in F). The corresponding flow/time diagram shows a diastolic retrograde flow (G). Three-chamber left ventricular cine image in diastole, confirming the transvalvular retrograde turbulence back to the left ventricle (the red line represents how panels A-F are aligned).

On the other hand, PC-CMR allows to calculated the regurgitant fraction (RF = backward volume/forward volume): an accurate estimation is achieved with an acquisition plane positioned just below the valve, where the backward velocity is higher, while a more reproducible estimation of AR is obtained with a plane positioned at the sino-tubular junction, where the regurgitant flow is laminar and the jet is exactly perpendicular to the imaging planes. In some cases, the excessive motion of the valve plane may interfere with the regurgitant volume measurement; acquisition of multiple PC-CMR planes at different levels may increase accuracy. PC-CMR demonstrated a high precision and reproducibility of flow measurements and correlated well with the degrees of severity assessed by TEE [25]. CMR may also measure the anatomic regurgitant orifice (ARO) by manually contouring the internal edge of valve leaflets in systole. In particular, ARO is strongly correlated with RF at CMR ($P < 0{,}001$) and highly accurate (AUC = 0.99) to detect moderately-severe and severe AR with a threshold of 0.28 cm2[26]. There is no unanimous consensus about the optimal threshold for classifying severe AR by CMR: AR may be classified into mild (RF < 20%), moderate (RF 20-29%, ARO: 0.3–0.5 cm2) and severe (RF ≥ 30%, ARO ≥ 0.5 cm2), when PC-MRI images are acquired at the sino-tubular junction[27]. However, other studies demonstrated that a RF >33% strongly predicted the need of surgery within 3 years, similarly to the value of 50% used in echocardiography[28].

Combined Aortic Valve Disease

Several patients are affected by concomitant aortic valve regurgitation and stenosis: a moderate combined aortic valve disease holds a prognosis similar to severe AS, and significantly poorer than patients with moderate isolated AS or AR [29]. Peak aortic velocity, which reflects both stenosis and regurgitant severity, is an important independent predicting factor for event-free survival [30, 31].

Only a few studies have been designed to specifically address the role of CMR in combined aortic valve disease, even though it can provide an accurate and independent evaluation of the two different components. A modification of PC-CMR is recommended in these patients: two axial planes are required, the first just below the aortic valve for measuring AR and the second at the tip of valve leaflets to quantify peak velocity.

Aortic Valve Masses and Pseudomasses

Aortic valvular masses are uncommon and include benign and malignant disease, vegetations, paravalvular abscesses and pseudoaneurysms. Primary cardiac tumors are rare, mostly benign (75% of cases)[32]. Papillary fibroelastoma is the most common cause of aortic valve tumor, accounting for 10% of all benign cardiac tumors (Figures 7, 8).

Other neoplasms may involve the aortic valvular apparatus such as myxoma, hamartoma, lipoma, as well as metastatic lesions. Generally, the first imaging of choice in the diagnosis and characterization of valvular masses is echocardiography, but CMR represents the reference imaging modality for tumor characterization, including location, size, tissue inhomogeneity, infiltration of adjacent compartments, pericardial or pleural effusion, contrast enhancement[33]. Compared to CT, an important limitation of CMR is the inability to study cardiac calcifications; compared to TTE and TOE, CMR presents a lower temporal resolution, making it difficult to assess highly mobile masses, such as vegetations and fibroelastomas.

Concerning other rare pseudolesions, such as pseudoaneurysms or valvular abscesses, CMR may be helpful in assessing the extent of the disease. Both pathologies are often related to post-SAVR infection or to native valve endocarditis. CMR may aid to characterize their localization and extension; particularly, cine-MR may evaluate the presence of communication between the abscess cavity and cardiac chambers. Finally, it is a non-invasive and accurate exam in the follow-up of patients with perivalvular diseases.

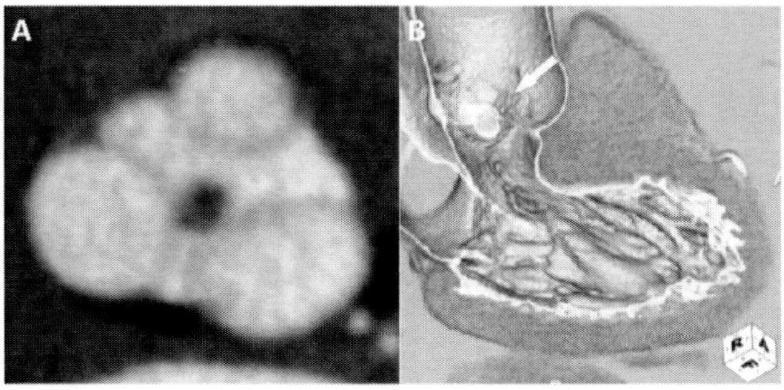

Figure 7. CCTA aortic valve axial plane (A) and 3D-volume rendering (B) images showing a papillary fibroelastoma (white arrow).

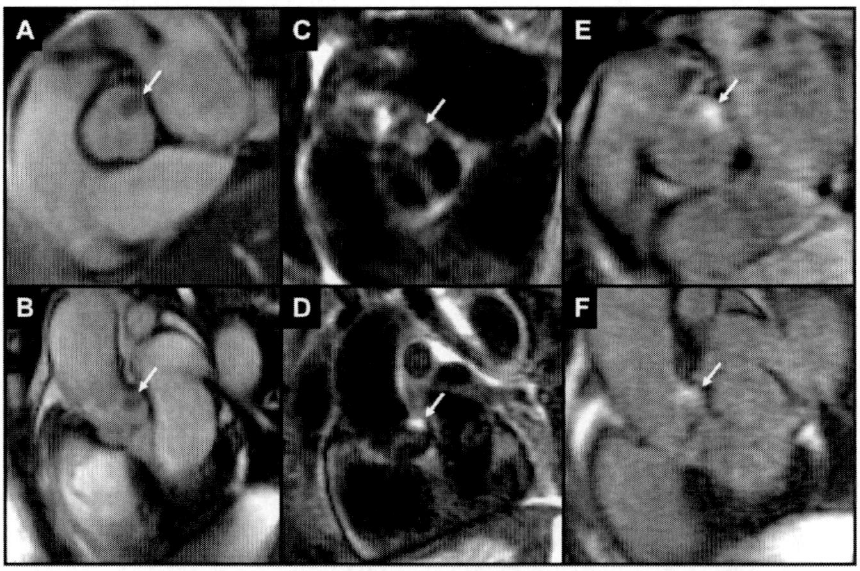

Figure 8. At CMR, a papillary fibroelastoma appears as a spherical mass attached to the left coronary cusp of the aortic valve (arrows). Steady-state free precession cine images (A, B). T1-weighted spin-echo sequence shows intermediate signal intensity of the mass (C). T2-weighted spin-echo sequence with fat inversion (short τ inversion recovery–STIR) shows high signal intensity of the mass (D). After gadolinium injection, the mass shows late enhancement (E, F). Modified from Carpenter et al.

CCTA can provide useful anatomic and functional information as an adjunct to echocardiography and CMR in the evaluation of cardiac masses. Thanks to its capability to identify calcification and fat infiltration, CCTA can serve as an ideal alternative to CMR imaging, especially in patients with CMR contraindications; it allows also an accurate definition of the vascular supply and of the cardiovascular extent of the mass and allows to rule out coronary artery disease prior to surgical intervention [34, 35].

VENTRICULAR REMODELLING AND DYSFUNCTION

CMR is the gold standard technique to measure biventricular volumes, mass, wall thickness and ejection fraction (EF), and is particularly useful in patients with nondiagnostic echocardiographic studies or complex congenital heart diseases. Volumes and mass are measured from a cine stack of short-axis biventricular contiguous slices. Modern cine sequences use breath-hold, electrocardiographic-gated, segmented steady-state free precession (SSFP) to produce images with high reproducibility, excellent myocardium-to-blood contrast, high spatial (1-2mm) and temporal (20-50 ms) resolution. CMR present a higher interstudy reproducibility than echocardiography for LV mass, LVEF and LV volumes [36]. Further CMR sequences allow to track myocardial deformation during the cardiac cycle and to calculate systolic and diastolic myocardial strain and strain rate from myocardial tagging, tissue phase contrast and feature tracking. The latter technique, in particular, is a post-processing analysis of conventional cineSSFP images and requires no extra acquisitions: the assessment of myocardial strain by CMR feature tracking, beyond traditional functional parameters, allows an accurate analysis of the myocardial deformation, resulting in an earlier and more sensitive recognition of LV contractile dysfunction with respect to LVEF [37].

Severe AS is usually associated with LV hypertrophy and with a variable degree of systolic dysfunction, which is not alwayes detected by a decline in LVEF. Feature tracking CMR allows to calculate earlier marker of systolic dysfunction such as strain and strain rate: severe AS has been associated with impaired longitudinal and circumferential strain values compared to controls, which was largely independent of symptoms and correlated with the postoperative functional recovery and clinical outcome [38].

Severe AR is considered a surgical indication in case of reduced LV function parameters (LVEF $<50\%$, LV end-diastolic dimension ≤ 70mm, LV end-systolic dimension ≤ 50 mm, and indexed LV end-systolic dimension <25 mm/m) [2]. Compared to linear measurements, LV volumes measured by CMR seems to better predict survival and outcome [28]. Assessment of LV end-diastolic and end-systolic volumes indexed for body surface area should be part of follow-up scans, because even in asymptomatic patients with normal LV function, LV progressive dilatation is a reasonable indication for surgery. CMR is a robust technique in providing accurate and reproducible assessment of regurgitation, LV volumes and systolic function at the same time, which is crucial for patient management and follow-up.

Patients are affected by concomitant aortic valve regurgitation and stenosis present an extreme LV remodelling, because the LV must adapt to accommodate both an elevated afterload (AS) and an increased preload (AR). In particular, LV mass and diastolic dysfunction are worse in patients with combined than single aortic valve disease [29].

Although CCTA is not recommended as the first-line modality for suspected myocardial diseases, CT allows the assessment of ventricular sizes, morphology, function, density, first pass perfusion defects and delayed-enhancement pattern in multiplanar reconstructions with high spatial resolution in short acquisition times. Therefore, CCTA is considered complementary to echocardiography and CMR in the diagnosis of LV myocardial diseases [39, 40].

Myocardial Tissue Characterization

CMR is the preferred imaging method to assess myocardial tissue changes, including edema using T2-STIR (short-tau inversion-recovery) sequences and fibrosis using late gadolinium enhancement (LGE) sequences. Contrast-enhanced CMR has become a first-line non-invasive exam to distinguish ischemic cardiomyopathy (characterized by subendocardial or transmural LGE, corresponding to a coronary territory) from primary nonischemic cardiomyopathies (characterized by patchy or mid-wall LGE), myocarditis (sub-epicardial LGE) and cardiac amyloidosis (diffuse subendocardial LGE in the early stages possibly evolving to diffuse biventricular and biatrial LGE in advanced disease) [41]. Myocardial fibrosis is an end-stage manifestation of aortic valvular pathology, triggered by pressure and/or volume overload and by an overexpression of profibrotic cytokines. Animal models of AS have shown that tissue fibrosis occurs in a late stage of the disease, following the initial myocyte hypertrophy which triggers the activation of myocardial fibroblasts [42]. In animal models of AR tissue fibrosis seems to occur earlier, during the initial phase of adaptive hypertrophy, in which more elastic forms of collagen are gradually replaced by inelastic matrix causing progressive heart failure [43]. Several clinical studies confirmed a relationship between fibrosis at histology and LGE at CMR, and demonstrated an inverse correlation between LV functional improvement after surgery and LGE presence, with a worse longterm survival after SAVR [44, 45].

Moreover, T1- and T2-mapping sequences allow direct signal quantification (in ms) from each myocardial voxel: they do not require regional differences, thus allowing quantification of diffuse myocardial changes. Native (pre-contrast) T1 mapping encompasses both intracellular and extracellular changes: regions of myocardial infarction, edema, fibrosis and amyloidosis all demonstrate prolonged pre-contrast T1 values compared with normal myocardium, while the accumulation of iron (in cardiac hemochromatosis) or lipids (as in Fabry disease) shortens pre-contrast T1 [46]. Native T2 mapping detects myocardial oedema, with higher sensitivity and reproducibility than T2-STIR [47]. Post-contrast T1 mapping allows calculation of myocardial extracellular volume (ECV): necrosis, interstitial edema, fibrosis and amyloidosis are the most common causes of ECV expansion [48]. Several studies have demonstrated the alteration of T1 mapping values compared to control cases, both in AS and AR [49, 50]. AS severity increases over time if left untreated, causing a parallel increase in left ventricular mass index, total amount of extracellular volume, and LGE mass; in particular, percentage ECV does not change, suggesting balanced increases in the size of the cellular and extracellular compartments as LV remodeling advances [51]. Moreover, in patients with severe aortic stenosis scheduled for aortic valve intervention, an increased ECV is a measure of left ventricular decompensation and a powerful independent predictor of mortality [52].

Stress perfusion CMR depicts contrast medium wash-in into the myocardium during a hyperemic state (induced by adenosine, dipyridamole or regadenoson): in territories supplied by significantly stenosed coronary arteries, the contrast wash-in is delayed and this results in hypointense areas within the myocardium in specific T1-weighted perfusion sequences [53]. Combined with LGE, stress CMR allows visualization of viable, ischaemic myocardium, thus providing diagnostic and prognostic information [54]. An important alternative to vasodilators is dobutamine stress CMR, which detects ischemia by monitoring regional wall motion during infusion of increasing doses of dobutamine. This technique is similar to stress echocardiography, but image quality is higher [55].

In the last few years, different CT techniques for detecting myocardial ischemia have emerged, such as CT-derived fractional flow reserve (FFR-CT), transluminal attenuation gradient (TAG), and myocardial CT perfusion (CTP) imaging. Myocardial CTP imaging can be performed with a single static scan during first pass of the contrast agent, with monoenergetic or dual-energy acquisition, or as a dynamic, time-resolved scan during stress by using coronary vasodilator agents (adenosine, dipyridamole, or regadenoson) [56]. CTP can obtain quantitative data of myocardial blood flow and coronary flow reserve to identify ischemia-associated lesions [57, 58].

Current guidelines recommend valvular replacement mainly for patient with symptomatic severe valvular disease, or LV function impairment. In the future, tissue characterization offered by CMR could be helpful in patient stratification by identifying those asymptomatic patients with subclinical interstitial myocardial fibrosis or with ovearload-induced myocardial ischaemia, that would benefit from an early treatment to prevent progression to symptomatc stages, heart failure and irreversible damages.

Aortic Remodelling and Dilation

Considering the valve defect and its related ascending aortopathy as a single "aortic disease complex," CCTA holds superior ability to anatomically evaluate the aortic root and thoracic aorta morphology over time, while CMR has the potential to merge morphological and functional valve features with the aortic anatomy and flow hemodynamics. In particular, 4D flow imaging identifies the regions of ascending aorta with increased wall shear stress, as shown in BAV patients [10, 11]. Indeed, in BAV patients without AS, the different cusp fusion phenotypes result in distinct wall shear stress patterns: right-left BAV patients exhibit increased wall shear stress by 9% to 34% ($P < 0.001$) at the aortic root and along the entire outer curvature of the ascending aorta, whereas right-noncoronary BAV patients show 30% wall shear stress increase ($P < 0.001$) at the distal portion of the ascending aorta. Viceversa, in patients with tricuspid aortic valve and no AS, aortic dilatation is associated with an aortic wall shear stress reduction by 21% to 33% ($P < 0.01$).

Aortic stenosis has been demonstrated to alter hemodynamics and wall shear stress in the ascending aorta, independently from aortic valve phenotype, overriding the previously described flow patterns associated with BAV [11]. In all patient groups, mild, moderate, and severe AS resulted in a marked increase in regional wall shear stress, while differences between valve phenotypes were no longer apparent.

Planning Surgical Interventions

Surgical aortic valve replacement (SAVR) is indicated in case of severe AS or AR, depending on symptoms and on ventricular function/remodelling[2]. The role of CMR in SAVR planning is growing since it allows to precisely assess the size of the aortic root, valve morphology, the associated aortic abnormalities, surgical access and relationships of aortic root with the surrounding structures. Moreover, the LV evaluation offered by CMR allows a more accurate estimate of the degree of hypertrophy, function and myocardial viability, which is particularly useful for potential candidates of a SAVR and coronary bypass combined procedure. However, the use of CMR in pre-surgical planning is still marginal in many centers, a secondary choice compared to echocardiogram and CT, generally limited to selected cases (young patients or those with renal failure).

Emerging applications of CMR include the investigation of the relationship between specific surgical techniques and resulting aortic hemodynamics, which could help to customize the intervention to the individual anatomy [59].

Planning Percutaneous Interventions

Transcatheter aortic valve implantation (TAVI, sometimes referred to as replacement, TAVR) is a minimally invasive alternative to conventional SAVR based on the transaortic, transfemoral, transsubclavian or transapical deployment of specific bioprosthetic valves. The procedure has shown to improve quality of life and survival not only in high risk individuals (non-eligible for SAVR), but also in intermediate and low risk subjects. A recent meta-analysis of all the currently available randomized controlled trials suggests that TAVI may even reduce 30-day and 1-year all-cause mortality compared with SAVR, independently from the surgical risk [60]. For these reasons, a steep increase in the number of TAVI procedures may soon be expected, accompanied by a rising demand of pre- and post-TAVI imaging examinations.

Pre-TAVI imaging is routinely performed for planning the preferred anatomic access and selecting the type and the size of implanted prosthesis [61] (Table 2).

CCTA is considered the gold-standard because of its wide availability, ease of use and comprehensiveness, covering the whole spectrum of required anatomical information, from the evaluation of the annular and aortic root to imaging of the coronary arteries and peripheral vascular vessels (Figure 9).

The systo-diastolic CCTA assessment of the aortic Virtual Basal Ring (VBT) allows to evaluate the stiffness of the fibro-muscular structures and their deformation related to the variation of the endocavitary pressures. The diameters and cross-sectional area on multiplanar reformatted CCTA images perpendicular to the median centerline of the aortic root are needful in identifying the correct device size to be released. The determination of the shape of the VBR allows to plan which type of interventional approach to adopt in case of replacement [62, 63] (Figure 10).

Table 2. Imaging methods for the evaluation of patients' anatomical suitability for TAVI according to current practice

	TTE/TOE	CCTA	CMR
AS severity	+++	++*	++
LV function	+++	++*	++
LV septal thickness	++	++*	+ ++
Concomitant valvular disease	+++	+	+++
AV annulus diameter	+++	+++	+++
AV anatomy	++	+++	++
AV calcification	++	+++	-
Aortic root measurements	++	+++	+++
AV annulus - coronary arteries distance	±	+++	+++
Coronary artery disease	-	+++	++
Coronary stenosis	-	+++	-
Peripheral arteries anatomy	-	+++	++
Peripheral arteries calcification	-	+++	-

AS, aortic stenosis; LV, left ventricular; AV, aortic annulus; TTE, transthoracic echocardiography; TOE, transoesophageal echocardiography; CCTA, Cardiac Computed Tomography Angiography; CMR, cardiac magnetic resonance. + + + Most frequentl used, + + less frequently used, + least used, - unsuitable. * related to the retrospective multiphasic acquisition.

In addition, CCTA in the same acquisition permits the evaluation of the thoracic aorta, the abdominal aorta and iliofemoral arteries in relation to the endovascular planning. The presence of kinking, luminal obstructions, intraluminal aortic thrombi, calcifications are always evaluable with the same CT scan as one-stop-shop option in planning percutaneous aortic valve replacement[64–66].

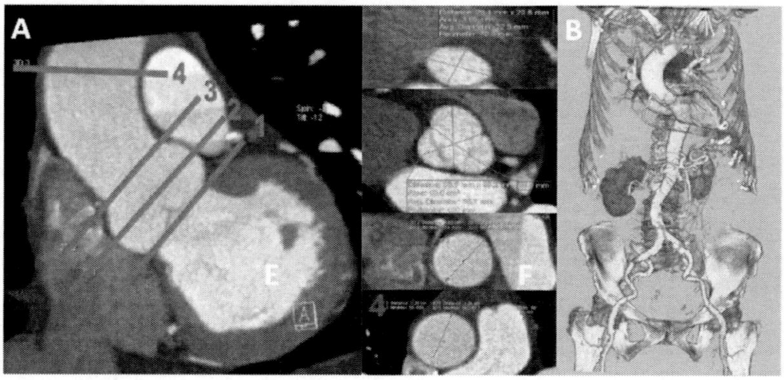

Figure 9. TAVI planning with CCTA scan. Coronal (A) and corresponding axial reconstructions (B) of the ECG-gated left ventricle and aortic root to be operated on. 3D-whole body vascular representation of the same scan (C), particularly useful to plan the percutaneous approach.

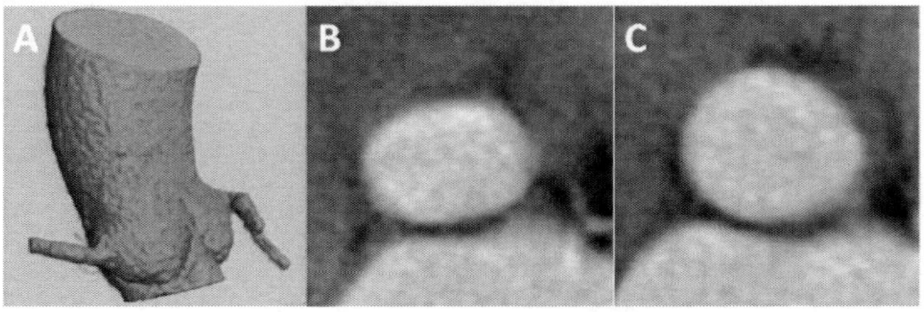

Figure 10. Three-dimensional CCTA reconstruction of the aortic root (A) and axial images at the level of the virtual basal ring (VBR) during diastole (B) and systole (C).

However, TAVI candidates, may be ineligible to CT in up to 20% of cases due to coexisting borderline renal function. In such cases, CMR may be a valid alternative to CT using non-contrast enhanced techniques, like the 3D-SSFP ECG-gated navigator-echo (so-called "whole heart") for thoracic aorta and the various MR-angiography sequences for the evaluation of the aorto-iliac arteries [67, 68]. CMR has shown an excellent correlation with CT for all the relevant pre-procedural parameters, including annulus size, aortic leaflet length, and coronary artery ostia height. It systemically underestimates the amount of leaflet calcifications, which have been demonstrated to be a negative predictor of post-procedural paravalvular leak, particularly when located in the so-called "landing zone." An additional strength of CMR is its higher temporal resolution than CT, which allows to obtain high quality motion-free images of the aortic root even in patients with higher heart rate. Precise measurements of aortic dimensions is crucial for procedural success, hence high-quality images are essential in order to provide reliable measurements.

Finally, still favouring CMR utilization in pre-TAVI planning, is the incremental prognostic value of assessing systo/diastolic LV function and tissue characterization, particularly for postoperative outcome prediction. In a study with tagging CMR, TAVI and SAVR procedures were associated with comparable declines in rotational LV mechanics at 6 months, with largely unchanged circumferential strain and strain rates. A reduced pre-operative mid LV circumferential strain was associated with post-operative mortality [38].

POST-PROCEDURAL IMAGING

Aortic Valve Complications

Sternal wire and valve prostheses are generally MR compatible, but they may degrade image quality: after mechanical valve implantation CMR is not recommended for the post-procedural assessment of valvular and paravalvular complications, while for most biological valves CMR allows to measure the effective orifice area (EOA) recognizing prosthesis-patient mismatch, to visualize the possible incomplete opening or closing of prosthetic cusps, sometimes to identify the underlying cause (e.g., pannus ingrowth or thrombosis) [69] (Figure 11).

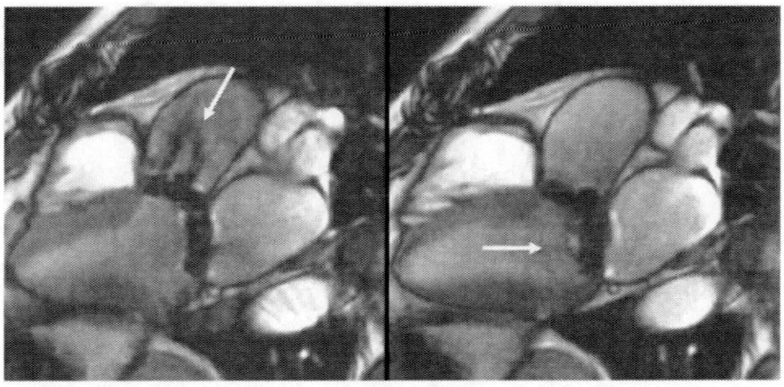

Figure 11. CMR Three-chamber cine view of a patient with mechanical aortic and mitral valves. In systole (left panel), please note the transaortic flow turbulence (arrow); in diastole (right panel), please note the transmitrali flow turbulence (arrow).

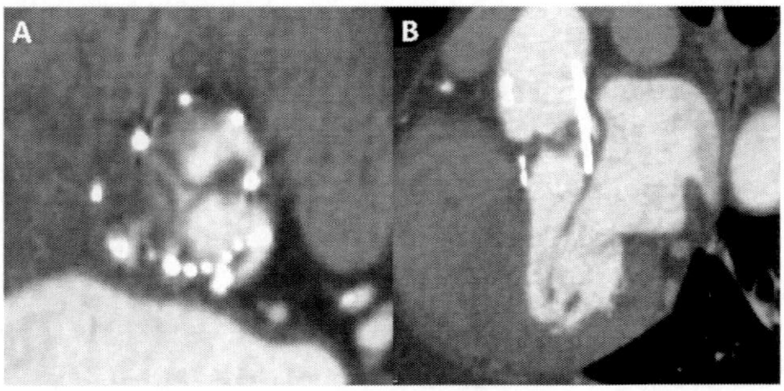

Figure 12. Sutureless aortic valve thrombosis formation evaluated with CCTA. Axial aortic valvular reconstruction (A) and tree-chambers view (B) showing the predominant involvement of the noncoronary (NC) and right coronary (RC) cusps with thrombus formation.

The implanted valve can be obstructed by thrombosis and pannus formation. The differential diagnosis cannot be easily performed by echocardiographic imaging modalities (TOE and TTE); only a few CMR studies have addressed this issue, while CT attenuation is the reference imaging modality to differentiate a thrombus (hypodense structure adhering to the prosthesis) from a pannus (its attenuation should be similar to the myocardium) [70] (Figures 12, 13).

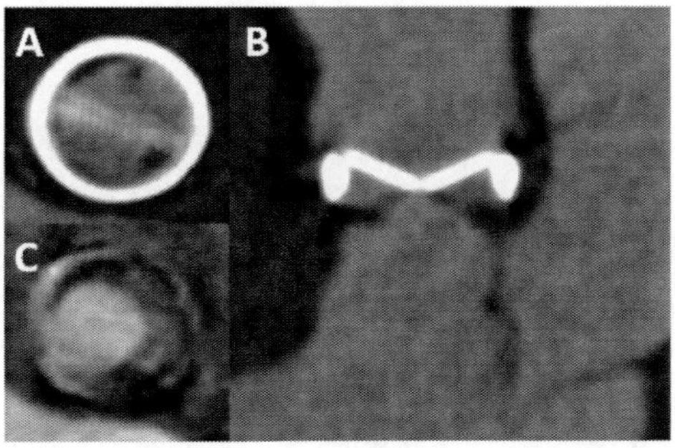

Figure 13. CCTA prosthetic aortic valve pannus formation identified as a small black circumferential low-attenuation (noncalcific) material with radial thickness >= 2 mm and encroachment on the valve cusps just below the suture ring extending into the housing (A-C).

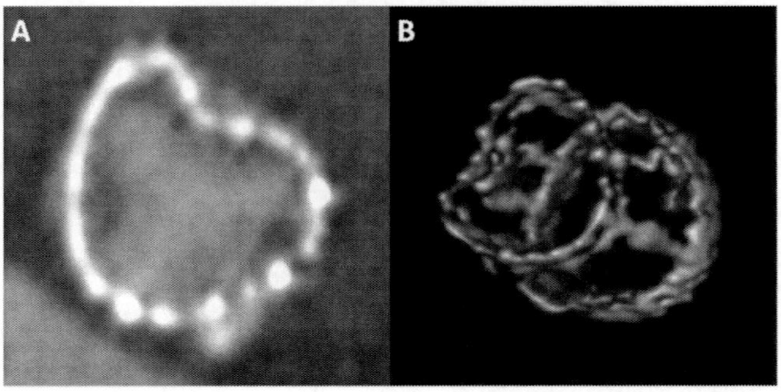

Figure 14. Sutureless valve after deployment (Perceval S, Livanova, London, UK). The double oblique axial multiplanar reconstraction image shows a tipical example of major valve stent deformation with minor thrombosis/pannus overgrowth at the basis of the prosthetic cusps, with aortic regurgitation attributed to the presence of a paravalvular leakage due to the invagination of the inflow stent (A, B) that is clearly visible at 1 o'clock (A).

When image quality is preserved, PC-CMR is also able to measure transprosthetic blood flow velocities and to estimate peak transprosthetic velocity, tranvalvular gradient and residual transvalvular regurgitation, as for native valves. Paravalvular leak refers to regurgitation between the prosthetic sewing ring and the surrounding anchoring tissue and represents a serious complication potentially related to valve dehiscence or malposition. In cine CMR images, a paravalvular leak appears as a signal-void artefact in the 3 chamber view and can be quantified using PC sequences, provided that the acquisition plane is positioned just below the valve, perpendicular to the jet direction; CMR grading of paravalvular leaks is more accurate than TTE, based on the regurgitation fraction (none/trivial, mild, moderate and severe AR defined as ≤8%, 9-20%, 21-39%, >40% regurgitant fractions respectively) [71]. At CCTA the paravalvular leak can be related to the stent deformation and underexpanded or incorrect size prosthesis (Figure 14).

Dehiscence is the spontaneous breakdown of the surgical sutures sewed between the prosthetic valve and the annulus and, besides the presence of a paravalvular leak, at CMR can be detected as a gap between the prosthetic valve and the annulus, using a stack of cine sequences parallel to the annular plane[70].

Aortic Complications

Stanford type A aortic dissection occurs in approximately 0.6% of post-SAVR patients but it appears to be more related to the intrinsic aortic wall abnormalities (aortic wall fragility, aortic regurgitation, and aortic wall thinning) rather than to the surgical procedure itself [70]. In case of clinical suspicion, a prompt TTE evaluation is mandatory, but only CMR and CT present a nearly 100% sensitivity and specificity to detect post-procedural aortic dissection. Pseudoaneurysm formation is more common in composite graft (7-25% of the patients), where the aortic root is replaced by a mechanical or biological valve pre-mounted on an tube graft, rather than in isolated aortic valve replacement. Both CCTA and CMR are helpful in the differential diagnosis between pseudoaneurysm and other pathological diverticular lesions and for assessing the patency of coronary ostia.

Ventricular Remodelling

Besides TTE, wich represents the cornerstone technique to track valvular and ventricular changes after aortic valve surgery, CMR may be needed in case of poor acoustic windows or for finer evaluations. In particular, CMR is able to accurately assess the LV reverse remodelling and the mass regression occuring immediately after SAVR, whici is related to good long-term prognosis. Following aortic valve replacement, native myocardial T1 has been demostrated to decrease towards normal values, associated with left ventricular mass regression and systolic function improvement; patients with persistent elevated native T1 after aortic valve replacement presented a worse outcome than those with T1 decrease [72]. Other studies have show on that, while LGE is not affected by SAVR, total extracellular volume decreases together with peak aortic-jet velocity and LV mass, confirming that diffuse interstitial fibrosis is indeed reversible; however, the accompanying rise (or unchange) in percentage ECV suggests that regression in cellular hypertrophy occurs faster and to a greater degree than the reduction of the extracellular component [51].

Technical Limitations

Nowadays advanced imaging is essential for a correct evaluation of the patient presenting a disease involving the aortic valve; however, both CCTA and CMR require a dedicated cardiac scanner and precise local skills, with higher costs compared with echocardiography. Technical limitations including tachyarrhythmias or breathing artefacts can be considered limited and relative contraindications together with claustrophobia. Selected patients may undergo a CMR scan under general anesthesia. Several metallic devices (including pacemakers and defibrillators) represent a limitation for CMR, but patients with newer CMR-conditional devices may safely undergo a CMR scan after device reprogramming; metallic devices can generate CT beam hardening artifacts and adequate sequences and parameters must be applied to avoid unsuitable diagnosis. Gadolinium-based and iodinated contrast agents are generally contraindicated in individuals with a glomerular filtration rate <30 mL/min/1.73 m2, even if the risk of nephrogenic systemic fibrosis is extremely low with newer cyclic gadolinium-based contrast agents (Woolen et al., 2020) and risk of iodinated contrast-induced nephropathy (CIN) is limited by the reduction in the amount of contrast media to be used [73].

Conclusion

Aortic valve disease is a complex group of different pathological entities requiring a multidisciplinary approach. From an imaging point of view, cardiac CT is the routinely used all-in-one method in the planning and follow-up of the surgical or interventional procedure from the sizing of the device to be implanted, passing through the study of the coronary artery disease to the anatomical relationship between the mediastinal structures and the whole chest anatomy, and studying the abdominal aorta and peripheral vascular accesses in a single-breath-hold with high accuracy. The advanced imaging parterre includes also CMR, which is able to investigate all the different aspects of the disease, ranging from early diagnosis to prognostic evaluation and pre- and post-treatment assessment. Although CMR is generally considered a second line tool by current guidelines, it is more reproducible than echocardiography concerning valve morphology, valve flow and ventricular function evaluation; furthermore, its unique ability to provide histologically in vivo information has a pivotal role in the detection of ventricular fibrosis and, therefore, in the prognostic patient stratification.

References

[1] Nkomo, V. T., J. M. Gardin, T. N. Skelton, J. S. Gottdiener, C. G. Scott, M. Enriquez-Sarano, Burden of valvular heart diseases: a population-based study, *Lancet.* 368 (2006) 1005–1011. doi:10.1016/S0140-6736(06)69208-8.

[2] Baumgartner, H., V. Falk, J. J. Bax, M. De Bonis, C. Hamm, P. J. Holm, B. Iung, P. Lancellotti, E. Lansac, D. Rodriguez Muñoz, R. Rosenhek, J. Sjögren, P. Tornos Mas, A. Vahanian, T. Walther, O. Wendler, S. Windecker, J. L. Zamorano, M. Roffi, O. Alfieri, S. Agewall, A. Ahlsson, E. Barbato, H. Bueno, J. P. Collet, I. M. Coman, M. Czerny, V. Delgado, D. Fitzsimons, T. Folliguet, O. Gaemperli, G. Habib, W. Harringer, M. Haude, G. Hindricks, H. A. Katus, J. Knuuti, P. Kolh, C. Leclercq, T. A. McDonagh, M. F. Piepoli, L. A. Pierard, P. Ponikowski, G. M. C. Rosano, F. Ruschitzka, E. Shlyakhto, I. A. Simpson, M. Sousa-Uva, J. Stepinska, G. Tarantini, D. Tchétché, V. Aboyans, S. Windecker, V. Aboyans, S. Agewall, E. Barbato, H. Bueno, A. Coca, J. P. Collet, I. M. Coman, V. Dean, V. Delgado, D. Fitzsimons, O. Gaemperli, G. Hindricks, B. Iung, P. Jüni, H. A. Katus, J. Knuuti, P. Lancellotti, C. Leclercq, T. McDonagh, M. F. Piepoli, P. Ponikowski, D. J. Richter, M. Roffi, E. Shlyakhto, I. A. Simpson, J. L. Zamorano, H. K. Kzhdryan, J. Mascherbauer, F. Samadov, V. Shumavets, G. Van Camp, D. Lončar, D. Lovric, G. M. Georgiou, K. Linhartova, N. Ihlemann, M. Abdelhamid, T. Pern, A. Turpeinen, E. Srbinovska-Kostovska, A. Cohen, Z. Bakhutashvili, H. Ince, M. Vavuranakis, A. Temesvári, T. Gudnason, D. Mylotte, R. Kuperstein, C. Indolfi, Y. Pya, G. Bajraktari, A. Kerimkulova, A. Rudzitis, V. Mizariene, F. Lebrun, D. C. Demarco, L. Oukerraj, B. J. Bouma, T. K. Steigen, M. Komar, L. M. De Moura Branco, B. A. Popescu, V. Uspenskiy, M. Foscoli, L. Jovovic, I. Simkova, M. Bunc, J. A. V. de Prada, M. Stagmo, B. A. Kaufmann, A. Mahdhaoui, E. Bozkurt, E. Nesukay, S. J. D. Brecker, 2017 ESC/EACTS Guidelines for the management of valvular heart disease, *Eur. Heart J.* 38 (2017) 2739–2791. doi:10.1093/eurheartj/ehx391.

[3] Piazza, N., P. de Jaegere, C. Schultz, A. E. Becker, P. W. Serruys, R. H. Anderson, Anatomy of the aortic valvar complex and its implications for transcatheter implantation of the aortic valve., *Circ. Cardiovasc. Interv.* 1 (2008) 74–81. doi:10.1161/CIRCINTERVENTIONS.108.780858.

[4] Looi, J. L., A. J. Kerr, R. Gabriel, Morphology of congenital and acquired aortic valve disease by cardiovascular magnetic resonance imaging, *Eur. J. Radiol.* 84 (2015) 2144–2154. doi:10.1016/j.ejrad.2015.07.022.

[5] Buchner, S., R. Kobuch, A. Luchner, K. Debl, Diagnosis of unicommissural unicuspid aortic valve stenosis by different imaging modalities, *J. Cardiovasc. Med.* 12 (2011) 347–348. doi:10.2459/JCM.0b013e3283403745.

[6] D. Muratori, P. Meani, G. Quattrocchi, P. Pedrotti, Association of unicuspid unicommissural aortic valve and complex congenital heart disease depicted by cardiac magnetic resonance., *Images Paediatr. Cardiol.* 18 (2016) 5–8. http://www.ncbi.nlm.nih.gov/pubmed/28405207 (accessed March 31, 2020).

[7] Liu, T., M. Xie, Q. Lv, Y. Li, L. Fang, L. Zhang, W. Deng, J. Wang, Bicuspid aortic valve: An update in morphology, genetics, biomarker, complications, imaging diagnosis and treatment, *Front. Physiol.* 10 (2019). doi:10.3389/fphys.2018.01921.

[8] Sievers, H. H., C. Schmidtke, A classification system for the bicuspid aortic valve from 304 surgical specimens, *J. Thorac. Cardiovasc. Surg.* 133 (2007) 1226–1233. doi:10.1016/j.jtcvs.2007.01.039.

[9] Wassmuth, R., F. von Knobelsdorff-Brenkenhoff, H. Gruettner, W. Utz, J. Schulz-Menger, Cardiac magnetic resonance imaging of congenital bicuspid aortic valves and associated aortic pathologies in adults., *Eur. Heart J. Cardiovasc. Imaging.* 15 (2014) 673–9. doi:10.1093/ehjci/jet275.

[10] Piatti, F., F. Sturla, M. M. Bissell, S. Pirola, M. Lombardi, I. Nesteruk, A. Della Corte, A. C. Alberto, E. Votta, 4D flow analysis of BAV-Related fluid-dynamic alterations: Evidences of wall shear stress alterations in absence of clinically-relevant aortic anatomical remodeling, *Front. Physiol.* 8 (2017). doi:10.3389/fphys.2017.00441.

[11] van Ooij, P., M. Markl, J. D. Collins, J. C. Carr, C. Rigsby, R. O. Bonow, S. Chris Malaisrie, P. M. McCarthy, P. W. M. Fedak, A. J. Barker, Aortic valve stenosis alters expression of regional aortic wall shear stress: New insights from a 4-dimensional flow magnetic resonance imaging study of 571 subjects, *J. Am. Heart Assoc.* 6 (2017) 1–14. doi:10.1161/JAHA.117.005959.

[12] Verma, S., S. C. Siu, Aortic dilatation in patients with bicuspid aortic valve, *N. Engl. J. Med.* 370 (2014) 1920–1929. doi:10.1056/NEJMra1207059.

[13] O. Tutarel, The quadricuspid aortic valve: A comprehensive review, *J. Heart Valve Dis.* 13 (2004) 534–537.

[14] Khan, S. K. A., S. S. Tamin, P. A. Araoz, Quadricuspid aortic valve by cardiac magnetic resonance imaging: A case report and review of the literature, *J. Comput. Assist. Tomogr.* 35 (2011) 637–641. doi:10.1097/RCT.0b013e318224a129.

[15] Gomel, M. A., R. Lee, K. J. Grande-Allen, Comparing the Role of Mechanical Forces in Vascular and Valvular Calcification Progression, *Front. Cardiovasc. Med.* 5 (2019). doi:10.3389/fcvm.2018.00197.

[16] Greenland, P., M. J. Blaha, M. J. Budoff, R. Erbel, K. E. Watson, Coronary Calcium Score and Cardiovascular Risk, *J. Am. Coll. Cardiol.* 72 (2018) 434–447. doi:10.1016/j.jacc.2018.05.027.

[17] Pawade, T., M. A. Clavel, C. Tribouilloy, J. Dreyfus, T. Mathieu, L. Tastet, C. Renard, M. Gun, W. S. A. Jenkins, L. MacRon, J. W. Sechrist, J. M. Lacomis, V. Nguyen, L. G. Gay, H. C. Calabria, I. Ntalas, T. R. G. Cartlidge, B. Prendergast, R. Rajani, A. Evangelista, J. L. Cavalcante, D. E. Newby, P. Pibarot, D. M. Zeitoun, M. R. Dweck, Computed Tomography Aortic Valve Calcium Scoring in Patients with Aortic Stenosis, *Circ. Cardiovasc. Imaging.* 11 (2018). doi:10.1161/CIRCIMAGING.117.007146.

[18] Clemente, A., I. Traghella, A. Mazzone, S. Sbrana, C. Vassalle, Vascular and valvular calcification biomarkers, in: *Adv. Clin. Chem.*, Academic Press Inc., 2020: pp. 73–103. doi:10.1016/bs.acc.2019.08.002.

[19] Nayak, K. S., J. F. Nielsen, M. A. Bernstein, M. Markl, P. D. Gatehouse, R. M. Botnar, D. Saloner, C. Lorenz, H. Wen, B. S. Hu, F. H. Epstein, J. N. Oshinski, S. V. Raman, Cardiovascular magnetic resonance phase contrast imaging, *J. Cardiovasc. Magn. Reson.* 17 (2015) 71. doi:10.1186/s12968-015-0172-7.

[20] Tanaka, K., A. N. Makaryus, S. D. Wolff, Correlation of aortic valve area obtained by the velocity-encoded phase contrast continuity method to direct planimetry using cardiovascular magnetic resonance, *J. Cardiovasc. Magn. Reson.* 9 (2007) 799–805. doi:10.1080/10976640701545479.

[21] Kupfahl, C., M. Honold, G. Meinhardt, H. Vogelsberg, A. Wagner, H. Mahrholdt, U. Sechtem, Evaluation of aortic stenosis by cardiovascular magnetic resonance imaging: Comparison with established routine clinical techniques, *Heart.* 90 (2004) 893–901. doi:10.1136/hrt.2003.022376.

[22] Paelinck, B. P., P. L. Van Herck, I. Rodrigus, M. J. Claeys, J. C. Laborde, P. M. Parizel, C. J. Vrints, J. M. Bosmans, Comparison of magnetic resonance imaging of aortic valve stenosis and aortic root to multimodality imaging for selection of transcatheter aortic valve implantation candidates, *Am. J. Cardiol.* 108 (2011) 92–98. doi:10.1016/j.amjcard.2011.02.348.

[23] Da Silveira, J. S., M. Smyke, A. V. Rich, Y. Liu, N. Jin, D. Scandling, J. A. Dickerson, C. E. Rochitte, S. V. Raman, L. C. Potter, R. Ahmad, O. P. Simonetti, Quantification of aortic stenosis diagnostic parameters: Comparison of fast 3 direction and 1 direction phase contrast CMR and transthoracic echocardiography, *J. Cardiovasc. Magn. Reson.* 19 (2017) 35. doi:10.1186/s12968-017-0339-5.

[24] Clavel, M. A., J. Malouf, D. Messika-Zeitoun, P. A. Araoz, H. I. Michelena, M. Enriquez-Sarano, Aortic valve area calculation in aortic stenosis by CT and doppler echocardiography, *JACC Cardiovasc. Imaging.* 8 (2015) 248–257. doi:10.1016/j.jcmg.2015.01.009.

[25] Cawley, P. J., C. Hamilton-Craig, D. S. Owens, E. V. Krieger, W. E. Strugnell, L. Mitsumori, C. L. D'Jang, R. G. Schwaegler, K. Q. Nguyen, B. Nguyen, J. H. Maki, C. M. Otto, Prospective comparison of valve regurgitation quantitation by cardiac magnetic resonance imaging and transthoracic echocardiography, *Circ. Cardiovasc. Imaging.* 6 (2013) 48–57. doi:10.1161/CIRCIMAGING.112.975623.

[26] Debl, K., B. Djavidani, S. Buchner, N. Heinicke, S. Fredersdorf, J. Haimerl, F. Poschenrieder, S. Feuerbach, G. A. Riegger, A. Luchner, Assessment of the anatomic regurgitant orifice in aortic regurgitation: a clinical magnetic resonance imaging study., *Heart.* 94 (2008) e8. doi:10.1136/hrt.2006.108720.

[27] Nadeau-Routhier, C., O. Marsit, J. Beaudoin, Current Management of Patients with Severe Aortic Regurgitation, *Curr. Treat. Options Cardiovasc. Med.* 19 (2017) 9. doi:10.1007/s11936-017-0508-8.

[28] Myerson, S. G., J. D'arcy, R. Mohiaddin, J. P. Greenwood, T. D. Karamitsos, J. M. Francis, A. P. Banning, J. P. Christiansen, S. Neubauer, Aortic regurgitation quantification using cardiovascular magnetic resonance: Association with clinical outcome, *Circulation.* 126 (2012) 1452–1460. doi:10.1161/CIRCULATIONAHA.111.083600.

[29] Egbe, A. C., S. A. Luis, R. Padang, C. A. Warnes, Outcomes in moderate mixed aortic valve disease: Is it time for a paradigm shift?, *J. Am. Coll. Cardiol.* 67 (2016) 2321–2329. doi:10.1016/j.jacc.2016.03.509.

[30] Zilberszac, R., H. Gabriel, M. Schemper, D. Zahler, M. Czerny, G. Maurer, R. Rosenhek, Outcome of combined stenotic and regurgitant aortic valve disease, *J. Am. Coll. Cardiol.* 61 (2013) 1489–1495. doi:10.1016/j.jacc.2012.11.070.

[31] Egbe, A. C., J. T. Poterucha, C. A. Warnes, Mixed aortic valve disease: midterm outcome and predictors of adverse events., *Eur. Heart J.* 37 (2016) 2671–8. doi:10.1093/eurheartj/ehw079.

[32] Burke, A., F. Tavora, The 2015 WHO Classification of tumors of the heart and pericardium, *J. Thorac. Oncol.* 11 (2016) 441–452. doi:10.1016/j.jtho.2015.11.009.

[33] Grebenc, M. L., M. L. Rosado De Christenson, A. P. Burke, C. E. Green, J. R. Galvin, Primary cardiac and pericardial neoplasms: Radiologic-pathologic correlation, *Radiographics.* 20 (2000) 1073–1103. doi:10.1148/radiographics.20.4.g00jl081073.

[34] Kassop, D., M. S. Donovan, M. K. Cheezum, B. T. Nguyen, N. B. Gambill, R. Blankstein, T. C. Villines, Cardiac Masses on Cardiac CT: A Review, *Curr. Cardiovasc. Imaging Rep.* 7 (2014) 1–13. doi:10.1007/s12410-014-9281-1.

[35] Kim, E. Y., Y. H. Choe, K. Sung, S. W. Park, J. H. Kim, Y. H. Ko, Multidetector CT and MR imaging of cardiac tumors, *Korean J. Radiol.* 10 (2009) 164–175. doi:10.3348/kjr.2009.10.2.164.

[36] Keenan, N. G., D. J. Pennell, CMR of ventricular function, *Echocardiography.* 24 (2007) 185–193. doi:10.1111/j.1540-8175.2007.00375.x.

[37] Andre, F., H. Steen, P. Matheis, M. Westkott, K. Breuninger, Y. Sander, R. Kammerer, C. Galuschky, E. Giannitsis, G. Korosoglou, H. A. Katus, S. J. Buss, Age- and gender-related normal left ventricular deformation assessed by cardiovascular magnetic resonance feature tracking, *J. Cardiovasc. Magn. Reson.* 17 (2015). doi:10.1186/s12968-015-0123-3.

[38] Al Musa, T., A. Uddin, P. P. Swoboda, T. A. Fairbairn, L. E. Dobson, A. Singh, P. Garg, C. D. Steadman, B. Erhayiem, A. Kidambi, D. P. Ripley, A. K. McDiarmid, P. Haaf, D. J. Blackman, S. Plein, G. P. McCann, J. P. Greenwood, Cardiovascular magnetic resonance evaluation of symptomatic severe aortic stenosis: association of circumferential myocardial strain and mortality, *J. Cardiovasc. Magn. Reson.* 19 (2017) 1–10. doi:10. 1186/s12968-017-0329-7.

[39] Hendel, R. C., M. R. Patel, C. M. Kramer, M. Poon, R. C. Hendel, J. C. Carr, N. A. Gerstad, L. D. Gillam, J. M. B. Hodgson, R. J. Kim, C. M. Kramer, J. R. Lesser, E. T. Martin, J. V. Messer, R. F. Redberg, G. D. Rubin, J. S. Rumsfeld, A. J. Taylor, W. G. Weigold, P. K. Woodard, R. G. Brindis, R. C. Hendel, P. S. Douglas, E. D. Peterson, M. J. Wolk, J. M. Allen, M. R. Patel, ACCF/ACR/SCCT/SCMR/ASNC/NASCI/SCAI/SIR 2006 Appropriateness Criteria for Cardiac Computed Tomography and Cardiac Magnetic Resonance Imaging* * Developed in accordance with the principles and methodology outlined by ACCF: Patel MR, Spertus JA, Brindis RG, Hendel RC, Douglas PS, Peterson ED, Wolk MJ, Allen JM, Raskin IE., *J. Am. Coll. Cardiol.* 48 (2006) 1475–1497. doi:10.1016/j.jacc.2006.07.003.

[40] Clayton, B., C. Roobottom, G. Morgan-Hughes, Assessment of the myocardium with cardiac computed tomography, *Eur. Hear. J. - Cardiovasc. Imaging.* 15 (2014) 603–609. doi:10.1093/ehjci/jeu028.

[41] Vöhringer, M., H. Mahrholdt, A. Yilmaz, U. Sechtem, Significance of late gadolinium enhancement in cardiovascular magnetic resonance imaging (CMR)., *Herz*. 32 (2007) 129–37. doi:10.1007/s00059-007-2972-5.

[42] Khan, R., R. Sheppard, Fibrosis in heart disease: Understanding the role of transforming growth factor-β1 in cardiomyopathy, valvular disease and arrhythmia, *Immunology*. 118 (2006) 10–24. doi:10.1111/j.1365-2567.2006.02336.x.

[43] Liu, S. K., N. R. Magid, P. R. Fox, S. M. Goldfine, J. S. Borer, Fibrosis, myocyte degeneration and heart failure in chronic experimental aortic regurgitation, *Cardiology*. 90 (1998) 101–109. doi:10.1159/000006827.

[44] Weidemann, F., S. Herrmann, S. Störk, M. Niemann, S. Frantz, V. Lange, M. Beer, S. Gattenlöhner, W. Voelker, G. Ertl, J. M. Strotmann, Impact of myocardial fibrosis in patients with symptomatic severe aortic stenosis., *Circulation*. 120 (2009) 577–84. doi:10.1161/CIRCULATIONAHA.108.847772.

[45] Podlesnikar, T., V. Delgado, J. J. Bax, Cardiovascular magnetic resonance imaging to assess myocardial fibrosis in valvular heart disease, *Int. J. Cardiovasc. Imaging*. 34 (2018) 97–112. doi:10.1007/s10554-017-1195-y.

[46] Sado, D. M., A. S. Flett, S. M. Banypersad, S. K. White, V. Maestrini, G. Quarta, R. H. Lachmann, E. Murphy, A. Mehta, D. A. Hughes, W. J. McKenna, A. M. Taylor, D. J. Hausenloy, P. N. Hawkins, P. M. Elliott, J. C. Moon, Cardiovascular magnetic resonance measurement of myocardial extracellular volume in health and disease., *Heart*. 98 (2012) 1436–41. doi:10.1136/heartjnl-2012-302346.

[47] Verhaert, D., P. Thavendiranathan, S. Giri, G. Mihai, S. Rajagopalan, O. P. Simonetti, S. V. Raman, Direct T2 quantification of myocardial edema in acute ischemic injury, *JACC Cardiovasc. Imaging*. 4 (2011) 269–278. doi:10.1016/j.jcmg.2010.09.023.

[48] Ugander, M., A. J. Oki, L. Y. Hsu, P. Kellman, A. Greiser, A. H. Aletras, C. T. Sibley, M. Y. Chen, W. P. Bandettini, A. E. Arai, Extracellular volume imaging by magnetic resonance imaging provides insights into overt and sub-clinical myocardial pathology., *Eur. Heart J*. 33 (2012) 1268–78. doi:10.1093/eurheartj/ehr481.

[49] Lee, S. P., W. Lee, J. M. Lee, E. A. Park, H. K. Kim, Y. J. Kim, D. W. Sohn, Assessment of diffuse myocardial fibrosis by using MR imaging in asymptomatic patients with aortic stenosis, *Radiology*. 274 (2015) 359–369. doi:10.1148/radiol.14141 120.

[50] Sparrow, P., D. R. Messroghli, S. Reid, J. P. Ridgway, G. Bainbridge, M.U. Sivananthan, Myocardial T1 mapping for detection of left ventricular myocardial fibrosis in chronic aortic regurgitation: pilot study., *AJR. Am. J. Roentgenol*. 187 (2006) W630-5. doi:10. 2214/AJR.05.1264.

[51] Everett, R. J., L. Tastet, M. A. Clavel, C. W. L. Chin, R. Capoulade, V. S. Vassiliou, J. Kwiecinski, M. Gomez, E. J. R. Van Beek, A. C. White, S. K. Prasad, E. Larose, C. Tuck, S. Semple, D. E. Newby, P. Pibarot, M. R. Dweck, Progression of hypertrophy and myocardial fibrosis in aortic stenosis: A multicenter cardiac magnetic resonance study, *Circ. Cardiovasc. Imaging*. 11 (2018). doi:10.1161/CIRCIMAGING.117. 007451.

[52] Everett, R. J., T. A. Treibel, M. Fukui, H. Lee, M. Rigolli, A. Singh, P. Bijsterveld, L. Tastet, T. Al Musa, L. Dobson, C. Chin, G. Captur, S. Y. Om, S. Wiesemann, V. M. Ferreira, S. K. Piechnik, J. Schulz-Menger, E. B. Schelbert, M. A. Clavel, D. E. Newby, S. G. Myerson, P. Pibarot, S. Lee, J. L. Cavalcante, S. P. Lee, G. P. McCann, J. P.

Greenwood, J. C. Moon, M. R. Dweck, Extracellular Myocardial Volume in Patients With Aortic Stenosis, *J. Am. Coll. Cardiol.* 75 (2020) 304–316. doi:10.1016/j.jacc.2019.11.032.

[53] Schwitter, J., A. E. Arai, Assessment of cardiac ischaemia and viability: role of cardiovascular magnetic resonance., *Eur. Heart J.* 32 (2011) 799–809. doi:10.1093/eurheartj/ehq481.

[54] Kwong, R. Y., Y. Ge, K. Steel, S. Bingham, S. Abdullah, K. Fujikura, W. Wang, A. Pandya, Y. Y. Chen, J. R. Mikolich, S. Boland, A. E. Arai, W. P. Bandettini, S. M. Shanbhag, A. R. Patel, A. Narang, A. Farzaneh-Far, B. Romer, J. F. Heitner, J. Y. Ho, J. Singh, C. Shenoy, A. Hughes, S. W. Leung, M. Marji, J. A. Gonzalez, S. Mehta, D. J. Shah, D. Debs, S. V. Raman, A. Guha, V. A. Ferrari, J. Schulz-Menger, R. Hachamovitch, M. Stuber, O. P. Simonetti, Cardiac Magnetic Resonance Stress Perfusion Imaging for Evaluation of Patients With Chest Pain, *J. Am. Coll. Cardiol.* 74 (2019) 1741–1755. doi:10.1016/j.jacc.2019.07.074.

[55] Nagel, E., H. B. Lehmkuhl, W. Bocksch, C. Klein, U. Vogel, E. Frantz, A. Ellmer, S. Dreysse, E. Fleck, Noninvasive diagnosis of ischemia-induced wall motion abnormalities with the use of high-dose dobutamine stress MRI: comparison with dobutamine stress echocardiography., *Circulation.* 99 (1999) 763–70. http://www.ncbi.nlm.nih.gov/pubmed/9989961 (accessed January 22, 2016).

[56] Cademartiri, F., S. Seitun, A. Clemente, L. La Grutta, P. Toia, G. Runza, M. Midiri, E. Maffei, Myocardial blood flow quantification for evaluation of coronary artery disease by computed tomography, *Cardiovasc. Diagn. Ther.* 7 (2017) 129–150. doi:10.21037/cdt.2017.03.22.

[57] S. S, D. L. C, C. F, B. A, T. N, B. M, B. GP, CT Myocardial Perfusion Imaging: A New Frontier in Cardiac Imaging, *Biomed Res. Int.* 2018 (2018). doi:10.1155/2018/7295460.

[58] Marini, C., S. Seitun, C. Zawaideh, M. Bauckneht, M. C. Morelli, P. Ameri, G. Ferrarazzo, I. Budaj, M. Balbi, F. Fiz, S. Boccalini, A. G. Pregliasco, A. Buschiazzo, A. Saracco, M. C. Bagnara, P. Bruzzi, C. Brunelli, C. Ferro, G. P. Bezante, G. Sambuceti, Comparison of coronary flow reserve estimated by dynamic radionuclide SPECT and multi-detector x-ray CT, *J. Nucl. Cardiol.* 24 (2017) 1712–1721. doi:10.1007/s12350-016-0492-5.

[59] Gaudino, M., F. Piatti, C. Lau, F. Sturla, J. W. Weinsaft, L. Weltert, E. Votta, N. Galea, I. Chirichilli, A. Di Franco, M. Francone, C. Catalano, A. Redaelli, L. N. Girardi, R. De Paulis, Aortic flow after valve sparing root replacement with or without neosinuses reconstruction, *J. Thorac. Cardiovasc. Surg.* 157 (2019) 455–465. doi:10.1016/j.jtcvs.2018.06.094.

[60] Takagi, H., Y. Hari, K. Nakashima, T. Kuno, T. Ando, Mortality after transcatheter versus surgical aortic valve replacement: an updated meta-analysis of randomised trials, *Netherlands Hear. J.* (2020). doi:10.1007/s12471-020-01378-1.

[61] Blanke, P., J. R. Weir-McCall, S. Achenbach, V. Delgado, J. Hausleiter, H. Jilaihawi, M. Marwan, B. L. Nørgaard, N. Piazza, P. Schoenhagen, J. A. Leipsic, Computed Tomography Imaging in the Context of Transcatheter Aortic Valve Implantation (TAVI)/Transcatheter Aortic Valve Replacement (TAVR): An Expert Consensus Document of the Society of Cardiovascular Computed Tomography, *JACC Cardiovasc. Imaging.* 12 (2019) 1–24. doi:10.1016/j.jcmg.2018.12.003.

[62] Hamdan, A., V. Guetta, E. Konen, O. Goitein, A. Segev, E. Raanani, D. Spiegelstein, I. Hay, E. Di Segni, M. Eldar, E. Schwammenthal, Deformation dynamics and mechanical properties of the aortic annulus by 4-dimensional computed tomography: Insights into the functional anatomy of the aortic valve complex and implications for transcatheter aortic valve therapy, *J. Am. Coll. Cardiol.* 59 (2012) 119–127. doi:10. 1016/j.jacc.2011.09.045.

[63] Blanke, P., M. Russe, J. Leipsic, J. Reinöhl, U. Ebersberger, P. Suranyi, M. Siepe, G. Pache, M. Langer, U. J. Schoepf, Conformational pulsatile changes of the aortic annulus: Impact on prosthesis sizing by computed tomography for transcatheter aortic valve replacement, *JACC Cardiovasc. Interv.* 5 (2012) 984–994. doi:10. 1016/j. jcin.2012.05.014.

[64] Kasel, A. M., S. Cassese, S. Bleiziffer, M. Amaki, R. T. Hahn, A. Kastrati, P. P. Sengupta, Standardized imaging for aortic annular sizing: Implications for transcatheter valve selection, *JACC Cardiovasc. Imaging.* 6 (2013) 249–262. doi:10.1016/j.jcmg. 2012.12.005.

[65] Delgado, V., A. C. T. Ng, N. R. van de Veire, F. van der Kley, J. D. Schuijf, L. F. Tops, A. de Weger, G. Tavilla, A. de Roos, L. J. Kroft, M. J. Schalij, J. J. Bax, Transcatheter aortic valve implantation: role of multi-detector row computed tomography to evaluate prosthesis positioning and deployment in relation to valve function., *Eur. Heart J.* 31 (2010) 1114–1123. doi:10.1093/eurheartj/ehq018.

[66] Achenbach, S., V. Delgado, J. Hausleiter, P. Schoenhagen, J. K. Min, J. A. Leipsic, SCCT expert consensus document on computed tomography imaging before transcatheter aortic valve implantation (TAVI)/transcatheter aortic valve replacement (TAVR), *J. Cardiovasc. Comput. Tomogr.* 6 (2012) 366–380. doi:10.1016/j.jcct.2012. 11.002.

[67] Jabbour, A., T. F. Ismail, N. Moat, A. Gulati, I. Roussin, F. Alpendurada, B. Park, F. Okoroafor, A. Asgar, S. Barker, S. Davies, S. K. Prasad, M. Rubens, R. H. Mohiaddin, Multimodality imaging in transcatheter aortic valve implantation and post-procedural aortic regurgitation: Comparison among cardiovascular magnetic resonance, cardiac computed tomography, and echocardiography, *J. Am. Coll. Cardiol.* 58 (2011) 2165–2173. doi:10.1016/j.jacc.2011.09.010.

[68] Pontone, G., D. Andreini, A. L. Bartorelli, E. Bertella, S. Mushtaq, P. Gripari, M. Loguercio, S. Cortinovis, A. Baggiano, E. Conte, V. Beltrama, A. Annoni, A. Formenti, G. Tamborini, M. Muratori, A. Guaricci, F. Alamanni, G. Ballerini, M. Pepi, Comparison of accuracy of aortic root annulus assessment with cardiac magnetic resonance versus echocardiography and multidetector computed tomography in patients referred for transcatheter aortic valve implantation, *Am. J. Cardiol.* 112 (2013) 1790–1799. doi:10.1016/j.amjcard.2013.07.050.

[69] von Knobelsdorff-Brenkenhoff, F., R. F. Trauzeddel, J. Schulz-Menger, Cardiovascular magnetic resonance in adults with previous cardiovascular surgery., *Eur. Heart J. Cardiovasc. Imaging.* 15 (2014) 235–48. doi:10.1093/ehjci/jet138.

[70] Pham, N., H. Zaitoun, T. L. Mohammed, E. Delapena-Almaguer, F. Martinez, G. M. Novaro, J. Kirsch, Complications of aortic valve surgery: Manifestations at CT and MR imaging, *Radiographics.* 32 (2012) 1873–1892. doi:10.1148/rg.327115735.

[71] Crouch, G., P. J. Tully, J. Bennetts, A. Sinhal, C. Bradbrook, A. L. Penhall, C. G. De Pasquale, R. A. Baker, J. B. Selvanayagam, Quantitative assessment of paravalvular

regurgitation following transcatheter aortic valve replacement, *J. Cardiovasc. Magn. Reson.* 17 (2015) 32. doi:10.1186/s12968-015-0134-0.

[72] Hwang, I. C., H. K. Kim, J. B. Park, E. A. Park, W. Lee, S. P. Lee, Y. J. Kim, D. W. Sohn, J. K. Oh, Aortic valve replacement-induced changes in native T1 are related to prognosis in severe aortic stenosis: T1 mapping cardiac magnetic resonance imaging study., *Eur. Heart J. Cardiovasc. Imaging*. (2019). doi:10.1093/ehjci/jez201.

[73] Isaka, Y., H. Hayashi, K. Aonuma, M. Horio, Y. Terada, K. Doi, Y. Fujigaki, H. Yasuda, T. Sato, T. Fujikura, R. Kuwatsuru, H. Toei, R. Murakami, Y. Saito, A. Hirayama, T. Murohara, A. Sato, H. Ishii, T. Takayama, M. Watanabe, K. Awai, S. Oda, T. Murakami, Y. Yagyu, N. Joki, Y. Komatsu, T. Miyauchi, Y. Ito, R. Miyazawa, Y. Kanno, T. Ogawa, H. Hayashi, E. Koshi, T. Kosugi, Y. Yasuda, Guideline on the use of iodinated contrast media in patients with kidney disease 2018, *Clin. Exp. Nephrol.* 24 (2020) 1–44. doi:10.1007/s10157-019-01750-5.

In: Perspectives in Aortic Valve Disease
Editor: Giovanni Concistrè ISBN: 978-1-53618-769-4

Chapter 5

DEGENERATIVE AORTIC VALVE DISEASE

Michele Emdin[1,2,*], Lucio Teresi[1], Samuele Cannas[1], Alberto Aimo[1] and Claudio Passino[1,2]

[1]Institute of Life Sciences, Scuola Superiore Sant'Anna, Pisa, Italy
[2]Fondazione G. Monasterio, Pisa, Italy

ABSTRACT

The spectrum of degenerative aortic valve disease ranges from aortic valve sclerosis to severe calcification with aortic stenosis. degenerative aortic valve disease is a progressive disease that affects about 30% of the population over 65 years in the United States and is the most common aortic valve pathology. It shares some pathophysiological mechanisms with atherosclerosis: most notably, mechanical stress triggers a local inflammation with lipid infiltration and calcification, and genetics may influence patient susceptibility, disease evolution and the response to treatment. Conversely, there are substantial differences in the process of calcification, which in degenerative aortic valve disease involves a switch of interstitial cells to an osteoblast-like phenotype together with non-osteogenic mechanisms, such as the mineralization of dead cells. Imaging techniques, including positron emission computed tomography and micro-optical coherence tomography, might allow to capture early disease manifestations, thus potentially allowing specific treatments. Despite the similarities with atherosclerotic disease, the efficacy of statins is controversial, while angiotensin converting enzyme inhibitors and molecules targeting inflammation, tissue remodeling or calcification are still under investigation. Aortic valve replacement or transcatheter aortic valve implantation are the treatments of choice for degenerative aortic valve disease, but prosthetic valves are susceptible to degeneration and thrombosis. Tissue engineering combines host cells and template materials to induce a natural regeneration of valve structures, either in vivo or in vitro, and is another potential approach under evaluation. This chapter will provide an overview of the pathophysiology of degenerative aortic valve disease, the role of imaging techniques for its management and the perspectives for treatment.

---

* Corresponding Author's Email: emdin@ftgm.it.

Keywords: aortic valve degenerative disease, calcific aortic valve, aortic stenosis, molecular imaging, tissue engineering

ABBREVIATIONS

ACE	Angiotensin converting enzyme
ACE-I	ACE inhibitors
ARBs	Angiotensin receptor blockers
AS	Aortic stenosis
BMP	Bone morphogenic protein
FDG	Fluorodeoxyglucose
LDL	Low-density lipoprotein
MGP	Matrix Gla protein
MMP	Metalloproteinase
mOCT	Micro-optical coherence tomography
NaF	Sodium fluoride
PET	Positron emission tomography
Pi	Phosphate
PPARγ	Peroxisome proliferator-activator γ
RAAVE	Rosuvastatin affecting aortic valve endothelium
RANK	Receptor activator of nuclear factor kappa B
RANKL	Receptor activator of nuclear factor kappa B ligand
ROS	Reactive oxygen species
TEHV	Tissue engineering of heart valves.

INTRODUCTION

Aortic valve disease is a major cause of morbidity and mortality worldwide, and its prevalence is increasing in parallel with population ageing [1]. The most common form is degenerative aortic valve disease. In populations above 65 years of age, the prevalence of aortic valve sclerosis, calcification, or thickening is reported to be 21–31% [2]. Moreover, in the older population there is a high prevalence (2–9%) of end-stage degenerative aortic valve disease with high-grade aortic stenosis (AS) often necessitating a therapeutic intervention [3]. The phenotypic spectrum of degenerative aortic valve disease ranges from a progressive thickening of valve cups (aortic sclerosis) to reduced leaflet motion that may limit forward blood flow (aortic stenosis) [4]. Far from being a simple deterioration of aortic valve cusps, degenerative aortic valve disease is now interpreted as the result of an active process including extracellular matrix remodeling and the activation of molecular pathways that promote calcification and angiogenesis. Some of these mechanisms are common to atherosclerosis, and many risk factors are shared between this process and coronary artery disease (CAD), including elderly age, male gender, diabetes, hypercholesterolemia, hypertension, and smoking. On the other hand, only 40-50% of patients with atherosclerosis develop degenerative aortic valve disease [5], suggesting an incomplete overlap between these two conditions.

In this chapter we will reappraise the pathophysiology of degenerative aortic valve disease, highlighting the similarities and differences with atherosclerosis, and some approaches proposed to prevent or relieve the degeneration of aortic cusps.

PATHOPHYSIOLOGY

Degenerative Aortic Valve Disease and Atherosclerosis

Degenerative aortic valve disease shares many characteristics with atherosclerotic disease, including a crucial role played by endothelial dysfunction in both conditions.

The aortic valve is chronically exposed to complex shear forces. It has been shown that directional shear stress is responsible for arterial endothelial alignment in vivo [6]. Cultured aortic endothelial cells dispose perpendicularly to flow direction, in contrast to the typical parallel alignment to flow seen in other endothelial culture studies [7]. Calcification occurs primarily on the aortic side of aortic valve leaflets, where flow is most turbulent, suggesting that shear stress and its interaction with valvular endothelium plays a role in calcification.

Following abnormal shear stress conditions, endothelial cells produce more reactive oxygen species and less nitric oxide. Oxidative stress promotes the expression of adhesion molecules such as vascular cell adhesion molecule 1 and intercellular adhesion molecule 1 (VCAM-1, ICAM-1) and chemokines such as monocyte chemoattractant protein-1 (MCP-1) by endothelial cells. Monocytes are recruited and activated into macrophages, which further amplify oxidative stress and inflammation [8]. Additionally, low density lipoproteins (LDLs) begin to accumulate in valve tissues. Both macrophages and LDLs display angiotensin-converting enzyme (ACE) activity, which converts angiotensin I to angiotensin II; the same activation may be catalyzed by chymase, which is released by mast cells. Angiotensin II type 1 receptor (AT1-R) is expressed constitutively by smooth muscle cells in vessels, and in pathologic conditions it is also expressed by fibroblasts in the aortic valve. Angiotensin II works as a chemotactic factor for monocytes, increases oxidative cellular stress, promotes LDLs uptake in the valve and the conversion of macrophages into foam cells [9-10] (Figure 1).

Early lesions in both atherosclerosis and degenerative aortic valve disease involves disruption of the basement membrane, macrophage and T-lymphocyte migration, and infiltration of lipoproteins. The inflammatory response drives activation of myofibroblasts, release of cytokines such as tumor necrosis factor alpha and transforming growth factor beta, and the expression of matrix metalloproteinases (MMPs).

However, specific cellular and genetic mechanisms of degeneration affect the aortic valve substrate. Shear stress forces are different in the aortic valve and arteries, because of the much more complex anatomy of the aortic valve. A bicuspid structure or the reduced elasticity and compliance of degenerated cusps are usually the mechanical triggers of the pathology [11], and calcification occurs primarily on the aortic side of the leaflets, where mechanical stress is higher [8]. Valvular endothelial cells are phenotypically different from other endothelial cells in the cardiovascular system as they tend to dispose perpendicularly to blood flow, instead of parallel. Therefore, also their response to pathological mechanical stimuli can be supposed to be different [8, 12].

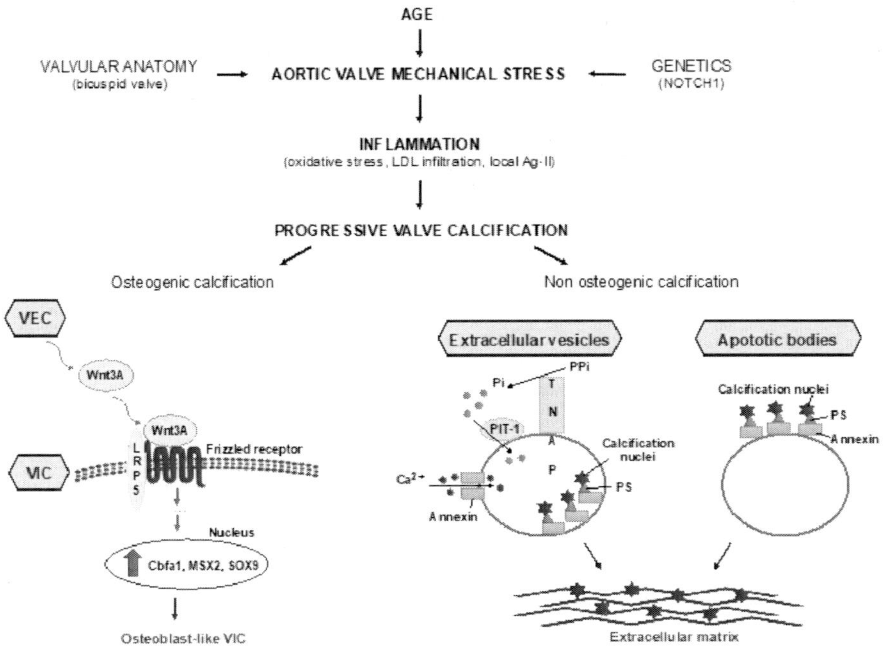

LRP5, LDL receptor-related protein 5; Pi phosphate; PIT-1, phosphate transporter-1; PPi, pyrophosphate; PS, phosphatidylserine; TNAP, tissue non-specific alkaline phosphatase; VEC, valvular endothelial cells; VIC, valvular interstitial cells.

Figure 1. Degenerative aortic valve disease pathophysiology.

Valves lack smooth muscle cells, which are an important feature of atherosclerotic lesions in the vasculature. By contrast, valves contain myofibroblasts that proliferate in response to decreased nitric oxide levels, angiotensin II; and local hormones, including tissue growth factor and platelet-derived growth factor.

There are as many smooth muscle cells in aortic valve leaflets as in vessels, but in the aortic valve there are also interstitial myofibroblasts that are activated and proliferate in response to inflammatory stimuli. They release tumor necrosis factor (TNF) α and transforming growth factor (TGF) β1, which promote calcification by up-regulating MMPs and the bone morphogenic protein (BMP). The calcification process is more pronounced and develops during an earlier disease stage than in atherosclerosis. Finally, neovascularization induced by inflammation is much less significant in degenerative aortic valve disease than in atherosclerosis [13].

Calcification

Calcification is a distinguishing feature of degenerative aortic valve disease. The osteogenic mechanism of calcification has been well characterized and is traditionally considered to be more relevant. It is driven by interstitial valve myofibroblasts switching their phenotype to bone-forming cells. This process starts with secretion of Wnt3a by valvular endothelial cell s into the sub-endothelial region in response to oxidative stress, inflammation and high cholesterol levels. Wnt3a binds LDL receptor-related proteins 5 (LRP-5) and the Frizzled receptor on the surface of the interstitial cells, forming a trimer. This elicits a transduction cascade including glycogen synthase kinase (GSK) 3β, and ultimately regulating the expression of transcription factors related to osteogenic bone formation (Cbfa1, Msx2 and Sox9) (Figure). This prompts the expression of osteopontin, osteonectin, osteocalcin, the receptor activator of nuclear factor kappa B (RANK) ligand, osteoprotegerin, bone alkaline phosphatase and BMP2. BMP2 is considered a major driver of valve calcification. These osteoblast-like cells proliferate and produce extracellular matrix resulting in ectopic osteogenesis [14].

Non-osteogenic calcification is less well known, but it could be as important as osteogenic calcification [15]. It was suspected thanks to the observation that some amorphous calcium deposits from calcified valves do not contain live cells. The proposed mechanisms are abnormal ions clearance and cell death secondary to local inflammation. Inflammation induces macrophages and valvular interstitial cells to release extracellular vesicles, which concentrate ions. On their membranes, annexin facilitates Ca2+ entrance in the lumen, while tissue non-specific alkaline phosphatase (TNAP) converts pyrophosphate (PPi) to phosphate (Pi) ions which goes into the lumen thanks to Na/Pi transporters (PiT-1). On the inner side of the membrane, complexes of annexin and phosphatidylserine bind Ca2+ and Pi, which can interact forming hydroxyapatite that accumulates and cause extracellular vesicles' rupture. On the extracellular space, amorphous hydroxyapatite forms structured crystals, because it accumulates in the extra-cellular matrix where there are charged fragments of collagen and proteoglycans, obtained after degradation by MMPs on the extracellular vesicles' surface (Figure 1). When systemic concentrations of Ca2+ and Pi are high as in chronic kidney disease this mechanism is promoted, because cells produce high density ions extracellular vesicles [15-16].

Apoptosis has a well-defined role in non-osteogenic calcification, while necrosis importance has not been clarified yet, but for sure it can promote inflammation [17]. Apoptotic bodies can concentrate ions as extracellular vesicles previously described, but some of them have phosphatidylserine also on the outer side of the membrane, so that they can form calcifications directly on the extracellular space [18] (Figure 1).

Osteogenic and non-osteogenic mechanisms of calcification are linked and promote each other. For example, extracellular vesicles contain dysfunctional miRNA as RUNX2 which can induce osteogenic switch of valvular interstitial cells [16]. It is possible that osteogenic calcification is prevalent in the early phases of degenerative aortic valve disease, while non-osteogenic mechanisms become more important in more advanced stages. However, it is important to remember that mechanisms for the prevention of local calcifications exist, but in the pathology they are no more sufficient. Among them, fetuin-A and matrix Gla protein have a major role. Fetuin-A is a circulating glycoprotein constitutively secreted by the liver. It binds small calcium-phosphate particles and promotes their phagocytosis and removal. However, in aortic lesions of degenerative aortic valve disease it is mostly degraded by MMPs overexpressed secondary to inflammation [19]. Matrix Gla protein (MGP) is a vitamin K-dependent protein, it prevents calcification by inhibiting BMP signaling and it is expressed by chondrocytes, vascular smooth muscle cells and by osteoblast-like myofibroblasts, as a negative control of the calcification process [20].

Genetic Factors

Many genetic factors are involved in degenerative aortic valve disease. Single-center studies have identified a role of several polymorphisms. Most notably, polymorphisms causing an overexpression of the LDL receptor and lipoprotein A display a strong association with calcification of arteries and valves [21].

In two families, loss-of-function mutations in the NOTCH1 gene have been linked both to a bicuspid anatomy and to the differentiation of mesenchymal cells toward an osteoblast-like phenotype [8-9]. In addition to influencing the development of degenerative aortic valve disease, genetic factors might also affect the response to therapies, but this point has not been investigated so far.

Role of Imaging

The natural history of degenerative aortic valve disease starts with microscopic calcific phenomena and culminates in severe valve stenosis. Conventional non-invasive imaging techniques have an average resolution of 1 mm, and detection of the earliest steps of valve degeneration requires novel, more sophisticated techniques.

Transthoracic echocardiography is an essential examination to assess valve structure and function, and valve characterization can be implemented by a transesophageal exam. Cardiac computed tomography (CT) allows to assess the anatomy of the aortic valve and the aortic root and the extent of calcification, and is essential to plan a percutaneous intervention. Cardiac magnetic resonance is not the optimal tool to assess calcified structures, and has a limited role in this setting. The use of gadolinium-containing immunomicelles targeting the macrophage scavenger receptor has been proposed to visualize the early stages of degenerative aortic valve disease [8].

The use of two positron emission tomography (PET) tracers has been proposed. 18F-fluorodeoxyglucose (18F-FDG) is typically trapped in inflammatory macrophages, whereas 18F-sodium fluoride (18F-NaF) is incorporated in hydroxyapatite during tissue calcification. 18F-NaF can detect early calcification (microcalcification) as an increased 18F-NaF activity was observed in 45% of patients with aortic sclerosis, 91% of those with mild or moderate AS, and 100% of those with severe AS [22]. In the same study, increased 18F-FDG activity was observed in 20% of patients with aortic sclerosis, 35% of those with mild or moderate AS, and 52% of those with severe AS. Interestingly, inflammation should be reduced in advanced degenerative aortic valve disease, but an increase in 18F-FDG is still detected. This could be explained by considering that, under hypoxic conditions, macrophages increase the uptake of glucose while reducing the release of inflammatory cytokines. On the other hand, 18F-FDG uptake by surrounding cardiomyocytes may interfere with signal detection; therefore, while 18F-NaF is a reliable marker of early calcification, the results of 18F-FDG imaging should be interpreted with more caution [23].

Optical molecular imaging employs near-infrared fluorescence imaging agents to assess the process of osteogenesis. Molecular imaging allows to clearly identify three stages of degenerative aortic valve disease, which are defined as initiation phase, propagation phase and late stage [8]. The late stage is characterized by irreversible changes in valve structure, which are easily detectable by conventional imaging techniques. Micro-optical coherence tomography (mOCT) has a spatial resolution of 1 μm. Molecular features, such as macrophages and calcium crystals, can be visualized with near-histological detail. Contrary to near-infrared molecular imaging, mOCT does not require the use of contrast agents. Both techniques are characterized by limited tissue penetration [24].

PHARMACOLOGICAL STRATEGIES

The medical management of AS is discussed in Chapter 12. Herein, we will present the possible approaches to modify the natural history of this condition, highlighting some experimental and clinical findings specifically related to degenerative aortic valve disease.

Lipid-Lowering Drugs

Studies in mice and rabbits showed that statins effectively slow down the degeneration of aortic valves, and results from some retrospective studies were in agreement with this conclusion. Among four clinical trials (SALTIRE [Scottish Aortic Stenosis and Lipid Lowering Trial], [25]; RAAVE [Rosuvastatin Affecting Aortic Valve Endothelium to Slow the Progression of Aortic Stenosis], [26]; SEAS [Simvastatin and ezetimibe in aortic stenosis], [27]; ASTRONOMER [Aortic Stenosis Progression Observation: Measuring the Effects of Rosuvastatin], [28]), only the RAAVE trial demonstrated an efficacy of statins on disease progression [8]. The relatively small size of these trials, the limited follow-up period, and the enrolment of patients with rather advanced degenerative aortic valve disease may contribute to these neutral results. Additionally, patients from retrospective cohorts were often on statins for hypercholesterolemia since many years. Therefore, statins could be effective in preventing disease progression only when started early [29], and a beneficial effect of statins could become appreciable only after many years of treatment. Research on statins and other lipid-lowering drugs, such as niacin, ISIS-APO(a)Rx, recombinant apolipoprotein A-1 Milano or Proprotein Convertase Subtilisin/Kexin-type 9 (PCSK9) inhibitors, is ongoing (30). To date, statin treatment is not recommended by European Society of Cardiology [31] and American College of Cardiology/American Heart Association guidelines [32] for the sole purpose of preventing disease progression.

Drugs Acting on the Renin-Angiotensin-Aldosterone System

ACEi and ARBs may exert beneficial effects on degenerative aortic valve disease progression by improving hemodynamics and then shear stress, and also by blunting the detrimental effects of angiotensin II and aldosterone on the valve tissue. On the other hand, this hypothesis has not been adequately explored in preclinical studies, and evidence from clinical trials that ACEi/ARBs can have a favorable impact on disease progression is limited (as discussed in Chapter 12).

Modulators of Valve Calcification

Some drugs modulating the calcification process have been evaluated. Denosumab is a promising inhibitor of RANK ligand (RANKL), which decreases calcium deposition up to 50% in in murine models [33]. Bisphosphonates have raised some expectations, also given their anti-inflammatory and lipid-lowering effects, but a retrospective analysis of 801 women with mild to moderate degenerative aortic valve disease did not show any positive effects. The SALTIRE II is testing the efficacy of denosumab or alendronic acid in degenerative aortic valve disease (Marquis-Gravel et al. 2016). Osteoprotegerin, a RANKL inhibitor used to treat osteoporosis, slowed the degeneration of aortic valve in mice, but studies in humans are lacking (Weiss et al. 2013). Vitamin D supplementation is another possible approach for reducing calcemia and is especially studied in patients with hyperparathyroidism or renal dysfunction [30]. Finally, vitamin K antagonists have emerged as risk factors for tissue calcification, possibly because of MGP inhibition. It has been proposed that they should be preferentially replaced by non-vitamin K antagonists, although evidence is currently lacking [20, 30].

Other Pharmacological Strategies

MMPs play an important role in valvular degeneration. Doxycycline at subantimicrobial doses acts as nonselective MMPs' inhibitor with a double action. It binds directly the MMPs' zinc domain, which is crucial for the interaction with substrates, and downregulate the transcription of MMPs mRNA [34]. However, when this drug was tested in apolipoprotein E−/− mice it did not slow degenerative aortic valve disease progression neither clinically nor histopatologically. Longer periods of treatment or the therapy with selective inhibitors have been considered as perspectives for future studies [35].

Pioglitazone is a peroxisome proliferator-activator γ (PPARγ) agonist. PPARγ is involved in cellular metabolism and its stimulation inhibits myofibroblasts switch to osteoblast-like cells, while promoting their switch to adipocyte-like cells. Pioglitazone seems to attenuate aortic valve degeneration in LDL receptor-/-/ApoB100/100 mice by decreasing lipid deposition, cell death and calcification. This drug has not been tested in humans [36].

Ectonucleotidases are membrane enzymes that metabolize secreted nucleotides into phosphate and pyrophosphate, which then accumulate in the extracellular spaces. They are overexpressed by pathologic myofibroblasts promoting calcification. In animal models, inhibitors of ectonucleotidases showed good results in slowing the aortic valve degeneration [37].

INTERVENTIONAL THERAPIES

Tissue Engineering

Aortic valve replacement and transcatheter aortic valve implantation are established therapeutic options for severe symptomatic AS, as extensively discussed in other chapters.

Valves implanted through either a surgical or percutaneous approach are susceptible to the same process of degeneration as native valves [8]. Tissue engineering of heart valves (TEHV) has been proposed as a possible alternative strategy. The general idea is an interaction between host cells and a template material to produce a native-like structures [5]. In vitro TEHV involves the culture and seeding of different types of autologous cells on a scaffold. The prosthesis is tailored to the heart anatomy of the patient, and after implantation behaves as a living tissue, responding to stressors and adapting to local environment. TEHV can be successfully placed percutaneously into the aortic valve position, thereby fully excluding the native leaflets while not compromising the coronary perfusion. Unfortunately, this approach is extremely time-consuming and expensive, does not exclude an immunogenic response, and carries a risk of neoplastic transformation [38]. In vivo TEHV is based on the percutaneous positioning of an acellular biodegradable scaffold in the aortic valve position to recruit endogenous cells. A transapical implantation technology is used by means of a transcatheter delivery system. After implantation of an in situ TEHV, the scaffold material is the main load-bearing structure. As the material is degraded and replaced by extra-cellular matrix and cells, the mechanical properties of the valve change, but integrity has to be maintained throughout the whole process. This process is more rapid, less invasive and less susceptible to infections than in vitro TEHV. The drawbacks of this approach include the low rate of recruitment of endogenous cells and possible toxic effects from scaffold degradation [39].

TEHVs have obtained a remarkable success in animal models even though they have not been yet tested in human patients. Dogs, primates, rodents, sheep and pigs have been all valuable models for the study of scaffold remodeling and recellularization. Hence, a future application in humans should be implemented [8].

Conclusion

Degenerative aortic valve disease is a major cause of mortality and morbidity that shares some mechanisms with atherosclerosis. Imaging techniques, including PET and mOCT, might allow to capture early disease manifestations, thus potentially allowing specific treatments. Despite the similarities with atherosclerosis, the efficacy of statins in degenerative aortic valve disease is controversial, while angiotensin converting enzyme inhibitors, molecules targeting inflammation, tissue remodeling or calcification are still under evaluation. Aortic valve replacement or transcatheter aortic valve implantation are the treatments of choice for degenerative aortic valve disease, but prosthetic valves are still susceptible to degeneration and thrombosis. TEHV combines host cells and template materials to induce a natural regeneration of valve structures, either in vivo or in vitro, and is another potential approach under evaluation.

References

[1] Nkomo, Vuyisile T, Julius M Gardin, Thomas N Skelton, John S Gottdiener, Christopher G Scott, and Maurice Enriquez-Sarano. 2006. "Burden of Valvular Heart

Diseases: A Population-Based Study." *The Lancet* 368 (9540). Elsevier: 1005–11. https://doi.org/10.1016/S0140-6736(06)69208-8.

[2] Otto, Catherine M., Ian G. Burwash, Malcolm E. Legget, Brad I. Munt, Michelle Fujioka, Nancy L. Healy, Carol D. Kraft, Carolyn Y. Miyake-Hull, and Rebecca G. Schwaegler. 1997. "Prospective Study of Asymptomatic Valvular Aortic Stenosis." *Circulation* 95 (9). American Heart Association: 2262–70. https://doi.org/10.1161/01.CIR.95.9.2262.

[3] Stritzke, Jan, Patrick Linsel-Nitschke, Marcello Ricardo Paulista Markus, Björn Mayer, Wolfgang Lieb, Andreas Luchner, Angela Döring, et al. 2009. "Association between Degenerative Aortic Valve Disease and Long-Term Exposure to Cardiovascular Risk Factors: Results of the Longitudinal Population-Based KORA/MONICA Survey." *European Heart Journal* 30 (16): 2044–53. https://doi.org/10.1093/eurheartj/ehp287.

[4] Lerman, Daniel Alejandro, Sai Prasad, and Nasri Alotti. 2015. "Calcific Aortic Valve Disease: Molecular Mechanisms and Therapeutic Approaches." *European Cardiology 10 (2). Radcliffe Cardiology:* 108–12. https://doi.org/10.15420/ecr.2015.10.2.108.

[5] Jover, Eva, Marco Fagnano, Gianni Angelini, and Paolo Madeddu. 2018. "Cell Sources for Tissue Engineering Strategies to Treat Calcific Valve Disease." *Frontiers in Cardiovascular Medicine* 5 (November). Frontiers Media S. A.: 155. https://doi.org/10.3389/fcvm.2018.00155.

[6] Flaherty, John T., Josephe Pierce, Victor J. Ferrans, Dali J. Patel, Kirk W. Tucker, and Donald L. Fry. 1972. "Endothelial Nuclear Patterns in the Canine Arterial Tree with Particular Reference to Hemodynamic Events." *Circulation Research* 30 (1). American Heart Association: 23–33. https://doi.org/10.1161/01.RES.30.1.23.

[7] Butcher, Jonathan T, Andrea M Penrod, Andrés J García, and Robert M Nerem. 2004. "Unique Morphology and Focal Adhesion Development of Valvular Endothelial Cells in Static and Fluid Flow Environments." *Arteriosclerosis, Thrombosis, and Vascular Biology* 24 (8): 1429–34. https://doi.org/10.1161/01.ATV.0000130462.50769.5a.

[8] Goldbarg, Seth H, Sammy Elmariah, Marc A Miller, and Valentin Fuster. 2007. "Insights into Degenerative Aortic Valve Disease." *Journal of the American College of Cardiology* 50 (13): 1205–13. https://doi.org/https://doi.org/10.1016/j.jacc.2007.06.024.

[9] O'Brien, Kevin D. 2006. "Pathogenesis of Calcific Aortic Valve Disease." *Arteriosclerosis, Thrombosis, and Vascular Biology* 26 (8). American Heart Association: 1721–28. https://doi.org/10.1161/01.ATV.0000227513.13697.ac.

[10] O'Brien, Kevin D., Shavelle David M., Caulfield Michael T., McDonald Thomas O., Olin-Lewis Katherine, Otto Catherine M., and Probstfield Jeffrey L. 2002. "Association of Angiotensin-Converting Enzyme with Low-Density Lipoprotein in Aortic Valvular Lesions and in Human Plasma." *Circulation* 106 (17). American Heart Association: 2224–30. https://doi.org/10.1161/01.CIR.0000035655.45453.D2.

[11] Robicsek, Francis, Mano J Thubrikar, and Alexander A Fokin. 2002. "Cause of Degenerative Disease of the Trileaflet Aortic Valve: Review of Subject and Presentation of a New Theory." *The Annals of Thoracic Surgery* 73 (4). Elsevier: 1346–54. https://doi.org/10.1016/S0003-4975(01)03001-6.

[12] Davies, Peter F., G. Passerini Anthony, and A. Simmons Craig. 2004. "Aortic Valve." *Arteriosclerosis, Thrombosis, and Vascular Biology* 24 (8). American Heart Association: 1331–33. https://doi.org/10.1161/01.ATV.0000130659.89433.c1.

[13] Sathyamurthy, I, and Shaji Alex. 2015. "Calcific Aortic Valve Disease: Is It Another Face of Atherosclerosis?" *Indian Heart Journal* 67 (5). Elsevier: 503–6. https://doi.org/10.1016/j.ihj.2015.07.033.

[14] Rajamannan, Nalini M. 2018. "*Osteocardiology: Calcific Aortic Valve Disease BT - Osteocardiology: Cardiac Bone Formation*." In, edited by Nalini M Rajamannan, 21–38. Cham: Springer International Publishing. https://doi.org/10.1007/978-3-319-64994-8_3.

[15] Weiss, Robert M, Jordan D Miller, and Donald D Heistad. 2013. "Fibrocalcific Aortic Valve Disease: Opportunity to Understand Disease Mechanisms Using Mouse Models." *Circulation Research* 113 (2): 209–22. https://doi.org/10.1161/CIRCRESAHA.113.300153.

[16] Bakhshian Nik, Amirala, Joshua D Hutcheson, and Elena Aikawa. 2017. "Extracellular Vesicles as Mediators of Cardiovascular Calcification." *Frontiers in Cardiovascular Medicine 4 (December). Frontiers Media* S. A.: 78. https://doi.org/10.3389/fcvm.2017.00078.

[17] Diane, Proudfoot, Skepper Jeremy N., Hegyi Laszlo, Bennett Martin R., Shanahan Catherine M., and Weissberg Peter L. 2000. "Apoptosis Regulates Human Vascular Calcification *In Vitro*." *Circulation Research* 87 (11). American Heart Association: 1055–62. https://doi.org/10.1161/01.RES.87.11.1055.

[18] Jahnen-Dechent, Willi, Alexander Heiss, Cora Schäfer, Markus Ketteler, and Dwight A Towler. 2011. "Fetuin-A Regulation of Calcified Matrix Metabolism." *Circulation* Research 108 (12): 1494–1509. https://doi.org/10.1161/CIRCRESAHA.110.234260.

[19] Zhang, Bin, Grace Casaclang-Verzosa, and Jordan D Miller. 2014. "*Mouse Models of Calcific Aortic Valve Disease BT - Molecular Biology of Valvular Heart Disease*." In, edited by Nalini M Rajamannan, 67–80. London: Springer London. https://doi.org/10.1007/978-1-4471-6350-3_10.

[20] Chiyoya, Mari, Kazuhiko Seya, Zaiqiang Yu, Kazuyuki Daitoku, Shigeru Motomura, Tadaatsu Imaizumi, Ikuo Fukuda, and Ken-Ichi Furukawa. 2018. "Matrix Gla Protein Negatively Regulates Calcification of Human Aortic Valve Interstitial Cells Isolated from Calcified Aortic Valves." *Journal of Pharmacological Sciences* 136 (4): 257–65. https://doi.org/https://doi.org/10.1016/j.jphs.2018.03.004.

[21] Smith, Gustav J, Kevin Luk, Christina-Alexandra Schulz, James C Engert, Ron Do, George Hindy, Gull Rukh, et al. 2014. "Association of Low-Density Lipoprotein Cholesterol-Related Genetic Variants with Aortic Valve Calcium and Incident Aortic Stenosis." *JAMA* 312 (17): 1764–71. https://doi.org/10.1001/jama.2014.13959.

[22] Dweck, Marc R, William S A Jenkins, Alex T Vesey, Mark A H Pringle, Calvin W L Chin, Tamir S Malley, William J A Cowie, et al. 2014. "18F-Sodium Fluoride Uptake Is a Marker of Active Calcification and Disease Progression in Patients With Aortic Stenosis." *Circulation: Cardiovascular Imaging* 7 (2): 371–78. https://doi.org/10.1161/CIRCIMAGING.113.001508.

[23] Dweck, Marc R, Jones Charlotte, Joshi Nikhil V., Fletcher Alison M., Richardson Hamish, White Audrey, Marsden Mark, et al. 2012. "Assessment of Valvular Calcification and Inflammation by Positron Emission Tomography in Patients with Aortic Stenosis." *Circulation* 125 (1). American Heart Association: 76–86. https://doi.org/10.1161/CIRCULATIONAHA.111.051052.

[24] Aikawa, Elena, and Otto Catherine M. 2012. "Look More Closely at the Valve." *Circulation* 125 (1). American Heart Association: 9–11. https://doi.org/10.1161/CIRCULATIONAHA.111.073452.

[25] Cowell, S Joanna, David E Newby, Robin J Prescott, Peter Bloomfield, John Reid, David B Northridge, and Nicholas A Boon. 2005. "A Randomized Trial of Intensive Lipid-Lowering Therapy in Calcific Aortic Stenosis." *New England Journal of Medicine* 352 (23): 2389–97. https://doi.org/10.1056/NEJMoa043876.

[26] Moura, Luis M, Sandra F Ramos, José L Zamorano, Isabel M Barros, Luis F Azevedo, Francisco Rocha-Gonçalves, and Nalini M Rajamannan. 2007. "Rosuvastatin Affecting Aortic Valve Endothelium to Slow the Progression of Aortic Stenosis." *Journal of the American College of Cardiology* 49 (5): 554–61. https://doi.org/10.1016/j.jacc.2006.07.072.

[27] Rossebø, Anne B, Terje R Pedersen, Kurt Boman, Philippe Brudi, John B Chambers, Kenneth Egstrup, Eva Gerdts, et al. 2008. "Intensive Lipid Lowering with Simvastatin and Ezetimibe in Aortic Stenosis." *New England Journal of Medicine* 359 (13): 1343–56. https://doi.org/10.1056/NEJMoa0804602.

[28] Chan, Kwan L, Koon Teo, Jean G Dumesnil, Andy Ni, and James Tam. 2010. "Effect of Lipid Lowering With Rosuvastatin on Progression of Aortic Stenosis." *Circulation* 121 (2): 306–14. https://doi.org/10.1161/CIRCULATIONAHA.109.900027.

[29] Rajamannan, Nalini M, Frank J Evans, Elena Aikawa, K Jane Grande-Allen, Linda L Demer, Donald D Heistad, Craig A Simmons, et al. 2011. "Calcific Aortic Valve Disease: Not Simply a Degenerative Process: A Review and Agenda for Research from the National Heart and Lung and Blood Institute Aortic Stenosis Working Group. Executive Summary: Calcific Aortic Valve Disease-2011 Update." *Circulation* 124 (16): 1783–91. https://doi.org/10.1161/CIRCULATIONAHA.110.006767.

[30] Marquis-Gravel, Guillaume, Björn Redfors, Martin B Leon, and Philippe Généreux. 2016. "Medical Treatment of Aortic Stenosis." *Circulation* 134 (22): 1766–84. https://doi.org/10.1161/CIRCULATIONAHA.116.023997.

[31] Baumgartner, Helmut, Volkmar Falk, Jeroen J Bax, Michele De Bonis, Christian Hamm, Per Johan Holm, Bernard Iung, et al. 2017. "2017 ESC/EACTS Guidelines for the Management of Valvular Heart Disease." *European Heart Journal* 38 (36): 2739–91. https://doi.org/10.1093/eurheartj/ehx391.

[32] Nishimura, Rick A., Catherine M. Otto, Robert O. Bonow, Blase A. Carabello, John P. Erwin, Robert A. Guyton, Patrick T. O'Gara, et al. 2014. "2014 AHA/ACC Guideline for the Management of Patients with Valvular Heart Disease: Executive Summary." *Circulation* 129 (23). American Heart Association: 2440–92. https://doi.org/10.1161/CIR.0000000000000029.

[33] Helas, Susann, Claudia Goettsch, Michael Schoppet, Ute Zeitz, Ute Hempel, Henning Morawietz, Paul J Kostenuik, Reinhold G Erben, and Lorenz C Hofbauer. 2009. "Inhibition of Receptor Activator of NF-KappaB Ligand by Denosumab Attenuates Vascular Calcium Deposition in Mice." *The American Journal of Pathology* 175 (2). American Society for Investigative Pathology: 473–78. https://doi.org/10.2353/ajpath.2009.080957.

[34] Castro, Michele M, Jose E Tanus-Santos, and Raquel F Gerlach. 2011. "Matrix Metalloproteinases: Targets for Doxycycline to Prevent the Vascular Alterations of

Hypertension." *Pharmacological Research* 64 (6): 567–72. https://doi.org/https://doi.org/10.1016/j.phrs.2011.04.002.

[35] Jung, Jae-Joon, Mahmoud Razavian, Hye-Yeong Kim, Yunpeng Ye, Reza Golestani, Jakub Toczek, Jiasheng Zhang, and Mehran M Sadeghi. 2016. "Matrix Metalloproteinase Inhibitor, Doxycycline and Progression of Calcific Aortic Valve Disease in Hyperlipidemic Mice." *Scientific Reports* 6 (1): 32659. https://doi.org/10.1038/srep32659.

[36] Chu, Yi, Donald D Lund, Robert M Weiss, Robert M Brooks, Hardik Doshi, Georges P Hajj, Curt D Sigmund, and Donald D Heistad. 2013. "Pioglitazone Attenuates Valvular Calcification Induced by Hypercholesterolemia." *Arteriosclerosis, Thrombosis, and Vascular Biology* 33 (3): 523–32. https://doi.org/10.1161/ATVBAHA.112.300794.

[37] Mathieu, Patrick, Ablajan Mahmut, Philippe Pibarot, Yohan Bossé, and Marie-Chloé Boulanger. 2014. "*Role of Ectonucleotidases and Purinergic Receptors in Calcific Aortic Valve Disease BT - Molecular Biology of Valvular Heart Disease*." In, edited by Nalini M Rajamannan, 117–26. London: Springer London. https://doi.org/10.1007/978-1-4471-6350-3_14.

[38] Sacks, Michael S, Frederick J Schoen, and John E Mayer. 2009. "Bioengineering Challenges for Heart Valve Tissue Engineering." *Annual Review of Biomedical Engineering* 11 (1): 289–313. https://doi.org/10.1146/annurev-bioeng-061008-124903.

[39] Kluin, Jolanda, Hanna Talacua, Anthal I P M Smits, Maximilian Y Emmert, Marieke C P Brugmans, Emanuela S Fioretta, Petra E Dijkman, et al. 2017. "In Situ Heart Valve Tissue Engineering Using a Bioresorbable Elastomeric Implant – From Material Design to 12 Months Follow-up in Sheep." *Biomaterials* 125: 101–17. https://doi.org/https://doi.org/10.1016/j.biomaterials.2017.02.007.

In: Perspectives in Aortic Valve Disease
Editor: Giovanni Concistrè

ISBN: 978-1-53618-769-4

Chapter 6

AORTIC VALVE ENDOCARDITIS: EPIDEMIOLOGY, TREATMENT AND OUTCOMES

Michele Danilo Pierri**, Mariano Cefarelli, Paolo Berretta, Jacopo Alfonsi, Luca Montecchiani and Marco Di Eusanio

Cardiac Surgery Department, Lancisi Cardiovascular Center,
Polytechnic University of Marche, Ancona, Italy

ABSTRACT

Infective endocarditis (IE) is an infrequent pathology, but burdened with high mortality. In recent years, it has been manifesting more frequently in older patients and relating to degenerative heart valve dysfunctions. Furthermore, it is increasingly linked to aggressive and antibiotic resistant microorganisms and to health related procedures. Localization of infection in the aortic valve is the most frequent. It can concern both native valve and artificial ones and, more recently, there have been many reported cases regarding percutaneously implanted valves. Frequently, aortic IE is complicated by an extension of the infection to the annulus with the formation of abscesses, fistulas and prostheses detachments.

The diagnosis of the aortic valve IE is based on clinical findings, culture tests and echocardiography examinations. New laboratory and radiological methods (also based on biological markers) have recently been proposed to increase the chances of having a more accurate diagnosis, especially in uncertain cases.

Aortic IE therapy is primarily based on antibiotic therapy; surgical therapy is indicated mainly in complicated forms with heart failure or uncontrolled infection. Early surgical therapy seems to have better results, but the question of the ideal timing remains unsolved, especially in patients with recent neurological damage.

Surgical treatment may consist in the replacement of the valve, with biological or mechanical prostheses, with the repair of abscesses and pseudoaneurysms with patches or, in the case of more destructive forms, in the replacement of the entire aortic root with homografts, stentless valves and conducts or valved conduits. Despite the increase in the age of the patients and the presence of comorbidities, outcome after surgical therapy have improved over time, even though mortality remains high and the rate of recurrences isn't

* Corresponding Author's Email: micheledanilo.pierri@ospedaliriuniti.marche.it.

negligible. Surgical mortality is particularly high in prosthetic valve endocarditis and percutaneously implanted valves.

Due to the complexity of the management and the challenges it poses, the creation of a multidisciplinary team devoted specifically to diagnosing and treating IE is recommended.

Keywords: endocarditis, aortic valve disease, surgical treatment

INTRODUCTION

Infective endocarditis (IE) is the infection of the endocardial surface, particularly the valves, implanted cardiac devices, prosthetic valves and intravascular conduit. It is an infrequent condition with high mortality rates, ranging between 15% and 30% [1].

IE was described initially by Osler in 1885 [2] when it was inevitably fatal. With the advent of antibiotic therapy, its mortality decreased, but still remained high; in more recent times, the diffusion of antibiotic-resistant and aggressive strains (frequently related to health care procedures) poses an additional challenge for its treatment. Early surgery was seen as a therapeutic option for IE especially in more aggressive and disruptive cases and, recently, a more aggressive surgical approach was suggested along with the expansion of the indications and anticipating the surgical timing in order to improve the prognosis. Often aortic valve IE is considered in the context of the so-called "Left heart endocarditis." However, number and anatomy of the leaflets, pressure differences across the valve and etiology, represent important differences in the characteristics of the two valves.

In this chapter we will focus on the aortic valve IE involvement, its epidemiology, treatment and outcome.

CLASSIFICATION

The above mentioned "left heart endocarditis" involving the left heart structures is opposed to the "right heart endocarditis" involving tricuspid and pulmonary valves.

Clinically, IEs are divided in sub-acute and acute forms, the first having more attenuated symptoms.

Another important classification differentiates between IE of native valve (NVE) and IE of implanted valvular prostheses (PVE). The latter is further sub-divided in early and late IE depending on whether they develop within a year after the implantation of the affected prosthesis or later. Alternatively, PVE can be classified as early-onset (within 60 days of surgery), intermediate-onset (from 60 to 365 days) and late-onset (over 1 year after surgery).

IE can also be classified as "community acquired" or related to "health care exposure": the former occurs more frequently and is related to streptococci while the latter frequently consists of staphylococci infections developed in the setting of health care with invasive procedures, intravenous lines, and implantable devices and frequently having an acute expression [3-6].

Epidemiology

The incidence of IE is of 3-10 cases every 100.000 units per year, but there are significative geographical differences [7-9].

In the USA, it is of 7.7 cases every 100.000 units per year in recent years [10]. A study based on the National Registry of Hospital Discharge reported a Spanish incidence of 5.56 cases per 100.000 units in 2014 [11]. During the same year, a Danish registry [12] reported 7.55 cases every 100.000 units while in Italy Cresti et al. [13] found 4.6 cases every 100.000 in the period between 1998 and 2014.

According to some [12, 14], there is an increasing trend of IE; some attribute these changes to the modified guideline suggestions about endocarditis prophylaxis [15], but the rise could also be a consequence of the aging population, increasing morbidity and expansion of health care invasive procedures.

Left side endocarditis are more frequent (90-95%) than right sided endocarditis and NVE are more common (90%) than PVE. Multiple valve endocarditis are infrequent.

The incidence of aortic involvement compared to the mitral one varies in different reports with conflicting results: Murdoch et al. [16] found an involvement of mitral valve in 41% of the cases and aortic valve in 37,6%; Olmos et al. [17] found no differences between the two valves; Ilaho Moreira et al. [18] reported a major incidence in aortic valve (55,7% vs 35%).

IE is associated with about half of cases with degenerative valve pathology (mainly mitral prolaxe and calcific aortic stenosis), but the number of cases with absence of previous valve disease is increasing, probably due to health care associated procedures and implantable devices. In recent times, there are increasing rates of IE reported on percutaneously implanted prostheses [19, 20].

Among the valvular congenital disease, bicuspid aortic valves play a prominent role, having a significant diffusion and increased susceptibility to IE in the adult population [21].

Physiopathology

The initial primer of IE is bacteremia. Microorganisms can enter the bloodstream as a consequence of multiple conditions both medical and not: tooth extraction, urinary catheterization, body piercing, procedures on the gastrointestinal, genitourinary o respiratory tracts. Bacteremia can occur frequently during daily activities [10]. Bacteremias resulting from health care are a growing cause of IE, accounting for an estimate 25% of cases in recent years [16].

The second phase is adhesion to cardiac structures: normally, endothelium is resistant to bacterial adhesion, but, given certain conditions, it becomes altered and vulnerable. In almost 50% of IE there is a previous, underlying predisposition, particularly a valve dysfunction [16]; in these cases there is an alteration of the blood flow that leads to endothelial damage as a consequence of shear stress and jet lesions. Damaged endothelium is the basis for micro thrombi formations, which, in turn, can be colonized by bacteria or fungi with the development of conglomerates that progressively grow due to bacterial multiplication and platelet and fibrin deposition. Some bacteria, particularly gram positive, can adhere to damaged endothelium with the mediation of proteins called adhesins. Platelet, fibrin, thrombus and colonizing bacteria grow to develop vegetations that are the "hallmark" of infective endocarditis [22, 23]. During this process, many microorganism (including staphylococci, streptococci and enterococci) produce biofilm, a polysaccharide slime-like matrix. Biofilm protects bacteria from the immunitary response and antibiotics [24, 25].

In native aortic valve endocarditis, vegetations are frequently found on the ventricular side of the valve. The extension of the infection beyond the aortic leaflets can lead to the formation of abscess (paravalvular cavity of a diameter of 1 cm or more), aorto-ventricular dehiscence, ventricular septal defect, fistula and extension to mitral or tricuspid valve.

In mechanical prostheses, the infective process initiates in the periannular site with frequent abscess formation while, in biologic valves, the process is mainly localized to the leaflets with rupture and perforation, but the annulus can be involved as well [26] (Figure 1).

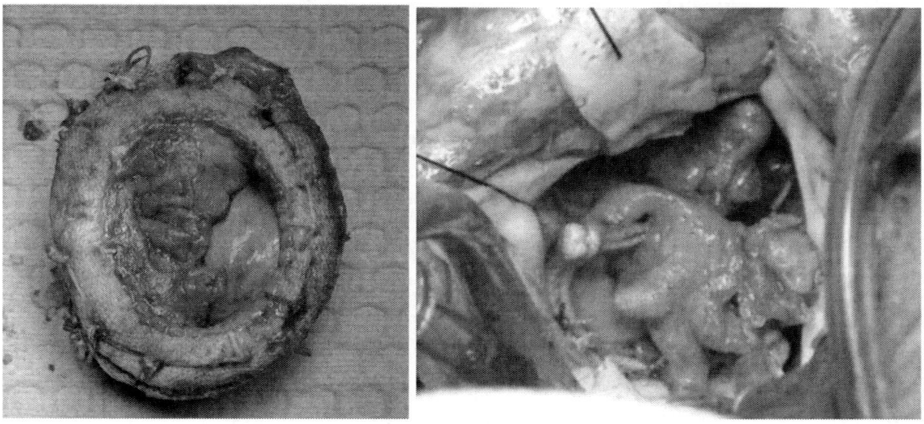

A B

Figure 1A and 1B. Large endocarditic vegetations on explanted (A) and in situ (B) biological valve prosthesis.

MICROBIOLOGY

Eighty-ninghty percent of IEs are caused by gram positive microorganism. Streptococci are a frequent cause of community acquired IEs; they cause subacute endocarditis, but, more recently and in compromised patients, can be clinically more aggressive. Enterococci are also frequent cause of IE and are more associated with health care related IE, but the most common cause of IE in developed country is Staphylococcus aureus that accounts for 30% of cases [16, 27] and causes an aggressive form, with high mortality and morbidity [28].

Coagulase negative staphylococci (CoNS) are frequent in PVE, but can also cause NVE [29] and are frequently methicillin resistant. 5-10% of IE are caused by gram negative bacteria of the HACECK group (Haemophilus, Actinobacillus, Cardiobacterium, Eikenella, Kingella) while fungi account for about 1% of cases.

The raise of antibiotic resistance in microorganisms responsible for IE has created more difficulty in their antibiotic management. Infection by methicillin resistant Staphylococcus aureus (MRSA) is now epidemic in many western countries and vancomycin resistance is also very frequent [30, 31].

The analysis of the Swedish register on infectious endocarditis (SRIE) published in 2019 [32] is one of the few publications that examines the data of the native endocarditis of the aortic valve separately from those of the mitral one. In this cohort, the major causative agent of endocarditis on the aortic valve is Streptococci alpha hemolytics, responsible for 33% of cases, followed by Staphylococcus aureus in 31%; enterococci are cause of 14% of aortic IEs. Mitral endocarditis have a different distribution with a greater and significant presence of staphylococcus aureus and a lower representation of enterococci. This difference is explained by the differences in pressure and calcification of the two valves with different strategies of aggression of the host tissue by Staphylococci and enterococci.

Symptoms

There are many variations in the modality of clinical presentation of IE: some patients rapidly develop sepsis (mainly in IE caused by Staphylococcus aureus) while others present nonspecific, subacute symptoms.

Cardiac symptoms are related to the valve incompetence or stenosis or both and to the disruption of left ventricular outflow tract. Patients may be asymptomatic or complaining asthenia and/or dyspnea, having more or less nuanced signs of decompensation up to frank decompensation and cardiogenic shock. Aortic valve endocarditis with annular extension can cause an atrioventricular block due to the disruption of conduction system [33].

Cerebral complications are the most severe extracardiac complications of IE, as well as the most frequent (occurring in 15 to 20% of patients) [34, 35]: macro or micro-emboli with ischemic or hemorrhagic strokes, transient ischemic attacks or asymptomatic embolisms or infection aneurysms. Emboli can also involve the lungs, spleen and the peripheral vessels [36].

Other symptoms occasionally occur as glomerulonephritis or rheumatic manifestations. Some of the "classic" systemic peripheral symptoms of IE, like Janeway lesions (hemorrhagic plaque on palm and soles) or Osler's node and splinter hemorrhage are now considered rare [16].

Diagnosis

Diagnosis of IE is difficult due to the high number of variations in clinical presentation with many nonspecific symptoms. It is based on the presence of clinical signs, microbiological findings and heart morphological examination (mainly performed with echocardiography).

Fever in patients with previous cardiac valve pathology and/or new or modified cardiac murmur can drive the diagnosis, same for the presence of vascular and immunological phenomena as emboli, Janeway lesion, Roth's spot, Osler nodes. Other generic non-specific clinical signs that occasionally occur are poor appetite and weight loss.

Blood cultures results represent an important point for the diagnosis of endocarditis. Culture tests should be multiple, at least 3, and taken before starting antibiotic therapy [37].

A relevant number IE have negative cultures: their rate range between 2 to 30% or more and are mainly related to assumption of antibiotic therapy before blood collection, but may also be consequence of infection caused by intracellular microorganism or fungi [21, 38, 39].

There are newer techniques that can allow causative diagnosis also when cultures are negative, as spectroscopy [40], serological test and the search for bacterial ribosomal RNA using the Polymerase Chain Reaction (PCR) [41].

In a recent literature review [42], it has been pointed out that sensitivity and specificity of PCR was 96% to 100%, greater than blood cultures, but the method is mainly applicable to valve tissue removed from patients who have undergone cardiac surgery.

Echocardiography is of paramount importance in IE diagnosis: the key finding for the echocardiography diagnosis of IE are vegetation, abscesses, and prostheses dehiscence. (Figures 2, 3)

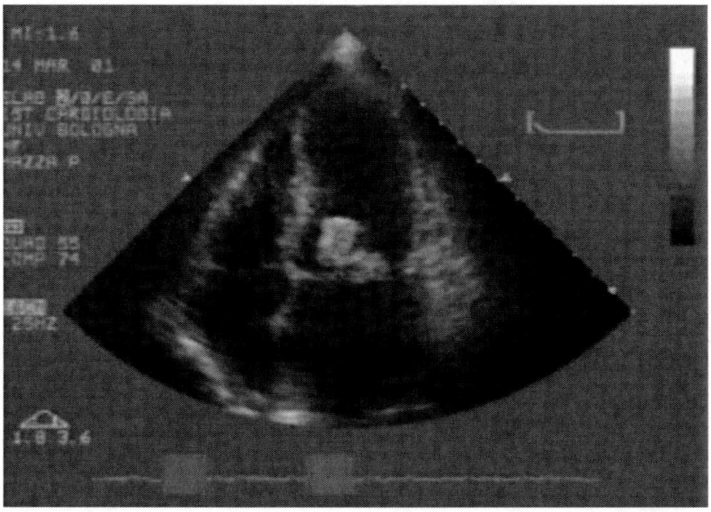

Figure 2. TEE shows a large aortic vegetation floating in left ventricle.

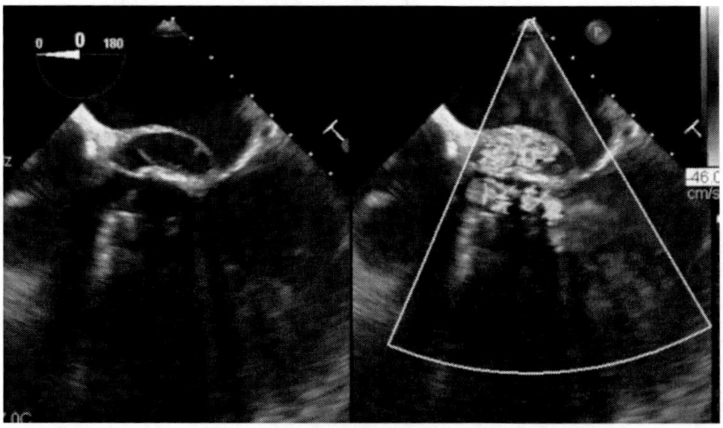

Figure 3. Aortic valve endocarditis with paravalvular psudoaneyrsm formation, transesophageal echocardiographic view.

The transthoracic echocardiography (TTE) is less invasive, but has low sensitivity, especially in the case of PVE for which the sensitivity is 40-70%. On the contrary, the transesophageal echocardiography (TEE) is more invasive and may require sedation or anesthesia, but has greater specificity in both NVE and PVE. TEE sensitivity and specificity in NVE vegetation's detection is respectively 90-100% and 100% and sensitivity of 77-90% in PVE diagnosis [43, 44].

The role of three-dimensional echocardiography is increasing. Its ability to reconstruct the volumes of irregular masses can be useful to evaluate the true dimensions of vegetations, perivalvular extension of the infection, prosthetic valve dehiscence, and valve perforation [45].

In uncertain cases, new diagnostic systems are emerging: computed tomography (CT) scans and combination of CT scan with metabolic imaging systems as 18-fluorodeoxyglucose positron emission tomography (18FDG-PET) or leukocyte scintigraphy (SPECT).

CT is useful in the study of anatomy, particularly in the paravalvular regions, in IE complication and in the cases of PVE when the artifacts caused by artificial valve can make echocardiography difficult [46, 47] (Figure 4).

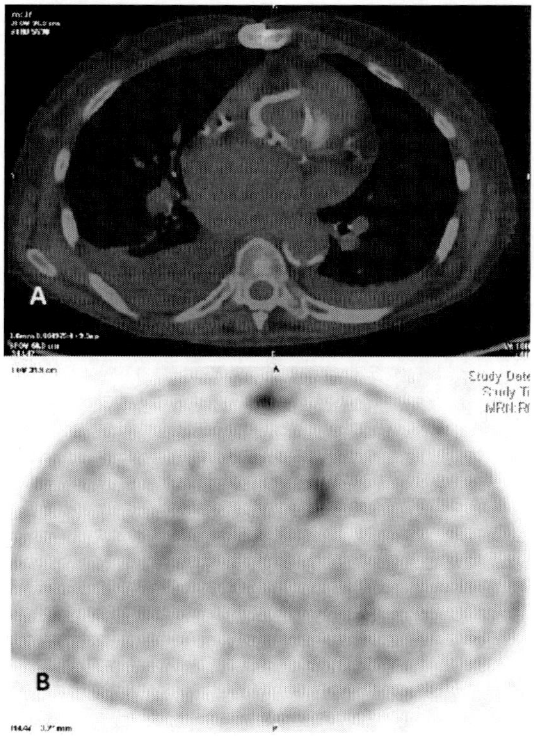

Figure 4. Transverse images from an 65-year-old woman with PVE: (A) integrated 18F-FDG-PET–CT; (B) 18F-FDG-PET–CT. High FDG uptake was observed at the level of the aortic prosthesis.

Metabolic tracers show areas of metabolic activity (PET) or inflammation (SPECT). In the cases of PVE, PET has a sensitivity and specificity of 70-80% and 80-90% respectively while for SPECT are reported values of 90% and 100%. [48-50]. Results are not good for the diagnosis of NVE: Ricciardi et al. examining 7 patients with suspected NVE found that 18F-

FDG-PET–CT failed to detect the infection in all cases [51]. Limits in the usefulness of metabolic imaging systems include the inability to discriminate between inflammation and infection, which leads to the risk of false positives in the first months after valve prostheses implantation, in the cases of post-pericardiotomy syndrome and prosthetic valve thrombosis.

Duke criteria are widely used as help for the diagnosis in the modified form to take into account the echocardiography morphological characteristics Duke algorithm, on the basis of a combination of major criteria (echocardiographic and microbiological) and minor criteria, grades the probability of having an endocarditis as defined, possible or rejected [52] (Table 1). Duke criteria has a sensitivity between 70 and 79% in IE diagnosis [53].

In a Spanish study [48] the integration of CT/PET data increased the sensitivity of Duke Criteria from 51% to 91% in cases of suspected PVE.

Table 1. Modified Duke criteria. Modified from Li JS et al.

Major Criteria	Blood colture positive		Typical micro-organisms consistent with IE from 2 separate blood cultures – S. aureus, S. viridans, S. bovis (gallolyticus), HACEK group, community acquired enterococci, in the absence of primary foci
		r	Persistently positive blood culture for organisms that are typical causes of IE: ≥2 positive blood cultures from blood samples drawn >12 hours apart
		r	For organisms that are more commonly skin contaminants: 3 or a majority of ≥4 separate blood cultures (with first and last drawn atleast 1 hour apart)
		r	Single positive blood culture for Coxiella burnetii or phase I IgG antibody titre >1:800
	Evidence of endocardial involvment	r	Positive echocardiogram (vegetation, abscess)
			New valvular regurgitation or dehiscence
Minor Criteria			Fever > 38°c
			Immunologic phenomena (glomerulonephritis, Osler's nodes, Roth's spots, Rheumatoid factor)
			Vascular phenomena (major arterial emboli, septic pulmonary infarcts, mycotic aneurysm, intracranial hemorrhage, conjuntival hemorrhage, Janeway lesions)
			Predisposition (preexistence of cardiac lesions or IV drug user)
			Positive blood culture but not meeting major criteria or serologic evidence of active infection with organism consistet with IE

TREATMENT

The treatment of patients with suspected or confirmed infective endocarditis should be provided by a multidisciplinary team with expertise in cardiology, cardiac surgery, and infectious disease. Successful treatment is dependent on eradication of the causative agent, which requires prolonged bactericidal antibiotic treatment. Guidelines indicate empiric and microorganism-specific antibiotic protocols [3, 54]. Because of the antibiotic resistance and tolerance and the drug's difficulty in penetrating vegetations and biofilm, treatment for IE should be prolonged for almost 4-6 weeks with endovcnous administration drugs in combination and at full dosage.

This entails an evident commitment of the health structures, with a significant impact on costs, also due to the need to keep the patient hospitalized.

For this reason, alternative antibiotic therapy modalities are being investigated, for example by switching to an oral antibiotic regimen after an initial phase of endovenous antibiotic therapy. A Danish multi center study [55] has recently used a mixed regimen of this sort with good results. The 400 patients examined had IE caused by Staphylococcus aureus, streptococci, enterococci, Staphylococci coagulase negative. However, patients with MRSA and those with cardiac abscesses and other infection sites were excluded.

Another promising field is that of long-acting lipoglycopeptide antibiotics such as dalbavancin and oritavancin which can be administered once a week [56].

SURGERY

Indication

Aggressive antibiotic therapy is essential to solve many cases of life-threatening endocarditis and is often able to eradicate the disease.

However, in many cases of ineffectiveness of medical therapy or complicated forms of IE, surgical therapy is required. The role of surgery for the treatment of bacterial endocarditis has gradually increased also thanks to the publication of encouraging surgery results. Indication for surgery are summarized in the periodically updated guidelines of American and European cardiology societies [3, 4] (Table 2).

A revision of reports about IE's surgical treatment (Imad M Tleyjeh et al. 2007) showed an increase in surgical cases of 7% per year from 1960 to 2000. Nonetheless, about 50% of patients with IE need surgery [57] and about 25% of patients with appropriate surgical indication according to current guidelines denied surgery [58].

The European cardiology society guidelines have indications relating to surgical timing [3]. Surgery is indicated on emergency bases (within 24 hours) in all cases complicated with refractory pulmonary edema or cardiogenic shock; urgent surgery (within few days) is indicated if there is evidence of poor hemodynamic tolerance; elective surgery when there aren't signs of cardiac decompensation.

Critical hemodynamic instability can be caused by acute aortic valve regurgitation or stenosis and fistula in cardiac chambers or pericardium. Since heart failure and cardiogenic shock are two of the strongest predictors of fatal outcome, early diagnosis and early surgery can be useful to lower the operative risk. Inability to control the infection despite optimal antibiotic therapy is indication of urgent treatment. Uncontrolled infection can have systemic expression as persistent fever o local expressions as increase volume of vegetation, development of pseudo aneurysms, fistula or perivalvular abscess. If the causative germ is difficult to eradicate, aggressive or with multiple antibiotic-resistances, surgery should be undertaken on elective or urgent basis.

Table 2. Indication to surgery

	2015 ESC Guidelines	Class	2014 AHA Guideline	Class
Heart failure	NVE o PVE causing refractory pulmonary oedema of cardiogenic shock	I	Valve dysfunction causing heart failure	I
	NVE o PVE causing symptoms of heart failure or ecochardiographic signs of poor haemodinamic tolerance	I		
Uncontrolled infection	Locally uncontrolled infection (abscess, false aneurysm, fistula, enlarging vegetation)	I	Hearth block or abscess	I
	Infection caused by fungi o multiresistant organisms	I	Resistant organysms	I
	Persisting positive blood cultures despite appropriate antibiotic therapy and adequate control of septic metastatic foci	IIa	Persistent infection/Relapsing infection	I
	PVE caused by staphylococci or non-HACEK gram-negative bacteria	IIa		
Prevention of embolysm	vegetations > 10 mm after one or more embolic episode despite appropriate antibiotic therapy	I	Recurrent emboli and persistent vegetation despite appropriate antibiotic therapy	Ia
	vegetations >10 mm, associated with severe valve stenosis or regurgitation, and low operative risk	IIa		
	isolated very large vegetations (>30 mm)	IIa		
	isolated large vegetations (>15 mm) and no other indication for surgery	IIb	Large mobile vegetation (native valve)	IIb

Embolic complications develop in 20 to 50% of the patients and are related to migration of vegetations [59, 60]. Vegetation's embolization can occur at any time, but seems to be more frequent during the initial weeks and before the beginning of the antibiotic therapy. There is a relation between vegetation's size and its mobility with risk of embolization [36].

Current guidelines indicate a class IIa recommendation for surgery in patients with vegetation > 10 mm when associated with severe valvular regurgitation or stenosis, but indicate that surgery in patients without valvular dysfunction and large vegetation (>15 mm) for the prevention of embolisms may be considered.

The concept of early surgery has gained popularity over time, also thanks to the improvement of surgical techniques and its good results. The topic was revived by the recent publication [61] of a prospective randomized study comparing early surgery versus conventional treatment in patients with left-sided IE. In this study, 37 patients underwent early surgery (within 48 hours after randomization) and 39 followed a conventional treatment timing. In the early surgery group, there was a reduced composite end point of death from any cause and embolic events, supported mainly by reduction in systemic embolisms.

There is no uniformity in the definition of "early surgery." Some define it as surgery performed in the "acute phase", during the course of antibiotic therapy, others as surgery within 7 days of diagnosis; others shift the timing to 10 days from diagnosis, others two weeks from diagnosis, while others define "early surgery" as surgery performed during the first hospitalization for IE [62-64].

Treatment in the acute phase with active or uncontrolled sepsis may lead to higher operative mortality and morbidity and risk of relapse [65] and the surgical operation could be more demanding due to the need to intervene on inflamed and infected tissue.

Although there are no prospectively randomized studies (excluding the one already mentioned, which however has several limitations), the advantages of early surgery have been highlighted by several observational studies, often enhanced by the propensity score technique [62-64]. Lalani et al. [64] studied the issue on a large multinational cohort of patients with definite IE. Effects of early surgery was assessed by propensity-based matching incorporating 25 clinically relevant covariates and 3 interaction terms. In subgroup analysis, surgery was found to confer a survival benefit compared with medical therapy among patients with a higher propensity for surgery (absolute risk reduction 10.9%) and those with paravalvular complications (17.3%), systemic embolization (12.9%), Staphylococcus aureus NVE (20.1%), and stroke (13%). Authors concluded that early surgery for NVE is associated with a significantly lower in-hospital mortality rate than medical therapy.

A recent meta-analisys analyzing 16 studies with 8141 patients [66] confirmed the connection between early surgery and better results in term of early and long-term results for NVE while the effectiveness of the "early surgery" approach in PVE was less clear.

While surgical therapy, especially early on, seems to give good results, there are cases in which it is believed that early intervention is impossible: patients with recent brain damage. In these cases, surgery can give a worsening of the neurological lesion with different mechanisms: heparinization, hypercoagulability and hypotension during extracorporeal circulation may contribute to further cerebral infarction into hamorrhagic or favor its extension.

This issue is particularly important because recently, using magnetic resonance imaging (MRI), it has been observed that there are many more patients with brain injuries than previously believed [34, 67] reaching up to 62%.

This group of patients has high mortality: in patients undergoing surgery with left side IE with pre-existing neurologic damage, mortality was 45% compared with 24% of those without [68, 69].

The STS guideline [3] suggests delaying operation for almost 4 weeks following neurologic damage.

However, in patients with complicated endocarditis, waiting 4 weeks may be impossible due to the presence of heart failure or other conditions that require urgent or emergency intervention. Furthermore, postponing the procedure exposes these patients to the risk of further cerebral embolic episodes.

Some studies have recently shown that surgery, even performed in the presence of ischemic brain damage, may not be as risky as expected [70-72].

In a retrospective study using magnetic resonance imaging as a tool to detect neurological damage, Yoshioka et al. [67] studied 64 patients with preoperative neurological damage. 34 were operated on within 14 days of neurological diagnosis (early group) and 30 after 14 days (late group). Worsening of the brain injury occurred in one patient from each group, while hemorrhagic transformation occurred only in one patient from the late group. The authors concluded that there are no benefits in delaying surgery beyond 14 days. However, the number and retrospective nature of the study do not allow generalizations.

A meta-analysis [68] including 27 studies found higher mortality in early surgery in the presence of ischemic or hemorrhagic brain damage (pooled relative risk 1.74, confidence interval 1.34-2.25) and a higher occurrence of worsening of the neurological damage. However, in the analysis of the subgroups, patients with ischemic stroke operated within 7 days did not worsen compared to those operated within 14 days; patients with hemorrhagic damage operated on within 21 days had an increase in mortality compared to those operated within the 28th day (pooled relative risk 1.77 vs 0.63) and a higher incidence of worsening of neurological damage (pooled relative risk 2.02 vs 0.44). The conclusion was that intervention in the presence of ischemic damage should be delayed by 7-14 days if possible and in the presence of hemorrhagic damage it should be delayed beyond 21 days.

It would be desirable, regarding this specific topic, to carry out randomized prospective studies that would allow a better definition of the optimal time for intervention while avoiding potential biases..

Techniques

Aims of IE surgery include: removal of all infected tissue and reconstruction of cardiac morphology and function.

In the achievement of these goals, we have to distinguish aortic valve IE in two principal groups:

- Infection limited to leaflet
- Infection extending beyond leaflet (or complex aortic valve endocarditis)

When only leaflets are involved, with both vegetation and perforation, the aortic valve surgery doesn't differ from the aortic valve replacement for non-infective aortic disease with valve replacement using mechanical or biological prostheses.

If abscess formations are detected upon removal of the cusps (or already known by means of preoperative diagnostic imaging), these must be debrided and the stitches, with pledgets, are placed to obliterate the cavity. When this is not possible due to extension of the disrupted tissue, an autologous or heterologous pericardium patch is sutured around the abscess cavity with the stitches passed on the healthy myocardial tissue and the aorta. The surface of the patch can be used as a hook for the sutures of the valve prosthesis.

Pericardial or Dacron patches are used also for the closure of structural defect in aorto-mitral continuity, left ventricle, atrium, mitral valve or ventricular septal defects.

When the infection extends beyond the annulus with paravalvular abscess formation and root destruction, the surgical treatment includes the resection of the infected tissue and reconstruction of the left ventricular outflow tract with coronary ostia reimplanted as buttons.

In these cases, use of cryopreserved homografts was historically considered as the gold standard [73]. Advantages in the homografts' use were the low recurrence of infection, good hemodynamic behavior with low gradient and low morbidity and mortality. The disadvantages were the demanding surgical techniques, the tendency to calcify and the limited availability [74, 75]. Recurrence of infection in the homograft has also been reported.

They were progressively substituted by stent less aortic valve, easier to implant and with similar characteristics [75-78]; furthermore stentless aortic valve are always available. They can be implanted in subcoronary position or be utilized for complete root replacement [79, 80].

Composite grafts using stented mechanical or biological valves were alternative to homograft and stentless valves.

Results

Early results of surgery for IE are inferior to elective non-infective valve surgery, ranging in recent series between 5 to 14%. Long term result are also inferior with a 10-year survival rate ranging between 40 to 60%. These results are partly due to patients' selection, as those operated frequently suffer from heart failure, uncontrolled infection, recurrent embolism, cardiac and systemic dysfunction and the potential presence of other infection's localization and persistence of microorganism in the biofilm complex.

Leontyev et coll. [81] retrospectively analyzed 172 patients operated for aortic valve IE with aortic root abscess at Herzzentrum, Universitat of Leipzig in Germany between 1996 and 2009. They had a 30 days mortality of 25% (35.5% in NVE vs 16.7% in NVE) and 1 and 5 years mortality were 55% and 50% respectively. Interestingly, they found a recurrence rate of 8.7% occurring mainly in the first 12-months following surgery.

In a recent single center report on 168 patients with aortic valve IE operated at Leuven University Hospital in Belgium between 2000 and 2013 [82] the operative mortality was 10.7%; there were no differences between treatment groups (stented graft, stented graft with patch, stentless valve, allograft and composite graft). During the 13-years follow up, there were other 47 deaths with survival at 10 years ranging from 55% to 75% in groups. Reinfection occurred in 23 patients and was significantly higher in patients treated with composite graft (33.3%) and lower in the patients treated with stentless valve (0%). Predictors of mortality were cardiogenic shock, septic shock, ejection fraction and concomitant mitral valve surgery while predictors of reinfection were mitral valve endocarditis and aortic root abscess.

The stented valves had an earlier re-infection peak compared to allographs in the group analyzed by Knosalla et coll. [83] while stentelss valve have a constant rate of reinfection without the initial risk increase [81, 82].

Prosthetic Valve Endocarditis

PVE accounts for 25% of the cases of IE and occurs in 1 to 6% of patients with valvular prostheses with high mortality rates ranging between 20 to 40% [84, 85].

PVE are traditionally divided in early and late on the basis of the interval between the valve implantation and the infection onset. Early PVE (within 12 months of the first surgery) accounts for the 43% of PVE while 57% has late PVE. The aortic valve is involved in 66.5% of cases [86].

This difference is important because the first form is directly linked to the surgical act and the perioperative period while the second has the same etiology as the NVE.

The time interval that defines the early from and late form is still object of debate to this day.

The guidelines indicate this time interval as 1 year [3, 4], but many reports indicate shorter intervals with almost 77% of cases occurring within 120 days. Lee et al. [87] found that the diagnosis of PVE occur in 46.4% in the first two months. The median time between surgery and infection ranged from 53 days and 129 days [88].

Moreover, after 120 days, a shift in causative microorganisms was observed: the most common agent causing early PVE is the Staphilocoloccus aureus (36%) and CoNS while late PVEs are more frequently caused by Enterococci and Streptococcus viridans. Staphylococcus aureus early PVE represent a subgroup with high risk of mortality and complication [89].

Some retrospective studies [90, 91] and a meta-analysis [92] have shown a greater risk of PVE for biological valves compared with mechanic ones, but this has not been confirmed in other studies.

In early PVE microorganisms invade prosthesis during valve replacement operation or via hamatogenic dissemination. In biological prostheses, PVE involves mainly leaflets with vegetation development and leaflet perforation. In mechanical prosthesis, the ring invasion is aided by the slow process of ring endothelization. From the ring, pathogens initially invade the perivalvular tissue causing abscess, pseudoaneurism, fistulas and valve dehiscence with extensive disruption [93, 94]. Periannular extension is present in 56-100% of PVE.

Symptoms of PVE don't differ from those of NVE and are frequently initially disregarded.

Diagnosis relies mainly on TEE while TTE is made difficult by artifacts caused by the prostheses.

Sensitivity of TEE in diagnosis of PVE ranges between 86% to 96% while TTE has a sensitivity of 17-36% [95]. CT/PET and CT-SPECT are useful in uncertain cases [46-49].

Antibiotic therapy is regarded as base treatment for PVE, but it frequently evolves into more complex forms requiring surgery.

Mortality decreased in recent years due the advancements in diagnostic and treatments, but still remains high. Surgery of PVE has high mortality 24-35% and frequently requires complex aortic root reconstruction.

In a large analysis involving 1313 patients operated on for IE at Deutsches Herzzentrum in Berlin [96], 349 were PVE (26,6%). The aortic valve prostheses endocarditis occurred in 215 cases (61.6%), 202 of which with abscess formation. The major causative agent was Staphilococcus aureus. The operative mortality within the whole group was of 28,4% and the 30-day, 1-, 5- and 10 year survival were 71,4 ± 2,4%, 58,7 ± 2,7%, 44,5 ± 3%, 31,7 ± 3,5%. Predictors of early mortality were: mechanical support, emergency operation, catecholamine support, mitral valve surgery and age. The main intervention performed on the aortic valve was aortic root replacement with homograft.

Habib et al. [97] identified the following mortality risk: severe heart failure, staphylococcal infection and PVE complications. Therefore, they suggested to aggressively treat patients with these three conditions. Luciani et al. [86] identified as mortality risk factors: female gender, shock status, surgical procedures within 3 months, multi valvular involvement and urgent surgery.

Moreover, many studies report high late mortality rate with 10 years survival of about 30% [96].

A new chapter in the field of prosthetic endocarditis has been opened with the spread of transcatheter valve implantation (TAVI) procedures: the incidence of endocarditis after TAVI is around 1% [19].

While some authors have indicated CoNS, Staphilococcus aureo, enterococci and streptococci as main causative agents [20], others have noted a higher incidence of bacteria normally present in the genitourinary and intestinal tract such as enterococci in trans femoral TAVI and a higher incidence of staphilococci in valve implanted using trans apical access [98]. In TAVI, the infection is mainly localized to the leaflet and less on the stent or the surrounding structures [19].

The majority of patients with TAVI IE are medically treated also if complications are present. In fact, rates of operative mortality within this subgroup of patients reaches 34% [99] as they had already been considered at high or very high operative risk when scheduled for TAVI.

Our Experience at the Lancisi Cardiovascular Center

We retrospectively analyzed the profile and outcome of surgically treated patients with aortic valve IE over a 4 years period, between January 2016 and December 2019.

One-hundred-seventeen endocarditis patients were operated upon. Of these, 76 (65%) patients (n = 53 men, median age 63 years) had aortic valve IE with 34 (44.7%) of them showing prosthetic endocarditis (PVE).

13 (17.1%) patients had mitral involvement and 2 (2.6%) tricuspid insufficiency requiring correction.

Periannular abscess was found in 21 (27.6%) patients and 9 (11.8%) of them developed pseudoaneurysms. Among patients with PVE, 24 (70.5%) had prostheses dehiscence.

Cultures were negatives in 42 (55.3%) patients. The most frequent causative microorganisms were streptococcus (15 patients), followed by staphylococci (11) and enterococci (6). Almost all patients underwent maximal antibiotic therapy immediately after the diagnosis of endocarditis was suspected and strict clinical followup with the cooperation of infective disease specialists and cardiologists. This likely justifies the high percentage of cases with negative cultures.

Emergency operation was performed in 11 (14.5%); 3 patients were in cardiogenic shock and 26 had severe cardiac failure at time of operation. Euroscore II was 7.2 (range 0.5 – 52).

Procedures performed included 58 aortic valve replacements (76.3%), 2 aortic root replacement with composite graft and 16 (21%) root replacement with stentless valved pericardial conduit implanted using a subannular suturing line (Biointegral) (Di Eusanio et al. 2019).

Associate procedures were mitral valve replacement or repair (n = 14), tricuspid valve repair (n = 2), pace-maker implantation (n = 9), abscess closure with pericardial or autologous patch (n = 6) and myocardial revascularization (n = 2).

Overall in-hospital mortality was 2.6% (n = 2): both patients had PVE and previous aortic root replacements. One had undergone aortic valve replacement with stented prostheses and root replacement with stentless valved conduit. The second patient was operated on in emergency due to cardiogenic shock and had a recent cerebral embolism. Both deaths occurred in the ICU, following multi-organ failure.

Despite its retrospective nature and the relatively limited number of patients taken into account, our case study shows that the mortality of patients with IE of the aortic valve can be significantly lowered with a combination of aggressive pre-operative antibiotic therapy, early surgery and by involving a diversified team of specialists in the handling of the patient.

Conclusion

Aortic valve IE is a complex disease with high mortality rate and its management presents many challenges.

Nowadays, there is an increasingly incidence of acute forms affecting elderly patients and with many comorbidities. The germs involved often exhibit antibiotic resistance and are more aggressive, also due to the emergence of health-care associated forms.

On the other hand, there are many fields in which innovations are being sought to improve treatments: new diagnostic techniques, new antibiotics and molecules to fight the biofilm and the shift toward early surgery.

New antibiotics could lead to better eradication of infections and new delivery strategies could incentivize hospitals let patients continue therapies at home. Molecules are tested to fight the biofilm. Surgical therapy, thanks to technical and anesthesiology improvements, moves towards early intervention in order to avoid the rise of complicated forms.

In any case, the various phases of the management of patients with endocarditis involve different medical professionals with diverse skills who must interface and cooperate in order to identify the best approach and timing for diagnosis and therapy.

The creation of multidisciplinary teams has been proposed in tertiary hospitals. Endocarditis teams should be trained by cardiologists, cardiac surgeons, infectious disease specialists and radiologists, pharmacologists and neurologists as needed. The team members should regularly meet in order to discuss their progress with endocarditis patients.

The implementation of these teams has been associated with a reduction in mortality [100, 101] and are strongly recommended in guidelines [4, 97].

References

[1] Cahill, Thomas J., and Bernard D. Prendergast. 2016. "Infective Endocarditis." *In The Lancet,* 387:882–93. Lancet Publishing Group. https://doi.org/10.1016/S0140-6736(15)00067-7.

[2] Osler, William. 1885. "The Gulstonian Lectures, on Malignant Endocarditis." *British Medical Journal* 1 (1264): 577–79. https://doi.org/10.1136/bmj.1.1264.577.

[3] Habib, Gilbert, Maria Grazia, Jean-paul Casalta France, Francesco Del, Gebrine El, Paola Anna, Bernard Iung France, et al. 2015. "2015 ESC Guidelines for the Management of Infective Endocarditis: The Task Force for the Management of

Infective Endocarditis of the European Society of Cardiology (ESC)." *European Heart Journal* 36 (1): 3075–3123. https://doi.org/10.1093/eurheartj/ehv319.

[4] Nishimura, Rick a, Catherine M Otto, Robert O Bonow, Blase a Carabello, John P Erwin, Robert a Guyton, Patrick T O'Gara, et al. 2014. "2014 AHA/ACC Guideline for the Management of Patients With Valvular Heart Disease: A Report of the American College of Cardiology/American Heart Association Task Force on Practice Guidelines." *Journal of the American College of Cardiology*, March. https://doi.org/10.1016/j.jacc.2014.02.536.

[5] Siniawski, Henryk, Onnen Grauhan, Michael Hofmann, Miralem Pasic, Yuguo Weng, Charles Yankah, Hans Lehmkuhl, and Roland Hetzer. 2005. "Aortic Root Abscess and Secondary Infective Mitral Valve Disease: Results of Surgical Endocarditis Treatment." *In European Journal of Cardio-Thoracic Surgery*, 27:434–40. https://doi.org/10.1016/j.ejcts.2004.12.001.

[6] Byrne, John G, Katayoun Rezai, Juan A Sanchez, Richard A Bernstein, Eric Okum, Marzia Leacche, Jorge M Balaguer, Shyam Prabhakaran, Charles R Bridges, and Robert S D Higgins. 2011. "Surgical Management of Endocarditis: The Society of Thoracic Surgeons Clinical Practice Guideline." *The Annals of Thoracic Surgery* 91 (6): 2012–19. https://doi.org/10.1016/j.athoracsur.2011.01.106.

[7] Hoen, Bruno, François Alla, Christine Selton-Suty, Isabelle Béguinot, Anne Bouvet, Serge Briançon, Jean Paul Casalta, et al. 2002. "Changing Profile of Infective Endocarditis: Results of a 1-Year Survey in France." *Journal of the American Medical Association* 288 (1): 75–81. https://doi.org/10.1001/jama.288.1.75.

[8] Berlin, J A, E Abrutyn, B L Strom, J L Kinman, M E Levison, O M Korzeniowski, R S Feldman, and D Kaye. 1995. "Incidence of Infective Endocarditis in the Delaware Valley, 1988-1990." *The American Journal of Cardiology* 76 (12): 933–36. https://doi.org/10.1016/s0002-9149(99)80264-1.

[9] Hogevik, Harriet, Lars Olaison, Rune Andersson, Johan Lindberg, and Kjell Alestig. 1995. "Epidemiologic Aspects of Infective Endocarditis in an Urban Population: A 5-Year Prospective Study." *Medicine* (United States) 74 (6): 324–39. https://doi.org/10.1097/00005792-199511000-00003.

[10] Sandoe, J. A. T., R. W. Watkin, T. S.J. Elliott, and M. J. Dayer. 2017. "Infective Endocarditis in the Adult Patient." Medicine (United Kingdom). Elsevier Ltd. https://doi.org/10.1016/j.mpmed.2017.08.004.

[11] Bustamante-Munguira, Juan, Carlos-A Mestres, Pablo Alvarez, Angels Figuerola-Tejerina, Rocio Eiros Bachiller, Esther Gómez-Sánchez, Francisco Javier Alvarez, Salvador Resino, Javier Castrodeza, and Eduardo Tamayo. 2018. "Surgery for Acute Infective Endocarditis: Epidemiological Data from a Spanish Nationwide Hospital-Based Registry." *Interactive Cardiovascular and Thoracic Surgery* 27 (4): 498–504. https://doi.org/10.1093/icvts/ivy127.

[12] Erichsen, Purnima, Gunnar H Gislason, and Niels Eske Bruun. 2016. "The Increasing Incidence of Infective Endocarditis in Denmark, 1994-2011." *European Journal of Internal Medicine* 35 (November): 95–99. https://doi.org/10.1016/j.ejim.2016.05.021.

[13] Cresti, Alberto, Mario Chiavarelli, Marco Scalese, Cesira Nencioni, Silvia Valentini, Francesco Guerrini, Incoronata D'Aiello, Andrea Picchi, Francesco De Sensi, and Gilbert Habib. 2017. "Epidemiological and Mortality Trends in Infective Endocarditis,

a 17-Year Population-Based Prospective Study." *Cardiovascular Diagnosis and Therapy* 7 (1): 27–35. https://doi.org/10.21037/cdt.2016.08.09.

[14] Slipczuk, Leandro, J Nicolas Codolosa, Carlos D Davila, Abel Romero-Corral, Jeong Yun, Gregg S Pressman, and Vincent M Figueredo. 2013. "Infective Endocarditis Epidemiology over Five Decades: A Systematic Review." *PloS One* 8 (12): e82665. https://doi.org/10.1371/journal.pone.0082665.

[15] Dayer, Mark J, Simon Jones, Bernard Prendergast, Larry M Baddour, Peter B Lockhart, and Martin H Thornhill. 2015. "Incidence of Infective Endocarditis in England, 2000-13: A Secular Trend, Interrupted Time-Series Analysis." *Lancet* (London, England) 385 (9974): 1219–28. https://doi.org/10.1016/S0140-6736(14)62007-9.

[16] Murdoch, David R., Ralph G. Corey, Bruno Hoen, M. Miró, Vance G. Fowler, Arnold S. Bayer, Adolf W. Karchmer, et al. 2009. "Clinical Presentation, Etiology, and Outcome of Infective Endocarditis in the 21st Century The International Collaboration on Endocarditis-Prospective Cohort Study." *Archives of Internal Medicine* 169 (5): 463–73. https://doi.org/10.1001/archinternmed.2008.603.

[17] Olmos, Carmen, Isidre Vilacosta, Cristina Fernández, Cristina Sarriá, Javier López, María Del Trigo, Carlos Ferrera, et al. 2014. "Comparison of Clinical Features of Left-Sided Infective Endocarditis Involving Previously Normal Versus Previously Abnormal Valves." *American Journal of Cardiology* 114 (2): 278–83. https://doi.org/10.1016/j.amjcard.2014.04.036.

[18] Ilhão Moreira, Rita, Madalena Coutinho Cruz, Luísa Moura Branco, Ana Galrinho, Luís Coutinho Miranda, José Fragata, and Rui Cruz Ferreira. 2018. "Infective Endocarditis: Surgical Management and Prognostic Predictors." *Revista Portuguesa de Cardiologia* 37 (5): 387–94. https://doi.org/10.1016/j.repc.2017.08.007.

[19] Amat-Santos, Ignacio J, Henrique B Ribeiro, Marina Urena, Ricardo Allende, Christine Houde, Elisabeth Bédard, Jean Perron, et al. 2015. "Prosthetic Valve Endocarditis after Transcatheter Valve Replacement: A Systematic Review." *JACC. Cardiovascular Interventions* 8 (2): 334–46. https://doi.org/10.1016/j.jcin.2014.09.013.

[20] Regueiro, Ander, Axel Linke, Azeem Latib, Nikolaj Ihlemann, Marina Urena, Thomas Walther, Oliver Husser, et al. 2016. "Association between Transcatheter Aortic Valve Replacement and Subsequent Infective Endocarditis and In-Hospital Death." *JAMA - Journal of the American Medical Association* 316 (10): 1083–92. https://doi.org/10.1001/jama.2016.12347.

[21] Lamas, C C, and S J Eykyn. 2000. "Bicuspid Aortic Valve--A Silent Danger: Analysis of 50 Cases of Infective Endocarditis." Clinical Infectious Diseases : *An Official Publication of the Infectious Diseases Society of America* 30 (2): 336–41. https://doi.org/10.1086/313646.

[22] Patti, J M, B L Allen, M J McGavin, and M Hook. 1994. "MSCRAMM-Mediated Adherence of Microorganisms to Host Tissues." *Annual Review of Microbiology* 48 (1): 585–617. https://doi.org/10.1146/annurev.mi.48.100194.003101.

[23] Werdan, Karl, Sebastian Dietz, Bettina Löffler, Silke Niemann, Hasan Bushnaq, Rolf Edgar Silber, Georg Peters, and Ursula Müller-Werdan. 2014. "Mechanisms of Infective Endocarditis: Pathogen-Host Interaction and Risk States." *Nature Reviews Cardiology*. https://doi.org/10.1038/nrcardio.2013.174.

[24] Elgharably, Haytham, Syed T Hussain, Nabin K Shrestha, Eugene H Blackstone, and Gösta B Pettersson. 2016. "Current Hypotheses in Cardiac Surgery: Biofilm in Infective Endocarditis." *Seminars in Thoracic and Cardiovascular Surgery* 28 (1): 56–59. https://doi.org/10.1053/j.semtcvs.2015.12.005.

[25] Chung, Pooi Y, and Yien S Toh. 2014. "Anti-Biofilm Agents: Recent Breakthrough against Multi-Drug Resistant Staphylococcus Aureus." *Pathogens and Disease* 70 (3): 231–39. https://doi.org/10.1111/2049-632X.12141.

[26] Habib, Gilbert, Franck Thuny, and Jean François Avierinos. 2008. "Prosthetic Valve Endocarditis: Current Approach and Therapeutic Options." *Progress in Cardiovascular Diseases* 50 (4): 274–81. https://doi.org/10.1016/j.pcad.2007.10.007.

[27] Selton-Suty, Christine, Marie Célard, Vincent Le Moing, Thanh Doco-Lecompte, Catherine Chirouze, Bernard Iung, Christophe Strady, et al. 2012. "Preeminence of Staphylococcus Aureus in Infective Endocarditis: A 1-Year Population-Based Survey." Clinical Infectious Diseases : *An Official Publication of the Infectious Diseases Society of America* 54 (9): 1230–39. https://doi.org/10.1093/cid/cis199.

[28] Fowler, Vance G., Jose M. Miro, Bruno Hoen, Christopher H. Cabell, Elias Abrutyn, Ethan Rubinstein, G. Ralph Corey, et al. 2005. "Staphylococcus Aureus Endocarditis: A Consequence of Medical Progress." *Journal of the American Medical Association* 293 (24): 3012–21. https://doi.org/10.1001/jama.293.24.3012.

[29] DeSimone, Daniel C., Imad M. Tleyjeh, Daniel D. Correa De Sa, Nandan S. Anavekar, Brian D. Lahr, Muhammad R. Sohail, James M. Steckelberg, Walter R. Wilson, and Larry M. Baddour. 2012. "Incidence of Infective Endocarditis Caused by Viridans Group Streptococci before and after Publication of the 2007 American Heart Association's Endocarditis Prevention Guidelines." *Circulation* 126 (1): 60–64. https://doi.org/10.1161/CIRCULATIONAHA.112.095281.

[30] Cuevas, Oscar, Emilia Cercenado, Ana Vindel, Jesús Guinea, Matilde Sánchez-Conde, Mar Sánchez-Somolinos, and Emilio Bouza. 2004. "Evolution of the Antimicrobial Resistance of Staphylococcus Spp. in Spain: Five Nationwide Prevalence Studies, 1986 to 2002." *Antimicrobial Agents and Chemotherapy* 48 (11): 4240–45. https://doi.org/10.1128/AAC.48.11.4240-4245.2004.

[31] Smith, T L, M L Pearson, K R Wilcox, C Cruz, M V Lancaster, B Robinson-Dunn, F C Tenover, et al. 1999. "Emergence of Vancomycin Resistance in Staphylococcus Aureus. Glycopeptide-Intermediate Staphylococcus Aureus Working Group." *The New England Journal of Medicine* 340 (7): 493–501. https://doi.org/10.1056/NEJM199902183400701.

[32] Vlasselaer, Abel Van, Magnus Rasmussen, Johan Nilsson, Lars Olaison, and Sigurdur Ragnarsson. 2019. "Native Aortic versus Mitral Valve Infective Endocarditis: A Nationwide Registry Study." *Open Heart* 6 (1): e000926. https://doi.org/10.1136/openhrt-2018-000926.

[33] DiNubile, Mark J., Stephen B. Calderwood, David M. Steinhaus, and Adolph W. Karchmer. 1986. "Cardiac Conduction Abnormalities Complicating Native Valve Active Infective Endocarditis." *The American Journal of Cardiology* 58 (13): 1213–17. https://doi.org/10.1016/0002-9149(86)90384-X.

[34] Snygg-Martin, Ulrika, Lars Gustafsson, Lars Rosengren, Asa Alsiö, Per Ackerholm, Rune Andersson, and Lars Olaison. 2008. "Cerebrovascular Complications in Patients with Left-Sided Infective Endocarditis Are Common: A Prospective Study Using

Magnetic Resonance Imaging and Neurochemical Brain Damage Markers." Clinical Infectious Diseases : *An Official Publication of the Infectious Diseases Society of America* 47 (1): 23–30. https://doi.org/10.1086/588663.

[35] Heiro, Maija, Jukka Nikoskelainen, Erik Engblom, Esa Kotilainen, Reijo Marttila, and Pirkko Kotilainen. 2000. "Neurologic Manifestations of Infective Endocarditis: A 17-Year Experience in a Teaching Hospital in Finland." *Archives of Internal Medicine* 160 (18): 2781–87. https://doi.org/10.1001/archinte.160.18.2781.

[36] Thuny, Franck, Giovanni Disalvo, Olivier Belliard, Jean François Avierinos, Valeria Pergola, Valerie Rosenberg, Jean Paul Casalta, et al. 2005. "Risk of Embolism and Death in Infective Endocarditis: Prognostic Value of Echocardiography - A Prospective Multicenter Study." *Circulation* 112 (1): 69–75. https://doi.org/10.1161/CIRCULATIONAHA.104.493155.

[37] Lee, Andrew, Stanley Mirrett, L Barth Reller, and Melvin P Weinstein. 2007. "Detection of Bloodstream Infections in Adults: How Many Blood Cultures Are Needed?" *Journal of Clinical Microbiology* 45 (11): 3546–48. https://doi.org/10.1128/JCM.01555-07.

[38] Brouqui, P., and D. Raoult. 2001. "Endocarditis Due to Rare and Fastidious Bacteria." *Clinical Microbiology Reviews*. https://doi.org/10.1128/CMR.14.1.177-207.2001.

[39] Fournier, Pierre-Edouard, Franck Thuny, Hervé Richet, Hubert Lepidi, Jean-Paul Casalta, Jean-Pierre Arzouni, Max Maurin, et al. 2010. "Comprehensive Diagnostic Strategy for Blood Culture-Negative Endocarditis: A Prospective Study of 819 New Cases." Clinical Infectious Diseases : *An Official Publication of the Infectious Diseases Society of America* 51 (2): 131–40. https://doi.org/10.1086/653675.

[40] Seng, Piseth, Michel Drancourt, Frédérique Gouriet, Bernard La Scola, Pierre-Edouard Fournier, Jean Marc Rolain, and Didier Raoult. 2009. "Ongoing Revolution in Bacteriology: Routine Identification of Bacteria by Matrix-Assisted Laser Desorption Ionization Time-of-Flight Mass Spectrometry." *Clinical Infectious Diseases : An Official Publication of the Infectious Diseases Society of America* 49 (4): 543–51. https://doi.org/10.1086/600885.

[41] Shrestha, Nabin K., Christopher S. Ledtke, Hannah Wang, Thomas G. Fraser, Susan J. Rehm, Syed T. Hussain, Gosta B. Pettersson, Eugene H. Blackstone, and Steven M. Gordon. 2015. "Heart Valve Culture and Sequencing to Identify the Infective Endocarditis Pathogen in Surgically Treated Patients." *Annals of Thoracic Surgery* 99 (1): 33–37. https://doi.org/10.1016/j.athoracsur.2014.07.028.

[42] Faraji, Reza, Mostafa Behjati-Ardakani, Seyed Mohammad Moshtaghioun, Seyed Mehdi Kalantar, Seyedeh Mahdieh Namayandeh, Mohammadhossien Soltani, Mahmood Emami, et al. 2018. "The Diagnosis of Microorganism Involved in Infective Endocarditis (IE) by Polymerase Chain Reaction (PCR) and Real-Time PCR: A Systematic Review." *Kaohsiung Journal of Medical Sciences*. Elsevier (Singapore) Pte Ltd. https://doi.org/10.1016/j.kjms.2017.09.011.

[43] Habib, Gilbert, Luigi Badano, Christophe Tribouilloy, Isidre Vilacosta, Jose Luis Zamorano, Maurizio Galderisi, Jens-Uwe Voigt, et al. 2010. "Recommendations for the Practice of Echocardiography in Infective Endocarditis." *European Journal of Echocardiography : The Journal of the Working Group on Echocardiography of the European Society of Cardiology* 11 (2): 202–19. https://doi.org/10.1093/ejechocard/jeq004.

[44] Evangelista, A., and M. T. González-Alujas. 2004. "Echocardiography in Infective Endocarditis." In *Heart*, 90:614–17. https://doi.org/10.1136/hrt.2003.029868.

[45] Sordelli, Chiara, Nunzia Fele, Rosa Mocerino, Sara Weisz, Luigi Ascione, Pio Caso, Antonio Carrozza, Carlo Tascini, Stefano De Vivo, and Sergio Severino. 2019. "Infective Endocarditis: Echocardiographic Imaging and New Imaging Modalities." *Journal of Cardiovascular Echography*. Wolters Kluwer Medknow Publications. https://doi.org/10.4103/jcecho.jcecho_53_19.

[46] Fagman, Erika, Sossio Perrotta, Odd Bech-Hanssen, Agneta Flinck, Carl Lamm, Lars Olaison, and Gunnar Svensson. 2012. "ECG-Gated Computed Tomography: A New Role for Patients with Suspected Aortic Prosthetic Valve Endocarditis." *European Radiology* 22 (11): 2407–14. https://doi.org/10.1007/s00330-012-2491-5.

[47] Habets, Jesse, Wilco Tanis, Lex A van Herwerden, Renee B A van den Brink, Willem P Th M Mali, Bas A J M de Mol, Steven A J Chamuleau, and Ricardo P J Budde. 2014. "Cardiac Computed Tomography Angiography Results in Diagnostic and Therapeutic Change in Prosthetic Heart Valve Endocarditis." *The International Journal of Cardiovascular Imaging* 30 (2): 377–87. https://doi.org/10.1007/s10554-013-0335-2.

[48] Pizzi, Mariá N., Albert Roque, Nuria Fernández-Hidalgo, Hug Cuéllar-Calabria, Ignacio Ferreira-González, Mariá T. Gonzàlez-Alujas, Gerard Oristrell, et al. 2015. "Improving the Diagnosis of Infective Endocarditis in Prosthetic Valves and Intracardiac Devices with 18F-Fluordeoxyglucose Positron Emission Tomography/Computed Tomography Angiography: Initial Results at an Infective Endocarditis Referral Center." *Circulation* 132 (12): 1113–26. https://doi.org/10.1161/CIRCULATIONAHA.115.015316.

[49] Erba, Paola A, Umberto Conti, Elena Lazzeri, Martina Sollini, Roberta Doria, Salvatore M De Tommasi, Francesco Bandera, et al. 2012. "Added Value of 99mTc-HMPAO-Labeled Leukocyte SPECT/CT in the Characterization and Management of Patients with Infectious Endocarditis." *Journal of Nuclear Medicine : Official Publication, Society of Nuclear Medicine* 53 (8): 1235–43. https://doi.org/10.2967/jnumed.111.099424.

[50] Bartoletti, Michele, Fabio Tumietto, Giovanni Fasulo, Maddalena Giannella, Francesco Cristini, Rachele Bonfiglioli, Luigi Raumer, et al. 2014. "Combined Computed Tomography and Fluorodeoxyglucose Positron Emission Tomography in the Diagnosis of Prosthetic Valve Endocarditis: A Case Series." *BMC Research Notes* 7 (1). https://doi.org/10.1186/1756-0500-7-32.

[51] Ricciardi, Alessandra, Pasquale Sordillo, Laura Ceccarelli, Gaetano Maffongelli, Giorgio Calisti, Barbara Di Pietro, Cristiana Ragano Caracciolo, et al. 2014. "18-Fluoro-2-Deoxyglucose Positron Emission Tomography-Computed Tomography: An Additional Tool in the Diagnosis of Prosthetic Valve Endocarditis." *International Journal of Infectious Diseases* 28 (November): 219–24. https://doi.org/10.1016/j.ijid.2014.04.028.

[52] Li, J. S., D. J. Sexton, N. Mick, R. Nettles, V. G. Fowler, T. Ryan, T. Bashore, and G. R. Corey. 2000. "Proposed Modifications to the Duke Criteria for the Diagnosis of Infective Endocarditis." *Clinical Infectious Diseases* 30 (4): 633–38. https://doi.org/10.1086/313753.

[53] Shrestha, Nabin, Sampurna Shakya, Syed Hussain, Gosta Pettersson, Brian Griffin, and Steven Gordon. 2017. "Sensitivity and Specificity of Duke Criteria for Diagnosis of Definite Infective Endocarditis: A Cohort Study." *Open Forum Infectious Diseases* 4 (suppl_1): S550–51. https://doi.org/10.1093/ofid/ofx163.1431.

[54] Baddour, Larry M., Walter R. Wilson, Arnold S. Bayer, Vance G. Fowler, Imad M. Tleyjeh, Michael J. Rybak, Bruno Barsic, et al. 2015. "Infective Endocarditis in Adults: Diagnosis, Antimicrobial Therapy, and Management of Complications: A Scientific Statement for Healthcare Professionals from the American Heart Association." *Circulation.* Lippincott Williams and Wilkins. https://doi.org/10.1161/CIR.0000000000000296.

[55] Iversen, Kasper, Nikolaj Ihlemann, Sabine U. Gill, Trine Madsen, Hanne Elming, Kaare T. Jensen, Niels E. Bruun, et al. 2019. "Partial Oral versus Intravenous Antibiotic Treatment of Endocarditis." *New England Journal of Medicine* 380 (5): 415–24. https://doi.org/10.1056/NEJMoa1808312.

[56] Tobudic, Selma, Christina Forstner, Heinz Burgmann, Heimo Lagler, Michael Ramharter, Christoph Steininger, Matthias G Vossen, Stefan Winkler, and Florian Thalhammer. 2018. "Dalbavancin as Primary and Sequential Treatment for Gram-Positive Infective Endocarditis: 2-Year Experience at the General Hospital of Vienna." *Clinical Infectious Diseases : An Official Publication of the Infectious Diseases Society of America* 67 (5): 795–98. https://doi.org/10.1093/cid/ciy279.

[57] Chu, Vivian H., Lawrence P. Park, Eugene Athan, Francois Delahaye, Tomas Freiberger, Cristiane Lamas, Jose M. Miro, et al. 2015. "Association between Surgical Indications, Operative Risk, and Clinical Outcome in Infective Endocarditis a Prospective Study from the International Collaboration on Endocarditis." *Circulation* 131 (2): 131–40. https://doi.org/10.1161/CIRCULATIONAHA.114.012461.

[58] Iung, Bernard, Thanh Doco-Lecompte, Sidney Chocron, Christophe Strady, François Delahaye, Vincent Le Moing, Claire Poyart, et al. 2016. "Cardiac Surgery during the Acute Phase of Infective Endocarditis: Discrepancies between European Society of Cardiology Guidelines and Practices." *European Heart Journal* 37 (10): 840–48. https://doi.org/10.1093/eurheartj/ehv650.

[59] Vilacosta, Isidre, Catherine Graupner, JoséAlberto SanRomán, Cristina Sarriá, Ricardo Ronderos, Cristina Fernández, Leonardo Mancini, Olga Sanz, Juan Victor Sanmartín, and Walter Stoermann. 2002. "Risk of Embolization after Institution of Antibiotic Therapy for Infective Endocarditis." *Journal of the American College of Cardiology* 39 (9): 1489–95. https://doi.org/10.1016/S0735-1097(02)01790-4.

[60] Steckelberg, J M, J G Murphy, D Ballard, K Bailey, A J Tajik, C P Taliercio, E R Giuliani, and W R Wilson. 1991. "Emboli in Infective Endocarditis: The Prognostic Value of Echocardiography." *Annals of Internal Medicine* 114 (8): 635–40. https://doi.org/10.7326/0003-4819-114-8-635.

[61] Kang, Duk Hyun, Yong Jin Kim, Sung Han Kim, Byung Joo Sun, Dae Hee Kim, Sung Cheol Yun, Jong Min Song, et al. 2012. "Early Surgery versus Conventional Treatment for Infective Endocarditis." *New England Journal of Medicine* 366 (26): 2466–73. https://doi.org/10.1056/NEJMoa1112843.

[62] Revilla, Ana, Javier López, Isidre Vilacosta, Eduardo Villacorta, María J Rollán, José R Echevarría, Yolanda Carrascal, et al. 2007. "Clinical and Prognostic Profile of Patients with Infective Endocarditis Who Need Urgent Surgery." *European Heart Journal* 28 (1): 65–71. https://doi.org/10.1093/eurheartj/ehl315.

[63] Tleyjeh, I M, J M Steckelberg, G Georgescu, H M K Ghomrawi, T L Hoskin, F B Enders, F Mookadam, W C Huskins, W R Wilson, and L M Baddour. 2008. "The Association between the Timing of Valve Surgery and 6-Month Mortality in Left-Sided Infective Endocarditis." *Heart* (British Cardiac Society) 94 (7): 892–96. https://doi.org/10.1136/hrt.2007.118968.

[64] Lalani, Tahaniyat, Christopher H Cabell, Daniel K Benjamin, Ovidiu Lasca, Christoph Naber, Vance G Fowler, G Ralph Corey, et al. 2010. "Analysis of the Impact of Early Surgery on In-Hospital Mortality of Native Valve Endocarditis: Use of Propensity Score and Instrumental Variable Methods to Adjust for Treatment-Selection Bias." *Circulation* 121 (8): 1005–13. https://doi.org/10.1161/CIRCULATIONAHA.109.864488.

[65] Thuny, Franck, Sylvain Beurtheret, Julien Mancini, Vlad Gariboldi, Jean-Paul Casalta, Alberto Riberi, Roch Giorgi, et al. 2011. "The Timing of Surgery Influences Mortality and Morbidity in Adults with Severe Complicated Infective Endocarditis: A Propensity Analysis." *European Heart Journal* 32 (16): 2027–33. https://doi.org/10.1093/eurheartj/ehp089.

[66] Liang, Fuxiang, Bing Song, Ruisheng Liu, Liu Yang, Hanbo Tang, and Yuanming Li. 2016. "Optimal Timing for Early Surgery in Infective Endocarditis: A Meta-Analysis." Interactive *Cardiovascular and Thoracic Surgery* 22 (3): 336–45. https://doi.org/10.1093/icvts/ivv368.

[67] Yoshioka, Daisuke, Taichi Sakaguchi, Takashi Yamauchi, Shuhei Okazaki, Shigeru Miyagawa, Hiroyuki Nishi, Yasushi Yoshikawa, Satsuki Fukushima, Shunsuke Saito, and Yoshiki Sawa. 2012. "Impact of Early Surgical Treatment on Postoperative Neurologic Outcome for Active Infective Endocarditis Complicated by Cerebral Infarction." *The Annals of Thoracic Surgery* 94 (2): 489–95; discussion 496. https://doi.org/10.1016/j.athoracsur.2012.04.027.

[68] Tam, Derrick Y., Bobby Yanagawa, Subodh Verma, Marc Ruel, Stephen E. Fremes, Amine Mazine, Seana Adams, and Jan O. Friedrich. 2018. "Early vs Late Surgery for Patients With Endocarditis and Neurological Injury: A Systematic Review and Meta-Analysis." *Canadian Journal of Cardiology*. Elsevier Inc. https://doi.org/10.1016/j.cjca.2018.05.010.

[69] García-Cabrera, Emilio, Nuria Fernández-Hidalgo, Benito Almirante, Radka Ivanova-Georgieva, Mariam Noureddine, Antonio Plata, Jose M Lomas, et al. 2013. "Neurological Complications of Infective Endocarditis: Risk Factors, Outcome, and Impact of Cardiac Surgery: A Multicenter Observational Study." *Circulation* 127 (23): 2272–84. https://doi.org/10.1161/CIRCULATIONAHA.112.000813.

[70] Piper, C., M. Wiemer, H. D. Schulte, and D. Horstkotte. 2001. "Stroke Is Not a Contraindication for Urgent Valve Replacement in Acute Infective Endocarditis." *Journal of Heart Valve Disease* 10 (6): 703–11.

[71] Ruttmann, Elfriede, Johann Willeit, Hanno Ulmer, Orest Chevtchik, Daniel Höfer, Werner Poewe, Günther Laufer, and Ludwig C Müller. 2006. "Neurological Outcome

of Septic Cardioembolic Stroke after Infective Endocarditis." *Stroke* 37 (8): 2094–99. https://doi.org/10.1161/01.STR.0000229894.28591.3f.

[72] Barsic, Bruno, Stuart Dickerman, Vladimir Krajinovic, Paul Pappas, Javier Altclas, Giampiero Carosi, José H Casabé, et al. 2013. "Influence of the Timing of Cardiac Surgery on the Outcome of Patients with Infective Endocarditis and Stroke." *Clinical Infectious Diseases : An Official Publication of the Infectious Diseases Society of America* 56 (2): 209–17. https://doi.org/10.1093/cid/cis878.

[73] Sabik, Joseph F., Bruce W. Lytle, Eugene H. Blackstone, Antonino G.M. Marullo, Gosta B. Pettersson, and Delos M. Cosgrove. 2002. "Aortic Root Replacement with Cryopreserved Allograft for Prosthetic Valve Endocarditis." *Annals of Thoracic Surgery* 74 (3): 650–59. https://doi.org/10.1016/S0003-4975(02)03779-7.

[74] Savage, Edward B, Paramita Saha-Chaudhuri, Craig R Asher, J Matthew Brennan, and James S Gammie. 2014. "Outcomes and Prosthesis Choice for Active Aortic Valve Infective Endocarditis: Analysis of the Society of Thoracic Surgeons Adult Cardiac Surgery Database." *The Annals of Thoracic Surgery* 98 (3): 806–14. https://doi.org/10.1016/j.athoracsur.2014.05.010.

[75] Schneider, Adriaan W, Mark G Hazekamp, Michel I M Versteegh, Eline F Bruggemans, Eduard R Holman, Robert J M Klautz, and Jerry Braun. 2016. "Stentless Bioprostheses: A Versatile and Durable Solution in Extensive Aortic Valve Endocarditis." *European Journal of Cardio-Thoracic Surgery : Official Journal of the European Association for Cardio-Thoracic Surgery* 49 (6): 1699–1704. https://doi.org/10.1093/ejcts/ezv463.

[76] Perrotta, Sossio, and Salvatore Lentini. 2010. "In Patients with Severe Active Aortic Valve Endocarditis, Is a Stentless Valve as Good as the Homograft?" *Interactive Cardiovascular and Thoracic Surgery* 11 (3): 309–13. https://doi.org/10.1510/icvts.2010.234831.

[77] Heinz, Anneliese, Julia Dumfarth, Elfriede Ruttmann-Ulmer, Michael Grimm, and Ludwig C Müller. 2014. "Freestyle Root Replacement for Complex Destructive Aortic Valve Endocarditis." *The Journal of Thoracic and Cardiovascular Surgery* 147 (4): 1265–70. https://doi.org/10.1016/j.jtcvs.2013.05.014.

[78] Miceli, Antonio, Mariagrazia Croccia, Simone Simeoni, Egidio Varone, Michele Murzi, Pier Andrea Farneti, Marco Solinas, and Mattia Glauber. 2013. "Root Replacement with Stentless Freestyle Bioprostheses for Active Endocarditis: A Single Centre Experience." *Interactive Cardiovascular and Thoracic Surgery* 16 (1): 27–30. https://doi.org/10.1093/icvts/ivs438.

[79] Perrotta, Sossio, and Salvatore Lentini. 2010. "In Patients with Severe Active Aortic Valve Endocarditis, Is a Stentless Valve as Good as the Homograft?" *Interactive Cardiovascular and Thoracic Surgery* 11 (3): 309–13. https://doi.org/10.1510/icvts.2010.234831.

[80] Di Eusanio, Marco, Paolo Berretta, Jacopo Alfonsi, and Mariano Cefarelli. 2019. "Aortic Root Endocarditis: A Biointegral Bioconduit Subannular Implantation." *Annals of Cardiothoracic Surgery* 8 (6): 713–14. https://doi.org/10.21037/acs.2019.09.02.

[81] Leontyev, Sergey, Michael A. Borger, Paul Modi, Sven Lehmann, Jörg Seeburger, Thorsten Doenst, and Friedrich W. Mohr. 2012. "Surgical Management of Aortic Root Abscess: A 13-Year Experience in 172 Patients with 100% Follow-Up." *Journal of*

Thoracic and Cardiovascular Surgery 143 (2): 332–37. https://doi.org/10.1016/j.jtcvs.2010.10.064.

[82] Elgalad, Abdelmotagaly, Amr Arafat, Tarek Elshazly, Mohamed Elkahwagy, Hossam Fawzy, Ehab Wahby, Abdel-Hady Taha, et al. 2019. "Surgery for Active Infective Endocarditis of the Aortic Valve With Infection Extending Beyond the Leaflets." *Heart, Lung & Circulation* 28 (7): 1112–20. https://doi.org/10.1016/j.hlc.2018.05.200.

[83] Knosalla, C, Y Weng, A C Yankah, H Siniawski, J Hofmeister, R Hammerschmidt, M Loebe, and R Hetzer. 2000. "Surgical Treatment of Active Infective Aortic Valve Endocarditis with Associated Periannular Abscess--11 Year Results." *European Heart Journal* 21 (6): 490–97. https://doi.org/10.1053/euhj.1999.1877.

[84] Mylonakis, Eleftherios, and Stephen B. Calderwood. 2001. "Infective Endocarditis in Adults." *New England Journal of Medicine*. https://doi.org/10.1056/NEJMra010082.

[85] Lalani, Tahaniyat, Vivian H Chu, Lawrence P Park, Enrico Cecchi, G Ralph Corey, Emanuele Durante-Mangoni, Vance G Fowler, et al. 2013. "In-Hospital and 1-Year Mortality in Patients Undergoing Early Surgery for Prosthetic Valve Endocarditis." *JAMA Internal Medicine* 173 (16): 1495–1504. https://doi.org/10.1001/jamainternmed.2013.8203.

[86] Luciani, N., E. Mossuto, D. Ricci, M. Luciani, M. Russo, A. Salsano, A. Pozzoli, et al. 2017. "Prosthetic Valve Endocarditis: Predictors of Early Outcome of Surgical Therapy. A Multicentric Study." *European Journal of Cardio-Thoracic Surgery* 52 (4). https://doi.org/10.1093/ejcts/ezx169.

[87] Lee, Jonathan H, Kimberly D Burner, Michael E Fealey, William D Edwards, Henry D Tazelaar, Thomas A Orszulak, Alan J Wright, and Larry M Baddour. 2011. "Prosthetic Valve Endocarditis: Clinicopathological Correlates in 122 Surgical Specimens from 116 Patients (1985-2004)." Cardiovascular Pathology : *The Official Journal of the Society for Cardiovascular Pathology* 20 (1): 26–35. https://doi.org/10.1016/j.carpath.2009.09.006.

[88] López, Javier, Ana Revilla, Isidre Vilacosta, Eduardo Villacorta, Carlos González-Juanatey, Itziar Gómez, María Jesús Rollán, and José Alberto San Román. 2007. "Definition, Clinical Profile, Microbiological Spectrum, and Prognostic Factors of Early-Onset Prosthetic Valve Endocarditis." *European Heart Journal* 28 (6): 760–65. https://doi.org/10.1093/eurheartj/ehl486.

[89] Tan, Hwee-Leong, Louis Y A Chai, Tiong-Cheng Yeo, Boon-Lock Chia, Paul A Tambyah, and Kian-Keong Poh. 2015. "Predictors of In-Hospital Adverse Events in Patients with Prosthetic Valve Infective Endocarditis." *Heart, Lung & Circulation* 24 (7): 705–9. https://doi.org/10.1016/j.hlc.2015.01.013.

[90] Brennan, J Matthew, Fred H Edwards, Yue Zhao, Sean O'Brien, Michael E Booth, Rachel S Dokholyan, Pamela S Douglas, Eric D Peterson, and DEcIDE AVR (Developing Evidence to Inform Decisions about Effectiveness–Aortic Valve Replacement) Research Team. 2013. "Long-Term Safety and Effectiveness of Mechanical versus Biologic Aortic Valve Prostheses in Older Patients: Results from the Society of Thoracic Surgeons Adult Cardiac Surgery National Database." *Circulation* 127 (16): 1647–55. https://doi.org/10.1161/CIRCULATIONAHA.113.002003.

[91] Østergaard, Lauge, Nana Valeur, Nikolaj Ihlemann, Morten Holdgaard Smerup, Henning Bundgaard, Gunnar Gislason, Christian Torp-Pedersen, Niels Eske Bruun, Lars Køber, and Emil Loldrup Fosbøl. 2018. "Incidence and Factors Associated with Infective Endocarditis in Patients Undergoing Left-Sided Heart Valve Replacement." *European Heart Journal* 39 (28): 2668–75. https://doi.org/10.1093/eurheartj/ehy153.

[92] Tao, Ende, Li Wan, WenJun Wang, YunLong Luo, JinFu Zeng, and Xia Wu. 2017. "The Prognosis of Infective Endocarditis Treated with Biological Valves versus Mechanical Valves: A Meta-Analysis." *PloS One* 12 (4): e0174519. https://doi.org/10.1371/journal.pone.0174519.

[93] Anguera, Ignasi, Jose M. Miro, Jose Alberto San Roman, Aristides de Alarcon, Manuel Anguita, Benito Almirante, Artur Evangelista, et al. 2006. "Periannular Complications in Infective Endocarditis Involving Prosthetic Aortic Valves." *American Journal of Cardiology* 98 (9): 1261–68. https://doi.org/10.1016/j.amjcard.2006.05.066.

[94] Wang, Andrew, Eugene Athan, Paul A. Pappas, Vance G. Fowler, Lars Olaison, Carlos Paré, Benito Almirante, et al. 2007. "Contemporary Clinical Profile and Outcome of Prosthetic Valve Endocarditis." *Journal of the American Medical Associatio*n 297 (12): 1354–61. https://doi.org/10.1001/jama.297.12.1354.

[95] Morguet, A. J., G. S. Werner, S. Andreas, and H. Kreuzer. 1995. "Diagnostic Value of Transesophageal Compared with Transthoracic Echocardiography in Suspected Prosthetic Valve Endocarditis." *Herz* 20 (6): 390–98.

[96] Musci, Michele, Michael Hübler, Aref Amiri, Julia Stein, Susanne Kosky, Rudolf Meyer, Yuguo Weng, and Roland Hetzer. 2010. "Surgical Treatment for Active Infective Prosthetic Valve Endocarditis: 22-Year Single-Centre Experience." European Journal of Cardio-Thoracic Surgery : *Official Journal of the European Association for Cardio-Thoracic Surgery* 38 (5): 528–38. https://doi.org/10.1016/j.ejcts.2010.03.019.

[97] Habib, Gilbert, C. Tribouilloy, F. Thuny, R. Giorgi, A. Brahim, M. Amazouz, J. P. Remadi, et al. 2005. "Prosthetic Valve Endocarditis: Who Needs Surgery? A Multicentre Study of 104 Cases." *Heart* 91 (7): 954–59. https://doi.org/10.1136/hrt.2004.046177.

[98] Eggebrecht, Holger, Sibylle Schelle, Miriam Puls, Björn Plicht, Ralph Stephan Von Bardeleben, Christian Butter, Andreas E. May, et al. 2015. "Risk and Outcomes of Complications during and after MitraClip Implantation: Experience in 828 Patients from the German TRAnscatheter Mitral Valve Interventions (TRAMI) Registry." *Catheterization and Cardiovascular Interventions* 86 (4): 728–35. https://doi.org/10.1002/ccd.25838.

[99] Chourdakis, Emmanouil, Ioanna Koniari, George Hahalis, Nicholas G. Kounis, and Karl Eugen Hauptmann. 2018. "Endocarditis after Transcatheter Aortic Valve Implantation: A Current Assessment." *Journal of Geriatric Cardiology. Science Press.* https://doi.org/10.11909/j.issn.1671-5411.2018.01.003.

[100] Carrasco-Chinchilla, Fernando, Gemma Sánchez-Espín, Josefa Ruiz-Morales, Isabel Rodríguez-Bailón, Jose M Melero-Tejedor, Rada Ivanova-Georgieva, Victoria García-López, Antonio Muñoz-García, Juan J Gómez-Doblas, and Eduardo de Teresa-Galván. 2014. "Influence of a Multidisciplinary Alert Strategy on Mortality Due to Left-Sided Infective Endocarditis." *Revista Espanola de Cardiologia* (English Ed.) 67 (5): 380–86. https://doi.org/10.1016/j.rec.2013.09.010.

[101] Chirillo, Fabio, Piergiorgio Scotton, Francesco Rocco, Roberto Rigoli, Elvio Polesel, and Zoran Olivari. 2013. "Management of Patients with Infective Endocarditis by a Multidisciplinary Team Approach: An Operative Protocol." *Journal of Cardiovascular Medicine* 14 (9): 659–68. https://doi.org/10.2459/JCM.0b013e32835ec585.

In: Perspectives in Aortic Valve Disease
Editor: Giovanni Concistrè
ISBN: 978-1-53618-769-4

Chapter 7

NEOPLASTIC DISORDERS INVOLVING THE AORTIC VALVE

Angela Pucci[1,*], *Alessandra Burini*[2,3], *Enrica Manzato*[2,3] *and Cristina Zucchinetti*[2,3]
[1]Histopathology Department, University Hospital of Pisa
[2]Sant'Anna School of Advanced Studies; Pisa, Italy
[3]University of Pisa, Faculty of Medicine and Surgery, Pisa, Italy

ABSTRACT

Aortic valve tumors are rare and mainly represented by benign and small masses, most commonly papillary fibroelastoma followed by myxoma. Malignant primary tumors are exceptionally reported and are mainly represented by sarcomas. The aortic valve may also present tumor-like lesions and pseudo-tumors, including thrombi, Lambl's excrescences and endocarditic vegetations. Although most aortic tumors are benign, small and often asymptomatic lesions, they may have dramatic clinical consequences, thus requiring surgical excision: embolic phenomena, outflow tract or coronary ostium occlusion. They may be incidentally discovered by echocardiography – the main diagnostic tool for cardiac masses. Computed tomography (CT) and cardiac magnetic resonance (CMR) may give additional information on tumor size, shape, location and characteristics, but definitive and differential diagnoses always require histology.

Keywords: cardiac tumors, magnetic resonance imaging, computed tomography

ABBREVIATIONS

CT	computed tomography
EMA	epithelial membrane antigen
FISH	fluorescence in situ hybridisation

* Corresponding Author's Email: angelapucci@libero.it.

H&E	hematoxylin/eosin
IE	infectious endocarditis
IMT	inflammatory myofibroblastic tumor
LE	Lambl's excrescences
CMR	cardiac magnetic resonance
MRI	magnetic resonance imaging
NBTE	non-bacterial thrombotic endocarditis
PAS	periodic acid-Schiff
PCR	polymerase chain reaction
PFE	papillary fibroelastoma
RT-PCR	retro transcription-polymerase chain reaction
TEE	transesophageal echocardiography
TTE	transthoracic echocardiography

INTRODUCTION

Primary cardiac tumors are rare, with a prevalence at autopsy of 0.001-0.03% versus 1.5-2.1% of secondary (metastatic) tumors. Valve tumors account for less than 10% of the heart tumors [1–5]. Although most cardiac valve tumors are benign and of small dimensions, they may have severe clinical sequelae and require surgical resection [1, 6, 7].

Cardiac valve tumors are more likely to occur in male (79% of cases) and adult patients, the average age being 52 years (range, 2 to 88 years). Each of the four cardiac valves may be involved with approximately equal frequency [4, 6, 7]. They are more commonly asymptomatic, with overt symptoms in about 38% of patients, depending also upon a variable risk of embolism, and including cardiac (angina, acute myocardial infarction, heart failure, syncope and even sudden death) and neurological (transitory ischemic attack, stroke, amaurosis) symptoms, but also mesenteric, renal, splenic or limb ischemia.

The most common aortic valve tumors are benign: papillary fibroelastoma (PFE), followed by myxoma, fibroma and hemangioma. Malignant tumors are exceptionally reported and almost exclusively represented by sarcomas and lymphomas, but both of them are more frequently found in the right side of the heart [5]. Average tumor size is 1.15 cm (range: 0.3 to 7 cm). A few cases have also been reported of secondary involvement of the aortic valve by tumors originating in different cardiac structures or other organs/tissues [1, 3, 5]. Although most tumor masses are nowadays identified in vivo by imaging techniques – first echocardiography for diagnosis, followed by computed tomography (CT) and cardiac magnetic resonance (CMR) for better definition of tumor characteristics – the definitive diagnosis of aortic valve tumors requires histology, which also represents the gold standard for the differential diagnosis of cardiac tumors [5].

Benign Tumors of the Aortic Valve

Papillary Fibroelastoma

Clinical Features

Papillary fibroelastoma (PFE) is the second most common primary cardiac tumor after myxoma and the most common valvular tumor, mainly affecting the aortic valve (in 52% cases) and accounting for three-quarters of cardiac valvular tumors [8–13]. Its estimated prevalence ranges between 0.02% and 0.45% in post-mortem and open heart surgery procedures, respectively [14]. With the increasing use of echocardiography, the diagnoses of PFE have been raising in asymptomatic patients, their actual prevalence being very likely underestimated [11, 13, 15]. PFE can be detected at all ages, but it is more common between the 4th and 8th decade (mean age 60 years) with a slight male preponderance (55%) [9]. It is nowadays recognized as a true neoplasia as supported by cytogenetic analyses, but in the past it has been considered a hamartoma, a giant form of Lambl's excrescence originating from a thrombus or an unusual response to infection or to hemodynamic injury [8, 12, 16].

In most patients, PFE is asymptomatic and incidentally diagnosed, but it carries a high risk of embolization and in up to 35% patients it can be clinically manifest [10, 14, 17, 18]. Because of the embolic risk, a few authors suggest that even incidentally diagnosed and asymptomatic PFEs should be surgically treated [13]. Surgical tumor resection is curative and usually allows valve sparing with an excellent outcome and almost no recurrence (maximum 1.6% of surgical cases) [13].

Another possible – although rare – mechanism of cardiac events is a transitory or permanent direct coronary ostium occlusion from a coronary cusp PFE [16, 17, 19].

Although PFE is usually a single tumor, in a few patients it may be multifocal, affecting the same or different sites of the heart [10]. It may be found on the aortic [9, 20–22] or the ventricular [18] side of a leaflet, the left coronary cusp being the least affected one.

Imaging

Historically, PFE mostly represented an incidental (post-mortem or surgical) finding, but it is now increasingly diagnosed by echocardiography, the best tool to study this lesion [12, 13, 23]. Trans-esophageal echocardiography (TEE) is more sensitive, but less accessible and more invasive than trans-thoracic echocardiography (TTE). TEE is also used during surgery, to guide tumor resection and to check the results [13, 21]. At echocardiography, PFE usually appears as a small (typically less than 2 cm), often mobile, pedunculated or sessile mass, with speckled appearance and a strippled pattern near the edges [23, 24]. The core (pedicle) is usually very echodense, thus enabling clinicians to differentiate it from vegetations and thrombi [25].

By CT, PFE shows as a hypodense mass with irregular borders, whereas by CMR it can be detected as a small, round, homogeneous mass with an intermediate signal intensity on T1- and a hyperintense one on T2-weighted images. It can be differentiated from a lipoma by fat-saturation sequences [24, 26].

Coronary angiography is used when PFE presents with angina symptoms or when a concomitant coronary artery disease is suspected. It can disclose occlusions or dilatations of coronary arteries due to embolism; moreover, a filling defect can be seen in cardiac chambers or in the first tract of ascending aorta because of the mass's presence. However, angiography is not recommended for PFE evaluation, because it is less sensitive than echocardiography and it carries a high risk of embolization due to catheter traumatism on the tumor surface [16].

Macroscopic Features

PFE diameter may be up to 70 mm, but it usually does not exceed 20 mm [9, 16]. It is a small, soft, sessile or – more often – pedunculated mass, this latter form being quite mobile and at higher risk of embolization [27]. The typical appearance of a surgical specimen of PFE (after immersion into water or saline solution) is commonly described as "sea anemone-like" because it is made of a central stalk with multiple papillary fronds [9, 28] (Figure 1A). Sometimes, organized thrombi attached to the tumor's surface can hide its typical papillary structure.

Microscopic Features

The definitive diagnosis of PFE relies on histology, which shows multiple papillary fronds radiating from a central stalk (Figure 1B). In each frond, three main layers can be observed: an inner central core of dense avascular matrix, with collagen, elastic fibers, and rare spindle cells; a loose myxoid tissue rich in acid mucopolysaccharides; and an external single layer of flat endothelial cells [28, 29]. Longitudinally oriented elastic fibers are a histological hallmark for the diagnosis [16].

These histological features allow the differential diagnosis from other valvular tumors, endocarditic vegetations, thrombi and Lambl's excrescences to be made [9, 21, 28, 30].

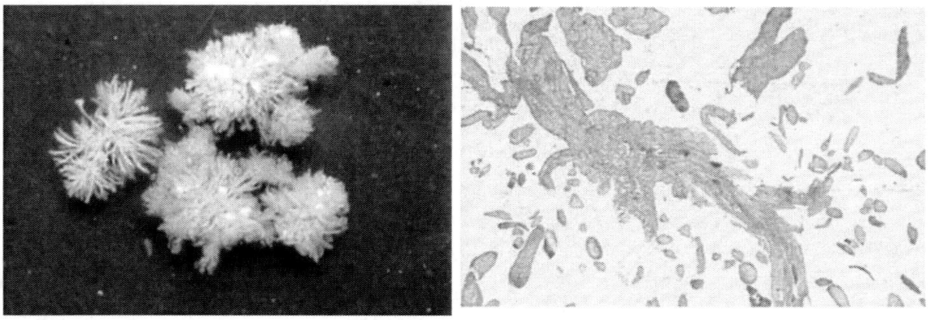

A B

Figure 1. A multifocal papillary fibroelastoma with fine papillary fronds that are displayed by water immersion (A). Histology shows that the papillary fronds are lined by an endothelial layer and have a connective tissue core with elastic fibers (B; Hematoxylin and Eosin staining, original magnification 2x).

Myxoma

Clinical Features

So far, less than twenty aortic valve myxomas have been reported [31–33]. Clinical presentation largely depends upon size, shape, mobility and mass surface characteristics. The most common symptoms are dyspnea and/or angina [32, 34–37]; signs of subaortic stenosis have also been reported in a case [31], but patients may also be asymptomatic [38, 39]. The right coronary and the non-coronary leaflets are more frequently involved, with the tumor located on the edge of the leaflet [32] or in fewer cases on the ventricular aspect [31, 33, 34, 36]. The mass may be polypoid and sessile or papillary, the first type often causing obstructive or heart failure symptoms and the latter one embolic phenomena [40–42] with distal ischemia, such as transient ischemic attacks or strokes [41, 43–45], lower limb ischemia [46, 47] and acute myocardial infarction [34].

Imaging

In most cases, the first diagnosis of the mass is done by TTE [32]. Aortic myxomas may show a heterogeneous core with necrosis, hemorrhages and calcifications which appear as cystic spaces and echo-lucent spots, respectively [21, 42], and the papillary forms may present multiple stretched villi [42]. Their brightness increases after administering contrast agents because of the tumor vascularity [47]. CT or CMR can give additional information about size, location and shape, tissue composition and anatomical characteristics for surgical planning [21, 25]. On non-contrast-enhanced CT images, a myxoma appears as a hypodense mass [48] and, after administration of contrast, as a filling defect, i.e., a hypodense region with non-homogeneous enhancement indicating areas of necrosis or hemorrhage [47, 48]. Using CMR, T1-weighted images show myxomas as isointense to the myocardium and T2-weighted images as hyperintense, since they have a great amount of extracellular water. As in CT, they can show non-homogeneous contrast enhancement [48]. Cine images are particularly useful as myxomas are often highly mobile, especially when pedunculated [48].

Macroscopic Features

Only single myxomas have been reported, the diameter ranging from 0,6 to 4 cm (most cases <1,5 cm) [32]. They appeared as myxoid (gelatinous) [36, 37, 44], sessile or more commonly pedunculated masses, with papillary and villous [43] or solid and smooth surfaces [35, 37–39, 41, 43, 47, 49]. Sometimes, they can present hemorrhagic areas [36, 44].

Microscopic Features

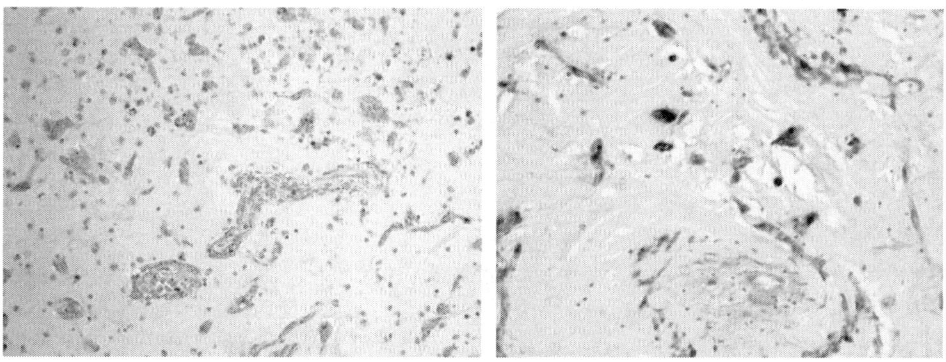

A B

Figure 2. A myxoma with the myxoid stroma and the lepidic cells in evidence (A; Hematoxylin and Eosin staining, original magnification 4x) that are immunoreactive for calretinin (B; Immunoperoxidase staining with Hematoxylin counterstaining, original magnification 10x).

Myxomas show an abundant myxoid, mucopolysaccharide-rich matrix embedding a variable number of stellate, oval, polygonal, or spindle (lepidic) cells without mitotic activity, immunoreactive for calretinin and S100, forming solid nests or perivascular cuffs as seen in the other cardiac myxomas (Figure 2A,B) [35, 36, 39, 44, 45, 47, 49–52].

The definitive diagnosis of aortic valve myxoma relies on histology, since its macroscopic features mimic PFE (Kim et al. 2012), LEs, endocarditic vegetations or thrombi [21, 45, 49, 53], but also hemangiomas and angiosarcomas [49].

Fibroma

Cardiac fibromas are the second most frequent cardiac tumors in the pediatric age after rhabdomyomas [5, 54, 55]. Cardiac fibromas are considered congenital tumors that may become clinically manifest later in life and are also known as cardiac fibromatosis. They have also been found in association with Gorlin syndrome [5].

Clinical Features

Cardiac fibromas are often associated with arrhythmias; moreover, they can cause hemodynamic compromise and congestive heart failure. They may also be found incidentally in asymptomatic patients. They usually arise in the left ventricular free wall, inter-ventricular septum or right ventricular free wall, but they can also infiltrate the myocardial wall. An exceptionally rare form of isolated fibroma has been described in the aortic valve of an elder woman [54]. Cardiac fibromas are benign lesions; nonetheless, most of them require surgery and even cardiac transplantation (when they are unresectable and diffusely infiltrating the myocardium) [5, 54, 55]. Sometimes, they obliterate the ventricular cavity. Aortic fibromas can cause outflow obstruction, thus requiring surgical excision.

Imaging

At echocardiography, a fibroma typically appears as a well-circumscribed, solitary mass. By CT, the mass shows low attenuation and it can also present calcifications, a helpful feature for diagnosis. By CMR, because of the fibrous nature of the tumor, the signal intensity is often reduced, compared to the adjacent uninvolved myocardium; contrast-enhanced imaging usually demonstrates a hypoperfused tumor core. In the single case report of aortic valve fibroma, TTE and TEE revealed a 9 x 7 mm, medium-echogenic mass on the right coronary cusp of the aortic valve, passively moving with the leaflet. CT showed no enhancement [54].

Macroscopic Features

Fibromas are well-defined, solitary lesions with smooth margins; their dimensions are usually great, ranging from 1 to 20 cm in diameter (average 3 cm). The typical appearance is of an elongated, lobulated or disc-shaped firm mass of a homogenous pearly-gray color. Calcifications are quite common, whereas cystic changes, hemorrhages, and necrosis are usually absent.

Microscopic Features

Cardiac fibromas are constituted by a fibroblastic (Figure 3) or a myofibroblastic proliferation interspersed among large amounts of collagen [5, 55]. Dystrophic calcifications are seen in approximately 25% of cases. The histological examination shows relatively bland stellate and spindle-shaped fibroblasts separated by a collagenous or collagenous-myxoid matrix. Mitotic activity is either absent or minimal. Some cells can have a myofibroblastic immuno-phenotype, with focal reactivity for muscle-specific and alpha-smooth muscle actin and/or cytokeratin in few cases. Desmin, S100 protein, and CD34 are usually not expressed [56].

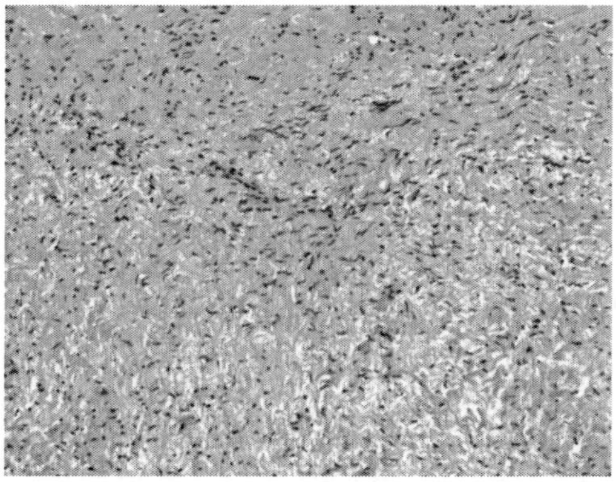

Figure 3. A fibroma, constituted by a fibrous stroma with scattered fibroblastic cells (Hematoxylin and Eosin staining, original magnification 4x).

Hemangioma

Cardiac hemangiomas or angiomas are benign vascular tumors or malformations, accounting for <5% of benign cardiac tumors, occurring at all ages (mean age 55 years) [5, 57]. Although most cardiac hemangiomas are found incidentally, patients may present with dyspnea, arrhythmias, signs of heart failure and pericardial effusion; they may be associated to vascular syndromes e.g., Kasabach-Merritt [57]. They have been rarely reported on the aortic valve [58–61], the most frequent locations being represented by the lateral wall of the left ventricle (21%), the anterior wall of the right ventricle (21%), the inter-ventricular septum (17%) and the right ventricular outflow tract [55, 57].

Imaging

By echocardiography, hemangiomas are usually hyperechoic, circumscribed, and often intra-cavitary masses [58]. With CT they are usually circumscribed and heterogeneous and are characterized by low attenuation and bright enhancement with contrast administration. With CMR, they may show intermediate to high intensity signal on T1 weighted images, very intense signal on T2 weighted images, and enhance brightly with contrast administration [57].

Macroscopic Features

These tumors are often large, and their gross appearance depends on the size of the vascular spaces within. They may be poorly circumscribed, slightly raised or infiltrating the surrounding tissue [62].

Microscopic Features

They are microscopically constituted by multiple dilated thin-walled vessels (cavernous type), smaller vessels resembling capillaries (capillary type) (Figure 4A), dysplastic malformed arteries and veins (arterio-venous hemangioma, cirsoid aneurysm), or often have combined features of cavernous, capillary and arteriovenous hemangiomas, and many contain fibrous tissue and fat [62]. Capillary hemangiomas present thin walled capillaries with scant, sometimes myxoid stroma whereas cavernous hemangiomas are usually non capsulated masses with infiltrative borders, constituted by large cavernous spaces separated by connective stroma and can show thrombosis and calcifications [62]. Immunostaining for endothelial cells such as CD31 (Figure 4B) and CD34 is strongly positive [61]. Those reported on the aortic valve are mainly constituted by capillary vessels and can be covered by normal endothelium [58], or by a thrombus [59].

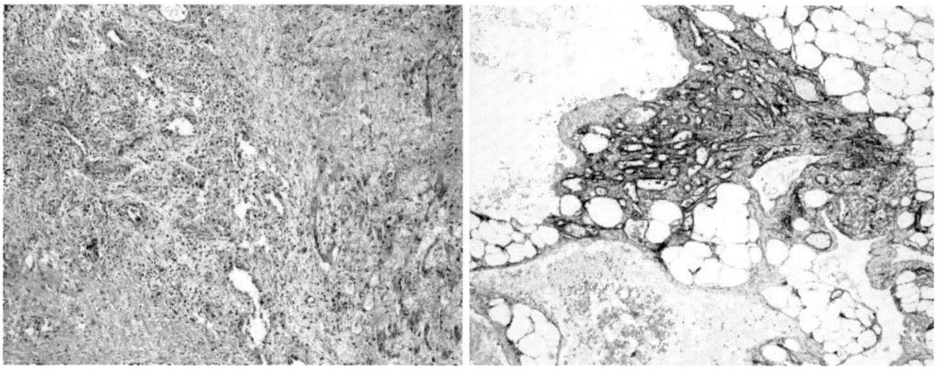

A B

Figure 4. A capillary hemangioma with a fibrous stroma (A; Hematoxylin and Eosin staining, original magnification 4x); the endothelial cells are immunoreactive for the CD31 endothelial antigen (B; Immunoperoxidase staining with Hematoxylin counterstaining, original magnification 10x).

Inflammatory Myofibroblastic Tumor

Initially described as an inflammatory pseudotumor, inflammatory myofibroblastic tumor (IMT) is nowadays considered a true tumor [5]. IMT is a ubiquitous neoplasia, but it is more frequently found in soft tissues and viscera of children and young adults (mean age 10 years). Cardiac IMTs are rare, clinical symptoms being related to their location within the heart: patients can be asymptomatic, present a constitutional syndrome (fever, weight loss, malaise) or cardiac symptoms such as chest pain, heart failure, arrhythmia, murmur, syncope and also sudden death, mainly due to coronary embolization [63, 64]. Lesions size ranges from 1 cm to 8.6 cm and they appear like a yellowish-white to gray mass, solid, glistening, nodular or polypoid, with or without a pedicle. Pathognomonic histologic features are spindled myofibroblastic cells with no cytologic atypia or nuclear pleomorphism and a chronic inflammatory infiltrate composed of lymphocytes, plasma cells and histiocytes. Immunohistochemistry show positivity for vimentin, smooth muscle actin, desmin (76% of cases), CD34, CD68, whereas ALK-1 is usually negative in cardiac IMTs [63, 65].

PRIMARY MALIGNANT TUMORS OF THE AORTIC VALVE

Primary malignant cardiac tumors are rare, cardiac metastases being the first malignancy of the heart [1, 3]. They are mainly represented by sarcomas, especially angiosarcomas and rhabdomyosarcomas, but also leiomyosarcomas, synovial and intimal sarcomas have been reported [5]. Primary or secondary lymphomas (almost exclusively non-Hodgkin lymphomas) have also been described in the heart [5]. Malignant tumors do not show any gender predominance nor age predilection, although some histotypes are prevalent at different ages (i.e., rhabdomyosarcoma in children and young adults); they grow progressively and most of them show poor prognosis [1, 3, 5]. Distant metastases may occur to sites such as liver, bone, and brain [3].

The diagnosis of the mass is usually done by TTE, but CT and CMR are useful for a better definition of tumor characteristics, the definitive diagnosis requiring histology and ancillary techniques such as immunohistochemistry and molecular techniques (fluorescence in situ hybridization (FISH) and/or PCR/RT-PCR). In the last decades, endomyocardial biopsy has been increasingly proved to be a valuable diagnostic tool for pre-operative diagnosis [66, 67].

Sarcoma

Sarcomas are the most frequent primary malignant tumors of the heart, but they exceptionally involve the left cardiac valves [1-5]. Their symptoms depend upon size and localization and the diagnosis of the mass is usually done by echocardiography, TEE first. An undifferentiated sarcoma of the aortic and mitral valves has been described in a 72-year-old woman [68]. Preoperative TEE highlighted the presence of masses on both left valves, the aortic valve showing a partially cystic tumor. After excisional surgery with dual valve replacement, histology showed an undifferentiated sarcoma. In the last decade, most undifferentiated cardiac sarcomas have been shown to be constituted by intimal sarcomas that have been described in the aorta [69] and major pulmonary vessels [70], as well as in cardiac chambers [69]. It is a highly pleomorphic neoplasia with high mitotic activity, showing no immunophenotypic cell differentiation and MDM2 overexpression (Figure 5).

A synovial sarcoma involving the right coronary aortic valve leaflet and the adjacent inter-ventricular septum has also been described [71]. Diagnosis is based on histological examination, which shows a monomorphic (spindle cells) or heterogeneous (spindle and epithelioid cytokeratin/epithelial membrane antigen (EMA)-immunoreactive cells) lesion. Additionally, exclusion criteria for other diseases must be met and the gene translocation t(X;18) (p11.2;q11.2) (present on approximately 90% of synovial sarcomas) can often be seen via FISH on histologic sections [5, 71–73]. Although chemotherapy can give short-term benefits in these patients, overall prognosis for cardiac sarcomas is poor [1, 3, 4, 72–74].

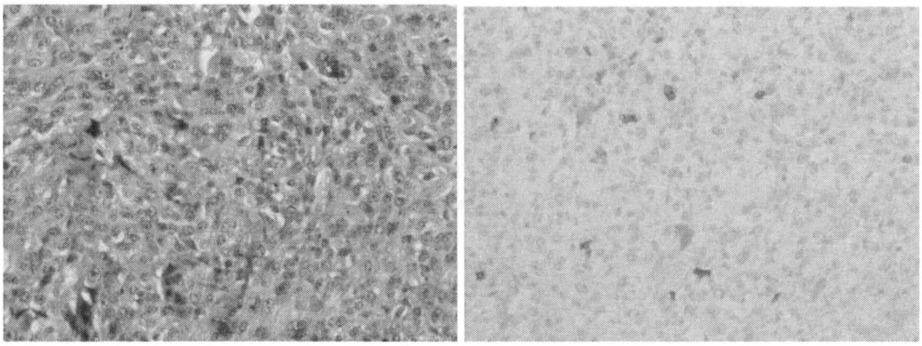

Figure 5. An intimal sarcoma of the aorta involving the aortic valve annulus and characterized by pleomorphic and undifferentiated cells (A; Hematoxylin and Eosin staining, original magnification 10x), a few of them expressing MDM2 (B; Immunoperoxidase staining with Hematoxylin counterstaining, original magnification 10x).

Non-Hodgkin Lymphoma

Cardiac involvement is not uncommon in lymphomas, but valvular involvement has only been exceptionally reported. In autopsy series, 18% of patients with systemic lymphomas had metastases to the heart, but only one had valvular involvement [75, 76]; and indeed there are isolated case reports of valve involvement in lymphoma cases [77], with only one describing a primary lymphoma affecting native valves [78] and the few others describing a primary lymphoma affecting prosthetic valves [79, 80]. Primary cardiac lymphomas (PCLs) represent less than 0.01% of all cardiac tumors, usually affect patients after the fifth decade of life and are almost exclusively represented by non-Hodgkin lymphomas [81, 82]. PCLs present in immunocompromised, immunosuppressed and HIV-positive patients, but it has also been described in immunocompetent patients [2, 83]. Symptoms are often sub-acute and nonspecific with few cases presenting with acute symptoms, including heart failure and even sudden death, diagnosis being very challenging [67]. Echocardiography may show an intracavitary mass or pericardial effusion, CT a heterogeneous contrast enhancement and CMR a variable signal intensity and contrast enhancement, but the differential diagnosis requires histology and immunophenotyping [66, 81]. The most frequent cardiac lymphoma is represented by the diffuse large B-cell non-Hodgkin lymphoma that is constituted by large CD20 immunoreactive cells, diffusely infiltrating the cardiac structures and showing a high proliferating (MIB1) index with or without EBV positivity [81,83].

The prognosis is usually poor because of the nonspecific symptoms and of the late diagnosis, but in patients with earlier diagnosis and appropriate treatment (chemotherapy) it is apparently improving in recent years [67, 84].

CARDIAC METASTASES

Cardiac metastases are more common than primary cardiac tumors, at least in adults. They usually have a poor prognosis, with survival after diagnosis ranging from 6 weeks to 15 months; moreover, they often are unrecognized without autopsy. They have been detected in autopsy studies of cancer patients in up to 15% of cases [85–87]. Valve metastases are very rare, probably because of the continuous cusps motion and absence of vessels on the cusps themselves. They can present with a neoplastic thrombotic endocarditis.

Most metastatic/secondary tumors are melanomas, sarcomas, lung, and haematological malignancies, but also breast and gastric carcinomas may secondarily involve cardiac structures, including cardiac valves. Because of improved survival of oncological patients, an increase in the incidence of metastatic cardiac tumors is likely to happen in the next future [85].

The clinical presentation includes shortness of breath, cough, anterior thoracic pain, pleuritic chest pain or peripheral edema.

Cardiac metastases can also be the first manifestation of the neoplastic disease and require differential diagnosis that usually relies on histological investigations, including immunohistochemistry and other ancillary techniques [88].

NON-NEOPLASTIC LESIONS (PSEUDOTUMORS) OF THE AORTIC VALVE

The aortic valve can show non-neoplastic masses that may be difficult to differentiate from true tumors. They are mainly represented by LEs, endocarditic vegetations, marantic endocarditis, thrombi and pannus (especially on prostheses), but also include blood cysts, rheumatoid nodules and calcifications [25, 89]. They can be differentiated from the site of origin, their number and definitely by histology [9, 30].

Thrombi appear as laminated masses with irregular or lobulated borders, micro-cavitations and no pedicle at the echocardiography. This latter element can help in differentiating them from PFEs (Figure 6).

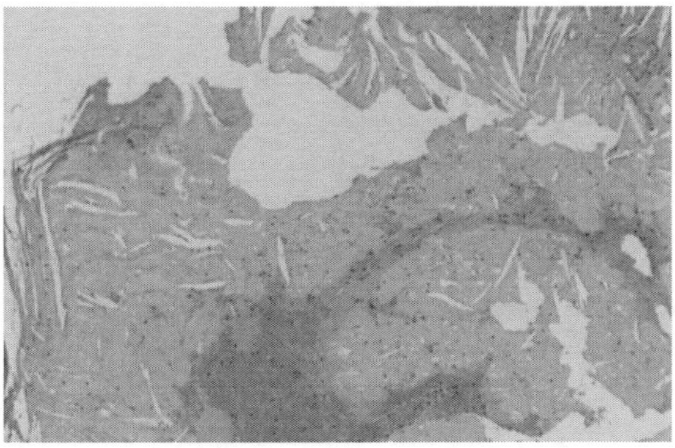

Figure 6. A thrombus of an aortic coronary cusp, showing fibrin and blood cells together with cholesterol clefts (Hematoxylin and Eosin staining, original magnification 10x).

Lambl's excrescences are filiform lesions occurring on the line of coaptation of cardiac valves due to wear and tear. Usually, they are smaller than PFEs and do not occur isolated (>90% are multiple lesions) [53]. They originate as small thrombi on endocardial surface and have the potential to embolize to distant organs, even if they usually remain asymptomatic. Microscopically, LEs consist of a dense core of collagenous and elastic fibrils enclosed by a single layer of endothelium; the densely hyalinized central core is lined by endocardial-type spindle cells. LEs localize on the ventricular side of aortic valve. Their dimensions are usually <2 mm in width and 5-10 mm in length, even if there have been case reports of giant LEs (>2 cm in diameter) that are more often associated with complications, such as ischemic stroke due to thromboembolic events [53, 90].

The current management of LEs includes close follow-up with TEE for asymptomatic lesions, whereas symptomatic cases undergo single or dual antiplatelet therapy or surgery, depending on first or subsequent episodes [90].

Hamartomas of the aortic valve are extremely rare. They consist of loose connective tissue and mature fat cells (in the lipomatous variant) or hyalinized fibrous tissue core with dense twisted clumps of elastin and abundant mucopolysaccharide content (fibroelastic variant) [91, 92]. A single case has also been reported of diffuse fatty infiltration in an insufficient bicuspid valve of a young male soccer player, the fatty tissue infiltrating the fibrous core of the leaflets [93] (Figure 7). Clinical presentation is variable, including asymptomatic cases and patients with severe valve regurgitation, symptoms of congestive heart failure or even fatal ischemic heart attack [91, 92].

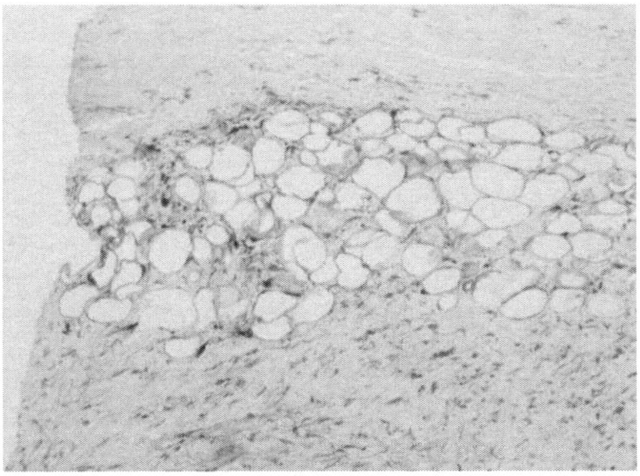

Figure 7. A lipomatous hamartoma of a bicuspid aortic valve, showing a leaflet with diffuse replacement of the fibrous core by adipose tissue that is S100 immunoreactive (Immunoperoxidase staining with Hematoxylin counterstaining, original magnification 20x).

Blood cysts are small (pinpoint to pinhead), rounded, reddish brown nodules, usually sessile but sometimes pedunculated. They are common findings in infants and seem to disappear with age (uncommon after 6 months); they more frequently occur on the mitral and tricuspid valves. Histologically, blood cysts consist in masses of red blood cells and few white blood cells packed in a spherical or ovoid cyst into the connective tissue and covered with a single layer of flat endothelium [94]. Rare cases are reported in children or adults, and the aortic valve is an unusual localization. In a case report, a 16-year-old girl with severe aortic regurgitation has been studied. Routine transthoracic echocardiography demonstrated the presence of a circular structure attached to the ventricular surface of the coronary cusp of the aortic valve, which needed surgery resection. The pathological examination recognized the lesion as a giant blood cyst [95].

Endocarditis

Valvular endocarditic vegetations are an important differential diagnosis with PFE since they can be very similar at the echocardiographic evaluation [25, 96]. They have an infectious origin, so they are generally associated with symptoms of endocarditis and their aspect can change quite quickly with time and therapies; they can also cause severe damage to the valvular leaflets. Valvular masses are an important finding in endocarditis, and they are called "vegetations" in this clinical setting. Depending on the infectious or non-infectious origin of endocarditis, vegetations can be sterile or not. Infective endocarditis (IE) is a cardiovascular infection of primary relevance because of the frequent complications on cardiac valves, devices and extracardiac complications. Etiology can be various, depending on epidemiology and localization of the vegetation (right or left heart), but in general there is a vast array of microorganisms that may cause IE: streptococci, staphylococci, enterococci, HACEK organisms, fungi. Vegetations are more commonly located on the mitral valve (41%), followed by the aortic valve (38%). The clinical presentation encompasses a broad spectrum of symptoms: fever, chills, weakness, dyspnea, cough and edema (cause to valve regurgitation and congestive heart failure), stroke and chest pain (cause to septic embolization). Signs must be find for the definition of IE with the modified Duke Criteria [25].

TTE imaging can characterize vegetations with sensitivity in the range of 90-100% and specificity of 90%, but in some cases TEE is necessary [25, 96]. One of the principal pathogenetic aspects of IE is the prior presence of non-bacterial thrombotic endocarditis (NBTE) characterized by endothelial disruption, platelet and fibrin deposition especially in points of cardiac structural abnormality that represent a nidus for subsequent adhesion by bacteria or fungi in the bloodstream.

NBTE or Marantic Endocarditis refers to the presence of sterile vegetations on the heart valves that are composed of an amorphous mixture of platelets and fibrin. Other than being susceptible to infections, these lesions can cause cardiac symptomatology or embolize to the pulmonary and systemic circulation (spleen, kidney, brain, coronary arteries). The diagnosis is more likely reached with TEE than with TTE [97–99].

Rheumatoid Nodules

Cardiac involvement in rheumatoid diseases is not uncommon, especially in rheumatoid arthritis [100]. In most cases, the involvement consists of non-specific inflammatory changes and specific granuloma formation that usually affects the pericardium. Specific rheumatoid nodules in the heart are not frequent, but there are cases reporting their localization also on the aortic valve and causing regurgitation and heart failure [100, 101]. Vegetations are more common in patients with systemic lupus erythematosus or primary antiphospholipid antibody syndrome and are called Libman-Sacks vegetations, usually evaluated with TEE [102]. These lesions are of variable shape and size, generally of soft tissue and located predominantly on the vessel side of aortic cusps. They have irregular borders, heterogeneous echogenicity and can complicate with thrombus and embolism or IE.

Conclusion

Although aortic valve tumors are rare, mainly benign and often asymptomatic, they may have severe clinical consequences because of embolic or obstructive phenomena, thus requiring surgical excision. Malignant primary tumors are only exceptionally reported and are mainly represented by sarcomas. The aortic valve can also present tumor-like lesions or pseudo-tumors, including thrombi, Lambl's excrescences and endocarditic vegetations. Even though TEE represents the main diagnostic tool and CT and CMR can add useful information about tumor size, shape, location and characteristics, definitive and differential diagnoses require histology.

References

[1] Burke A. Primary malignant cardiac tumors. *Semin Diagn Pathol*. 2008;25:39–46.
[2] Bruce CJ. Cardiac tumours: Diagnosis and management. *Heart.* 2011;97:151–60.
[3] Al-Mamgani A, Baartman L, Baaijens M, De Pree I, Incrocci L, Levendag PC. Cardiac metastases. *Int J Clin Oncol*. 2008;13:369–72.
[4] Edwards FH, Hale D, Cohen A, Thompson L, Pezzella AT, Virmani R. Primary cardiac valve tumors. Ann Thorac Surg [Internet]. *The Society of Thoracic Surgeons*; 1991;52:1127–31. Available from: http://dx.doi.org/10.1016/0003-4975(91)91293-5.
[5] Travis W, Brambilla E, Burke A, Marx A, Nicholson A, editors. WHO classification of the tumours of the lung, pleura, thymus and heart. 4th ed. Lyon, France: International agency for research on cancer; 2015.
[6] Li T, Liu C, Luo Y, Gong S, Xiao Y, Wang X, et al. Retrospective analysis of 11 cases of primary cardiac valve tumors. *Anatol J Cardiol*. 2019;21:11–7.
[7] Huang Z, Sun L, Du M, Ruan Y, Wang H. Primary Cardiac Valve Tumors: Early and Late Results of Surgical Treatment in 10 Patients. *Ann Thorac Surg*. 2003;76:1609–13.
[8] Ikegami H, Andrei AC, Li Z, McCarthy PM, Malairie SC. Papillary Fibroelastoma of the Aortic Valve: Analysis of 21 Cases, Including a Presentation with Cardiac Arrest. *Texas Hear Inst J*. 2015;42:131–5.
[9] Gowda RM, Khan IA, Nair CK, Mehta NJ, Vasavada BC, Sacchi TJ. Cardiac papillary fibroelastoma: A comprehensive analysis of 725 cases. *Am Heart J.* 2003;146:404–10.
[10] Duarte Rodrigues J, Ferreira J, Almeida J, Campelo M, Júlia M, Pinho P. Cardiac papillary fibroelastoma : Report of a surgical series. Rev Port Cardiol [Internet]. *Sociedade Portuguesa de Cardiologia;* 2019; 37:981–6.
[11] Saxena P, Lee A, Konstantinov IE, Newman MAJ. Papillary Fibroelastoma of Aortic Valve: Diagnosis and Surgical Management. *Hear Lung Circ*. 2008;17:349–51.
[12] Darvishian F, Farmer P. Papillary fibroelastoma of the heart: Report of two cases and review of the literature. *Ann Clin Lab Sci.* 2001;31:291–6.
[13] Tamin SS, Maleszewski JJ, Scott CG, Khan SK, Edwards WD, Bruce CJ, et al. Prognostic and bioepidemiologic implications of papillary fibroelastomas. *J Am Coll Cardiol* [Internet]. Elsevier Inc; 2015; 65:2420–9.
[14] Iqbal I, Ullah W, Khan MAA, Haq S, Cheema A. A Case of Fibroelastoma with Widespread Embolism to the Brain, Kidney, and Spleen. *Cureus*. 2019;11:1–9.

[15] Maludum O, Ugoeke N, Mahida H, Ajam F. Papillary fi broelastoma on the aortic valve presenting as multiple cardiac arrests from electrical storm due to ischemia in patient without previous cardiac history. *Hear Rhythm Case Reports* [Internet]. Elsevier Inc.; 2018;5:134–7.

[16] Eftekhari H, Islam A, Slawsky M. Aortic valve fibroelastoma presenting with myocardial infarction. *Catheter Cardiovasc Interv*. 2011;77:716–9.

[17] Logan N, Islam MS, Chughtai JZ, Murphy NF. An atypical cause of myocardial infarction: Case report of an obstructing papillary fibroelastoma of the aortic valve. *Eur Hear J - Case Reports*. 2019;3:1–5.

[18] Kolek M, Dvorackova J, Motyka O, Brat R. Cardiac papillary fibroelastomas: A 10-year single-center surgical experience and long-term echocardiographic follow-up study. *Biomed Pap. Biomedical Papers*; 2019;164:84–91.

[19] Zull DN, Diamond M, Beringer D. Angina and sudden death resulting from papillary fibroelastoma of the aortic valve. *Ann Emerg Med*. 1985;14:470–3.

[20] Kanarek SE, Wright P, Liu J, Boglioli LR, Bajwa AS, Hall M, et al. Multiple fibroelastomas: A case report and review of the literature. *J Am Soc Echocardiogr*. 2003;16:373–6.

[21] Rana BS, Monaghan MJ, Ring L, Shapiro LS, Nihoyannopoulos P. The pivotal role of echocardiography in cardiac sources of embolism. *Eur J Echocardiogr.* 2011. p. 25–31.

[22] Karaağaç A, Olsun A, Can T, Yeşilkaya MI, Kaplan M. An aortic valve papillary fibroelastoma: A case report. *Turkish J Thorac Cardiovasc Surg*. 2018;26:146–9.

[23] Jha NK, Khouri M, Murphy DM, Salustri A, Khan JA, Saleh MA, et al. Papillary fibroelastoma of the aortic valve - a case report and literature review. *J Cardiothorac Surg* [Internet]. BioMed Central Ltd; 2010;5:84.

[24] Han J, Xiang H, Ridley WE, Ridley LJ. Anemone appearance : Papillary fibroelastoma Journal of Medical Imaging and Radiation Oncology. *J Med Imaging Radiat Oncol.* 2018;62:2018.

[25] Mann DL, Zipes DP, Libby P, Bonow RO, Braunwald E. Braunwald's heart disease: A textbook of cardiovascular medicine. Tenth. Braunwald's Hear. Dis. A Textb. Cardiovasc. Med. Philadelphia: Elsevier/Saunders; 2015.

[26] Kumbala D, Sharp T, Kamalesh M. "Perilous pearl" - Papillary fibroelastoma of aortic valve: A case report and literature review. *Angiology.* 2008;59:625–8.

[27] Taha ME, Kumaresan J. Aortic Valve Papillary Fibroelastoma: A Sea Anemone in the Heart, A Case Report. *Cardiol Res.* 2019;10:378–81.

[28] Yamamoto S, Fuchimoto K, Tanaka A, Matsumoto M, Yamamoto T. Papillary fibroelastoma of the aortic valve: Report of a Case. Surg Today. 2002;32:354–8.

[29] Mignogna C, Amorosi A, Mastroroberto P. Sea Anemone Tumor: Macroscopic Diagnosis of Cardiac Papillary Fibroelastoma. *Int J Surg Pathol* [Internet]. 2019;27:185–6.

[30] Chu A, Aung TT, Sahalon H, Choksi V, Feiz H. Lambl's excrescence associated with cryptogenic stroke: A case report and literature review. *Am J Case Rep*. 2015;16:876–81.

[31] Gorlach G, Hagel K, Mulchl J, Scheld H, Moosdorf R, Fitz H, et al. Myxoma of the aortic valve in a child. *J Cardiovasc Surg*. 1986;6:679–80.

[32] Espinosa-Queb NN, Luna-Sánchez JA, Revilla-Casaos H, Domínguez-Rodríguez JA, Lara-Valdés ÁJ, Tarelo-Saucedo JM. Aortic valve myxoma. Systematic review and a new case report. Cirugia Cardiovascular. 2019;26:283–8.

[33] Zumer-Meulenbelt A, Deleuze P, Lefort J, Perchet H, Vaury P, Fischer M, et al. Aortic valve myxoma: conservative valvular surgery. *Arch Mal Coeur Vaiss.* 1999;92: 1515–8.

[34] Dyk W, Konka M. Unusual Complication of Aortic Valve Grape-Like Myxoma. *Ann Thorac Surg.* 2009;88:1022.

[35] Kim HY, Kwon SU, Jang WI, Kim HS, Kim JS, Lee HS, et al. A rare case of aortic valve myxoma: Easy to confuse with papillary fibroelastoma. *Korean Circ J.* 2012;42:281–3.

[36] Prifti E, Ademaj F, Kajo E, Baboci A. A giant myxoma originating from the aortic valve causing severe left ventricular tract obstruction: A case report and literature review. *World J Surg Oncol.* 2015;13:4–7.

[37] Changwe GJ, Zhang T, Zhang H, Zou C. Non-syndromic aortic valve myxoma in a teen, cause of angina symptoms. *J Cardiothorac Surg.* 2019;14:4–6.

[38] Watarida S, Katsuyama K, Yasuda R, Magara T, Onoe M, Nojima T, et al. Myxoma of the aortic valve. *Ann Thorac Surg.* 1997;63:234–6.

[39] Laguna G, Carrascal Y, Arce N, Martínez G. Incidental aortic valve myxoma: Tumour excision and aortic valve repair. *Eur J Cardio-thoracic Surg.* 2015;48:510–1.

[40] Vaideeswar P, Butany JW. Benign cardiac tumors of the pluripotent mesenchyme. *Semin Diagn Pathol.* 2008;25:20–8.

[41] Koyalakonda SP, Mediratta NK, Ball J, Royle M. A rare case of aortic valve myxoma: An unusual cause of embolic stroke. *Cardiology.* 2011;118:101–3.

[42] Mankad R, Herrmann J. Cardiac tumors: Echo assessment. *Echo Res Pract.* 2016;3:R65–77.

[43] Ramsheyi A, Deleuze P, Attelis N, Bical O, Lefort JF. Aortic valve myxoma. *J Card Surg.* 1998;13:491–3.

[44] Fernández AL, Vega M, El-Diasty MM, Suárez JM. Myxoma of the aortic valve. *Interact Cardiovasc Thorac Surg.* 2012;15:560–2.

[45] Alkuwaiti FA, Elghoneimy Y, Ghazal S. Aortic valve Myxoma presenting with a stroke: A case report and review of the literature. *Sultan Qaboos Univ Med J.* 2018;18:e537–40.

[46] Kennedy P, Parry AJ, Parums D, Pillai R. Myxoma of the aortic valve. *Ann Thorac Surg.* 1995;59:1221–3.

[47] Javed A, Zalawadiya S, Kovach J, Afonso L. Aortic valve myxoma at the extreme age: A review of literature. *BMJ Case Rep.* 2014;2013–5.

[48] Liddy S, McQuade C, Walsh KP, Loo B, Buckley O. The Assessment of Cardiac Masses by Cardiac CT and CMR Including Pre-op 3D Reconstruction and Planning. *Curr Cardiol Rep.* 2019;21(9):103.

[49] Okamoto T, Doi H, Kazui T, Suzuki M, Koshima R, Yamashita T, et al. Aortic valve myxoma mimicking vegetation: Report of a case. *Surg Today.* 2006;36:927–9.

[50] Pucci A, Gagliardotto P, Zanini C, Pansini S, Di Summa M, Mollo F. Histopathologic and clinical characterization of cardiac myxoma: Review of 53 cases from a single institution. *Am Heart J.* 2000;140:134–8.

[51] Bianchi G, Margaryan R, Kallushi E, Cerillo AG, Farneti PA, Pucci A, et al. Outcomes of Video-assisted Minimally Invasive Cardiac Myxoma Resection. *Heart Lung Circ.* 2019; 28:327–33.

[52] Pucci A, Mattioli C, Matteucci M, Lorenzini D, Panvini F, Pacini S, et al. Cell differentiation in cardiac myxomas: confocal microscopy and gene expression analysis after laser capture microdissection. *Heart Vessels.* 2018; 33:1403–10.

[53] Aziz F, Baciewicz FA. Lambl's excrescences: Review and recommendations. *Texas Hear Inst J.* 2007;34:366–8.

[54] Zhu Y, Zhang X, Guan X, Wang L. Collagenous fibroma of the right coronary cusp: A case report and literature review. *Echocardiography.* 2015;32:390–2.

[55] Pucci A, Botta G, Sina N, Tibaldi M, Valori A, Grosso E, et al. Life-threatening tumors of the heart in fetal and postnatal age. *J Pediatr.* 2013; 162:964-969.

[56] Fukunaga M, Ushigome S. Collagenous Fibroma (Desmoplastic Fibroelastoma): A Distinctive Fibroblastic Soft Tissue Tumor. *Adv Anat Pathol.* 1999;6:275–80.

[57] Li W, Teng P, Xu H, Ma L, Ni Y. Cardiac hemangioma: A comprehensive analysis of 200 cases. *Ann Thorac Surg.* 2015;99:2246–52.

[58] Vivirito M, Boldorini R, Rossi L, Caimmi PP, Bernardi M, Teodori G. Capillary hemangioma of the aortic valve: False preoperative diagnosis of endocarditis. *J Thorac Cardiovasc Surg.* 2006;132:690–1.

[59] Cotier P, Bruneval P, Amemiya K. Vascular malformation in a bicuspid aortic valve. *Cardiovasc Pathol.* 2019; 38:39–41.

[60] van Broekhoven A, Krijnen PAJ, Niessen HWM, Vonk ABA. Hemangioma of the Atherosclerotic Changed Aortic Valve. *Case Reports Cardiol.* 2019;2019:1–4.

[61] Val-Bernal JF, Cuadrado M, Garijo MF, Revuelta JM. Incidental in vivo detection of an isolated hemangioma of the aortic valve in a man with a history of renal transplantation. *Virchows Arch.* 2006;449:121–3.

[62] Cotran R, Kumar V, Robbins S, Abbas AK, Aster JC. *Robbins and Cotran pathologic basis of disease.* Philadelphia, PA Saunders, Ipswich, MA. 2015.

[63] Eilers AL, Nazarullah AN, Shipper ES, Jagirdar JS, Calhoon JH, Husain SA. Cardiac Inflammatory Myofibroblastic Tumor: A Comprehensive Review of the Literature. *World J Pediatr Congenit Hear Surg.* 2014;5:556–64.

[64] Butany J, Dixit V, Leong SW, Daniel LB, Mezody M, David TE. Inflammatory myofibroblastic tumor with valvular involvement: a case report and review of the literature. *Cardiovasc Pathol.* 2007;16:359–64.

[65] Li L, Burke A, He J, Chang L, Zielke HR, Fowler DR. Sudden unexpected death due to inflammatory myofibroblastic tumor of the heart: A case report and review of the literature. *Int J Legal Med.* 2011;125:81–5.

[66] Leone O, Veinot JP, Angelini A, Baandrup UT, Basso C, Berry G, et al. 2011 Consensus statement on endomyocardial biopsy from the Association for European Cardiovascular Pathology and the Society for Cardiovascular Pathology. *Cardiovasc* Pathol. 2012;21:245–74.

[67] De Martino A, Del Re F, Barzaghi C, Bortolotti U, Papi L, Pucci A. Occult primary cardiac lymphomas causing unexpected/sudden death or acute heart failure. *Virchows Arch.* 2020;1–5.

[68] Ramos RB, Branco LM, Galrinho AI, Cunha J, Oliveira MF, Fragata J, et al. Primary Undifferentiated Sarcoma of the Mitral and Aortic Valves. *J Heart Valve Dis.* 2008;17:348–51.

[69] Pucci A, De Martino A, Levantino M, Berchiolli R, Basolo F, Bortolotti U. Intimal sarcoma of the descending aorta mimicking aortitis. *Aorta.* 2016;4:142–5.

[70] Restrepo CS, Betancourt SL, Martinez-Jimenez S, Gutierrez FR. Tumors of the Pulmonary Artery and Veins. *Semin Ultrasound.* 2012;33:580–90.

[71] Okoro KU, Roby MD, Sane DC, Budin RE. Infiltrating Cardiac Synovial Sarcoma Presenting as Acute Cerebrovascular Accident. *Case Rep Med.* 2017;2017:11–4.

[72] Talukder M, Joyce L, Marks R, Kaplan K. Primary cardiac synovial sarcoma. Interact *Cardiovasc Thorac Surg.* 2010;11:490–2.

[73] Lange S, Kremer J, Schenone A, Shultze M, Van Tine B. Current Management and Molecular Targets of Synovial Sarcoma. *Austin J Cancer Clin Res.* 2014;1:1–9.

[74] Shirani S, Soleymanzadeh-Ardabili M, Arami M. Intimal sarcoma of the descending aorta. *Arch Iran Med.* 2007;10:253–4.

[75] Roberts WC, Glancy DL, Devita VT. Heart in malignant lymphoma (Hodgkin's disease, lymphosarcoma, reticulum cell sarcoma and mycosis fungoides). A study of 196 autopsy cases. *Am J Cardiol.* 1968;22:85–107.

[76] McDonnell PJ, Mann RB, Bulkley BH. Involvement of the heart by malignant lymphoma: a clinicopathologic study. Cancer. 1982; 49:944-951.

[77] Lin YS, Chu PH, Kuo MC, Jung SM, Lim KE, Kuo CT, et al. Use of a B-type natriuretic peptide in evaluating the treatment response of a relapsed lymphoma with cardiac involvement. *Int J Hematol.* 2006;83:44–6.

[78] Yazar O, Muyldermans T, Mees U, Achten R, Geukens R, Hendrikx M. Aortic valve lymphoma presenting as acute coronary syndrome. *J Heart Valve Dis.* 2008;17:130–2.

[79] Bagwan IN, Desai S, Wotherspoon A, Sheppard MN. Unusual presentation of primary cardiac lymphoma. *Interact Cardiovasc Thorac Surg.* 2009;9:127–9.

[80] Dürrleman NM, El-Hamamsy I, Demaria RG, Carrier M, Perrault LP, Albat B. Cardiac lymphoma following mitral valve replacement. *Ann Thorac Surg.* 2005;79:1040–2.

[81] Burke A, Tavora F. The 2015 WHO Classification of tumors of the heart and pericardium. *J. Thorac. Oncol.* 2016.

[82] Miguel CE, Bestetti RB. Primary cardiac lymphoma. *Int J Cardiol.* 2011; 149:358–63.

[83] Carras S, Berger F, Chalabreysse L, Callet-Bauchut E, Cordier JF, Salles G, et al. Primary cardiac lymphoma: diagnosis, treatment and outcome in a modern series. *Hematol Oncol.* 2017;35:510–9.

[84] Oliveira GH, Al-Kindi SG, Hoimes C, Park SJ. Characteristics and survival of malignant cardiac tumors a 40-year analysis of >500 patients. *Circulation.* 2015;132:2395–402.

[85] Burazor I, Aviel-Ronen S, Imazio M, Goitein O, Perelman M, Shelestovich N, et al. Metastatic cardiac tumors: From clinical presentation through diagnosis to treatment. *BMC Cancer*; 2018; 18:1–9.

[86] Goldberg AD, Blankstein R, Padera RF. Tumors metastatic to the heart. *Circulation.* 2013;128:1790–4.

[87] Reynen K, Köckeritz U, Strasser RH. Metastases to the heart. *Ann Oncol.* 2004;15:375–81.

[88] Bussani R, De-Giorgio F, Abbate A, Silvestri F. Cardiac metastases. *J Clin Pathol.* 2007;60:27–34.

[89] Yuan S-M, Jing H, Lavee J. Tumors and tumor-like lesions of the heart valves. *Rare Tumors.* 2009;1:105–9.

[90] Ammannaya GKK. Lambl's Excrescences: Current Diagnosis and Management. *Cardiol Res.* 2019;10:207–10.

[91] Wada T, Miyamoto S, Anai H, Zaizen H, Hadama T. Aortic valve lipomatous hamartoma in a young woman. *Japanese J Thorac Cardiovasc Surg.* 2005;53:577–9.

[92] Rona G, Feeney N, Kahn DS. Fibroelastic hamartoma of the aortic valve producing ischemic heart disease. *Am J Cardiol.* 1963;12:869–74.

[93] De Martino A, Blasi S, Lorenzini D, Fornaro M, Basolo F, Bortolotti U, Pucci A. Lipomatous hamartoma-like lesion of a bicuspid aortic valve: an incidental surgical finding. *Cardiovasc Pathol.* 2016; 25:500–2.

[94] Boyd TAB. Blood cysts on the heart valves of infants. *Am J Pathol.* 1949;25:757–9.

[95] DeGroff C, Silberbach M, Sahn DJ, Droukas P. Giant blood cyst of the aortic valve. *J Am Soc Echocardiogr.* 1995;8:543–5.

[96] Stewart JA, Silimperi D, Harris P, Wise NK, Fraker TD, Kisslo JA. Echocardiographic documentation of vegetative lesions in infective endocarditis: Clinical implications. *Circulation.* 1980;61:374–80.

[97] Young RSK, Zalneraitis EL. Marantic endocarditis in children and young adults: Clinical and pathological findings. *Stroke.* 1981;12:635.

[98] Borowski A, Ghodsizad A, Cohnen M, Gams E. Recurrent embolism in the course of marantic endocarditis. *Ann Thorac Surg.* 2005;79:2145–7.

[99] Salzberg SP, Nemirovsky D, Goldman ME, Adams DH. Aortic Valve Vegetation Without Endocarditis. *Ann Thorac Surg.* 2009; 88:267–9.

[100] Chand EM, Freant LJ, Rubin JW. Aortic valve rheumatoid nodules producing clinical aortic regurgitation and a review of the literature. *Cardiovasc Pathol.* 1999;8:333–8.

[101] Roldan CA, DeLong C, Qualls CR, Crawford MH. Characterization of Valvular Heart Disease in Rheumatoid Arthritis by Transesophageal Echocardiography and Clinical Correlates. *Am J Cardiol.* 2007;100:496–502.

[102] Roldan CA, Shively BK, Crawford MH. An echocardiographic study of valvular heart disease associated with systemic lupus erythematosus. *N Engl J Med.* 1996;335:1424–30.

In: Perspectives in Aortic Valve Disease
Editor: Giovanni Concistrè
ISBN: 978-1-53618-769-4

Chapter 8

AORTIC ROOT INVOLVEMENT IN CONGENITAL HEART DEFECTS: SPECIAL SURGICAL TOPICS

Vitali Pak, Elisa Barberi and Duccio Federici*
Pediatric Cardiac Surgery, Heart Hospital,
Monasterio Foundation, Massa, Italy

ABSTRACT

The aortic root can be involved in many complex congenital heart diseases. Valvular anomalies, along with structural diseases of the aortic root, can present themselves as integral part of the congenital defect or might be the expression of secondary injury starting from another cardiac lesion. In this chapter we wish to describe three conditions in which structural and functional anomalies of the aortic root imply special surgical considerations. Aortic regurgitation secondary to restrictive ventricular septal defect, aortic valve anomaly in the setting of Truncus Arteriosus and the Aortico-Left Ventricular Tunnel are here elucidated in terms of pathophysiology, clinical picture and surgical management. Surgical results, long-term outcomes and current perspectives of each of these conditions are provided according to the most recent literature.

Keywords: congenital aortic disease, aortic regurgitation, ventricular septal defect, truncus arteriosus, aortic-left ventricular tunnel

TRUNCUS ARTERIOSUS AND TRUNCAL VALVE REGURGITATION

Vitali Pak

Introduction

Anatomy and Classification

Truncus arteriosus accounts for fewer than 3% of all congenital heart defects. Truncus arteriosus is an anomaly of the conotruncus and characterized by the presence of one vessel

* Corresponding Author's Email: federici@ftgm.it.

arises from the base of both ventricles with single truncal valve, a high large subarterial ventricular septal defect and by the origination of the pulmonary arteries from the truncus.

Anatomy of the truncus arteriosus includes description of the origin of the pulmonary arteries, type of ventricular septal defect, morphology of truncal valve, pathway of the coronary arteries and associated malformation. There are two classification systems in use: one from Collett and Edwards and another from Van Praagh and Van Praagh. (Figure 1). Collett and Edwards divide truncus arteriosus in types I–IV. In type I a short main pulmonary artery arise from the truncus and then bifurcates into a right and left pulmonary artery. In type II the right and left pulmonary artery arise as separate orifices from posterior aspect of the truncus. In type III the right and left pulmonary artery arise from the opposite sides of the truncus. In type IV there is no main pulmonary artery and the lungs are supplied by aortopulmonary collaterals [1, 2].

Van Praagh and Van Praagh divide truncus arteriosus according to the existence or absence of the conotruncal septum and define type A as cases with and type B as cases without ventricular septal defect. In type A1 a common origin of pulmonary arteries from the truncus. In type A2 two separate right and left branch pulmonary arteries from the dorsal truncus. In type A3 only one branch pulmonary artery arises from the truncus, the other orginates from a ductus-like structure from the aortic arch. Type A4, the truncus continues via a ductus arteriosus into the descending aorta. The right and left pulmonary arteries come off the truncus before the ductus. The ascending aorta is small. It appears to arise from the main pulmonary artery. The aortic arch is interrupted [1, 2].

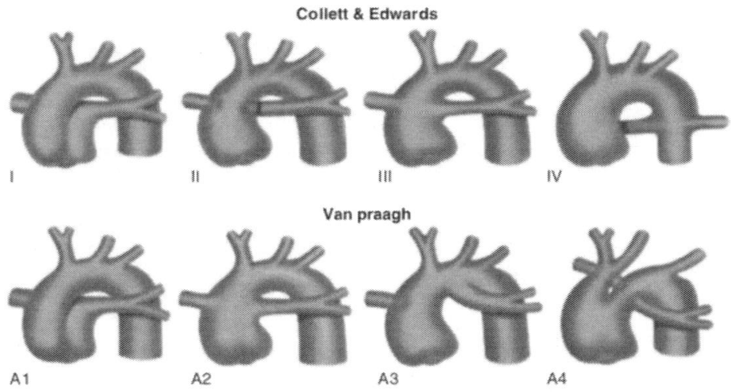

Figure 1. Truncus arteriosus classifications.

Most commonly an intermediate type of these two forms (type I-II and type A1-A2) is found and the central and peripheral pulmonary arteries are well developed without stenosis in most clinical cases. Another more practical classification of truncus arteriosus include three types: truncus arteriosus with confluent pulmonary arteries, truncus arteriosus with absence of one pulmonary artery and truncus arteriosus with associated interrupted aortic arch or aortic coarctation.

The ventricular septal defect in truncus arteriosus is located usually under the truncus and usually separated from the tricuspid valve by the posterior limb of the septal band. Two types of arrangement can be seen posteriorly. In approximately 80% of patients with truncus arteriosus, the posterior margin of the defect is muscular, completely separated from the anterior leaflet of the tricuspid valve (infundibular subarterial defect), so that risk of complete heart block at the time of surgical closure is small. The other 20% of patients have a perimembranous infundibular defect, the posterior margin of which extends back to the anterior leaflet of the tricuspid valve. In rare cases, when the ventricular septal defect is very small, closure can create left ventricular outflow tract obstruction [3, 4].

Often the origin of the coronary arteries is abnormal, there is wide variability of coronary arterial ostial location, number, angle of takeoff and degree of patency.

Lenox et al. published a high incidence of coronary ostial and arterial abnormalities in a study of 30 pathologic specimens of truncus arteriosus. They found following types of abnormalities: left coronary ostium in a posterior and high position; close relation of the left coronary ostium to the pulmonary artery segment in three-leaflet truncal valves; stenosis of the coronary ostium or the location of the ostium above or in a commissure; the acute angle takeoff of the coronary artery; the position of the left anterior descending artery as it courses posteriorly and close to the truncal wall; the size and course of the conal and diagonal arteries from the right coronary artery across the right ventricular outflow area; a single coronary artery or ostium with branches crossing the right ventricle below the truncus, the circumflex arising from the right coronary artery and coursing behind the truncus, and the right coronary artery originating from the left anterior descending artery. The ostial location of the coronary arteries can be located very close to the truncal valve commissures and to the origins of the right and left pulmonary arteries [5]. There are usually two coronary arteries, but a single coronary artery is not uncommon. Sometimes the left coronary artery originates high from the posterior wall of the truncus [3]. Although the distal branching of the coronary arteries is usually normal. The anomalous anterior descending coronary artery can originate from the right coronary artery and run across the infundibulum of the right ventricle, like in tetralogy of Fallot [6, 7, 8, 11]. Surgeons should keep in mind that the coronary arteries can be located essentially anywhere around the truncal root.

The aortic arch is left-sided in about 60%, right-sided in about 25-30% and interrupted in about 10%-15% of cases of persistent truncus arteriosus. The interruption is usually of type B (interruption distal to the origin of the left carotid artery). In up to 90% of patients with truncus arteriosus, a DiGeorge syndrome can be found [9, 10].

Truncal Valve

The truncal valve has a variable number of leaflets and variable morphology. The number of cusps varies from two to six. Rarely there are more than four individual cusps [2]. The truncal valve is tricuspid in approximately 50%, bicuspid in about 30% and quadricuspid in about 15 – 20% of cases of persistent truncus arteriosus. In exceptional cases, the valve is unicuspid. Various degrees of truncal valve dysplasia with abnormal leaflets and inadequate commissural support are often present, resulting in important truncal valve regurgitation. It is rare for a truncal valve to be structurally stenotic. There is always continuity between the truncal valve and the mitral valve. The truncal valve overrides the ventricular septal defect and relates equally to the two ventricles in about 50% of cases. In the other cases, the truncal valve originates predominantly from the right ventricle but in some instances from the left ventricle [1, 3].

Methods

Surgical Repair of Truncal Valve Regurgitation

Truncal valve regurgitation remains a challenging problem and estimated to occur in 25–50% of patients with truncus arteriosus.

The presence of truncal valve regurgitation usually evaluate by preoperative transthoracic echocardiography and colour Doppler imaging using standard echocardiographic criteria, including M-mode assessment of left ventricular function, diastolic flow reversal in the descending aorta (mild = brief diastolic reversal flow; moderate = intermediate diastolic reversal flow; severe = holodiastolic reversal flow), colour-flow regurgitant jet size (mild = small central jet <25% of left outflow tract; moderate = intermediate jet greater than mild but no signs of severe; severe = large central jet >65% of left outflow tract) and measurements of the truncal regurgitant jet width: annulus ratio (mild < 25; moderate = 25–64; severe ≥65).[15]. Traditional strategies for the operative management of these patients have included temporization of this problem or attempts at valve replacement with a homograft valve or a mechanical prosthesis. However, none of these options have been shown to be very successful or desirable. Thus, repair of the moderate or severe regurgitant truncal valve constitutes the optimal surgical strategy, particularly in the neonatal period [12, 13].

The significant regurgitant truncal valve is almost always amenable to various repair techniques. The reported techniques can be summarized as approximation, resection, or extension of the leaflets, remodeling of the valvar support, and external annuloplasty and etc. In this chapter we try to describe the techniques of surgical repair of the truncal valve insufficiency currently used by pediatric cardiac surgeons.

In case when regurgitation of truncal valve seemed to be peripheral at the commissures can be used a commissuroplasty, as described by Trusler, to suspend a prolapsed cusp (Figure 2) [14].

Naimo et al. describe a subcommissural annuloplasty in patients with a large truncal valve annulus and relatively normal leaflets by placement of 5-0 Ti-Cron (Medtronic, Minneapolis, MN, USA) sutures pledgeted with autologous pericardium to the subcommissural region of the truncal valve. If the sino-tubular junction and annulus were dilated, they were also plicated with a full-thickness pledgeted suture. (Figure 3) [15]. Another technique can be used is the approximation technique, based on the fact that many patients will have a quadricuspide valve. The valve can be converted to a trileaflet or bileaflet structure by approximating one or two of the cusps (Figure 4) [16].

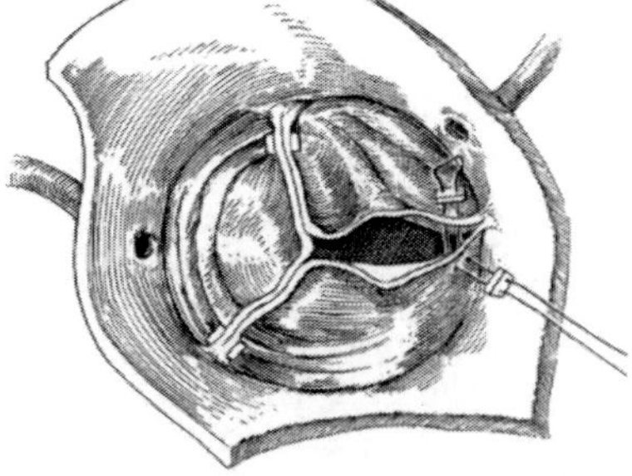

Figure 2. Commissuroplasty and commissural suspension performed for prolapsing leaflet.

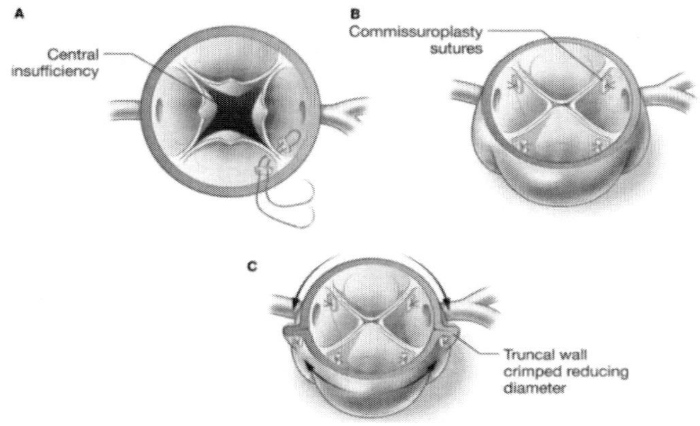

Figure 3. Subcommissural annuloplasty.

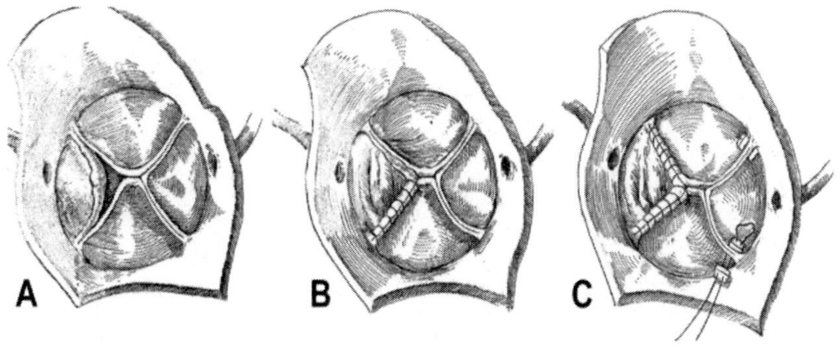

Figure 4. Approximation of the leaflets for correction of truncal valvar insufficiency. (A) Quadricuspid truncal valve with a deficient leaflet. (B) Repair is accomplished using leaflet union to create either a tricuspid or bicuspid valve. (C) Additional commissuroplasty sutures are utilized as needed to provide additional support at the commissural posts.

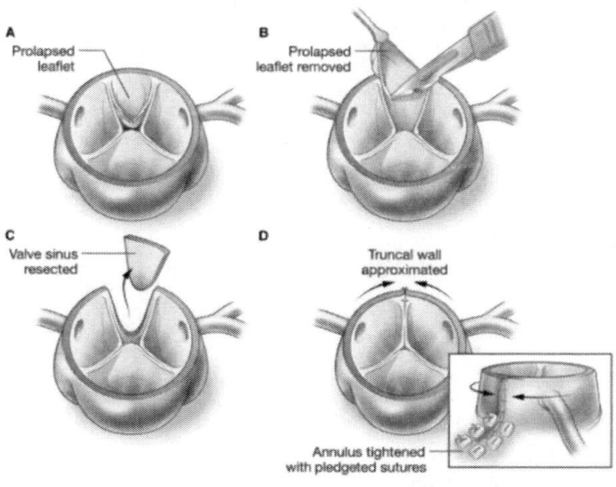

Figure 5. Cusp resection and annular reduction. (A) The quadrileaflet truncal valve with one prolapsed leaflet. (B) Resection and remove of the smaller of the four leaflets (C) Resection of the truncal valve sinus. (D) Remodelling of the annular support with pledget-based sutures to reduce the diameter of the outflow tract. The truncal wall is closed with running polypropylene suture in two layers.

Imamura et al. described other technique to resect the leaflets with tricuspidisation of a quadricuspid truncal valve. The smallest/incompetent leaflet is excised, along with the corresponding segment of the annulus. The remaining annular edges are sutured together to approximate the size of the ascending aorta (Figure 5) [17].

The same procedure performed in a patient in whom the prolapsing small leaflet arises from a truncal sinus that gives rise to a coronary artery (Figure 6).

Those working at the Cleveland Clinic have also reported a valvoplasty technique for insufficient aortic valves but this type of repair is suitable even in case of truncal valve insufficiency with presence of one prolapsed cuspid. They performed surgery on 28 patients, threequarters with bifoliate valves. They carried out triangular resection of the free edge of the prolapsing leaflet, coupled with plication of the peripheral attachments of the zones of apposition between the leaflets at the sinutubular junction (Figure 7) [18].

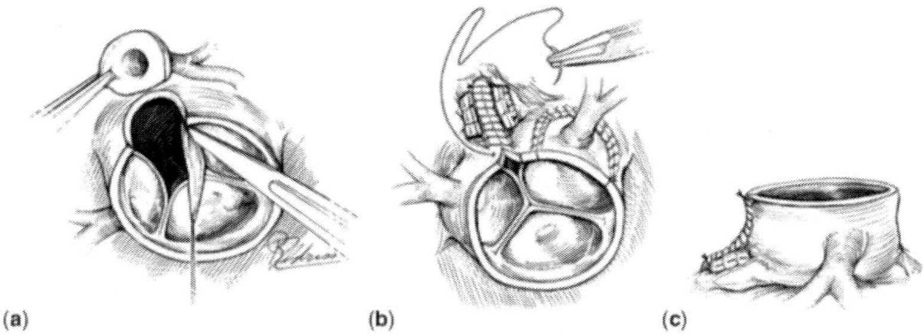

Figure 6. (a) A coronary arterial button has been excised, and the leaflet being removed. (b) The coronary arterial button has been reimplanted into the adjacent sinus of the truncal root. The annular support of the leaflets has been remodeled with pledget-supported sutures, and the truncal wall is being closed. (c) The completed result.

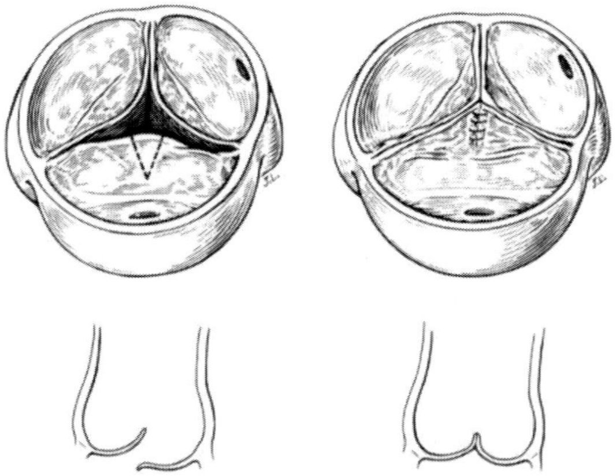

Figure 7. Aortic valvoplasty technique. Upper panel, a triangular shaped wedge of the prolapsed leaflet is excised (dashed lines). The leaflet is then reapproximated with interrupted polypropylene suture. The left lower panel shows the prolapsed leaflet, causing aortic insufficiency, which is then corrected by the wedge resection, resulting in a competent valve (right lower panel).

In some cases when insufficiency of the truncal valve with normal anatomy of the cusps caused only by dilation of the annulus, to improve central coaptation a circumferential annuloplasty can be used. The subvalvar suture is tied over an appropriate-sized probe to aid in reduction annuloplasty (Figure 8) [16].

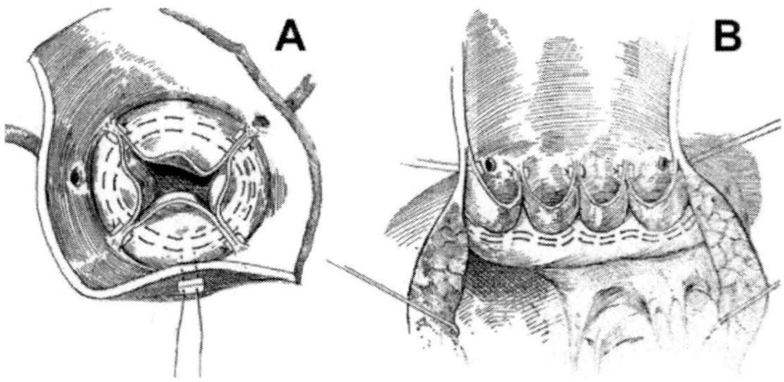

Figure 8. (A) Subvalvar annuloplasty technique. (B) Lateral view of repaired valve.

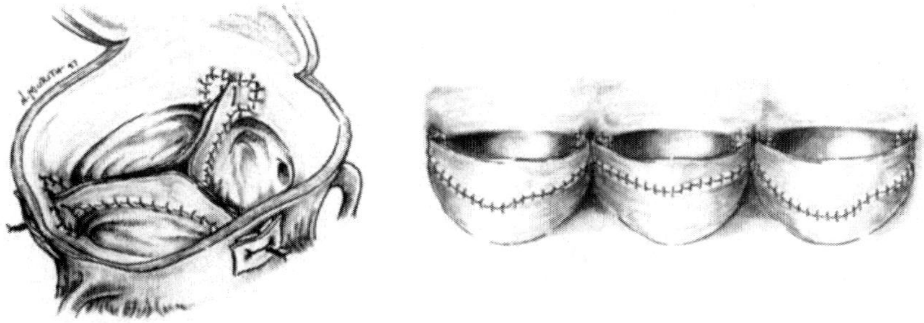

Figure 9. Surgical technique of extending aortic leaflets with fresh autologous pericardium.

Another technique of repair of the truncal valve is the extension of leaflets with pericardium was described. The principle is to utilize glutaraldehyde-preserved autologous pericardium to augment the valvar leaflets. Pericardial strips are sutured to the leading edge of the leaflets, and anchored to the aortic wall. In general, the strips are tailored so as to be slightly redundant, thus allowing approximation of the leaflets (Figure 9) [19, 20, 21].

In cases of inability to preserve the truncal valve, only unique solution is its replacement with a mechanical prosthesis or with a homograft [22, 23].

Other surgical techniques such as leaflet-base-preserving truncal valve repair with ethanol-treated autologous pericardium or aortic valve neocuspidization (Ozaki) procedure, recently been published. Until midterm results are available, however, these procedures cannot be recommended for the truncal valve repair [24, 25].

Discussion

Outcomes of Truncal Valve Surgery and Current Perspectives

Truncal valve regurgitation remains a risk factor for early and late morbidity and mortality of patients with truncus arteriosus. Previous studies have reported initial moderate or severe truncal valve insufficiency as a risk factor for truncal valve reoperation [26, 27]. A review of the Society of Thoracic Surgeons Congenital Heart Surgery Database results, reporting 572 truncus arteriosus repairs from 2000 to 2009, included 27 patients with truncal valve surgeries (23 at truncus arteriosus repair, 4 later). The mortality of truncus repair with a concomitant truncal valve procedure (30%) was significantly increased compared with controls without truncal valve surgery at truncus arteriosus repair (10%, $p = 0.0002$), while all 4 patients who had delayed truncal valve procedures died. The association of truncus arteriosus repair, IAA repair and TVR had a mortality of 60%. Postoperative mechanical circulatory support was utilized in 45 patients (7.8%) in the overall cohort, and was significantly more common in the truncal valve surgery group versus the isolated common arterial trunk repair group (18% versus 7%, $p = 0.002$). Postoperative length of stay was also longer in the common arterial trunk plus truncal valve surgery group (Table 1) [28].

The association of truncal valve insufficiency with mortality risk has been noted by multiple authors. The report by Ebert and colleagues in 1984 of 100 patients with common arterial trunk undergoing repair in the first 6 months of life revealed a mortality rate of 11%. In that series, 8 of the 11 deaths had evidence of preoperative truncal valve insufficiency; 1 patient underwent truncal valve replacement [29]. Hanley and colleagues published a series of 63 patients undergoing repair of common arterial trunk at Children's Hospital Boston. They found that severe truncal valve insufficiency before surgery was a significant risk factor for early death in both univariate and multi- variate analyses [30]. Rajasinghe and colleagues reported the long-term follow-up of patients undergoing repair of common arterial trunk in infancy and found severe truncal insufficiency to be a risk factor for late death among initial hospital survivors (n = 27, 30% mortality) [31]. Di Donato and colleagues from the Mayo Clinic found moderate or severe truncal valve regurgitation to be associated with poor long term survival in a study of 167 patients over a 17-year period (n = 62, 50% mortality) [32]. Pearl and associates at the University of California, Los Angeles, reviewed their experience of 32 patients who underwent common arterial trunk repair in infancy and similarly concluded that truncal valve insufficiency is an incremental risk factor for early and late mortality [33].

Table 1. Outcomes (CAT- common arterial trunk; IAA- interrupted aortic arch; TVS - truncal valve surgery)

	Overall (n = 572)	Isolated CAT Repair (n = 545)	CAT Repair + TVS (n = 27)	*p* Value
In-hospital mortality				
Overall	61 (11%)	53 (10%)	8 (30%)	0.0002
Without IAA repair	50 (9%)	45 (9%)	5 (23%)	0.003
With IAA repair	11 (28%)	8 (24%)	3 (60%)	0.41
Postoperative mechanical circulatory support	45 (8%)	40 (7%)	5 (18%)	0.002
Postoperative length of stay, days	16 (10–29)	15.5 (10–29)	29 (14–83)	0.02

In contrast to these reports, some recent single-center series have not shown truncal valve regurgitation to be associated with increased mortality at the time of primary repair. Bove and associates reported a series of 46 neonates undergoing repair of common arterial trunk at the University of Michigan. Five patients required truncal valve replacement, but neither truncal valve regurgitation nor truncal valve replacement was related to death. A recent report by

Hawkins and associates showed that in their institution's experience (n = 42), complex cases with truncal valve insufficiency, interrupted aortic arch, or both, were associated with greater utilization of resources but not with a higher rate of operative mortality [34].

Myers and colleagues published a series of 36 patients underwent truncal valve repair during correction of common arterial trunk at Children's Hospital Boston from 1997 to 2012. Valve repair improved regurgitation in 31 of 36 repairs (86%) and was less than moderate in 27 patients (75%) after repair. There were 3 early deaths (8%), all of which were in neonates. During a mean follow-up of 38.3 ± 44.9 months (range 1 month—15 years), there was 1 late death, 16 patients required reoperation on the truncal valve and 1 required a second reoperation. Freedom from reoperation for truncal valve insufficiency was 91.4 ± 4.8% at 1 year, 87.2 ± 6.1% at 2 years, 55.0 ± 10.4% at 5 years and 22.9 ± 12.2% at 10 years (Figure 10) [27].

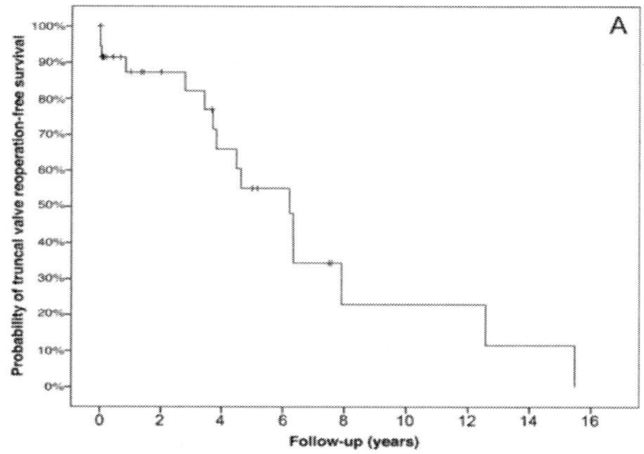

Figure 10. Kaplan–Meier estimates of freedom from truncal valve reoperation after truncal valve repair. (A-Entire cohort).

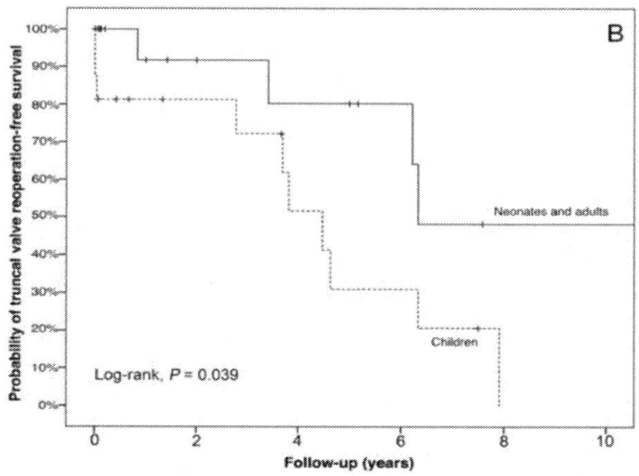

Figure 11. Kaplan–Meier estimates of freedom from truncal valve reoperation after truncal valve repair. (B-Analysis stratified by age).

In that series, 22 patients had a quadricuspid, 13 a tricuspid and 1 a bicuspid truncal valve before repair. The Kaplan–Meier survival analysis stratified by age category showed that neonates and adults had significantly more reoperations than children (P = 0.039). (Figure 11) A quadricuspid anatomy after repair tended to have worse freedom from reoperation, however, not to a significant level (P = 0.15), and tricuspidization also tended towards better freedom from reoperation (P = 0.19) (Figure 12) [27].

Similarly, Ivanov et al. found that overall freedom from truncal valve reoperation at 10 years was 83.9 ± 5.9 (95% CI 72.2–95.5). Freedom from truncal valve reoperation at 10 years in patients with initial tricuspid valve morphology was 93.8 ± 6.1 (95% CI 81.9–100.0); with a quadricuspid valve, it was 66.8 ± 11.6 (95% CI 44.1–89.5) and none of the patients with a bicuspid valve required reoperation at 8 years. Initial significant truncal valve regurgitation was associated with a later truncal valve reoperation (hazard ratio 17.2, 95% CI 2.1–145.0; P = 0.008) (Table 2) [37].

Kaza et al. reviewed their single-centre experience in truncal valve repair in 17 patients from 1995 to 2008. This study, although on a more limited number of patients, has the advantage of including 3 non-neonatal patients and follow-up data. Three patients had 1 re-repair, and 1 had 2 re-repairs before undergoing a prosthetic valve replacement at age 13 years. Freedom from reintervention on the truncal valve is 70% at 5 years and 50% at 7 years after the initial valve repair. Freedom from truncal valve replacement is 100% at 10 years (Figure 13) [35].

Table. 2. Analysis of variables for truncal valve reoperation

Variables	TrV reoperation (%)	Univariable HR (95% CI)	*P*-value
Number of TrV cusps			
2	0% (0/9)		
3	1.9% (1/52)	0.001 (0.001-2.0)	0.98
4	16.7% (6/36)	0.1 (0.01-1.0)	0.054
Significant TrV insufficiency	25% (6/24)	17.4 (2.1-145.0)	0.008

CI: confidence interval; HR: hazard ratio; TrV: truncal valve.

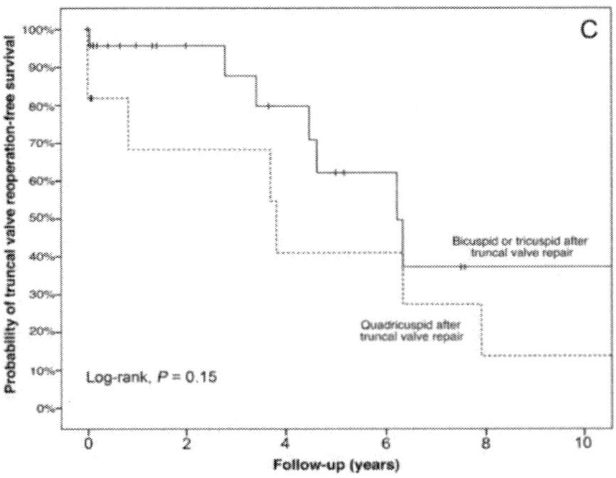

Figure 12. Kaplan–Meier estimates of freedom from truncal valve reoperation after truncal valve repair. (C- Analysis stratified by truncal valve anatomy).

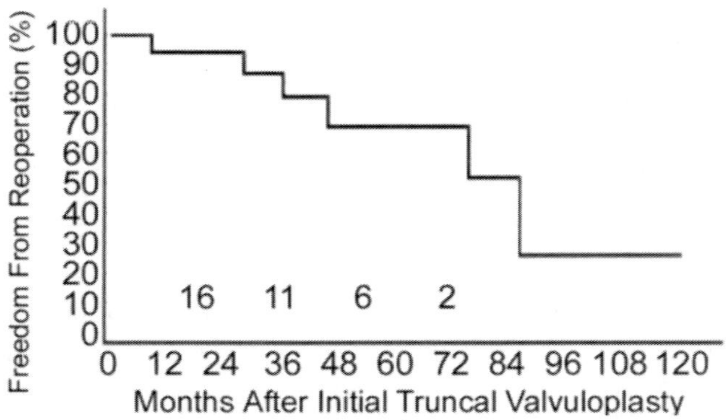

Figure 13. Kaplan-Meier graph demonstrating freedom from repeat valvuloplasty.

Henaine and colleagues reported a contemporary review of 153 patients who underwent repair of truncus arteriosus at Marie-Lannelongue Hospital. This series included 9 patients who underwent truncal valve intervention at the time of the primary repair (valvuloplasty in 6, valve replacement in 3). There were 4 early deaths in this series, and 2 patients were noted to have a competent native truncal valve at follow-up. Authors found that freedom from truncal valve reoperation was 96%, 82% and 63% at 1, 10 and 18 years respectively (Figure 14) [36].

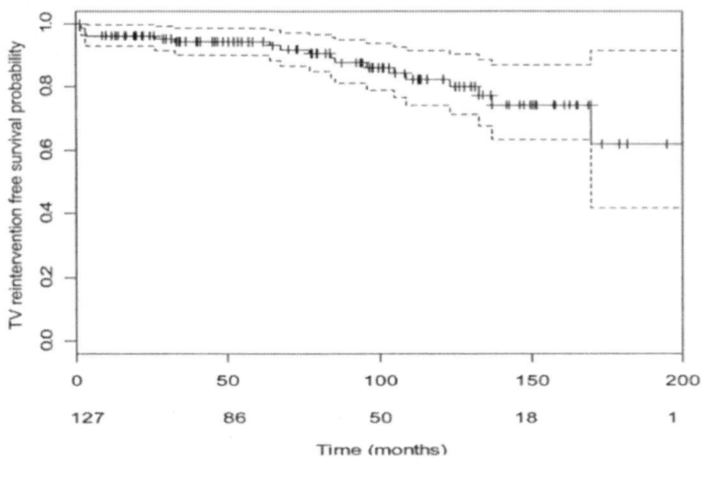

Figure 14. Freedom from truncal valve reintervention after correction of truncus arteriosus.

Naimo et al. focused on 80 patients with truncus arteriosus and truncal valve regurgitation. Sixty-one (76%) had mild, 17 (21%) had moderate and 2 (2.5%) patients had severe truncal valve regurgitation in the preoperative echocardiography. Patients with moderate or severe regurgitation showed more frequently quadricuspid valves. Sixty-three percent of patients with moderate or severe regurgitation underwent concomitant truncal valve surgery with a 25% early mortality and 81% of patients required truncal valve reparation at a median follow-up time of 20 years [15]. Truncal valve insufficiency has been reported in approximately 25% of truncus arteriosus patients. The optimal surgical approach to management of truncal valve insufficiency remains controversial.

The following procedures and guidelines to be helpful:

- Trivial or mild truncal valve regurgitation has in general a good outcome without any concomitant valve surgery.
- For moderate to severe truncal valve insufficiency, truncal valve repair is the most desirable and first choice. Severe regurgitation should be addressed at the primary valve repair in any age.
- Multiple leaflets (more than three) require careful attention. In cases when a quadricuspid truncal valve is found in truncus arteriosus patients with moderate truncal valve regurgitation the repair is especially recommended.
- The truncal valve replacement for treatment of truncal valve insufficiency remains as a second option especially at the initial operation.
- Anomalies associated with truncus arteriosus such as significant truncal valve regurgitation, interrupted aortic arch and/or coronary anomalies remain a risk factor for morbidity and mortality.
- The truncal valve repair could be lifesaving and can also be performed in the neonates without increasing operative mortality but it has limited durability.
- Initial moderate or severe truncal valve insufficiency is a risk factor for late truncal valve reoperation. Truncal valve reintervention procedures can be performed with good early-term and mid-term results.

The main advantages of truncal valve repair include the natural postoperative valve hemodynamics and the avoidance of oral anticoagulation. Although they do not exist on the best truncal valve repair surgery, understanding the mechanisms of truncal valve insufficiency is believed to be very important for the choice of individualized surgical approach for each patient.

Ventricular Septal Defect and Aortic Valve Regurgitation

Elisa Barberi

Introduction

Description

The International Society for Nomenclature of Paediatric and Congenital Heart Disease (ISNPCHD) has defined ventricular septal defect (VSD) as a congenital cardiac malformation in which there is a hole or pathway between the ventricular chambers [38]. VSD is a common congenital heart disease with an incidence of approximately 1.5–6.0 per 1000 newborns.

The scheme proposed by the ISNPCHD classifies VSDs as central perimembranous, inlet, trabecular muscular, and outlet defects, using a geographic approach as the starting point of classification while highlighting the importance of describing the borders to facilitate better understanding [39].

Central perimembranous defects are usually adjacent to the area of fibrous continuity between the septal leaflet of the tricuspid valve and the aortic valve, and they are located below and behind the postero-inferior limb of the septal band.

Inlet defects open into the right ventricle (RV) inlet below the postero-inferior limb of the septal band and the medial papillary muscle, whereas outlet defects open into the RV outlet between the 2 limbs of the septal band. Inlet defects can be associated with malalignment of the atrial septum and ventricular septum, typically with a straddling tricuspid valve.

In contrast, outlet defects are often associated with malalignment of the muscular or fibrous outlet septum relative to the limbs of the septal band. The conduction pathway is located along the postero-inferior border of all perimembranous defects and juxta-arterial defects with a fibrous postero-inferior rim.

Trabecular muscular defects are embedded within the apical muscular ventricular septum and can occupy any of its geographic components.

All VSDs can occur in isolation, as confluent combinations of two or more types, or as integral components of other CHDs. Early diagnosis for such defect using echocardiography is routine, even in early fetal life. With exact fetal diagnosis, it will almost certainly prove possible to identify those defects that are the most likely to close, as opposed to those which will require interventional or surgical treatment. For those requiring treatment, use of anatomic information permits an accurate assessment of any individual defect relative to the atrioventricular conduction axis without fear of inducing atrioventricular block. Thus, proper diagnosis, particularly of the doubly committed defect, should now be the prelude to timely successful management, and hopefully a normal post-interventional or postoperative outcome [40].

A subset of patients with VSDs will develop aortic insufficiency (AI). These VSDs may be located in the subarterial (also referred to as supracristal, subpulmonary, doubly committed subarterial, conal septal, or infundibular position), perimembranous (also referred to as subcristal, conotruncal, or paramembranous position), or outlet muscular positions [41].

AI complicates doubly committed subarterial VSDs about five times more often than perimembranous VSDs [42]. Several mechanisms may be responsible for the development of AI: lack of structural support and forces for leaflets adjacent to the VSD, abnormal commissural suspension, loss of continuity between the aortic media and aortic annulus but the Venturi effect is the predominant pathogenetic factor in the development of AI associated with a VSD. Surgical management of this VSDs should be based on knowledge of its anatomic features, natural history and the incidence of aortic valvar prolapse (AVP) and AI.

Epidemiology

Outlet type VSDs include doubly committed juxta-arterial, perimembranous outlet type, and muscular outlet type. Doubly committed juxta-arterial VSDs account for approximately 5-7% of VSDs in the Western Hemisphere. In the Eastern Hemisphere, although the overall incidence of VSDs is no greater in Asians than in other groups, doubly committed VSDs account for approximately 30% of VSDs in Asians. This type is paramount importance because accounts for approximately one-quarter of all VSDs cases requiring surgical closure.

Higher occurrence of the condition in this population has not been adequately explained, but one may assume that it is genetically determined [43].

The association of juxta-arterial type VSD with aortic valve prolapse, mainly right coronary cusp prolapse, and aortic regurgitation (AR) has been defined. According to previous reports, the incidence of AVP in juxta-arterial VSD was 36% to 79% [44]. The peak age for AVP was around 7 years, and that for AR was between 5 and 10 years [45]. In contrast, study about AVP and AR in perimembranous outlet and muscular outlet VSDs is limited.

Methods

Etiology, Pathophysiology and Clinical Description

In 1921, Laubry and Pezzi were the first to report the valvular complications of the aortic valve and aortic regurgitation in VSDs.

Van Praagh and McNamara's report [46], based on morphological findings of autopsied heart specimens, and additional data resulting from the study of a ruptured aneurysm of the sinus of Valsalva allowed to describe the major factors that contribute to AVP and AI into the VSDs.

Two major, conceptually distinct but functionally interdependent factors contribute to the AVP and AI into the VSD: anatomical factor and hemodynamic factor.

Anatomical Factor

Aortic valve regurgitation complicates the course of patients with subarterial VSDs five times as often as it does patients with perimembranous VSDs. The fundamental hemodynamic forces at work seem to be similar between the two types of VSDs, and therefore other anatomic factors must be modifying the development of AI.

For example in the doubly committed subarterial VSDs, the crucial phenotypic feature of this defect is the altered morphology of the arterial trunks with respect to the normally structured heart. This defect can only exist in absence of the "septal" component of the free-standing infundibular sleeve which normally supports the pulmonary trunk, a trait seen in hearts with common arterial trunk. It is no coincidence, therefore, that both these lesions are found in the setting of 22q11 deletion, pointing to their similar genetic background which itself is more prevalent in far Eastern populations [47].

In the normal heart, the pulmonary root is lifted away from the base of the heart by the free-standing infundibulum. In consequence of the deficient infundibulum, there is a fibrous continuity between the leaflets of the aortic and pulmonary valves, with the defect not only committed to the aorta, but also to the pulmonary trunk, hence its doubly committed phenotype (Figure 15). Owing to the lack of anatomical muscular support provided by the subpulmonary infundibulum, the right coronary leaflet, and occasionally the non-coronary leaflet of the aortic valve tend to prolapse through the defect.

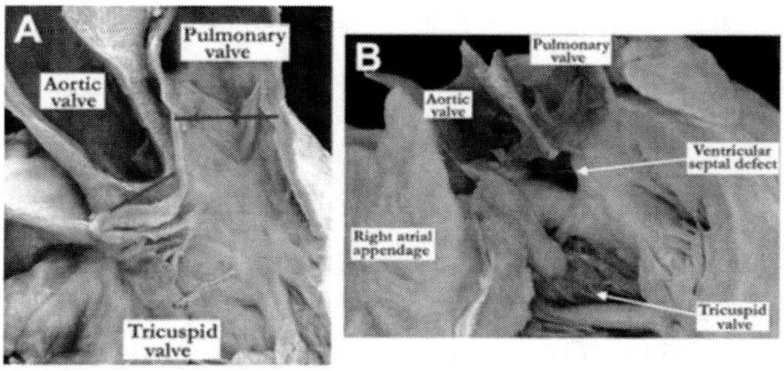

Fig 1. (A) In the normal heart, the free-standing muscular subpulmonary infundibulum lifts the pulmonary trunk away from the base of the heart. The leaflets of the aortic and pulmonary valves are separated, and are at different levels. (B) This subpulmonary infundibular sleeve is not present in the heart with the doubly committed juxtaarterial ventricular septal defect, pictured at right, a feature that brings the aortic and pulmonary valves into alignment, and allows for the fibrous continuity between the leaflets of the two valves.

Figure 15. Reprinted from Devlin et al. Ann Thorac Surg 2014; 97:2134–41 [52].

Aortic insufficiency can be partially explained by a lack of infundibular conal septal support from below.

Most large perimembranous defects are closely related to the aortic valve and very few are associated with aortic valve prolapse with or without incompetence. There is probably an intrinsic structural abnormality of the aortic valve that, in addition to the VSD, predisposes one or more cusps to progressively prolapse. Yacoub and associates postulated that this basic structural abnormality is a progressive discontinuity between the aortic valve annulus and the aortic media [48]. There is no pathologic data to support this theory and it's difficult to determine if this was the result of progressive cusp deformity or the cause of cusp prolapse. Two additional factors, drag forces and the differences in anatomy between subarterial and perimembranous VSDs, may play a role in the development of AI. The superior border of the subarterial VSD is adjacent to the hinge point of right coronary cusp and the VSD has a shallow, half-moon shape. As a result, the jet of blood through the defect is maximally exposed to the right coronary cusp. In contrast, perimembranous VSDs have a more circular shape and appear to need additional anatomic conditions such as override of the non-coronary cusp for the development of AI [49].

Abnormal commissural structures have been observed in some cases of AI associated with a VSD. The partial fusion of the commissures, resulting in a bicuspid aortic valve, contributes to the development of AI when present, but is not a satisfactory explanation for most cases. A lack of special forces has been implicated as a cause of AI in this group of patients. With the progressive deformity of the cusp, a point is reached where the appropriate surfaces of the opposite cusps cannot meet. This is the beginning of AI [50].

Hemodynamic Factor

Proposed mechanisms leading to AI in patients with a VSDs include several mechanisms but a review of literature [51, 52] suggest that hemodynamic factors also probably aggravate the tendencies toward the development of AI. These effects are present throughout the entire cardiac cycle and depend on the Venturi effect.

The Venturi effect explains the pathogenesis of aortic valve prolapse and AI in a subset of patients with a VSD. Giovanni Venturi, a professor of physics, expanded on Bernoulli's observation that as the velocity of a fluid increases a low-pressure zone is created. As a fluid passes through conduits of varying diameter, changes in velocity and pressure will occur, so that as the caliber of the conduit decreases, the fluid velocity will increase and the pressure will decrease. This low-pressure zone within a restrictive VSD can impact the adjacent cusp of the aortic valve.

One way to gauge the size of a VSD is by the velocity of blood flow through it and this is in part a function of the size of the VSD relative to the aortic root. If there is restriction to flow through the VSD and an aortic valve cusp is adjacent to the defect then the increase in velocity of blood through the defect could adversely affect the adjacent cusp.

A Venturi effect is created by the left-to-right shunting through the VSD during early systole. This turbulent flow tends to displace the aortic cusp, especially unsupported right coronary leaflet, into the right ventricle (Figure 16A). Later in systole the aortic cusp prolapses into the VSD and is acted on by direct pressure from the cavity of the left ventricle (Figure 16C), which tends to displace both the cusp and the anulus further into the right ventricle (Figure 16E). During diastole the high pressure in the aortic root distends the dilated sinus with further displacement of the aortic anulus toward the right ventricle (Figure 16B). The intra-aortic pressure forces the aortic valvar leaflet to close, but the unsupported prolapsed leaflet is pushed down into the VSD, away from the opposed coronary leaflet, resulting eventually in AI (Figure 16D-F). The increasing aortic regurgitation and the existing left-to-right shunt cause left ventricular volume overload, which could cause potentially irreversible changes in the left ventricular wall structure and function.

This mechanism was proposed by Tatsuno et al. [53] in 1973 and hypothesizing that the Venturi effect is the mechanism that results in AI, the VSD must be restrictive: smaller the defect is, higher will be the gradient across it and it will cause the blood to shunt across more vigorously thus drawing the nearby cusp in it and causing it to prolapse and then the AI.

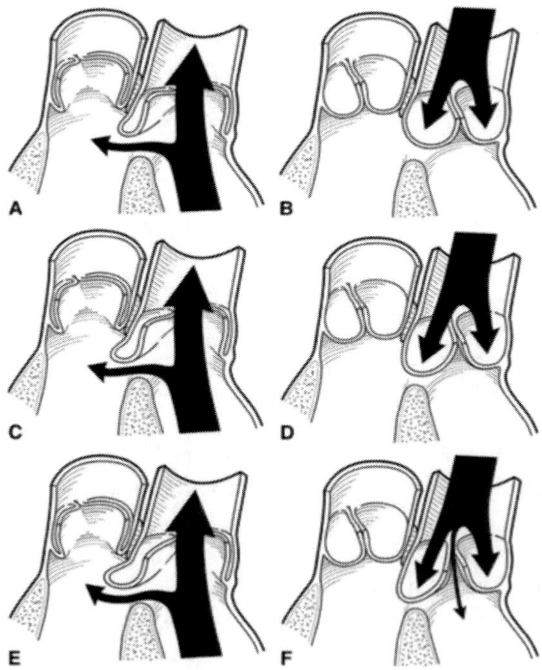

Figure 16. Reprinted from Tweddell et al. [51].

VSD is commonly diagnosed in the neonatal period, but neither AVP nor AI are present at birth. The physiological triggering factors act after birth due to the decrease in pulmonary vascular resistance which therefore results in a high-velocity jet across the VSD and AVP precedes the development of AI [54].

The observations supporting these points are that VSDs associated with AI are restrictive is the older age of the patients undergoing surgery for VSD/AI, between 5 and 10 years of age [55]. Chiu et al. from the National Taiwan University, reported a series of 677 patients with subarterial, perimembranous, and outlet muscular VSDs with AVP. There was no difference in the Qp/Qs associated with AVP among the three types and the average Qp/Qs among 373 patients who developed AVP was about 1.62 and pulmonary artery pressures are at most only mildly elevated. A review of the literature indicates that for patients with VSD and AI the VSD is restrictive with a Qp/Qs 2 and an absence of pulmonary artery hypertension depends on the Venturi effect as the predominate mechanism for the development of AI associated with a VSD [51].

Diagnosis

Congestive heart failure does not occur in patients with an isolated, small VSD. General examination findings consist of a long harsh systolic murmur and no signs of respiratory distress or growth failure. Second heart sound findings depend on volume of shunt flow as well as pulmonary artery pressure and resistance.

Physical examination should focus on whether AI is present. Blood pressure must be carefully evaluated for pulse pressure (ie, the difference between systolic and diastolic blood pressures) and pulse amplitude, as these increase with increasing AI unless heart failure also occurs. Significant AI may cause a late diastolic murmur at the apex resulting from atrial contraction augmenting late ventricular filling. This is the Austin Flint murmur.

Chest radiography is normal in infancy if the left-to-right shunt is small. Radiography in the older child or adult with progressive AI may reveal left heart enlargement and prominence of the ascending aorta. Shunt volume is generally smaller, thus pulmonary arterial vascularity is generally normal.

Although the diagnosis is usually made by the presence of a diastolic murmur in a patient known to have a VSD, recent refinement in echocardiographic techniques allows accurate recognition and quantification of the various components of the AVP and AI.

The position, presence and size of the defects were determined by echocardiography, with careful attention to distinguish the truly doubly committed VSDs from perimembranous defects with outlet extension, using meticulous echocardiographic observation of the short-axis view of the right ventricular outflow tract at the level of the aortic root. The size of the defect was graded as being small, moderate or large in relation to the dimensions of the aortic valvar orifice, using values of less than 25%, between 25 and 50% or greater than 50%, respectively. When measuring the size of the defect, no account was taken of any portion occluded by a prolapsing leaflet of the aortic valve.

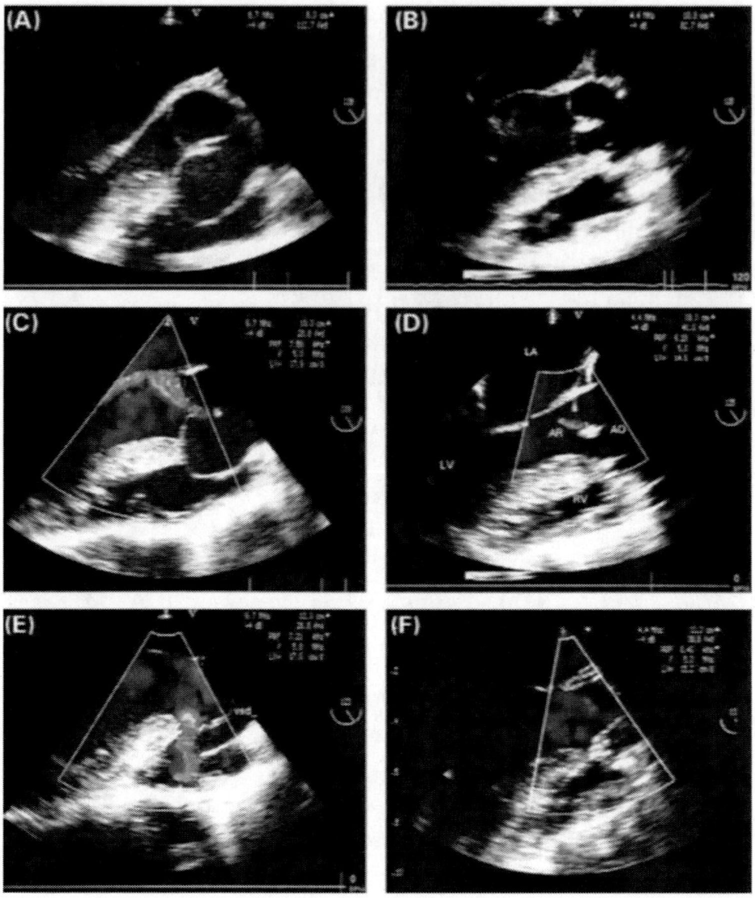

Figure 17. Reprinted from Evdokia Petropoulou, Stergios Theodoropoulos, and Magdi H. Yacoub [57].

The diagnosis of AVP and AI was made according to the echocardiographic findings that were confirmed by angiographic or surgical findings. AI was diagnosed by two-dimensional and color doppler echo in parasternal long-axis view and was graded as absent, mild (AR jet reaching just beneath the aortic valve), moderate (AR jet reaching beyond the anterior cusp of the mitral valve but not reaching the left ventricular apex), or severe (AR jet reaching the left ventricular apex) [56].

Three-dimensional (17D) echocardiographic imaging of VSDs closely correlates with surgical findings.

Figure 3A shows the discontinuity between the aortic media and the crest of the septum, the dilatation of the sinus of Valsalva and the prolapse of the cusp. This was associated with moderate AI with a jet towards the anterior mitral leaflet (Figure 17C). During systole the VSD shunt was visible (Figure 17E), while in diastole the prolapsing cusp obstructed the VSD (Figure 3C). After surgical correction (Figure 3B) AI was trivial (Figure 17D) and there were no shunts during systole (Figure 17F) or diastole (Figure 17D) [57].

Advances in prenatal diagnosis could also now permit anticipation of the diagnosis and allow for a better follow-up, with more appropriate timing for closure of the defect.

Surgical Management

Heart failure, a large shunt, poor growth, or elevated pulmonary artery pressure would all be indications for VSD closure regardless of presence of AI. Development of AI may occurs even in the absence of congestive heart failure and the indications of surgery become more complicated. The primary indications for closure of these defects, therefore, are AVP and AI. Secondary indications include the degree of left-to-right shunting, and the known potential for AVP.

Closure of the VSD, with or without aortic valve repair, is indicated for both perimembranous and subarterial VSDs when more than trivial AI is identified because AI is progressive [58].

For patients with a subarterial VSD and AVP, VSD closure is indicated because of the high likelihood of progression of AVP and development of AI, furthermore spontaneous closure is difficult. Lun et al. [59] suggested that all subarterial VSDs of 5 mm should be closed regardless of the presence of AVP to prevent the development of AI.

For the patient with a hemodynamically insignificant perimembranous VSD with AVP but without AI, indications for surgery are less clear. Progression of AI is variable but the closure of the VSD reduces the risk for AVP even if the surgical closure for perimembranous VSDs places the conduction system at risk. Therefore, in the absence of AI, prophylactic closure of restrictive perimembranous VSDs with AVP is probably not justified [53].

Elgamal et al. recommend closure of VSDs, regardless of the type, the size, or the apparent absence of AVP, when any degree of AI is identified [58]. Of the various repair techniques existing they perform in a Trusler's aortic valve repair where the excess lenght of the prolapsed aoric valve cusp is plicated against the aortic wall using a horizontal suture reinforced with a Teflon or pericardial pledgets. The adequacy of the initial repair is the determinant of long-term results: the excessive elongation and prolapse of the aortic valve need more plication sutures and valvuloplasty failure may occur. Okita and colleagues confirmed, in their multivariate analysis, that the number of plication sutures represent an independent risk factor for valve repair [60].

Surgical closure, with or without simultaneous repair of the aortic valve, is still considered the gold standard for the treatment of this congenital heart defect [53]. The approach through a right atriotomy, does not always allow for adequate exposure of the upper part of the doubly committed VSDs. This means that either a longitudinal right ventriculotomy, or a longitudinal incision in the pulmonary trunk, or an oblique incision of the ascending aorta, will likely be needed, with the last approach also allowing direct repair of the aortic valve [61]. It is very important to repair the defect with a patch that realigns the ventricular septum and provides support for the leaflets of the aortic valve, possibly avoiding further surgery.

Figure 18A shows the typical operative view of the doubly committed VSD through the opened pulmonary trunk. After cross-clamping the aorta, and delivering cold blood cardioplegic solution, we placed interrupted pledgeted supported sutures around the defect. A critical part of the process of closure involves placing sutures directly in the base of the pulmonary valvar leaflets as an anchoring point where there is no muscular septum separating the aortic and pulmonary valves, as shown in Figure 18B. All defects were closed with a round polytetrafluoroethylene patch, which supports the leaflets of the aortic valve.

Some studies have observed that once AI develops, it will progress even after closure of VSD. It may end up in need of aortic valve replacement. Chauvaud [62] observed 16% need of aortic valve replacement even after VSD closure. Other studies [63] found closure of VSD or aortic valve repair will halt the process of further damage to aortic valve.

The optimal timing for surgical treatment remains controversial. The closure of the defect, with or without repair of the aortic valve, should be performed at the first appearance of, or if there is progression of previously observed trivial AI [64]. The seeming presence of a 'functionally' restrictive defect on echocardiography, with most of the area of the morphologically large defect closed by the prolapsing aortic valve leaflet, can be misleading and can cause a dangerous delay in referral for treatment. The relatively low risk of cardiopulmonary bypass needs to overcome the benefits of preventing aortic valve complications.

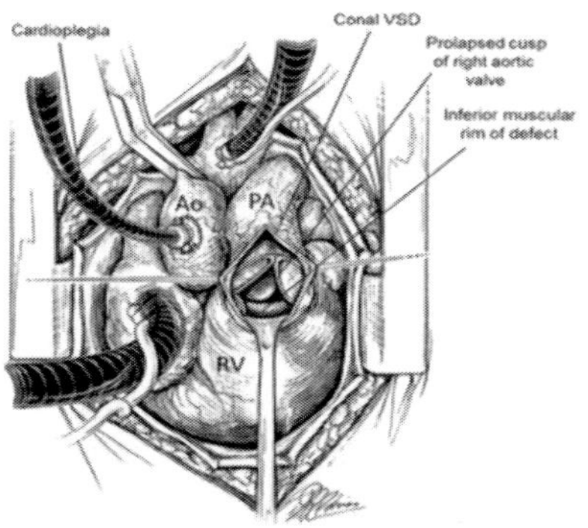

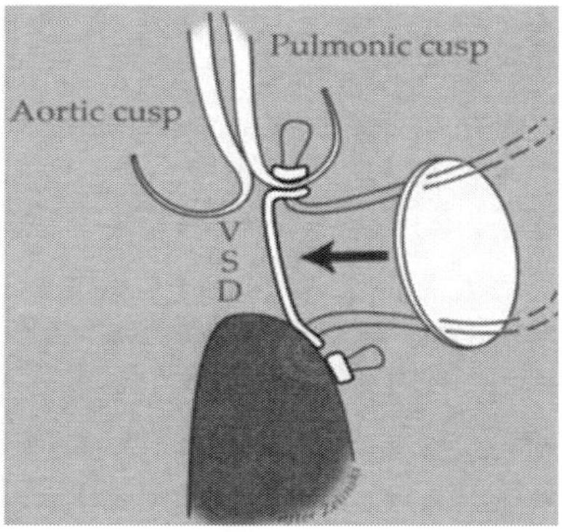

Figure 18A. Figure 18B. Reprinted from Devlin et al. [52].

A distinct relationship has been shown between the age of the patients and the development of AVP [15]. In a series of 209 patients with doubly committed and juxtaarterial VSD, 100% of patients had aortic valve prolapse by age 15 years, the mean age of onset of aortic valve prolapse was 4.9 years [65]. In a series of 395 patients with doubly committed juxtaarterial VSD, half had AI by the age of 8 and almost nine tenths by the age of 20 [66]. Aneurysm of the sinus of Valsalva was not found before the age of 10 years, but began to develop during the second decade of life, and was diagnosed most frequently in the third decade of life.

Discussion

Outcome and Perspectives

Early detection of these type of VSDs and early accurate assessment of anatomical morphology of aortic valve are crucial to prevent further progression of the disease.

Optimal operation timing may be important to achieve better outcomes after repair and prevent the development of aortic valve complications.

Patch closure remains the gold standard in managing these defects. The morbidity and mortality associated with VSD closure even combined with aortic valvuloplasty is low. Okita and colleagues reported a hospital mortality of 1.6% with no late deaths, resulting in a 15-

year actuarial survival of 98.3% [23]. Trusler and associates experienced no hospital deaths with two late deaths, yielding a 10-year actuarial survival of 96% [67]. Elgamal et al. reported 15-year actuarial freedom from repair failure of 81% compares favorably with other published series, where estimates range from 85% at 10 years to 64% at 15 years [58]. Rhodes and colleagues reported an 18-year freedom from reoperation of 51% [68].

Jung et al. observed that AI progression occurred in only one of our patients after VSD closure, which was unexpectedly low (0.98%). Moreover, 95.1% (98 patients) of the patients had less than faint degree AI in preoperative echo, showing an unexpectedly low prevalence of preoperative AI in subarterial VSD patients who underwent surgical closure. Only the patients with aortic valve abnormalities or delayed operation had AI progression or persisting more than mild degree AI [69].

In summary, patients with a doubly committed VSD and AVP should undergo surgery to prevent the development of AI because this complicates about half of subarterial VSDs with AVP and spontaneous closure is rare. Patients with perimembranous VSDs with AVP should be followed with serial echocardiography and undergo VSD closure if more than trivial AI develops [51].

Aortico-Left Ventricular Tunnel (ALVT)

Duccio Federici

Introduction

Description and Anatomical Considerations

The aortico-left ventricular tunnel, firstly described by Levy et al. in 1963 [70], is a rare congenital malformation characterized by a paravalvular communication between the ascending aorta and the left ventricle. It's incidence is estimated around 1 in 1000 infants born with congenital heart disease [71]. Associated defects, usually involving the proximal coronary arteries, or the aortic or pulmonary valves, are present in nearly half of the cases.

The aortic-left ventricular tunnel typically originates from an aortic orifice cephalad to the right coronary artery, at the level or just above the sino-tubular junction. In rare cases the tunnel may originate above the left coronary artery or may open into the right ventricle. The tunnel follows a descending route along the aorto-pulmonary interspace entering just below the left-right commissure of the aortic valve. A buldge is typically visible along the anterolateral aspect of the ascending aorta and represents the anterior wall of the tunnel. The posterior wall is constituted by the true aortic wall and the tunnel's floor usually involves the muscle of the right ventricular outflow tract [72].

ALVT is classified into four types (Figure 19) according to Hovaguimian classification [73]:

Type I: Slit-like aortic orifice without valvular distorsion

Type II: Oval-shaped aortic orifice with aneurysmal extracardiac component

Type III: Oval aortic orifice with aneurismal intracardiac component
Type IV: Combination of type II and III

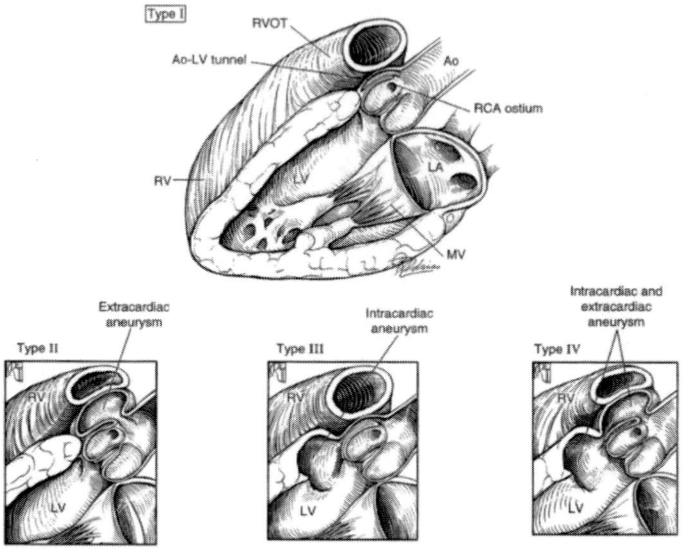

Figure 19. For types of aortic-left ventricular tunnel. LV (left ventricle); RV (right ventricle); RVOT (right ventricular outflow tract); RCA (right coronary artery); MV (mitral valve): LA (left atrium). Reprinted from Kim RW et al. [74].

In addition to the aforementioned classification, Ho et al. [71] suggested that the tunnels never cross the interventricular septum but travel downsward into the fibrofatty plane between the aortic root and the subpulmonary infundibulum, entering in the left ventricular outflow tract immediately above the aortic-ventricular junction in the subcomimsural triangle of the left and right valvular cups [74] (Figure 20).

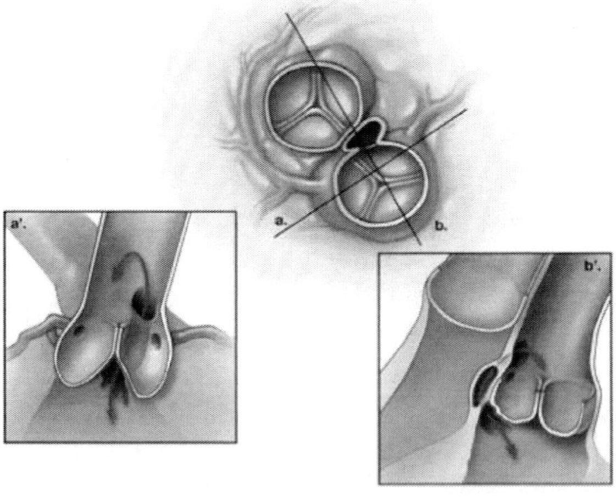

Figure 20. Schematic representation of the most common type of aorto-vetricular tunnel. Note its course along the fibrofatty plane between aortic root and subpulmonary infundibulum. Reprinted from Mckay R. [90].

Etiology

Etiology of aortic-ventricular tunnel is unknown. However, the substrate for its formation and that of the associated valvular and coronary artery anomalies may be inferred from developmental anatomy. The cushions forming the facing aortic and pulmonary sinuses with their respective valvar leaflets normally become separated by an extracardiac tissue plane. The coronary arteries, also initially encased by this cuff of myocardium, grow through it to connect with the aortic sinuses. Failure of this tissue plane development might result in a tunnel above one of the facing aortic sinuses and explain also the potential involvement of the proximal coronary arteries and the aortic leaflets [75, 76].

Pathophysiology and Clinical Description

The aortico-left ventricular tunnel, by virtue of its anatomic features, is a pathophysiological model of massive aortic insufficiency.

In AVLT a loud "to and fro" murmur radiating over the entire precordium is typical, usually with systolic and diastolic thrills. Bounding pulses indicate rapid aortic run-off. In older patients, these signs may suggest aortic valve stenosis with incompetence, but the second heart sound should have a normal aortic components in uncomplicated ALVT. Most patients develop sympoms of heart failure during the first year of life, tipically in the first six months. The onset, severity and progression of heart failure is, however quite variable, ranging from many years of asymptomatic status [77-79] to a rapid decompensation [80], sudden death or death in utero [81]. Generally is not possible to correlate clinical course to specific morphology of the tunnel, but the wide clinical spectrum could reflect variable degree of coronary artery involvement, left ventricular outflow tract obstruction or right ventricular outflow obstruction.

Diagnosis

Echocardiography is the modality of choice for the diagnosis of ALVT [82, 83]. Transthoracic cross-sectional imaging in a parasternal long-axis view demonstrates the tunnel, as well as its aortic origin and left ventricular opening (Figure 21). Both two dimensional and real-time three dimensional echocardiography have also established reliable fetal diagnosis [71, 84]. Color-doppler study typically shows diastolic flow passing laterally from the aorta to the left ventricle (Figure 22). Left ventricle, best assessed in short axis cuts, usually shows some degree of hypertrophy and dilatation. MRI is also used as a second-level modality for diagnosis of ALVT. Cardiac catheterization is actually indicated only when associated lesions or coronary artery origins cannot be evaluated on non-invasive studies.

Differential diagnosis is crucial, considering that ALVT must be distinguished from other lesions which cause rapid diastolic run-off of blood from aorta into left ventricle and produce cardiac failure. Among these must be mentioned:

- Sinus of Valsalva fistula
- Truncus Arteriosus with valvular regurgitation
- Aorto-pulmonary window
- Ventricular septal defect with aortic regurgitation
- Coronary artery fistula

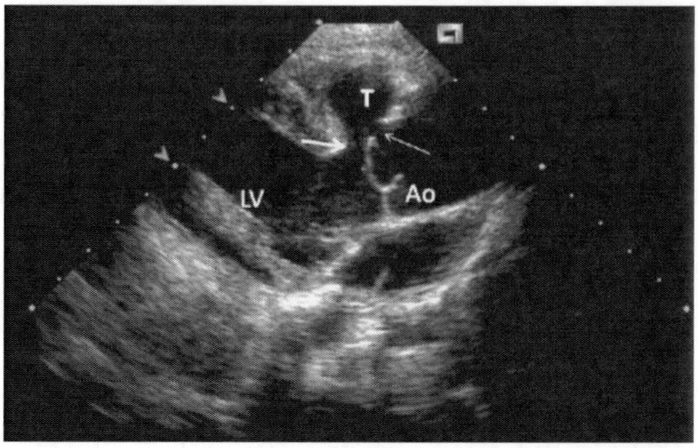

Figure 21. Parasternal long-axis view showing aorto-left ventricular tunnel. Ao (aorta); LV (left ventricle); T (tunnel). Reprinted from Kathare P et al. [85].

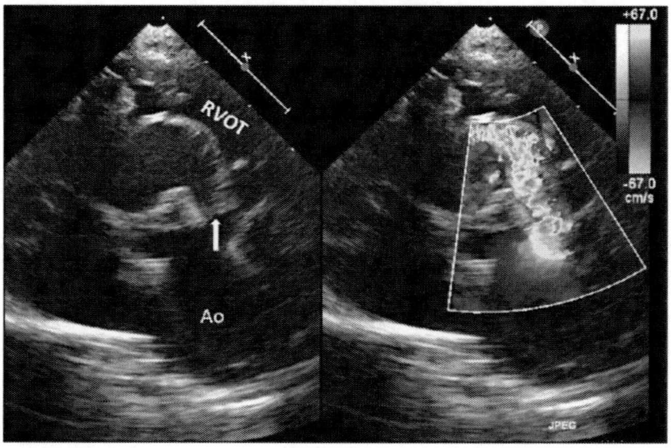

Figure 22. Modified Parasternal long-axis view showing aorto-left ventricular tunnel and its diastolic run-off into left ventricle. Ao (aorta); LV (left ventricle); RVOT (right ventricular outflow tract); T (tunnel). Reprinted from Kathare P et al. [85].

Methods

Principles of Surgical Management

Without intervention, most of the patients die early in life for congestive heart failure. Optimal surgical timing is within the first six months of life, due to the evidence of normalization of left ventricular size and function if correction is performed in that time window. Lack of support to the right or left aortic leaflet can result in progressive aortic regurgitation, although surgical technique may importantly influence the long-term aortic valve function.

Principles of surgical correction include:

- Closure of the aortic and ventricular openings
- Restoration of aortic valve function
- Ensuring normal coronary perfusion
- Relief of left or right ventricular outflow tract obstruction

Several techniques has been proposed in surgical management of ALVT, as direct closure of tunnel openings eventually associated with additional measures like external tunnel ligation or obliteration [86, 87]. Currently, the best surgical approach is a separate patch closure of both the aortic and ventricular opening, through tran-aortic and trans-infundibular approach, along with internal plication and reduction of the lateral tunnel wall [88]. The rationale of this strategy lies in these keypoints:

- Closing the ventricular opening in order to avoid an open blind-ending pouch with high pressure. This condition might create a rightward buldging of the lateral tunnel wall generating right ventricular outflow tract obstruction.
- Restoring an adeguate anatomical support to the aortic valve and anulus by means of two separate patches
- Closing the ventricular opening of the tunnel from the right side excluding its thin lateral wall.
- Maintaining integrity of the aortic root avoiding external opening of the tunnel

The Two-Patch Technique

Surgery is performed on cardiopulmonary bypass (CPB) under mild hypothermia. The tunnel is externally compressed during antegrade cold blood cardioplegia delivery in order to avoid left ventricular run-off. If a coronary arise from the tunnel, so as to preclude external compression, retrograde cardioplegia may be delivered.

A transverse aortotomy is performed. The aortic valve and coronary ostia are carefully inspected to exclude anomalies. An additional dose of selective cardioplegia is delivered in the coronary ostia.

A transverse ventriculotomy is carried in the sub-pulmonary infundibulum around 1 cm below the ventriculo-arterial junction.

The aortic and ventricular openings of the tunnel are identified. A right angled clamp is then passed through the aortic opening of the tunnel and an incision is made into its lateral wall, thus creating a tunnel to right ventricular communication which is essentially a iatrogeninc sub-aortic ventricular septal defect (Figure 23).

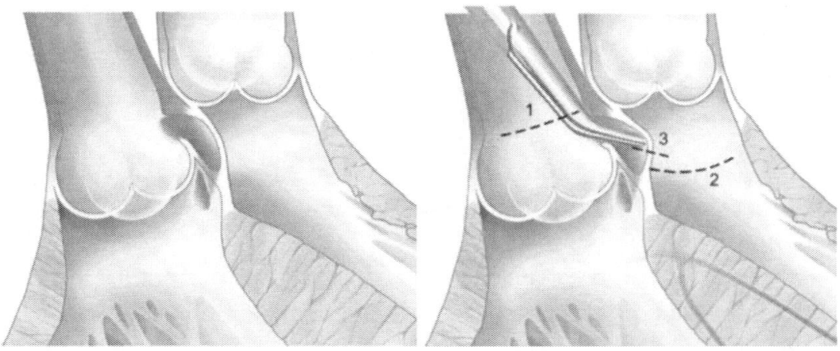

Figure 23. Schematic view of ALVT showing aortic and left ventricular openings and the tunnel course (right panel). Right-angled clamp passed through the tunnel (left panel). Reprinted from Mueller C et al. [88].

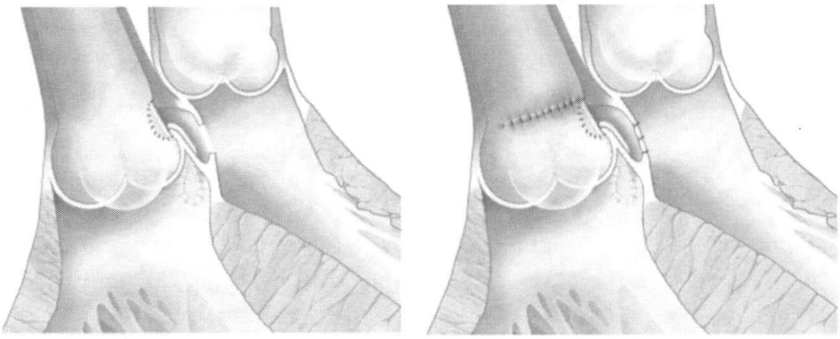

Figure 24. Two-patch technique for ALVT correction: The aortic opening is closed through the aortotomy and the ventricular opening through the right ventriculotomy The latera tunnel wall is plicated and deduced (left panel). Reprinted from Mueller C et al. [88].

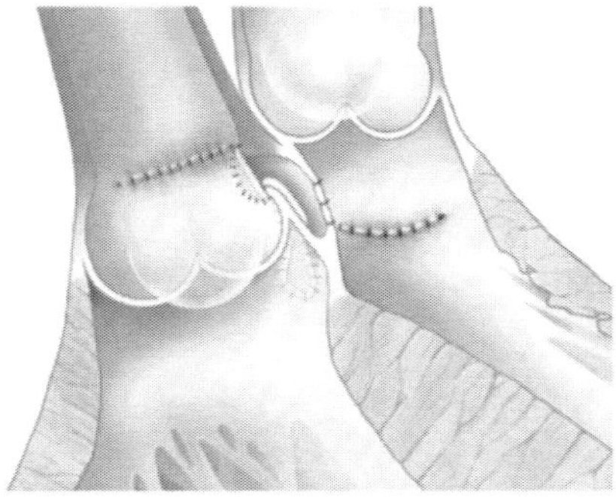

Figure 25. Final result of two-patch technique. Note the direct closure of aortotomy and right ventriculotomy. Reprinted from Mueller C. et al. [88].

The opened lateral wall of the tunnel is then exposed from the right ventricular side.

The aortic opening is closed through the aortotomy using xenopericardial patch secured with polipropilene running suture.

The ventricular opening is closed through the infundibular approach using the same material and technique of the aortic opening (Figure 24). The thin lateral wall of the tunnel is then plicated and reduced by means of direct suture.

Aortotomy and right ventriculotomy are closed by direct suture (Figure 25).

The aortic cross-clamp is removed and surgical result is checked by echocardiography.

Associated Anomalies

Coronary origin from the tunnel pose a surgical challenge. The orifice of a coronary artery can be displaced above or below the origin of the tunnel, or it may lie within the tunnel. When the coronary ostium arise proximally within the tunnel a patch closure of the aortic opening distally so as to ensure coronary pefsusion of the aortic root has been described [87]. More distal origin of the coronary artery from the tunnel needs detachment of coronary botton and its reimplantation in higher position into the ascending aorta.

Atresia of the left or right coronary artery has also been reported. More than two orifices, single coronary ostium, and intramural course in the posterior wall of the tunnel have all been observed [89].

Bicuspid aortic valve, with or without stenosis, is present in about 20% of cases. Pulmonary valve stenosis is reported in 5% of cases [89].

Discussion

Outcome and Current Perspectives

Operative outcome, overall survival and freedom from reintervention after ALVT have been recently elucidated in a multicentric study performed by the European Congenital Heart Surgeons Association and the World Society for Pediatric and Congenital Heart Surgery (ECHSA – WSPCHS) [89]. Data were collected from 15 participating centers. The cohort was represented by 42 patients (85% with ALVT) who underwent surgical correction of aortic-left/right ventricular tunnel between 1987 and 2018.

Median age at diagnosis and operation in ALVT group was 25 days, with 77.8% of patients undergoing surgery before six months of age. In 30% of ALVT patients, preoperative moderate to severe aortic regurgitation (AR) was present.

In patients with right ventricular tunnels the median age at diagnosis and correction was 6 years.

Perioperative (30 days) mortality for the ALVT group was 8.3%. The median follow-up of the ALVT survivors was 22 years and the freedom from reintervention was 90%. 10% underwent reoperation for residual aortic stenosis (AS). The overall mortality of the entire cohort of patients was 9.5%: The cause of death was mainly related to residual AS, thus emphasizing the importance of fixing the aortic valve at the time of initial repair.

Surgical technique employed was not uniform in the ALVT group, with only 33% of patients who underwent closure of both aortic and ventricular ends of tunnel (two-patch technique).

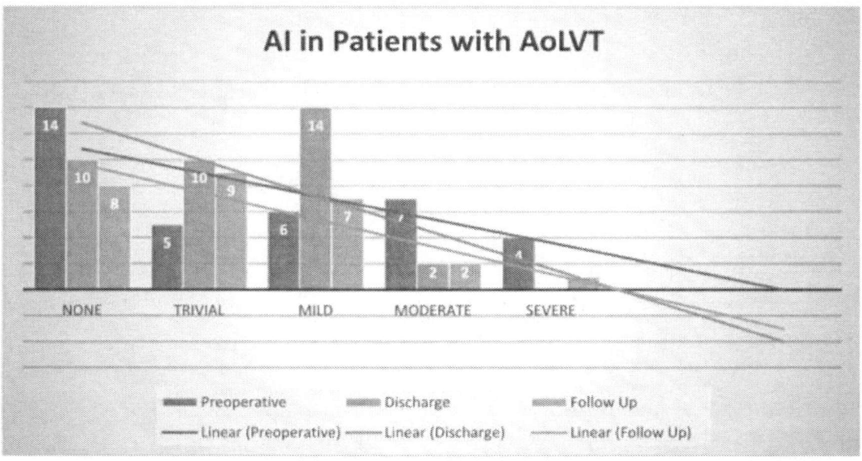

Figure 26. Graphic representation of preoperative prevalence and postoperative evolution of AR in ALVT patients. AR degree remains stable at late follow-up in 85% of patients, with only three patients showing severe aortic regurgitation. AI (aortic regurgitation); AoLVT (aortico-left ventricular tunnel). Reprinted from Protopapas ME et al. [89].

Aortic regurgitation, probably due to turbulence-related damage of the leaflets, is a major concern in ALVT management. In this cohort preoperative AR, ranging from mild to severe, was present preoperatively in 42% of patients. Interestingly, at late follow-up, 85% of patients had stable or improved AR with only three patients showing severe regurgitation (Figure 26). The simple ALVT repair seems to fix aortic regurgitation in most cases. However, this is in contrast with the results of Martins et al. who found that half of the ALVT patients required late aortic valve replacement [71].

The ECHSA-WSPCHS study [89] is actually the large retrospective multicentric series on surgical management of aorto-ventricular tunnel, and three important "take home messages" can be extrapolated from it:

1. Early surgical repair, immediately after diagnosis, is recommended even in asymptomatic patients.
2. Coexistence of significant aortic stenosis requires aggressive treatment, even with Ross procedure if needed, since a more conservative approach is associated with high early mortality and higher reoperation rate
3. Preoperative AR is a frequent finding in ALVT but remains stable postoperatively in most cases later in life. ALVT repair alone seems sufficient to prevent evolution of valvular regurgitation.

REFERENCES

[1] Jonas, A. Richard. 2004. *Comprehensive Surgical Management of Congenital Heart Disease*. London: Hodder Arnold. (Jonas 2004, 429–439).

[2] Ziemer, Gerhard, and Haverich Axel. 2017. *Cardiac Surgery: Operations on the Heart and Great Vessels in Adults and Children.* Berlin: Springer. (Ziemer and Haverich 2017, 597-605).

[3] Stark, Jaroslav F., de Leval, Marc R., Tsang, Victor T. 2006 *Surgery for Congenital Heart Defects.* London: John Wiley&Sons, Ltd. (Stark, de Leval and Tsang 2006, 515-529).

[4] Crupi, G., Macartney, F. J., Anderson, R. H. 1977 "*Persistent truncus arteriosus. A study of 66 autopsy cases with special reference to definition and morphogenesis.*" *Am J Cardiol* 40:569–578.

[5] Rodefeld, Mark D., Hanley, Frank L. 2002 *"Neonatal truncus arteriosus repair: surgical techniques and clinical management." Pediatric Cardiac Surgery Annual of the Seminars in Thoracic and Cardiovascular Surgery,* 5:212-217.

[6] Suzuki, A., Sy, H., Anderson, R. H., Deanfield, J. E. 1989 "*Coronary arterial and sinusal anatomy in hearts with a common arterial trunk."Ann Thorac Surg* 48:792–797.

[7] Lenox, C. C., Debich, D. E., Zubebuhler, J. R. 1992*"The role of coronary artery abnormalities in the prognosis of truncus arteriosus."J Thorac Cardiovasc Surg* 104:1728–1742.

[8] delaCruz, M. V., Cayre, R., Angelini, P., Noriega-Ramos, N., Sadowinski, S. 1990 *"Coronary arteries in truncus arteriosus." Am J Cardiol* 66:1482–1486.

[9] Jahangiri, M., Zurakowski, D., Mayer, J. E., del Nido, P. J., Jonas, R. A. 2000 *"Repair of the truncal valve and associated interrupted arch in neonates with truncus arteriosus." J Thorac Cardiovasc Surg* 119:508– 514.

[10] Sano, S., Brawn, W. J., Mee, R. B. 1990 *"Repair of truncus arteriosus and interrupted aortic arch." J Cardiac Surg* 5:157–162.

[11] Lenox, Cora C., Debich, Diane E., and Zuberbuhler, James R. 1992 *"The role of coronary artery abnormalities in the prognosis of truncus arteriosus." J. Thorac Cardiovasc Surg* 104: 1728-1742.

[12] De Leval, M. R., McGoon, D. C., Wallace, R. B., Danielson, G. K., Mair, D. D. 1974 *"Management of truncal valvular regurgitation." Ann Surg* 180:427–432.

[13] 13. Elkins, R. C., Steinberg, J. B., Razook, J. D., Ward, K. E., Overholt, E. D., Thompson, W. M. Jr. 1990 *"Correction of truncus arteriosus with truncal valvar stenosis or insufficiency using two homografts." Ann Thorac Surg* 50:728–733.

[14] Trusler, G. A., Moes, C. A., Kidd, B. S. 1973 *"Repair of ventricular septal defect with aortic insufficiency." J Thorac Cardiovasc Surg* 66:394–403.

[15] Naimo, P. S., Fricke, T. A., d'Udekem, Y., et al. 2018 *"Impact of truncal valve surgery on the outcomes of the truncus arteriosus repair." Eur J Cardiothorac Surg* 54:524-31.

[16] Kaza, Aditya K., Burch, Phillip T., Pinto, Nelangi, LuAnn Minich, L., Tani, Lloyd Y., and Hawkins, John A. 2010 *"Durability of truncal valve repair."Ann Thorac Surg* 90:1307–12.

[17] Imamura, M., Drummond-Webb, J. J., Sarris, G. E., Mee, R. B. 1999 *"Improving early and intermediate results of truncus arteriosus repair: a new technique of truncal valve repair." Ann Thorac Surg* 67:1142–1146.

[18] Cosgrove, D. M., Rosenkranz, E. R., Hendren, W. G., Bartlett, J. C., Stewart, W. J. 1991 *"Valvuloplasty for aortic insufficiency." J Thorac Cardiovasc Surg* 102: 571–576.

[19] Duran, C., Kumar, N., Gometza, B., al Halees, Z. 1991 *"Indications and limitations of aortic valve reconstruction." Ann Thorac Surg* 52: 447–453.

[20] Kalangos, A., Beghetti, M., Baldovinos, A., et al. 1999 *"Aortic valve repair by cusp extension with the use of fresh autologous pericardium in children with rheumatic aortic insufficiency." J Thorac Cardiovasc Surg* 118: 225–236.

[21] Backer, Carl L. 2005 *"Techniques for repairing the aortic and truncal valves." Cardiol Young* 15 (Suppl.1): 125-131.

[22] Bobylev, D., Sarikouch, S., Tudorache, I., Cvitkovic, T., Soylen, B., Boethig, D. et al. 2018 "Double semilunar valve replacement in complex congenital heart disease using decellularized homografts." *Interact CardioVasc Thorac Surg* 1-7 doi:10.1093/icvts/ivy212. .

[23] Yoshitake, Shuichi, Kaneko,Yukihiro, Yakuwa, Kazuki, and Achiwa, Ikuya 2019 *"Successful Truncal Valve Replacement With a Mechanical Valve After Bilateral Pulmonary Artery Banding" World Journal for Pediatric and Congenital Heart Surgery* Vol. 10(3): 384-387

[24] Fujita, Shuhei, Yamagishi, Masaaki, Miyazaki, Takako, and Yaku, Hitoshi. 2018 *"Leaflet-base–preserving truncal valve repair with ethanol-treated autologous pericardium. J Thorac Cardiovasc Surg* 1-3. https://doi.org/10.1016/j.jtcvs.2018.08.103

[25] Baird, Christopher W., Sefton, Brenda, Chavez, Mariana, Sleeper, Lynn A., Marx, Gerald R. and del Nido, Pedro J. 2020 *"Congenital aortic and truncal reconstruction*

utilizing the Ozaki technique:short-term clinical results" The Journal of Thoracic and Cardiovascular Surgery. https://doi.org/10.1016/j.jtcvs.2020.01.087.

[26] Jahangiri, M., Zurakowski, D., Mayer, J. E., del Nido, P. J., Jonas, R. A. 2000 *"Repair of the truncal valve and associated interrupted arch in neonates with truncus arteriosus." J Thorac Cardiovasc Surg* 119:508–514.

[27] Myers, Patrick O., Bautista-Hernandez, Victor, del Nido, Pedro J., Marx, Gerald R., Mayer, John E., Pigula, Frank A. and Baird, Christopher W. 2013 *"Surgical repair of truncal valve regurgitation." European Journal of Cardio-Thoracic Surgery* 44: 813–820.

[28] Russell, H. M., Pasquali, S. K., Jacobs, J. P., Jacobs, M. L., O'Brien, S. M., Mavroudis, C. et al. 2012 *"Outcomes of repair of common arterial trunk with truncal valve surgery: a review of the society of thoracic surgeons congenital heart surgery database." Ann Thorac Surg* 93:164–169.

[29] Ebert, P.A., Turley, K., Stanger, P., Hoffman, J., Heymann, M.A., Rudolph, A.M. 1984 *"Surgical treatment of truncus arteriosus in the first 6 months of life." Ann Surg* 200:451–456.

[30] Hanley FL, Heinemann MK, Jonas RA, et al. 1993 *"Repair of truncus arteriosus in the neonate." J Thorac Cardiovasc Surg* 105:1047–56.

[31] Rajasinghe, H. A., McElhinney, D. B., Reddy, V. M., Mora, B. N., Hanley, F. L. 1997 "*Long-term follow-up of truncus arteriosus repaired in infancy: a twenty-year experience." J Thorac Car- diovasc Surg* 113:869–79.

[32] Di Donato, R. M., Fyfe, D. A., Puga, F. J., et al. 1985 *"Fifteen-year experience with surgical repair of truncus arteriosus." J Thorac Cardiovasc Surg* 89:414–422.

[33] Pearl, J. M., Laks, H., Drinkwater, D.C., et al. 1991 *"Repair of truncus arteriosus in infancy."Ann Thorac Surg* 52:780 –786.

[34] Bove, E. L., Lupinetti, F. M., Pridjian, A. K., et al. 1993 *"Results of a policy of primary repair of truncus arteriosus in the neonate." J Thorac Cardiovasc Surg* 105:1057–1066.

[35] Kaza, Aditya. K, Burch, Phillip. T, Pinto, Nelangi, Minich, LuAnn L., Tani, Lloyd. Y, and Hawkins, John.A. 2010 *"Durability of truncal valve repair." Ann Thorac Surg* 90:1307–1312.

[36] Henaine, R., Azarnoush, K., Belli, E., et al. 2008 *"Fate of truncal valve in truncus arteriosus." Ann Thorac Surg* 85:172–178.

[37] Ivanov, Y., Mykychak, Y., Fedevych, O., Motrechko, O., Kurkevych, A., Yemets, I. 2019 *"Single-centre 20-year experience with repair of truncus arteriosus. Interact CardioVasc Thorac Surg 1-8.* https:// doi:10.1093/icvts/ivz007.

[38] Franklin RC, Be land MJ, Colan SD, et al. Nomenclature for congenital and paediatric cardiac disease: the International Paediatric and Congenital Cardiac Code (IPCCC) and the Eleventh Iteration of the International Classification of Diseases (ICD-11). Cardiol Young 2017; 27: 1872–938.

[39] Leo Lopez et al. Classification of Ventricular Septal Defects for the Eleventh Iteration of the International Classification of Diseases—Striving for Consensus: A Report From the International Society for Nomenclature of Paediatric and Congenital Heart Disease. *Ann Thorac Surg* 2018; 106:1578.

[40] KP McCarthy, SY Ho, and RH Anderson. Ventricular Septal Defects: Morphology of the Doubly Committed Juxtaarterial and Muscular Variants. *Images Paediatr Cardiol.* 2000 Jul-Sep; 2(3): 5–23.

[41] Jacobs JP, Burke RP, Quintessenza JA, et al: Congenital Heart Surgery Nomenclature and Database Project: Ventricular septal defect. *Ann Thorac Surg* 69:S25-S35, 2000 (suppl 4).

[42] Eroglu AG, Oztunc F, Saltik L, et al: Aortic valve prolapse and aortic regurgitation in patients with ventricular septal defect. *Pediatr Cardiol* 24:36-39, 2003.

[43] McDaniel NL, Gutgesell HP. Ventricular septal defects. Allen HD, Driscoll DJ, Shaddy RE, Feltes TF. Moss and Adams' Heart Disease in Infants, Children, and Adolescents. 7th ed. Philadelphia: Wolters Kluwer/ Lippincott Williams & Wilkins; 2008. 667-682.

[44] Momma K, Toyama K, Takao A, et al. Natural history of juxta-arterial infundibular ventricular septal defect. *Am Heart J* 1984;108:1312–7.

[45] Lue HC, Sung TC, Hou SH, et al. Ventricular septal defect in Chinese with aortic valve prolapse and aortic regurgitation. *Heart Vessels* 1986;2:111– 6.

[46] Van Praagh R, McNamara JJ. Anatomic types of ventricular septal with aortic insufficiency. *Am Heart J* 1968;75:604–19.

[47] McElhinney DB, Anderson RH. Developmental anomalies of the outflow tracts and aortic arch: towards an understanding of the role of deletions within the 22nd chromosome. *Cardiol Young*. 1999;9:451–457.

[48] Yacoub MH, Khan H, Stauri G, Shinebourne E, Radley- Smith R. Anatomic correction of the syndrome of prolapsing right coronary aortic cusp, dilatation of the sinus of Valsalva, and ventricular septal defect. *J Thorac Cardiovasc Surg* 1997; 113:253– 61.

[49] Chiu SN, Wang JK, Lin MT, et al: Aortic valve prolapse associated with outlet-type ventricular septal defect. *Ann Thorac Surg* 79:1366-1371, 2005.

[50] Trusler GA, Williams WG, Smallhorn JF, et al: Late results after repair of aortic insufficiency associated with ventricular septal defect. *J Thorac Cardiovasc Surg* 103:276-281, 1992.

[51] Tweddell JS, Pelech AN, Frommelt PC. Ventricular septal defect and aortic valve regurgitation: pathophysiology and indications for surgery. *Semin Thorac Cardiovasc Surg Pediatr Card Surg Ann* 2006;9:147–52.

[52] Devlin Paul J. Devlin, BA, Hyde M. Russell, MD, Michael C. Monge, MD, Angira Patel, MD, John M. Costello, MD, MPH, Diane E. Spicer, BS, Robert H. Anderson, MD, and Carl L. Backer, MD. Doubly Committed and Juxtaarterial Ventricular Septal Defect: Outcomes of the Aortic and Pulmonary Valves. *Ann Thorac Surg* 2014;97:2134–41.

[53] Tatsuno K, Konno S, Ando M, et al: Pathogenetic mechanisms of pro- lapsing aortic valve and aortic regurgitation associated with ventricular septal defect. Anatomical, angiographic, and surgical considerations. *Circulation* 48:1028-1037, 1973.

[54] Tomita H, Arakaki Y, Ono Y, et al: Severity indices of right coronary cusp prolapse and aortic regurgitation complicating ventricular septal defect in the outlet septum: Which defect should be closed? *Circ J* 68:139-143, 2004.

[55] Chiu SN, Wang JK, Lin MT, et al: Aortic valve prolapse associated with outlet-type ventricular septal defect. *Ann Thorac Surg* 79:1366-1371, 2005.

[56] Cheung Y-f, Chiu CS, Yung T-c, Chau AK (2002) Impact of pre- operative aortic cusp prolapse on long-term outcome after surgical closure of subarterial ventricular septal defect. *Ann Thorac Surg* 73:622–627.

[57] Evdokia Petropoulou, Stergios Theodoropoulos, and Magdi H. Yacoub. Repair of all the components of the syndrome of aortic regurgitation and VSD. doi:10.1093/eurheartj/ehi524.

[58] Elgamal MA, Hakimi M, Lyons JM, et al: Risk factors for failure of aortic valvuloplasty in aortic insufficiency with ventricular septal defect. *Ann Thorac Surg* 68:1350-1355, 1999.

[59] Lun K, Li H, Leung MP, et al: Analysis of indications for surgical closure of subarterial ventricular septal defect without associated aortic cusp prolapse and aortic regurgitation. *Am J Cardiol* 87:1266-1270, 2001.

[60] Okita Y, Miki S, Kusuhara K, et al. Long-term results of aortic valvuloplasty for aortic regurgitation associated with ventricular septal defect. *J Thorac Cardiovasc Surg* 1988;96: 769–74.

[61] Gabriels C, Gewillig M, Meyns B, Troost E,Van De Bruaene A, Van Damme S et al. Doubly committed ventricular septal defect: single-centre experi- ence and midterm follow-up. *Cardiology* 2011;120:149–56.

[62] Chauvaud S, Serraf A, Mihaileanu S, Soyer R, Blondeau P, Dubost C, et al. Ventricular septal defect associated with aortic valve incompetence: results of two surgical managements. *Ann Thorac Surg*. 1990;49(6):875-880.

[63] Tariq Waqar, Muhammad Farhan Ali Rizvi, Ahmad Raza Baig. Doubly committed Subarterial Ventricular Septal defect repair: An experience of 51 cases. *Pak J Med Sci.* 2017;33(5):1112-1116.

[64] Ahmad Mahir Shamsuddin, Yen Chuan Chen, Abdul Rahim Wong, Trong-Phi Le, Robert H. Anderson and Antonio F. Corno Surgery for doubly committed ventricular septal defects. *Interactive CardioVascular and Thoracic Surgery* 23 (2016) 231–234.

[65] Chiu S-N, Wang J-K, Lin M-T. Aortic valve prolapse associated with outlet-type ventricular septal defect. *Ann Thorac Surg* 2005;79:1366–71.

[66] Momma K, Toyama K, Takao A, et al. Natural history of subarterial infundibular ventricular septal defect. *Am Heart J* 1984;108:1312–7.

[67] Trusler GA, Williams WG, Smallhorn JF, Freedom RM. Late results after repair of aortic insufficiency associated with ventricular septal defect. *J Thorac Cardiovasc Surg* 1992;103: 276– 81.

[68] Leung MP, Beerman LB, Siewers RD, Bahnson HT, Zuber- buhler JR. Long-term follow-up after aortic valvuloplasty and defect closure in ventricular septal defect with aortic regurgitation. *Am J Cardiol* 1987;60:890–4.

[69] Hanna Jung, Yoon Yong Cho, Youngok Lee. Progression of Aortic Regurgitation After Subarterial Ventricular Septal Defect Repair: Optimal Timing of the Operation. *Pediatric Cardiology* (2019) 40:1696–1702.

[70] Levy MJ, Lillehei CW, Anderson RC, Amplatz K, Edwards JE: Aortico-left ventricular tunnel. *Circulation* 1963, 27: 841-53.

[71] Martins JD, Sherwood MC, Mayer JE et al: Aortic-left ventricular tunnel: 35-year experience. *J Am Coll Cardiol* 44:446-450,2004.

[72] Ho SY, Mulago M, Cook AC, et al: Surgical anatomy of aorto-left ventricular tunnel. *Ann Thorac Surg* 65:509-514, 1998.

[73] Hovaguimian H, Cobanoglu A, Starr A: Aortic-left ventricular tunnel:A clinical review and new surgical classification. *Ann Thorac Surg* 45: 106-12, 1988.
[74] Kim RW, Spray TL: Surgical correction of aortic-left ventricular tunnel. *Semin Thorac Cardiovasc Surg Pediatr card Surg Ann* 9:177-179, 2006.
[75] Bernanke DH, Velkey JM: Development of the coronary blood supply: Changing concepts and current ideas. *Anat Rec* 2002, 269 (4): 198-208.
[76] Ya J, Van Der Hoff MJ, De Boer PA, et al. normal development of the outflow tract in the rat. *Circ Res* 1998, 82:464-72.
[77] Akalin H, Erol C, Oral D et al. Aortico-left ventricular tunnel: Successful diagnostic and surgical approach to the oldest patients in the literature. *J Thorac Cardiovasc Surg* 1989, 97: 804-5.
[78] Kafka H, Chan KL, Leach AJ. Asymptomatic aortico-left ventricular tunnel in adulthood. *Am J Cardiol* 1989, 63: 1021-2.
[79] Serino W, Andrade JL, Ross D, De Leval M, Sommerville J. Aorto-left ventricular communication after closure. Late postoperative problems. *Br Heart J* 1983, 49: 501-6.
[80] Bove KE, Swartz DC. Aortico-left ventricular tunnel. A new concept. *Am J Cardiol* 1967, 19: 696-709.
[81] Sousa-Uva M, Touchot A, Fermont L, Piot D, Delezoide AL, Serraf A, Lacour-Gayet F, Roussin R, Bruniaux J, Planché C. Aortico-left ventricular tunnel in fetuses and infants. *Ann Thorac Surg* 1996, 61: 1805-10.
[82] Cook AC, Fagg NKL, Ho SY, Groves AMM, Sharland GK, Anderson RH, Allen LD. Echocardiographic-anatomical correlation in aorto-left ventricular tunnel. *Br Heart J* 1995, 74: 443-8.
[83] Grab D, Paulus WE, Terinde R, Lange D. Prenatal diagnosis of an aortico-left ventricular tunnel. *Ultrasound Obstet Gynecol* 2000, 15:435-8.
[84] Sreeram M, Franks R, Arnold R, Walsh K. Aortico-left ventricular tunnel: Long-term outcome after surgical repair. *J Am Coll Cardiol* 1991, 17: 950-5.
[85] Kathare P, Subramanyam RG, Dash TK, Muthusvamy KS, Raghu K, Koneti NR. Diagnosis and management of aorto-left-ventricular tunnel. *Ann Pediatr Cardiol* 2015 May-Aug 8 (2): 103-7.
[86] Nezafati MH, Maleki MH, Javan H, Zirak N. epair of aorto-left ventricular tunnel arising from the left sinus of Valsalva. *J Card Surg* 2010;25: 245-6.
[87] Ono M, Goerler H, Boethig D, Breymann T. Surgical repair of aorto-left ventricular tunnel arisning from the left aortic sinus. *Interact Cardiovasc Thorac Surg* 2008;7: 510-1.
[88] Mueller C, Dave H, Pretre R. Surgical repair of aorto-ventricular tunnel. *Multimed Man cardiothorac Surg* 2012 Jan 1;2012.
[89] Protopapas EM, Anderson RH, Backer CL et al. European Congenital heart Surgeons Association – *World Society for Pediatric and Congenital Heart Surgery* (ECHSA – WSPCHS) study group. Surgical management of aorto-ventricula tunnel. A multicenter study. *Semin Thorac Cardiovasc Surg* 2020 Feb (article in press).
[90] Mckay R. Aorto-ventricular tunnel. *Orphanet J Rare Dis* 2007, 2-41.

In: Perspectives in Aortic Valve Disease
Editor: Giovanni Concistrè
ISBN: 978-1-53618-769-4

Chapter 9

ADULT BICUSPID AORTIC VALVE

Alessandro Della Corte** and Federica Lo Presti
Department of Translational Medical Sciences,
University of Studies of Campania "L. Vanvitelli",
Unit of Cardiac Surgery and Transplant, Monaldi Hospital, Naples, Italy

ABSTRACT

Bicuspid aortic valve (BAV) is the most common congenital defect of the heart, occurring in 0.5-2% of live births. It is estimated to be responsible for a relevant burden of valvular and vascular disease in the adulthood (bicuspid valvulo-aortopathy). The present chapter focuses on the aspects of valvular morbidity (aortic valve stenosis, regurgitation, endocarditis) and complications of the thoracic aorta in the adult (aortic dilatation, aortic dissection), trying to underscore similarities and unique features of BAV-related conditions compared to the respective diseases in tricuspid aortic valve patients. Epidemiological aspects, pathogenetic theories, risk stratification strategies and treatment principles will be briefly reviewed.

Keywords: bicuspid aortic valve, aortic valve stenosis, aortic valve regurgitation, infective valve endocarditis, aortopathy, aortic aneurysm, aortic dissection

INTRODUCTION

Bicuspid aortic valve (BAV) is the most common congenital defect of the heart, occurring in 0.5-2% of live births and uniquely predisposing the subject to chronic or acute complications either in infancy or in adulthood [1]. Most cases are isolated, non-syndromic conditions, however the BAV can also be a part of complex clinical disorders, including Turner syndrome (about one third of Turner patients have a BAV), Shone complex, Loeys-Dietz syndrome, etc. generally diagnosed in pediatric age [2]. Notably, even the non-syndromic forms of BAV carry risks not only related to the aortic valve, but also to the

* Corresponding Author's Email: aledellacorte@libero.it.

thoracic aorta: BAV is indeed best defined as a peculiar valvulo-aortopathy. This chapter will focus on the implications of BAV in adulthood, therefore the main phenotypic expressions and valvulo-aortic diseases occurring in the isolated non-syndromic forms will be the object of the following paragraphs.

PHENOTYPES OF BICUSPID AORTIC VALVE

A BAV is defined as an aortic valve with two instead of three functional cusps, as a result of congenital "fusion" or "non-separation" of two underdeveloped leaflets [1]: according to which cusps are involved by the malformation, different types of BAV can result (Figure 1). Traditionally, BAV morphological phenotypes (or morphotypes) are referred to according to the Sievers classification [3], which takes into account the number of raphes and the pattern of cusp fusion. The number of raphes defines the main category, being type 0 without a raphe ("pure" bicuspid valves), type 1 with one raphe (the most frequent, accounting for nearly 90% of cases) and type 2 with two raphes (better termed as unicuspid valves). The pattern of cusp fusion defines the first sub-category: type 0 encompasses all circumferential orientations of a BAV, among which either antero-posterior or latero-lateral variants exist, due to fusion of right- and left-coronary cusps (RL) or right- and non-coronary cusps (RN), respectively. Among type 1 BAVs, the most frequent pattern of fusion is the RL (nearly 70%), followed by RN (15%) and the rarer LN (around 3%). Notably there seem to be differences in those prevalence figures according to ethnicity: in particular the RN and LN forms seem more frequent in Asian ethnicities compared to the western people [4]. Although widely employed for several years this classification is only simplistically descriptive and has been criticized as not useful in clinical and surgical practice: several attempts have been made to systematize the morphological variability of the BAV with clinically-oriented methods, i.e., in radiology [5], in interventional cardiology [6], in reparative surgery [7]. A consensus of experts has very recently agreed upon a new classification of the BAV, which avoids misnomers (e.g., type 0 BAV for unicuspid; "true" BAV for the valve with 2 leaflets and 2 sinuses) and indicates the different categories with descriptive denominations in English language rather than with numbers and letters (unpublished).

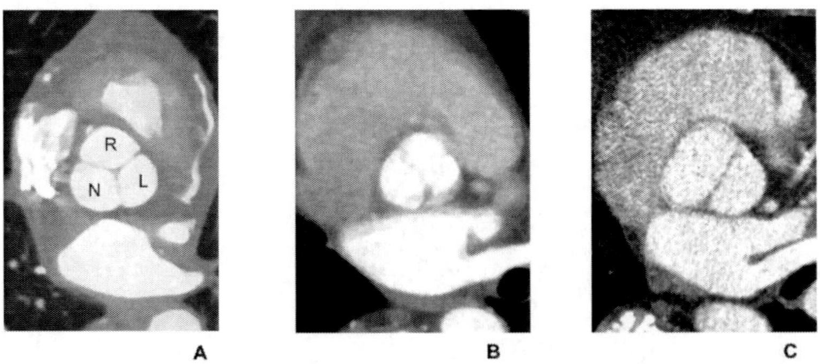

Figure 1. Computed tomography scans of: A) a normal tricuspid aortic valve (R= right coronary cusp, L= left coronary cusp, N= noncoronary cusp); B) a congenital bicuspid aortic valve of the RL morphotype; C) a congenital bicuspid aortic valve of the RN morphotype. Note the relative dimesions of the cusps: the non-fused cusp (N in panel B and L in panel C) cover a larger surface area than they would in the normal tricuspid aortic valve whereas the fused cusp is the result of two underdeveloped cusps joint together.

Embryogenesis and Hemodynamic Effects of Different Morphotypes

A study carried out in adult and embryonic hearts of eNOS knock-out mice and inbred Syrian hamsters, animal models with a high incidence of RN- and RL-type BAV, respectively, presented evidence suggesting that different genetic substrates could underlie the diverse valve morphotypes [8]. RN-BAVs could be the product of a defect occurring before the left ventricular outflow tract (LVOT) septation, probably due to an exaggerated NO-dependent endothelial to mesenchymal transition, whereas RL-BAVs could result from the anomalous septation of the proximal outflow tract, likely due to neural crest cells disorders [8]. However, a subsequent large cross-sectional study of BAV human families found that the 2 most frequent BAV morphotypes could be interchangeably inherited within the same family, with a morphologic concordance of nearly 70% in family members [9]. Therefore, it remains likely that different dys-embryogenetic mechanisms underlie the different valve morphotypes, but the genetic bases could overlap, and inheritance could be complex and multigenic.

Four-dimensional flow magnetic resonance imaging (4D flow MRI) studies highlighted differences in ascending aortic flow directions and severity of derangements among different valve fusion patterns. RL-BAVs give rise to a helical jet flow directed toward the right anterior aortic wall [10], with higher axial WSS at the aortic root and proximal ascending [11]. The RN-BAVs, instead, generate a flow jet initially directed toward the posterior aorta [10], with higher circumferential WSS in mid and distal ascending aorta related to more severe rotational flow [11]. Cusps fusion pattern and valvular dysfunction can also affect the severity of flow derangements: in RN-BAVs there are more severe flow abnormalities and larger aortas than in RL-BAVs, as well as in valvular stenosis compared to regurgitation [12].

Different Inherent Risks?

Whether the abovementioned different morphotypes of BAV imply different risks of valve or aorta complications has been investigated in several studies. The RN type was reported to be associated with more rapid progression towards aortic valve stenosis in the pediatric age [13]; others have confirmed the higher frequency of BAV stenosis and lower frequency of BAV insufficiency in patients with the latero-lateral orientation of the cusps or RN-coronary fusion [14, 15].

Clinical follow-up investigations have yielded contrasting results regarding the differences in aortopathy risk between the two main morphotypes: in a pediatric population the RN type was significantly associated in univariate analysis with faster growth of the ascending aorta (not confirmed however in multivariable analysis) [16]. However, according to another study enrolling adult BAV patients, the RL type was a predictor of greater velocity of size increase over time [17]. Such investigations might have been jeopardized by the inclusion of a limited number of phenotypic variables: Della Corte et al., by including among the explored covariates also the aortic phenotype (pattern of dilatation of the aorta) found no significant association of either valve morphotype with faster growth of the aorta, whereas the root phenotype (aortic dilation predominantly at the sinuses, with normal or less dilated ascending tract – a phenotype in which the valve is almost exclusively of the RL type) was a significant predictor [18]. So far the evidence on associations of the BAV morphotypes with different risk of aortopathy is considered inconclusive; once aortopathy develops, however, there is unique association of the RL type with more proximal localization of the dilatation and of the RN type with more distal involvement (possibly extending into the proximal arch): the consistency of these findings with the different patterns of post-valvular flow and interaction of flow with the aortic wall with different morphotypes, as reported above, is striking [19, 20].

Bicuspid Aortic Valve Stenosis

Although echocardiographically normo-functional, in most BAVs the two cusps exhibit asymmetric anatomy and therefore asymmetric systolic excursion, generating geometrically abnormal transvalvular-flow patterns (systolic transvalvular jet not parallel to the vessel's axis), causing an intrinsic degree of subclinical stenosis: the tangential forces exerted on the aortic wall, namely wall shear stresses (WSSs), are uneven compared to the normal laminar flow [12, 21, 22].

Once diagnosed, the BAV requires echocardiographic follow-up, with shorter intervals between subsequent controls once valve dysfunction has developed. Since in BAV subjects the LVOT diameter is larger than in TAV counterparts and ejective jets may be particularly eccentric, guidelines recommend to estimate the severity of the stenosis by exploring the transaortic peak velocity and mean gradient in multiple windows, whereas valve area represents a secondary parameter [23].

Currently, the available knowledge and tools to predict progression of BAV stenosis remain limited, although an echocardiography-based valve degeneration score, taking into account calcification, thickening and mobility reduction, proved to predict need for surgery in the follow-up, thus identifying a higher-risk subgroup of patients who may require more frequent assessments [24]. Further computed tomography-based indexes or genetic tests could be helpful in the future in predicting the evolution of an initially borderline valve function [25].

BAV is a Relevant Cause of Aortic Valve Stenosis

In the majority of adults with a congenital BAV, the malformation is sooner or later complicated by valve dysfunction necessitating aortic valve replacement (AVR), reported to be necessary in 53% of patients within 25-years of diagnosis [26]. Calcific aortic stenosis (AS) represents the most common fate of a BAV [24, 27], typically occurring earlier in life than in a TAV subject [28]. As a consequence, after age-matching, BAV-AS patients exhibit lower prevalence of systemic cardiovascular risk factors than TAV-AS subjects [29]. In causing the predisposition of a BAV to AS, possible mutations affecting valve tissue array and calcium deposition, e.g., those in the *NOTCH1* gene [30] and intrinsically increased leaflet stress and turbulent flow [12, 21, 22] may trump the effect of further acquired and modifiable cardiovascular risk factors. However, total cholesterol and hypertension have been found associated with AS onset in BAV patients [31]. The mechanisms of AS progression, including inflammation, calcium deposition and ossification are shared between BAV and

TAV patients [32]. Despite higher transvalvular gradient with a similar degree of valve stenosis, BAV-AS patients exhibit lower degree of cardiac impairment, in terms of diastolic function, stroke volume, left ventricular ejection fraction, left atrial size, and pulmonary hypertension, than TAV-AS counterparts [29]. A subgroup of BAV patients may exhibit early valve degeneration, i.e., calcification, thickening and decreased mobility, independent of valve hemodynamics: in this subgroup, the risk of AVR at 12 years is as high as 70% [24].

AVR for AS represents the second most common cardiac operation in the adult population, preceded only by coronary artery bypass grafting. Data from a large study of adults undergoing aortic valve replacement for stenosis underscored the great contribution of BAV condition to the epidemiology of AS, inasmuch as congenitally malformed aortic valves are slightly more frequent than normal tricuspid ones, at least in male patients [33]. In younger patients unicuspid valves are more prevalent: only 15% of patients requiring surgery under 60 years had a TAV, conversely representing the majority (52%) of stenotic valves in older patients [33].

Invasive Treatment of BAV Stenosis

Surgical treatment of BAV-AS follows current guidelines for the management of valvular heart disease, which do not distinguish between TAV and BAV [23, 34]. However, as already mentioned, the BAV population faces severe AS and subsequent surgery one or two decades earlier than TAV subjects, implying longer exposure to prosthesis-related complications (e.g., prosthetic infective endocarditis, degeneration of biological prostheses, valve thrombosis and so on) and greater impact on lifestyle (e.g., physical activity or sports, lifelong anticoagulant therapy for mechanical prostheses, and so on) [25].

Notwithstanding the younger age at operation, early outcomes of aortic valve replacement (AVR) for BAV patients are similar to those for tricuspid counterparts, in terms of both in-hospital/30-days mortality and complications [35, 36]. Long-term outcomes in BAVs are satisfactory too, with a reported 15-years survival after isolated valve surgery ranging between 68% and 78% [35, 37], with no substantial difference after age-matching with TAVs [35]. The good long term results are probably in part explained also by BAV stenosis patients receiving on average larger size prostheses, due to their inherent larger LVOT dimensions, thus making patient prosthesis mismatch, associated with poorer outcomes after AVR [38, 39], a relatively uncommon condition [29]. BAV women undergoing AVR present more frequently with AS and with more advanced AS than BAV men [40]. Although they often receive smaller prostheses, associated with higher transvalvular gradients and lower degrees of ventricular postoperative remodeling [41], short- and long-term outcomes after AVR in women are similar to men [40].

Transcatheter aortic valve replacement (TAVR) has widespread as a therapy for severe symptomatic AS in tricuspid patients whose risk with conventional surgery was deemed high or unacceptable [42, 43]. An usually asymmetric annulus and an uneven distribution of calcium in the setting of BAV stenosis [44] led to the exclusion of BAV patients from both TAVR trials [43] and current guidelines recommendations [23, 34, 45], due to concerns of possible noncircular deployment of the prosthesis and consequent dysfunction.

Although initially off-label TAVR procedures in BAV patients resulted in higher incidence of valve malposition and malfunction, significant paravalvular leaks (PVL), more conversion to surgery, more pacemaker requirements and less overall procedural success than conventional surgery [46], there is mounting interest in improving TAVR outcomes in BAV-AS patients, given the lowering of age and surgical-risk class thresholds for transcatheter procedures in tricuspid counterparts. Recent analyses, however, confirmed lower device success and higher rates of PVL - with a clear reduction by latest generation device implant [47, 48, 49] -, similar in-hospital/30 days mortality compared either with TAVR performed on TAV-AS [47, 48] or with surgical AVR [48]. CT-angiography remains the gold standard for careful annulus analysis and TAVR planning [50, 51]. Further studies are warranted to compare long-term efficacy and safety of transcatheter vs conventional replacement.

Bicuspid Aortic Valve Regurgitation

Minimal degrees of aortic regurgitation (AR) are common among congenitally BAV subjects. Pure AR was reported as significantly less common than stenosis (30% vs 70%) in echocardiographic cohorts [46], as well as in surgical and autoptic series [52]. Nonetheless, a purely regurgitant BAV with a dysfunction severe enough to require surgery is known to cause almost the 7% of AVR due to primary AR, i.e., not secondary to aortic dilatation/dissection or endocarditis [53]. In TTE examinations, the parasternal long axis view can show in diastolic frames how one or both cusps prolapse, usually generating a hyper-eccentric AR jet. Alternatively, secondary AR can be identified as a central jet associated with dilatation of one or more of the valve-root complex components, including the annulus, one or more sinuses, and the sino-tubular junction.

The Regurgitant BAV

BAV patients affected by pure degenerative aortic regurgitation have unique clinical features: the majority of them are males [54], taller and younger than those who suffer from AS [55, 56, 57], more often with a RL cusp fusion pattern, whereas the aorta is commonly affected by dilatation mainly involving the sinuses of Valsalva, in the so-called “root phenotype” [58].

Once valvular dysfunction reaches thresholds for surgical treatment [23], the valve should be replaced or, when feasible in experienced centers repaired: pre-operative echocardiography plays a pivotal role in assessing reparability of the regurgitant BAV [46] and today several preoperative measurements of the valve-root complex configuration can predict the durability of the repair.

Principles of BAV Repair

At the beginning of the BAV repair experience, excellent short-term results were reached, however in mid-term follow-up a relevant incidence of recurrent regurgitation was recorded [59, 60, 61]. Repair techniques for regurgitant BAVs and valve-preserving surgery for BAV-related aneurysms have evolved considerably over the past 20 years: nowadays, most non-calcified BAVs are preserved or repaired – even more frequently than TAVs –, with a cumulative reoperation incidence of 20% at 15 years when combined with root surgery [62].

The improvement in repair results was achieved by means of both accurate understanding of pathogenetic mechanisms and identification of morphologic predictors of reparability, leading to more standardized and reproducible correction of all pathologic components of valve and root at the time of surgery [63, 64]. The most important mechanisms underlying BAV regurgitation are [65]:

- cusp prolapse, almost always of the fused cusp, sometimes involving also the non-fused cusp, possibly as a result of long-standing regurgitation;
- annular dilatation;
- root dilatation (sinuses, sino-tubular junction).

Free margin plication of the prolapsing cusp represents a milestone in BAV repair, already introduced in the early 90's [59]. Over the years, it became clear that the underestimation of the extent of prolapse (e.g., of both fused and non-fused cusp) and the intraoperative finding of an insufficient cusp tissue amount were among the reasons of repair failure and/or withdrawal. Therefore, echocardiographic and intra-operative measurements were introduced of both cusp geometric height, useful to assess the amount of leaflet tissue available as repair substrate, and cusp effective height, useful to quantify the amount of prolapse independently of each leaflet [66, 67].

Aortic annular stabilization/reduction is also fundamental to improve the durability of repair, and it is mandatory with an annular diameter exceeding 26-27 mm [68, 69, 70]. Subcommissural plication sutures [69] have been quit in favor of annuloplasty performed by either circular suture [68] or external ring [70] or of valve-sparing reimplantation.

Whenever the aortic root is enlarged, its replacement is necessary, either with valve reimplantation or root remodeling completed with annuloplasty [71, 72]. Some Authors suggested lowering the threshold for aortic root replacement in this setting to a diameter exceeding 42-43 mm [63].

Recently, with the spreading of the repair techniques and the increased experience of reference Centers, the anatomy of the regurgitant BAV has been more and more recognized to encompass a spectrum of different morphologies, from the symmetric BAV with two sinuses and two seamless cusps, through the BAV forms with two underdeveloped and fused cusps and one non-fused cusp, to the more asymmetric forms with incomplete raphe in the fused cusp [7, 73]. The symmetry of the two cusps (evenness of the respective portions of total valve surface area covered) has been quantified as the angle of commissural orientation (CO), whereas 180° indicates the symmetric BAV with two equally sized cusps [7]. The height of the sub-commissural triangle below the raphe or pseudo-commissure is lower than the one of the normal commissures: this height decreases with increasing symmetry of the valve configuration. Also, the annulus (virtual basal ring) is more circular in the symmetric forms, more elliptic in the asymmetric ones [73]. Symmetrical valves benefit from cusp plication alone, asymmetrical BAVs may need commissural re-orientation towards 180° during root surgery [74, 75], whereas the very asymmetrical BAVs are probably best treated as TAVs.

In patients presenting with cusp retraction/perforation, calcification of the raphe or a very asymmetric BAV, the choice should tend towards AVR rather than repair [76]. However, in treating a BAV-AR, surgeons must keep in mind that survival after repair is similar to that of gender- and age-matched BAV controls [77, 78].

ENDOCARDITIS OF THE BAV

Infective endocarditis (IE) is a rare but serious disease involving heart valves, with high morbidity and mortality. Patients with structural abnormalities of cardiac valves, such as BAV, are known to be exposed to a higher risk of IE. Although the linearized incidence of endocarditis in BAV adults is low, about 0.3%/year in several estimates [24, 79], the high BAV prevalence within the adult population implies that adequate attention must be paid to the risk of infective complications of BAV.

Indications for Prophylaxis, Risks and Treatments

Published systematic reports of clinical features and surgical treatments of IE in adults with BAV have been few [80, 81]. Patients with IE on BAV are younger, with less comorbidity [82, 83] and more frequently male [84] than TAV counterparts. A multicenter study estimated in BAV subjects a 23-fold higher adjusted relative risk (RR) of aortic valve IE than TAV subjects [83].

Based on the risk of both IE and its complications, predisposing cardiac conditions are officially classified as low-, intermediate-, and high-risk. Currently, IE antibiotic prophylaxis (IEAP) is recommended by guidelines only for high-risk conditions, which do not include the BAV [85, 86]. Some investigators showed higher rates of IE from either verified *viridans group streptococci* etiology or suspected dental origin in a BAV subgroup than in the remaining endocarditis patients [87], whereas others authors observed a lower incidence of *Sthaphylococcus aureus* infection in BAV IE [83]. Several studies underscored a higher frequency of perivalvular abscess in the BAV IE group compared with the TAV IE group [82-84]. The underlying mechanism for this phenomenon remains unclear. However, the high frequency of BAV cusps calcifications possibly extending to the perivalvular area and the histologic derangements occurring in the BAV aortic media might explain an increased susceptibility to infection spreading to the structures adjacent to the valve, resulting in a perivalvular abscess and/or mycotic root involvement [84]. Perivalvular involvement is a known factor increasing postoperative mortality in surgery for IE [88], only in part explained by a greater technical complexity of the operation, that has to include abscess cavity opening, draining and repairing [84]. Notably, in multivariate analysis, BAV was the only independent predictor associated with an increased risk of aortic perivalvular abscess [84]. The observation of a clinical profile similar to that of high-risk IE patients suggested to reconsider the case for IEAP in BAV subjects [87]: anyway, the recommendation is still being debated [89, 90]. BAV IE patients are 2-fold likely to undergo valve replacement than TAV IE counterparts within the 5 years subsequent to the onset of the disease [83]. Prompt diagnosis leads to timely surgery, that might prevent the formation and extension of perivalvular abscess.

Despite the younger age of the BAV patients at surgery, no significant difference was found in terms of in-hospital mortality between BAV and TAV IE patients, the two groups thereafter showing similar age-adjusted postoperative 1-year and 5-year mortality [83, 84]. Further studies are needed to evaluate clinical features and surgical outcomes of IE among BAV and TAV patients, in order to identify high-risk subgroups earlier, thus improving surgical results [84].

BAV AORTOPATHY

Besides valve dysfunction or infection, the most common complications of BAV include dilation or dissection of the ascending aorta [91]. BAV-associated aortopathy, thought to occur in 30 to 80% of BAV patients, is a heterogeneous disease, both in terms of natural history and anatomo-clinical forms of the disease [18, 58]. The natural course can vary, ranging from indolent aortic diameter growth to rapid progression or earlier occurrence of life-threatening complications [91]. The velocity of growth of the aorta in BAV patients can be in absolute terms similar to the one observed in Marfan syndrome patients at the level of the Valsalva sinuses, although the segment experiencing the fastest growth rate in BAV is the tubular ascending [92].

Two main phenotypes of aortic dilatation can be observed: the most common one is the "ascending phenotype" - predominant dilatation located at the tubular tract, distal to the sinotubular junction -, encountered in 60-70% of dilated BAV aortas and usually associated with aortic stenosis (AS) and advanced age [58]. The rarer "root phenotype" - a dilated aorta with diameter at Valsalva sinuses exceeding the diameter of the tubular tract - represents the 20-25% of BAV aneurysms. It is uniquely associated with male sex, aortic regurgitation (AR), RL-BAV and younger age at presentation: this type of dilatation, occurring earlier in life and independently of hemodynamics, has been suggested to be a phenotypic marker of more diffuse and more severe disease of the whole ascending aorta [56].

Pathogenetic Hypotheses

Historically, two hypotheses on the pathogenesis of BAV aortopathy have been juxtaposed against each other: the genetic one and the hemodynamic one.

Arguments in favor of the first have included: aortic diameters being greater in BAV than in age-matched TAV subjects already in childhood, especially at the ascending tubular tract [93]; BAV patients with the same degree of AS having greater aortic diameters than TAV counterparts [94]; progressive dilatation after isolated AVR in BAV patients with normal aortic dimensions at the time of surgery [95]; non-BAV first degree relatives of aortic dilation BAV patients exhibiting aneurismal aortic disease [96]. Genes associated so far with BAV (with or without its complications) include the NOTCH1 (encoding for a heterodimeric transmembrane receptor involved into development of the cardiac outflow tract), ACTA2 (smooth muscle actin alpha 2), GATA5 (encoding for a mediator of nitric oxide synthase activation and endocardial cell differentiation), NKX2.5 (involved in cardiovascular morphogenesis and modulation of vascular wall homeostasis), SMAD6 (that negatively regulates both the bone morphogenetic protein pathway and the transforming growth factor-β1 signaling) and ROBO4 (encoding for a protein expressed in endothelial cells of the normal ascending aorta). Although these pathways could be relevant in the pathogenesis of the disease, to date, no major gene explaining a high rate of BAV/TAA cases has emerged. Possible obstacles to progress in this field of research include: extreme locus heterogeneity; incomplete penetrance; sex bias; environmental and/or epigenetic modifications of the clinical course of the disease [97, 98].

Arguments forwarded by other Authors in favor of the hemodynamic theory included: the evidence of altered flow patterns distal to the BAV even with normal echocardiographic function [22, 99]; the striking correlation between site of dilatation of the aorta and location of the highest wall stresses with different BAV morphologies (RL vs RL) [19]; the typical asymmetric expression of aortic wall alterations (more severe at the convexity, or greater curvature of the ascending aorta, where the skewed flow-jet from the malformed valve impinges on the vessel wall, than at the concavity, or lesser curvature) [58, 100, 101, 102]. Indeed, outward vascular remodeling is known to be a well conserved adaptive mechanism, in response to increased wall shear stress (WSS), aimed at bringing it back to physiological levels [103]. Histological analysis of aortic wall samples harvested during surgery in BAV patients subjected to pre-operative 4D flow MRI for WSS mapping showed more pronounced elastic fiber loss and disarray in regions of aortic wall exposed to elevated WSS compared with those subjected to normal WSS within the same aorta [101].

There is mounting evidence supporting that both pathogenic factors (gene variants and hemodynamic derangements) can be considered as culprits in the onset and progression of bicuspid aortopathy and the respective predominance of either factor in the determinism of the disease can vary across the different anatomo-clinical forms of the disease [14]. Clinical heterogeneity may be subtended by diverse combinations of coexisting genetic and hemodynamic causative factors: the ascending phenotype may be a form of disease in whom hemodynamic factors are predominant in determining aortic wall abnormalities and dilation; the root phenotype is suggested to be the form in whom the role of some genetic defect trumps the hemodynamic derangements [58, 104, 105].

Indications to Treatment: Wavering Guidelines

Elective surgery on BAV dilated aortas is performed in order to prevent life-threatening complications such as aortic rupture or dissection, whose age-adjusted relative risk in BAV subjects is almost 8-fold higher than in the general population [91]. From 1998 to 2017, 11 international official guidelines documents have been issued on thoracic aortic aneurysms [106]: the thresholds for elective repair of BAV aortas ranged from the initial 5.5 cm to a more aggressive nadir of 4.0 to 4.5 cm reached in 2010 [107], to return back to a conservative cut-off of 5.5 cm since 2012 [108].

The wavering of recommendations reflected shifting perspectives in the etiology of BAV aortopathy [109]. Aggressive approaches (both in terms of timing and extension of resection) derived by the old assumption that in BAV patients an inherited frailty involves potentially the entire aorta exposing it to life-long risk of dilatation and rupture. This widespread belief led ten years ago to surgical indications similar to those for Marfan syndrome patients [104], including BAV among connective tissue disorders [107]. On the other hand, the only two natural history studies performed on the BAV population showed a much lower risk of acute aortic events than in Marfan syndrome [24, 79]. On these bases, more conservative approaches were suggested [108, 110], considering that not all BAV patients are exposed to an equally high risk of aortic complications [109]. An interesting survey of 100 Canadian cardiac surgeons [111] revealed that in real-world practice the operative approaches to BAV aortopathy are highly variable both in terms of thresholds diameters and extent of the resection. Finally in 2018, an American Association for Thoracic Surgery (AATS) consensus document addressed uniquely BAV aortopathy [105]: repair of the ascending aorta/root was recommended for an aortic diameter:

- ≥55 mm in patients without risk factors;
- ≥50 mm in patients with risk factors (e.g., root phenotype or predominant AR, uncontrolled hypertension, family history of aortic dissection/sudden death, coarctation, aortic growth >3 mm/year);
- ≥50 mm when the patients are at low surgical risk and operated on by an experienced aortic team in a center with established surgical results;
- ≥45 mm in patients undergoing concomitant cardiac surgery.

The Risk of Aortic Dissection

Traditionally, aortic dissection has been interpreted as the result of mechanical aortic wall failure, exclusively related to dilatation. The risk of dissection was cumulated with the risk of rupture in old studies [112], and a critical diameter of 60 mm was found to represent the "hinge point" at which this risk increased abruptly, therefore a diameter of 55 mm was reasonable for elective surgery to prevent such acute complications of aortopathies. However, data from a retrospective analysis from the International Registry of Acute Aortic Dissections (IRAD) undermined the value of the aortic diameter as a predictor of acute aortic dissection, since this complication occurred at diameters less than 50 mm in about 40% of affected patients [113]. In BAV patients, in particular, the degree of medial degeneration in the aortic wall seemed independent from the vessel diameter [114] and less severe than in diameter-matched TAV controls [115]. Notably, when the phenotypic heterogeneity of BAV aortopathy was accounted for in analyses, studies suggested a greater risk of dissection with the root phenotype dilatation compared to the more frequent ascending phenotype [116] and the "hinge point" of the risk of dissection at presentation was at 50 mm for the root and 53 mm for the ascending tract in a large study from the Cleveland Clinic [117]. Several reports consistently found significantly greater diameters at the time of acute dissection in BAV than in TAV patients [118, 119, 120]: this finding, apparently in contrast with the evidence of greater risk of dissection in BAV subjects, moreover at a younger mean age, remains unexplained and yet it stresses the idea that the risk of dissection in general is only in part related to the size of the aorta [121].

Certainly, there is a critical need to develop individualized risk assessment beyond size and growth criteria, with an approach involving precision medicine. This could include quantification of wall remodeling phenomena by assessment of circulating biomarkers [102], estimation of wall biomechanical properties including stiffness and distensibility by techniques of functional imaging [122], measurement of flow patterns and creation of WSS maps by 4D flow MRI [11] and identification of genetic alterations by specific tests [98].

REFERENCES

[1] Michelena, H. I., Della Corte, A., Prakash, S. K., Milewicz, D. M., Evangelista, A. & Enriquez-Sarano, M. (2015). "Bicuspid aortic valve aortopathy in adults: Incidence, etiology, and clinical significance." *Int J Cardiol.*, *201*, 400-7. doi: 10.1016/j.ijcard.2015.08.106.

[2] Niaz, T., Poterucha, J. T., Johnson, J. N., Craviari, C., Nienaber, T., Palfreeman, J., Cetta, F. & Hagler, D. J. (2017). "Incidence, morphology, and progression of bicuspid aortic valve in pediatric and young adult subjects with coexisting congenital heart defects." *Congenit Heart Dis.*, *12*, 261-9. doi: 10.1111/chd.12429.

[3] Sievers, H. H. & Schmidtke, C. (2007). "A classification system for the bicuspid aortic valve from 304 surgical specimens." *J Thorac Cardiovasc Surg.*, *133*(5), 1226-33. doi: 10.1016/j.jtcvs.2007.01.039.

[4] Kong, W. K. F., Regeer, M. V., Poh, K. K., Yip, J. W., van Rosendael, P. J., Yeo, T. C., Tay, E., Kamperidis, V., van der Velde, E. T., Mertens, B., Marsan, N. A., Delgado, V. & Bax, J. J. (2018). "Inter-ethnic Differences in Valve Morphology., Valvular Dysfunction, and Aortopathy Between Asian and European Patients With Bicuspid Aortic Valve." *Eur Heart J.*, *39*(15), 1308-1313. doi: 10.1093/eurheartj/ehx562.

[5] Buchner, S., Hülsmann, M., Poschenrieder, F., Hamer, O. W., Fellner, C., Kobuch, R., Feuerbach, S., Riegger, G. A., Djavidani, B., Luchner, A. & Debl, K. (2010). "Variable phenotypes of bicuspid aortic valve disease: classification by cardiovascular magnetic resonance." *Heart.*, *96*(15), 1233-40. doi: 10.1136/hrt.2009.186254.

[6] Jilaihawi, H., Chen, M., Webb, J., Himbert, D., Ruiz, C. E., Rodés-Cabau, J., Pache, G., Colombo, A., Nickenig, G., Lee, M., Tamburino, C., Sievert, H., Abramowitz, Y., Tarantini, G., Alqoofi, F., Chakravarty, T., Kashif, M., Takahashi, N., Kazuno, Y., Maeno, Y., Kawamori, H., Chieffo, A., Blanke, P., Dvir, D., Ribeiro, H. B., Feng, Y., Zhao, Z. G., Sinning, J. M., Kliger, C., Giustino, G., Pajerski, B., Imme, S., Grube, E., Leipsic, J., Vahanian, A., Michev, I., Jelnin, V., Latib, A., Cheng, W. & Makkar, R. (2016). "A Bicuspid Aortic Valve Imaging Classification for the TAVR Era." *JACC Cardiovasc Imaging.*, *9*(10), 1145-1158. doi: 10.1016/j.jcmg.2015.12.022.

[7] de Kerchove, L., Mastrobuoni, S., Froede, L., Tamer, S., Boodhwani, M., van Dyck, M., El Khoury, G. & Schäfers, H. J. (2019). "Variability of repairable bicuspid aortic valve phenotypes: towards an anatomical and repair-oriented classification." *Eur J Cardiothorac Surg.*, *ezz033*. doi: 10.1093/ejcts/ezz033. Online ahead of print.

[8] Fernández, B., Durán, A. C., Fernández-Gallego, T., Fernández, M. C., Such, M., Arqué, J. M. & Sans-Coma, V. (2009). "Bicuspid aortic valves with different spatial orientations of the leaflets are distinct etiological entities." *J Am Coll Cardiol.*, *54*, 2312–2318. doi: 10.1016/j.jacc.2009.07.044.

[9] Robeldo-Carmona, J., Rodriguez-Bailòn, I., Carrasco-Chinchilla, F., Fernàndez, B., Jimènez-Navarro, M., Porras-Marin, C., Montiel-Trujillo, A., García-Pinilla, J. M., Such-Martínez, M. & De Teresa-Galván, E. (2013). "Hereditary patterns of bicuspid

aortic valve in a hundred families." *Int J Cardiol.*, *168*, 3443–3449. doi: 10.1016/j.ijcard.2013.04.180.

[10] Hope, M. D., Hope, T. A., Meadows, A. K., Ordovas, K. G., Urbania, T. H., Alley, M. T. & Higgins, C. B. (2010). "Bicuspid Aortic Valve: Four-dimensional MR Evaluation of Ascending Aortic Systolic Flow Patterns." *Radiology.*, *255*(1), 53–61.doi: 10.1148/radiol.09091437.

[11] Rodríguez-Palomares, J. F., Dux-Santoy, L., Guala, A., Kale, R., Maldonado, G., Teixidó-Turà, G., Galian, L., Huguet, M., Valente, F., Gutiérrez, L., González-Alujas, T., Johnson, K. M., Wieben, O., García-Dorado, D. & Evangelista, A. (2018). "Aortic flow patterns and wall shear stress maps by 4D-flow cardiovascular magnetic resonance in the assessment of aortic dilatation in bicuspid aortic valve disease." *J Cardiovasc Magn Reson.*, *20*(1), 28. doi: 10.1186/s12968-018-0451-1.

[12] Bissell, M. M., Hess, A. T., Biasiolli, L., Glaze, S. J., Loudon, M., Pitcher, A., Davis, A., Prendergast, B., Markl, M., Barker, A. J., Neubauer, S. & Myerson, S. G. (2013). "Aortic dilation in bicuspid aortic valve disease: flow pattern is a major contributor and differs with valve fusion type." *Circ Cardiovasc Imaging.*, *6*(4), 499-507. doi: 10.1161/CIRCIMAGING.113.000528.

[13] Fernandes, S. M., Khairy, P., Sanders, S. P. & Colan, S. D. (2007). "Bicuspid aortic valve morphology and interventions in the young." *J Am Coll Cardiol.*, *49*(22), 2211-2214. doi:10.1016/j.jacc.2007.01.090.

[14] Della Corte, A., Bancone, C., Dialetto, G., Covino, F. E., Manduca, S., D'Oria, V., Petrone, G., De Feo, M. & Nappi, G. (2014). "Towards an Individualized Approach to Bicuspid Aortopathy: Different Valve Types Have Unique Determinants of Aortic Dilatation." *Eur J Cardiothorac Surg.*, *45*(4), e118-24. doi: 10.1093.ejcts/ezt601.

[15] Toufan Tabrizi, M., Rahimi Asl, R., Nazarnia, S. & Pourafkari, L. (2018). "Evaluation of relationship between bicuspid aortic valve phenotype with valve dysfunction and associated aortopathy." *J Cardiovasc Thorac Res.*, *10*(4), 236-242. doi:10.15171/jcvtr.2018.41.

[16] Holmes, K. W., Lehmann, U. C., Dalal, D., Nasir, K., Dietz, H. C., Ravekes, W. J., Thompson, W. R. & Spevak, P. J. (2007). "Progressive Dilation of the Ascending Aorta in Children With Isolated Bicuspid Aortic Valve." *Am J Cardiol.*, *99*(7), 978-83. doi: 10.1016/j.amjcard.2006.10.065.

[17] Thanassoulis, G., Yip, J. W. L., Filion, K., Jamorski, M., Webb, G., Siu, S. C. & Therrien, J. (2008). "Retrospective Study to Identify Predictors of the Presence and Rapid Progression of Aortic Dilatation in Patients With Bicuspid Aortic Valves." *Nat Clin Pract Cardiovasc Med.*, *5*(12), 821-8. doi: 10.1038/ncpcardio1369.

[18] Della Corte, A., Bancone, C., Buonocore, M., Dialetto, G., Covino, F. E., Manduca, S., Scognamiglio, G., D'Oria, V. & De Feo, M. (2013). "Pattern of ascending aortic dimensions predicts the growth rate of the aorta in patients with bicuspid aortic valve." *JACC Cardiovasc Imaging.*, *6*(12), 1301-1310. doi:10.1016/j.jcmg.2013.07.009.

[19] Mahadevia, R., Barker, A. J., Schnell, S., Entezari, P., Kansal, P., Fedak, P. W. M., Malaisrie, S. C., McCarthy, P., Collins, J., Carr, J. & Markl, M. (2014). "Bicuspid Aortic Cusp Fusion Morphology Alters Aortic Three-Dimensional Outflow Patterns, Wall Shear Stress, and Expression of Aortopathy." *Circulation.*, *129*(6), 673-82. doi: 10.1161/CIRCULATIONAHA.113.003026.

[20] Verma, S. & Siu, S. C. (2014). "Aortic dilatation in patients with bicuspid aortic valve." *N Engl J Med.*, *370*(20), 1920-1929. doi:10.1056/NEJMra1207059.

[21] Robicsek, F., Thubrikar, M. J., Cook, J. W. & Fowler, B. (2004). "The Congenitally Bicuspid Aortic Valve: How Does It Function? Why Does It Fail?" *Ann Thorac Surg.*, *77*(1), 177-85. doi: 10.1016/s0003-4975(03)01249-9.

[22] Barker, A. J., Markl, M., Bürk, J., Lorenz, R., Bock, J., Bauer, S., Schulz-Menger, J. & von Knobelsdorff-Brenkenhoff, F. (2012). "Bicuspid aortic valve is associated with altered wall shear stress in the ascending aorta." *Circ Cardiovasc Imaging.*, *5*(4), 457-66. doi: 10.1161/CIRCIMAGING.112.973370.

[23] Nishimura, R. A., Otto, C. M., Bonow, R. O., Blase, A., Carabello, B. A., Erwin, 3rd J. P., Guyton, R. A., O'Gara, P. T., Ruiz, C. E., Skubas, N. J., Sorajja, P., Sundt, 3rd T. M., Thomas, J. D. & ACC/AHA Task Force Members. (2014). " 2014 AHA/ACC guideline for the management of patients with valvular heart disease: a report of the American College of Cardiology/American Heart Association Task Force on Practice Guidelines [published correction appears in J Thorac Cardiovasc Surg. 2014 Oct 21;64(16):1763. Dosage error in article text]." *J Thorac Cardiovasc Surg.*, *148*(1), e1-e132. doi:10.1016/j.jtcvs.2014.05.014.

[24] Michelena, H. I., Desjardins, V. A., Avierinos, J. F., Russo, A., Nkomo, V. T., Sundt, T. M., Pellikka, P. A., Tajik, A. J. & Enriquez-Sarano, M. (2008). "Natural history of asymptomatic patients with normally functioning or minimally dysfunctional bicuspid aortic valve in the community." *Circulation.*, *117*(21), 2776-84. doi: 10.1161/CIRCULATIONAHA.107.740878.

[25] Della Corte, A., Body, S. C., Booher, A. M., Schaefers, H. J., Milewski, R. K., Michelena, H. I., Evangelista, A., Pibarot, P., Mathieu, P., Limongelli, G., Shekar, P. S., Aranki, S. F., Ballotta, A., Di Benedetto, G., Sakalihasan, N., Nappi, G., Eagle, K. A., Bavaria, J. E., Frigiola, A. & Sundt, T. M. (2014). International Bicuspid Aortic Valve Consortium (BAVCon) Investigators. "Surgical treatment of bicuspid aortic valve disease: knowledge gaps and research perspectives." *J Thorac Cardiovasc Surg.*, *147*(6), 1749-57., 1757.e1. doi: 10.1016/j.jtcvs.2014.01.021.

[26] Michelena, H. I., Prakash, S. K., Della Corte, A., Bissell, M. M., Anavekar, N., Mathieu, P., Bossé, Y., Limongelli, G., Bossone, E., Benson, D. W., Lancellotti, P., Isselbacher, E. M., Enriquez-Sarano, M., Sundt, T. M., 3rd. Pibarot, P., Evangelista, A., Milewicz, D. M. & Body, S. C. (2014). BAVCon Investigators. "Bicuspid aortic valve: identifying knowledge gaps and rising to the challenge from the International Bicuspid Aortic Valve Consortium (BAVCon)." *Circulation.*, *129*(25), 2691-704. doi: 10.1161/CIRCULATIONAHA.113.007851.

[27] Fedak, P. W. M., Verma, S., David, T. E., Leask, R. L., Weisel, R. D. & Butany, J. (2002). "Clinical and Pathophysiological Implications of a Bicuspid Aortic Valve." *Circulation.*, *106*(8), 900-4. doi: 10.1161/01.cir.0000027905.26586.e8.

[28] Vahanian, A. & Otto, C. M. (2010). "Risk Stratification of Patients With Aortic Stenosis." *Eur Heart J.*, *31*(4), 416-23. doi: 10.1093/eurheartj/ehp575.

[29] Huntley, G. D., Thaden, J. J., Alsidawi, S., Michelena, H. I., Maleszewski, J. J., Edwards, W. D., Scott, C. G., Pislaru, S. V., Pellikka, P. A., Greason, K. L., Ammash, N. M., Malouf, J. F., Enriquez-Sarano, M., Nkomo, V. T. (2018). "Comparative Study of Bicuspid vs. Tricuspid Aortic Valve Stenosis." *Eur Heart J Cardiovasc Imaging.*, *19*(1), 3-8. doi: 10.1093/ehjci/jex211.

[30] Mathieu, P., Bossé, Y., Huggins, G. S., Della Corte, A., Pibarot, P., Michelena, H. I., Limongelli, G., Boulanger, M. C., Evangelista, A., Bédard, E., Citro, R., Body, S. C., Nemer, M. & Schoen, F. J. (2015). "The pathology and pathobiology of bicuspid aortic valve: State of the art and novel research perspectives." *J Pathol Clin Res.*, *1*(4), 195-206. doi: 10.1002/cjp2.21.

[31] Chan, K. L., Ghani, M., Woodend, K. & Burwash, I. G. (2001). "Case-controlled Study to Assess Risk Factors for Aortic Stenosis in Congenitally Bicuspid Aortic Valve." *Am J Cardiol.*, *88*(6), 690-3. doi: 10.1016/s0002-9149(01)01820-3.

[32] Wallby, L., Janerot-Sjöberg, B., Steffensen, T. & Broqvist, M. (2002). "T Lymphocyte Infiltration in Non-Rheumatic Aortic Stenosis: A Comparative Descriptive Study Between Tricuspid and Bicuspid Aortic Valves." *Heart.*, *88*(4), 348-51. doi: 10.1136/heart.88.4.348.

[33] Roberts, W. C. & Ko, J. M. (2005). "Frequency by decades of unicuspid, bicuspid, and tricuspid aortic valves in adults having isolated aortic valve replacement for aortic stenosis, with or without associated aortic regurgitation." *Circulation.*, *111*(7), 920-5. doi: 10.1161/01.CIR.0000155623.48408.C5.

[34] Baumgartner, H., Falk, V., Bax, J. J., De Bonis, M., Hamm, C., Holm, P. J., Iung, B., Lancellotti, P., Lansac, E., Rodriguez Muñoz, D., Rosenhek, R., Sjögren, J., Tornos Mas, P., Vahanian, A., Walther, T., Wendler, O., Windecker, S., Zamorano, J. L. & ESC Scientific Document Group. (2017). "2017 ESC/EACTS Guidelines for the management of valvular heart disease." *Eur Heart J.*, *38*(36), 2739-2791. doi:10.1093/eurheartj/ehx391.

[35] Girdauskas, E., Disha, K., Borger, M. A. & Kuntze, T. (2014). "Long-term prognosis of ascending aortic aneurysm after aortic valve replacement for bicuspid versus tricuspid aortic valve stenosis." *J Thorac Cardiovasc Surg.*, *147*(1), 276-282. doi:10.1016/j.jtcvs.2012.11.004.

[36] Aicher, D., Fries, R., Rodionycheva, S., Schmidt, K., Langer, F. & Schäfers, H. J. 2010. "Aortic valve repair leads to a low incidence of valve-related complications." *Eur J Cardiothorac Surg.*, *37*(1), 127-132. doi:10.1016/j.ejcts.2009.06.021.

[37] Goland, S., Czer, L. S., De Robertis, M. A., Mirocha, J., Kass, R. M., Fontana, G. P., Chang, W. & Trento, A. (2007). "Risk factors associated with reoperation and mortality in 252 patients after aortic valve replacement for congenitally bicuspid aortic valve disease." *Ann Thorac Surg.*, *83*(3), 931-937. doi:10.1016/j.athoracsur. 2006.10.047.

[38] Pibarot, P. & Dumesnil, J. G. (2009). "Prosthetic heart valves: selection of the optimal prosthesis and long-term management." *Circulation.*, *119*(7), 1034-1048. doi:10.1161/CIRCULATIONAHA.108.778886.

[39] Blais, C., Dumesnil, J. G., Baillot, R., Simard, S., Doyle, D. & Pibarot, P. (2003). "Impact of valve prosthesis-patient mismatch on short-term mortality after aortic valve replacement." *Circulation.*, *108*(8), 983-988. doi:10.1161/01.CIR.0000085167. 67105.32.

[40] Andrei, A. C., Yadlapati, A., Malaisrie, S. C., Puthumana, J. J., Li, Z., Rigolin, V. H., Mendelson, M., Clennon, C., Kruse, J., Fedak, P. W. M., Thomas, J. D., Higgins, J. A., Rinewalt, D., O Bonow, R. & McCarthy, P. M. (2015). "Comparison of outcomes and presentation in men-versus-women with bicuspid aortic valves undergoing aortic valve replacement." *Am J Cardiol.*, *116*(2), 250-255. doi:10.1016/j.amjcard.2015.04.017.

[41] González-Juanatey, J. R., García-Acuña, J. M., Vega Fernandez, M., Amaro Cendón, A., Castelo Fuentes, V., García-Bengoechea, J. B. & de la Peña, M. G. (1996). "Influence of the size of aortic valve prostheses on hemodynamics and change in left ventricular mass: implications for the surgical management of aortic stenosis." *J Thorac Cardiovasc Surg.*, *112*(2), 273-280. doi:10.1016/s0022-5223(96)70249-0.

[42] Smith, C. R., Leon, M. B., Mack, M. J., Miller, D. C., Moses, J. W., Svensson, L. G., Tuzcu, E. M., Webb, J. G., Fontana, G. P., Makkar, R. R., Williams, M., Dewey, T., Kapadia, S., Babaliaros, V., Thourani, V. H., Corso, P., Pichard, A. D., Bavaria, J. E., Herrmann, H. C., Akin, J. J., Anderson, W. N., Wang, D., Pocock, S. J. PARTNER Trial Investigators. (2011). "Transcatheter versus surgical aortic-valve replacement in high-risk patients." *N Engl J Med.*, *364*(23), 2187-2198. doi:10.1056/NEJMoa1103510.

[43] Leon, M. B., Smith, C. R., Mack, M., Miller, D. C., Moses, J. W., Svensson, L. J., Tuzcu, E. M., Webb, J. G., Fontana, G. P., Makkar, R. R., Brown, D. L., Block, P. C., Guyton, R. A., Pichard, A. D., Bavaria, J. E., Herrmann, H. C., Douglas, P. S., Petersen, J. L., Akin, J. J., Anderson, W. N., Wang, D., Pocock, S. & PARTNER Trial Investigators. (2010). "Transcatheter aortic-valve implantation for aortic stenosis in patients who cannot undergo surgery." *N Engl J Med.*, *363*(17), 1597-1607. doi:10.1056/NEJMoa1008232.

[44] Philip, F., Faza, N. N., Schoenhagen, P., Desai, M. Y., Tuzcu, E. M., Svensson, L. G. & Kapadia, S. R. (2015). "Aortic annulus and root characteristics in severe aortic stenosis due to bicuspid aortic valve and tricuspid aortic valves: implications for transcatheter aortic valve therapies." *Catheter Cardiovasc Interv.*, *86*(2), E88-E98. doi:10.1002/ccd.25948.

[45] Holmes, D. R., Jr. Mack, M. J., Kaul, S., Kaul, S., Agnihotri, A., Alexander, K. P., Bailey, S. R., Calhoon, J. H., Carabello, B. A., Desai, M. Y., Edwards, F. H., Francis, G. S., Gardner, T. J., Kappetein, A. P., Linderbaum, J. A., Mukherjee, C., Mukherjee, D., Otto, C. M., Ruiz, C. E., Sacco, R. L., Smith, D. & Thomas, J. D. (2012). "2012 ACCF/AATS/SCAI/STS expert consensus document on transcatheter aortic valve replacement." *J Am Coll Cardiol.*, *59*(13), 1200-1254. doi:10.1016/j.jacc.2012.01.001.

[46] Michelena, H. I., Chandrasekaran, K., Topilsky, Y., Messika-Zeitoun, D., Della Corte, A., Evangelista, A., Schäfers, H. J., Enriquez-Sarano, M. & BAVCon. (2018). "The Bicuspid Aortic Valve Condition: The Critical Role of Echocardiography and the Case for a Standard Nomenclature Consensus." *Prog Cardiovasc Dis.*, *61*(5-6), 404-415. doi:10.1016/j.pcad.2018.11.003.

[47] Bob-Manuel, T., Heckle, M. R., Ifedili, I. A., Wang, J. & Ibebuogu, U. N. (2019). "Outcomes of transcatheter aortic valve replacement in bicuspid aortic valve stenosis." *Ann Transl Med.*, *7*(5), 102. doi:10.21037/atm.2019.02.04.

[48] Elbadawi, A., Saad, M., Elgendy, I. Y., Barssoum, K., Omer, M. A., Soliman, A., Almahmoud, M. F., Ogunbayo, G. O., Mentias, A., Gilani, S., Jneid, H., Aronow, H. D., Kleiman, N. & Abbott, J. D. (2019). "Temporal Trends and Outcomes of Transcatheter Versus Surgical Aortic Valve Replacement for Bicuspid Aortic Valve Stenosis." *JACC Cardiovasc Interv.*, *12*(18), 1811-1822. doi:10.1016/j.jcin.2019.06.037.

[49] Ueshima, D., Nai Fovino, L., Brener, S. J., et al. (2020). "Transcatheter aortic valve replacement for bicuspid aortic valve stenosis with first- and new-generation

bioprostheses: A systematic review and meta-analysis." *Int J Cardiol.*, 2020, 298, 76-82. doi:10.1016/j.ijcard.2019.09.003.

[50] Yoon, S. H., Bleiziffer, S., De Backer, O., et al. (2017). "Outcomes in Transcatheter Aortic Valve Replacement for Bicuspid Versus Tricuspid Aortic Valve Stenosis." *J Am Coll Cardiol.*, *69*(21), 2579-2589. doi:10.1016/j.jacc.2017.03.017.

[51] Perlman, G. Y., Blanke, P., Dvir, D., et al. (2016). "Bicuspid Aortic Valve Stenosis: Favorable Early Outcomes With a Next-Generation Transcatheter Heart Valve in a Multicenter Study." *JACC Cardiovasc Interv.*, *9*(8), 817-824. doi:10.1016/j.jcin.2016.01.002.

[52] Roberts, W. C. (1970). "The congenitally bicuspid aortic valve. A study of 85 autopsy cases." *Am J Cardiol.*, *26*(1), 72-83. doi:10.1016/0002-9149(70)90761-7.

[53] Roberts, W. C., Morrow, A. G., McIntosh, C. L., Jones, M. & Epstein, S. E. (1981). "Congenitally bicuspid aortic valve causing severe, pure aortic regurgitation without superimposed infective endocarditis. Analysis of 13 patients requiring aortic valve replacement." *Am J Cardiol.*, *47*(2), 206-209. doi:10.1016/0002-9149(81)90385-4.

[54] Roberts, W. C., McCullough, S. P. & Vasudevan, A. (2018). "Characteristics of Adults Having Aortic Valve Replacement for Pure Aortic Regurgitation Involving a Congenitally Bicuspid Aortic Valve Unaffected by Infective Endocarditis or Aortic Dissection." *Am J Cardiol.*, *122*(12), 2104-2111. doi:10.1016/j.amjcard.2018.08.063.

[55] Fernandes, S., Khairy, P., Graham, D. A., et al. (2012). "Bicuspid aortic valve and associated aortic dilation in the young." *Heart.*, *98*(13), 1014-1019. doi:10.1136/heartjnl-2012-301773.

[56] Della Corte, A. (2014). "Phenotypic heterogeneity of bicuspid aortopathy: a potential key to decode the prognosis?" *Heart.*, *100*(2), 96-7. doi: 10.1136/heartjnl-2013-305004.

[57] Evangelista, A., Gallego, P., Calvo-Iglesias, F., Bermejo, J., Robledo-Carmona, J., Sanchez, V., Saura, D., Arnold, R., Carro, A., Maldonado, G., Sao-Aviles, A., Teixido, G., Galian, L., Rodriguez-Palomares, J. & Garcia-Dorado, D. (2018). "Anatomical and clinical predictors of valve dysfunction and aortic dilation in bicuspid aortic valve disease." *Heart.*, *104*, 566–573. doi: 10.1136/heartjnl-2017-311560.

[58] Della Corte, A., Bancone, C., Quarto, C., Dialetto, G., Covino, F. E., Scardone, M., Caianiello, G. & Cotrufo, M. (2007). "Predictors of ascending aortic dilatation with bicuspid aortic valve: a wide spectrum of disease expression." *Eur J Cardiothorac Surg*, *31*, 397-405. doi: 10.1016/j.ejcts.2006.12.006.

[59] Cosgrove, D. M., Rosenkranz, E. R., Hendren, W. G., Bartlett, J. C. & Stewart, W. J. (1991). "Valvuloplasty for aortic insufficiency." *J Thorac Cardiovasc Surg.*, *102*(4), 571-577.

[60] Fraser, C. D., Jr. Wang, N., Mee, R. B., et al. (1994). "Repair of insufficient bicuspid aortic valves." *Ann Thorac Surg.*, *58*(2), 386-390. doi:10.1016/0003-4975(94)92212-8.

[61] Casselman, F. P., Gillinov, A. M., Akhrass, R., Kasirajan, V., Blackstone, E. H. & Cosgrove, D. M. (1999). "Intermediate-term durability of bicuspid aortic valve repair for prolapsing leaflet." *Eur J Cardiothorac Surg.*, *15*(3), 302-308. doi:10.1016/s1010-7940(99)00003-2.

[62] Schneider, U., Feldner, S. K., Hofmann, C., et al. (2017). "Two decades of experience with root remodeling and valve repair for bicuspid aortic valves." *J Thorac Cardiovasc Surg.*, *153*(4), S65-S71. doi:10.1016/j.jtcvs.2016.12.030.

[63] Ehrlich, T., de Kerchove, L., Vojacek, J., Boodhwani, M., El-Hamamsy, I., De Paulis, R., Lansac, E., Bavaria, J. E., El Khoury, G. & Schäfers, H. J. (2020). "State-of-the art bicuspid aortic valve repair in 2020." *Prog Cardiovasc Dis.*, *4*, S0033-0620(20)30082-7. doi: 10.1016/j.pcad.2020.04.010. Online ahead of print.

[64] Lansac, E., Di Centa, I., Raoux, F., Al Attar, N., Acar, C., Joudinaud, T. & Raffoul, R. (2008). "A lesional classification to standardize surgical management of aortic insufficiency towards valve repair." *Eur J Cardiothorac Surg.*, *33*(5), 872-8. doi: 10.1016/j.ejcts.2007.12.033.

[65] Aicher, D., Kunihara, T., Abou Issa, O., Brittner, B., Gräber, S. & Schäfers, H. J. (2011). "Valve configuration determines long-term results after repair of the bicuspid aortic valve." *Circulation.*, *123*(2), 178-185. doi:10.1161/CIRCULATIONAHA. 109.934679.

[66] Schäfers, H. J., Bierbach, B. & Aicher, D. (2006). "A new approach to the assessment of aortic cusp geometry." *J Thorac Cardiovasc Surg.*, *132*(2), 436-438. doi:10.1016/j.jtcvs.2006.04.032.

[67] Schäfers, H. J., Schmied, W., Marom, G. & Aicher, D. (2013). "Cusp height in aortic valves." *J Thorac Cardiovasc Surg.*, *146*(2), 269-274. doi:10.1016/j.jtcvs.2012.06.053.

[68] Schneider, U., Hofmann, C., Aicher, D., Takahashi, H., Miura, Y. & Schäfers, H. J. (2017). "Suture Annuloplasty Significantly Improves the Durability of Bicuspid Aortic Valve Repair." *Ann Thorac Surg.*, *103*(2), 504-510. doi:10.1016/j.athoracsur. 2016.06.072.

[69] Navarra, E., El Khoury, G., Glineur, D., et al. (2013). "Effect of annulus dimension and annuloplasty on bicuspid aortic valve repair." *Eur J Cardiothorac Surg.*, *44*(2), 316-323. doi:10.1093/ejcts/ezt045.

[70] Lansac, E., Di Centa, I., Sleilaty, G., et al. (2016). "Long-term results of external aortic ring annuloplasty for aortic valve repair." *Eur J Cardiothorac Surg.*, *50*(2), 350-360. doi:10.1093/ejcts/ezw070.

[71] Kayatta, M. O., Leshnower, B. G., McPherson, L., Zhang, C., Lasanajak, Y. & Chen, E. P. (2019). "Valve Sparing Root Replacement Provides Similar Midterm Outcomes in Bicuspid and Trileaflet Valves." *Ann Thorac Surg.*, *107*(1), 54-60. doi: 10.1016/j.athoracsur.2018.07.045.

[72] Lenoir, M., Maesen, B., Stevens, L. M., et al. (2018). "Reimplantation versus remodelling with ring annuloplasty: comparison of mid-term outcomes after valve-sparing aortic root replacement." *Eur J Cardiothorac Surg.*, *54*(1), 48-54. doi:10.1093/ ejcts/ezy016.

[73] Chirichilli, I., Irace, F. G., Weltert, L. P., et al. (2020). "A direct correlation between commissural orientation and annular shape in bicuspid aortic valves: a new anatomical and computed tomography classification." *Interact Cardiovasc Thorac Surg.*, *30*(5), 666-670. doi: 10.1093/icvts/ivz325.

[74] Schneider, U., Schmied, W., Aicher, D., Giebels, C., Winter, L. & Schäfers, H. J. (2017). "Sinus Plication to Improve Valve Configuration in Bicuspid Aortic Valve Repair-Early Results." *Ann Thorac Surg.*, *103*(2), 580-585. doi:10.1016/j.athoracsur. 2016.06.064.

[75] de Kerchove, L., Boodhwani, M., Glineur, D., et al. (2011). "Valve sparing-root replacement with the reimplantation technique to increase the durability of bicuspid

aortic valve repair." *J Thorac Cardiovasc Surg., 142*(6), 1430-1438. doi:10.1016/ j.jtcvs.2011.08.021.

[76] Miyahara, S., Schneider, U., Morgenthaler, L. & Schäfers, H. J. (2019). "(Almost) All Nonstenotic Bicuspid Aortic Valves Should Be Preserved or Repaired." *Semin Thorac Cardiovasc Surg., 31*(4), 656-660. doi: 10.1053/j.semtcvs.2019.03.008.

[77] Schneider, U., Hofmann, C., Schöpe, J., et al. "Reconstruction of bicuspid aortic valves – Long-term results of a differentiated anatomic repair concept." *JAMA Cardiology*. In press.

[78] Lansac, E., Bouchot, O., Arnaud Crozat, E., Hacini, R., Doguet, F., Demaria, R., et al. (2015). "Standardized approach to valve repair using an expansible aortic ring versus mechanical Bentall: early outcomes of the CAVIAAR multicentric prospective cohort study." *J Thorac Cardiovasc Surg., 149*(2 Suppl), S37-45. doi: 10.1016/ j.jtcvs.2014.07.105.

[79] Tzemos, N., Therrien, J., Yip, J., et al. (2008). "Outcomes in adults with bicuspid aortic valves." *JAMA., 300*(11), 1317-1325. doi:10.1001/jama.300.11.1317.

[80] Lamas, C. C. & Eykyn, S. J. (2000). "Bicuspid aortic valve--A silent danger: analysis of 50 cases of infective endocarditis." *Clin Infect Dis., 30*(2), 336-341. doi:10.1086/313646.

[81] Tribouilloy, C., Rusinaru, D., Sorel, C., et al. (2010). "Clinical characteristics and outcome of infective endocarditis in adults with bicuspid aortic valves: a multicentre observational study." *Heart., 96*(21), 1723-1729. doi:10.1136/hrt.2009.189050.

[82] Becerra-Muñoz, V. M., Ruíz-Morales, J., Rodríguez-Bailón, I., Sánchez-Espín, G., López-Garrido, M. A., Robledo-Carmona, J., Guijarro-Contreras, A., García-López, M. V., Ivanova-Georgieva, R., Mora-Navas, L., Gómez-Doblas, J. J. & de Teresa-Galván, E. (2017). "Infective Endocarditis in Patients With Bicuspid Aortic Valve: Clinical Characteristics, Complications, and Prognosis." *Enferm Infecc Microbiol Clin., 35*(10), 645-650. doi: 10.1016/j.eimc.2016.06.017.

[83] Kiyota, Y., Della Corte, A., Montiero Vieira, V., et al. (2017). "Risk and outcomes of aortic valve endocarditis among patients with bicuspid and tricuspid aortic valves." *Open Heart., 4*(1), e000545. Published 2017 May 16. doi:10.1136/openhrt-2016-000545.

[84] Chen, J., Lu, S., Hu, K., et al. (2017). "Clinical Characteristics and Surgical Treatment of Infective Endocarditis With Bicuspid Aortic Valve." *Int Heart J., 58*(2), 220-224. doi:10.1536/ihj.16-284.

[85] Wilson, W., Taubert, K. A., Gewitz, M., et al. (2007). "Prevention of infective endocarditis: guidelines from the American Heart Association: a guideline from the American Heart Association Rheumatic Fever, Endocarditis, and Kawasaki Disease Committee, Council on Cardiovascular Disease in the Young, and the Council on Clinical Cardiology, Council on Cardiovascular Surgery and Anesthesia, and the Quality of Care and Outcomes Research Interdisciplinary Working Group [published correction appears in *Circulation.*, 2007, Oct 9, *116*(15), e376-7]." Circulation. 116(15):1736-1754. doi:10.1161/CIRCULATIONAHA.106.183095.

[86] Habib, G., Hoen, B., Tornos, P., et al. (2009). "Guidelines on the prevention, diagnosis, and treatment of infective endocarditis (new version 2009): the Task Force on the Prevention, Diagnosis, and Treatment of Infective Endocarditis of the European Society of Cardiology (ESC). Endorsed by the European Society of Clinical

Microbiology and Infectious Diseases (ESCMID) and the International Society of Chemotherapy (ISC) for Infection and Cancer." *Eur Heart J.*, *30*(19), 2369-2413. doi:10.1093/eurheartj/ehp285.

[87] Zegri-Reiriz, I., de Alarcón, A., Muñoz, P., et al. (2018). "Infective Endocarditis in Patients With Bicuspid Aortic Valve or Mitral Valve Prolapse." *J Am Coll Cardiol.*, *71*(24), 2731-2740. doi:10.1016/j.jacc.2018.03.534.

[88] Di Mauro, M., Dato, G. M. A., Barili, F., et al. (2017). "Corrigendum to "A predictive model for early mortality after surgical treatment of heart valve or prosthesis infective endocarditis. The EndoSCORE". [Int. J. Cardiol. 241 (Aug 15 2017) 97-102]." *Int J Cardiol.*, *258*, 337. doi: 1 0.1016/j.ijcard.2018.01.019.

[89] Dayer, M. J., Jones, S., Prendergast, B., Baddour, L. M., Lockhart, P. B. & Thornhill, M. H. (2015). "Incidence of infective endocarditis in England, 2000-13: a secular trend, interrupted time-series analysis." *Lancet.*, *385*(9974), 1219-1228. doi:10.1016/S0140-6736(14)62007-9.

[90] Dayer, M. J., Jones, S., Prendergast, B., Baddour, L. M., Lockhart, P. B. & Thornhill, M. H. (2015). "Infective endocarditis and antibiotic prophylaxis - Authors' reply." *Lancet.*, *386*(9993), 531-532. doi:10.1016/S0140-6736(15)61471-4.

[91] Michelena, H. I., Khanna, A. D., Mahoney, D., Margaryan, E., Topilsky, Y., Suri, R. M., Eidem, B., Edwards, W. D., Sundt, T. M. 3rd. & Enriquez-Sarano, M. (2011). "Incidence of Aortic Complications in Patients With Bicuspid Aortic Valves." *JAMA*, *306*(10), 1104-1112. doi: 10.1001/jama.2011.1286.

[92] Detaint, D., Michelena, H. I., Nkomo, V. T., Vahanian, A., Jondeau, G. & Sarano, M. E. (2013). "Aortic dilatation patterns and rates in adults with bicuspid aortic valves: a comparative study with Marfan syndrome and degenerative aortopathy." *Heart.*, *100*(2), 126–134.doi:10.1136/heartjnl-2013-304920.

[93] Beroukhim, R. S., Kruzick, T. L., Taylor, A. L., Gao, D. & Yetman, A. T. (2006). "Progression of aortic dilation in children with a functionally normal bicuspid aortic valve." *Am J Cardiol.*, *98*, 828-830. doi: 10.1016/j.amjcard.2006.04.022.

[94] Keane, M. G., Wiegers, S. E., Plappert, T., Pochettino, A., Bavaria, J. E. & Sutton, M. G. (2000). "Bicuspid Aortic Valves Are Associated With Aortic Dilatation Out of Proportion to Coexistent Valvular Lesions." *Circulation.*, *102*, III-35–III-39. doi: 10.1161/circ.102.suppl_3.III-35. 25.

[95] Yasuda, H., Nakatani, S., Stugaard, M., Tsujita-Kuroda, Y., Bando, K., Kobayashi, J., Yamagishi, M., Kitakaze, M., Kitamura, S. & Miyatake, K. (2003). "Failure to prevent progressive dilation of ascending aorta by aortic valve replacement in patients with bicuspid aortic valve: comparison with tricuspid aortic valve." *Circulation.*, *108*, Suppl 1, II291-4. doi: 10.1161/01.cir.0000087449.03964.fb.

[96] Loscalzo, M. L., Goh, D. L., Loyes, B., Kent, K. C., Spevak, P. J. & Dietz, H. C. (2007). "Familial thoracic aortic dilation and bicommissural aortic valve: a prospective analysis of natural history and inheritance." *Am J Med Genet Part A.*, *143A*, 1960-1967. doi: 10.1002/ajmg.a.31872.

[97] Gould, R. A., Aziz, H., Woods, C. E., Seman-Senderos, M. A., Sparks, E., Preuss, C., Wünnemann, F., Bedja, D., Moats, C. R., McClymont, S. A., Rose, R., Sobreira, N., Ling, H., MacCarrick, G., Kumar, A. A., Luyckx, I., Cannaerts, E., Verstraeten, A., Björk, H. M., Lehsau, A. C., Jaskula-Ranga, V., Lauridsen, H., Shah, A. A., Bennett, C. L., Ellinor, P. T., Lin, H., Isselbacher, EM., Lino Cardenas, C. L., Butcher, JT.,

Hughes, G. C. & Lindsay, M. E. (2019). Baylor-Hopkins Center for Mendelian Genomics; MIBAVA Leducq Consortium, Mertens L, Franco-Cereceda A, Verhagen JMA, Wessels M, Mohamed SA, Eriksson P, Mital S, Van Laer L, Loeys BL, Andelfinger G, McCallion AS, Dietz HC. "ROBO4 variants predispose individuals to bicuspid aortic valve and thoracic aortic aneurysm." *Nat Genet.*, *51*(1), 42-50. doi: 10.1038/s41588-018-0265-y.

[98] Prakash, S. K., Bossé, Y., Muehlschlegel, J. D., Michelena, H. I., Limongelli, G., Della Corte, A., Pluchinotta, F. R., Russo, M. G., Evangelista, A., Benson, D. W., Body, S. C., Milewicz, D. M. & on behalf of the BAVCon Investigators. (2014). "A Roadmap to Investigate the Genetic Basis of Bicuspid Aortic Valve and its Complications: Insights From the International BAVCon (Bicuspid Aortic Valve Consortium)" *J Am Coll Cardiol.*, *64* (8), 832-839. doi: 10.1016/j.jacc.2014.04.073.

[99] Della Corte, A., Bancone, C., Conti, C. A., Votta, E., Redaelli, A., Del Viscovo, L. & Cotrufo, M. (2012). "Restricted cusp motion in right-left type of bicuspid aortic valves: a new risk marker for aortopathy." *J Thorac Cardiovasc Surg.*, *144*(2), 360-9, 369.e1. doi: 10.1016/j.jtcvs.2011.10.014.

[100] Forte, A., Della Corte, A., Grossi, M., Bancone, C., Provenzano, R., Finicelli, M., De Feo, M., De Santo, L. S., Nappi, G., Cotrufo, M., Galderisi, U. & Cipollaro, M. (2013). "Early cell changes and TGFbeta pathway alterations in the aortopathy associated with bicuspid aortic valve stenosis." *Clin Sci.*, *124*, 97–108. doi: 10.1042/CS20120324.

[101] Guzzardi, D. G., Barker, A. J., van Ooij, P., Malaisrie, S. C., Puthumana, J. J., Belke, D. D., Mewhort, H. E. M., Svystonyuk, D. A., Kang, S., Verma, S., Collins, J., Carr, J. O., Bonow, R., Markl, M., Thomas, J. D., McCarthy, P. M. & Fedak, P. W. M. (2015). "Valve-Related Hemodynamics Mediate Human Bicuspid Aortopathy. Insights From Wall Shear Stress Mapping." *J Am Coll Cardiol.*, *66*(8), 892-900. doi: 10.1016/j.jacc.2015.06.1310.

[102] Hardikar, A. A. & Marwick, T. H. (2015). "The natural history of guidelines: The case of aortopathy related to bicuspid aortic valves." *Int J Cardiol.*, *199*, 150–153. doi: 10.1016/j.ijcard.2015.06.059.

[103] Forte, A., Bancone, C., Cobellis, G., Buonocore, M., Santarpino, G., Fischlein, T. J. M., Cipollaro, M., De Feo, M. & Della Corte, A. (2017). "A Possible Early Biomarker for Bicuspid Aortopathy: Circulating Transforming Growth Factor β-1 to Soluble Endoglin Ratio." *Circ Res.*, *120*(11), 1800-1811. doi: 10.1161/CIRCRESAHA.117.310833.

[104] van Ooij, P., Markl, M., Collins, JD., MD; Carr, JC., Rigsby, C., Bonow, R. O., Malaisrie, S. C., McCarthy, P. M., Fedak, P. W. M. & Barker, A. J. (2017). "Aortic Valve Stenosis Alters Expression of Regional Aortic Wall Shear Stress: New Insights From a 4-Dimensional Flow Magnetic Resonance Imaging Study of 571 Subjects." *J Am Heart Assoc.*, *6*, e005959. doi: 10.1161/JAHA.117.005959.

[105] Girdauskas, E., Schulz, S., Borger, M. A., Mierzwa, M. & Kuntze, T. (2011). "Transforming growth factor-beta receptor type II mutation in a patient with bicuspid aortic valve disease and intraoperative aortic dissection." *Ann. Thorac. Surg.*, *91*, e70–e71. doi: 10.1016/j.athoracsur.2010.12.060.

[106] Borger, M. A., Fedak, P. W. M., Stephens, E. H., et al. (2018). "The American Association for Thoracic Surgery consensus guidelines on bicuspid aortic valve-related aortopathy: Full online-only version." *J Thorac Cardiovasc Surg.*, *156*(2), e41-e74. doi:10.1016/j.jtcvs.2018.02.115.

[107] Hardikar, A. A. & Marwick, T. H. (2015). "The natural history of guidelines: The case of aortopathy related to bicuspid aortic valves." *Int J Cardiol.*, *199*, 150–153. doi: 10.1016/j.ijcard.2015.06.059.

[108] Hiratzka, L. F., Bakris, G. L., Beckman, J. A., Bersin, R. M., Carr, V. F., Casey, D. E. Jr. Eagle, K. A., Hermann, L. K., Isselbacher, E. M., Kazerooni, E. A., Kouchoukos, N. T., Lytle, B. W., Milewicz, D. M., Reich, D. L., Sen, S., Shinn, J. A., Svensson, L. G. & Williams, D. M. (2010). American College of Cardiology Foundation/American Heart Association Task Force on Practice Guidelines; American Association for Thoracic Surgery; American College of Radiology; American Stroke Association; Society of Cardiovascular Anesthesiologists; Society for Cardiovascular Angiography and Interventions; Society of Interventional Radiology; Society of Thoracic Surgeons; Society for Vascular Medicine. "2010 ACCF/AHA/AATS/ACR/ASA/SCA/ SCAI/SIR/STS/SVM Guidelines for the diagnosis and management of patients with thoracic aortic disease. Task Force on Practice Guidelines, American Association for Thoracic Surgery, American College of Radiology, American Stroke Association, Society of Cardiovascular Anesthesiologists, Society for Cardiovascular Angiography and Interventions, Society of Interventional Radiology, Society of Thoracic Surgeons, and Society for Vascular Medicine." *Circulation.*, *121*, e266–e369. doi: 10.1016/j.jacc.2010.02.015.

[109] Vahanian, A., Alfieri, O., Andreotti, F., Antunes, M. J., Baron-Esquivias, G., Baumgartner, H., Borger, M. A., Carrel, T. P., De Bonis, M., Evangelista, A., Falk, V., Iung, B., Lancellotti, P., Pierard, L., Price, S., Schafers, H. J., Schuler, G., Stepinska, J., Swedberg, K., Takkenberg, J., Von Oppell, U. O., Windecker, S., Zamorano, J. L. & Zembala, M. (2013). Joint Task Force on the Management of Valvular Heart Disease of the European Society of Cardiology (ESC) and the European Association for Cardio-Thoracic Surgery (EACTS). "Guidelines on the management of valvular heart disease (version 2012). The Joint Task Force on the Management of Valvular Heart Disease of the European Society of Cardiology (ESC) and the European Association for Cardio-Thoracic Surgery (EACTS)." *G Ital Cardiol* (Rome)., *14*(3), 167-214. doi: 10.1714/1234.13659.

[110] Fedak, P. W. M., Barker, A. J. & Verma, S. (2016). "Year in Review: Bicuspid Aortopathy." *Curr Opin Cardiol.*, *31*(2), 132–138. doi:10.1097/ HCO.0000000000000258.

[111] Erbel, R., Aboyans, V., Boileau, C., Bossone, E., Di Bartolomeo, R., Eggebrecht, H., Evangelista, A., Falk, V., Frank, H., Gaemperli, O., Grabenwöger, M., Haverich, A., Iung, B., Manolis, A. J., Meijboom, F., Nienaber, C. A., Roffi M., Rousseau, H., Sechtem, U., Sirnes, P. A., Allmen, R. S. & Vrints, C. J. (2014). ESC Committee for Practice Guidelines. "2014 ESC Guidelines on the diagnosis and treatment of aortic diseases: Document covering acute and chronic aortic diseases of the thoracic and abdominal aorta of the adult. The Task Force for the Diagnosis and Treatment of Aortic Diseases of the European Society of Cardiology (ESC)." *Eur Heart J.*, *35*(41), 2873-926. doi: 10.1093/eurheartj/ehu281.

[112] Verma, S., Yanagawa, B., Kalra, S., Ruel, M., Peterson, M. D., Yamashita, M. H., Fagan, A., Currie, M. E., White, C. W., Wai Sang, S. L., Rosu, C., Singh, S., Mewhort, H., Gupta, N. & Fedak, P. W. (2013). "Knowledge, attitudes, and practice patterns in surgical management of bicuspid aortopathy: a survey of 100 cardiac surgeons." *J Thorac Cardiovasc Surg.*, *146*(5), 1033-1040.e4. doi: 10.1016/j.jtcvs.2013.06.037.

[113] Coady, M. A., Rizzo, J. A., Hammond, G. L., Mandapati, D., Darr, U., Kopf, G. S. & Elefteriades, J. A. (1997). "What is the appropriate size criterion for resection of thoracic aortic aneurysms?" J Thorac Cardiovasc Surg.113(3):476-91; discussion 489-91. doi: 10.1016/S0022-5223(97)70360-X.

[114] Pape, L. A., Tsai, T. T., Isselbacher, E. M., Oh, J. K., O'gara, P. T., Evangelista, A., Fattori, R., Meinhardt, G., Trimarchi, S., Bossone, E., Suzuki, T., Cooper, J. V., Froehlich, J. B., Nienaber, C. A. & Eagle, K. A. (2007). International Registry of Acute Aortic Dissection (IRAD) Investigators. "Aortic diameter > or = 5.5 cm is not a good predictor of type A aortic dissection: observations from the International Registry of Acute Aortic Dissection (IRAD)." *Circulation.*, *116*, 1120–1127. doi: 10.1161/CIRCULATIONAHA.107.702720.

[115] Leone, O., Biagini, E., Pacini, D., Zagnoni, S., Ferlito, M., Graziosi, M., Di Bartolomeo, R. & Rapezzi, C. (2012). "The elusive link between aortic wall histology and echocardiographic anatomy in bicuspid aortic valve: implications for prophylactic surgery." *Eur J Cardiothorac Surg.*, *41*, 322–327. doi: 10.1016/j.ejcts.2011.05.064.

[116] Heng, E., Stone, J. R., Kim, J. B., Lee, H., MacGillivray, T. E. & Sundt, T. M. (2015). "Comparative histology of aortic dilatation associated with bileaflet versus trileaflet aortic valves." *Ann Thorac Surg.*, *100*(6), 2095-101; discussion 2101. doi: 10.1016/j.athoracsur.2015.05.105.

[117] Girdauskas, E., Rouman, M., Disha, K., Espinoza, A., Misfeld, M., Borger, M. A. & Kuntze, T. (2015). "Aortic Dissection After Previous Aortic Valve Replacement for Bicuspid Aortic Valve Disease." *J Am Coll Cardiol.*, *66*(12), 1409-11. doi: 10.1016/j.jacc.2015.07.022.

[118] Wojnarski, C. M., Svensson, L. G., Roselli, E. E., Idrees, J. J., Lowry, A. M., Ehrlinger, J., Pettersson, G. B., Gillinov, A. M., Johnston, D. R., Soltesz, E. G., Navia, J. L., Hammer, D. F., Griffin, B., Thamilarasan, M., Kalahasti, V., Sabik, J. F. 3rd, Blackstone, E. H. & Lytle, B. W. (2015). "Aortic Dissection in Patients With Bicuspid Aortic Valve-Associated Aneurysms." *Ann Thorac Surg.*, *100*(5), 1666-73, discussion 1673-4. doi: 10.1016/j.athoracsur.2015.04.126.

[119] Etz, C. D., von Aspern, K., Hoyer, A., et al. (2015). "Acute type A aortic dissection: characteristics and outcomes comparing patients with bicuspid versus tricuspid aortic valve." *Eur J Cardiothorac Surg.*, *48*(1), 142-150. doi:10.1093/ejcts/ezu388.

[120] Eleid, M. F., Forde, I., Edwards, W. D., et al. (2013). "Type A aortic dissection in patients with bicuspid aortic valves: clinical and pathological comparison with tricuspid aortic valves." *Heart.*, *99*(22), 1668-1674. doi:10.1136/heartjnl-2013-304606.

[121] Rylski, B., Blanke, P., Beyersdorf, F., et al. 2014. "How does the ascending aorta geometry change when it dissects?." *J Am Coll Cardiol.*, *63*(13), 1311-1319. doi:10.1016/j.jacc.2013.12.028.

[122] Della Corte, A. (2015). "The conundrum of aortic dissection in patients with bicuspid aortic valve: the tissue, the mechanics and the mathematics." *Eur J Cardiothorac Surg.*, *48*(1), 150-151. doi:10.1093/ejcts/ezu418.

[123] Nistri, S., Grande-Allen, J., Noale, M., et al. (2008). "Aortic elasticity and size in bicuspid aortic valve syndrome." *Eur Heart J.*, *29*(4), 472-479. doi:10.1093/eurheartj/ehm528.

In: Perspectives in Aortic Valve Disease
Editor: Giovanni Concistrè
ISBN: 978-1-53618-769-4

Chapter 10

MANAGEMENT OF AORTIC VALVE DISEASE IN LVADS

A. Montalto[1,*], C. Amarelli[2], K. Hopkins[3], V. Piazza[4] and F. Musumeci[1]

[1]Department of Cardiac Surgery and Heart Transplantation, San Camillo Hospital, Rome, Italy
[2]Department of Cardiac Surgery and Heart Transplant, Monaldi Hospital, Azienda dei Colli, Neaples, Italy
[3]Department of Pediatrics, Division of Pediatric Cardiology, Northwestern University Feinberg School of Medicine, Chicago, IL, US
[4]Division of Cardiology Department of Cardiac Surgery and Heart Transplantation, San Camillo Hospital, Rome, Italy

ABSTRACT

Aortic regurgitation in patients implanted with a left ventricle assist device (LVAD) compromises effective left ventricle unloading by creating a closed blood recirculatory loop between the pump, the incompetent aortic valve, the left ventricle, and back to the pump again. Regurgitation through the aortic valve (AV) reduces antegrade LVAD output, diminishes systemic organ perfusion and elevates left heart filling pressure. Increase in filling pressure can lead to worsening of mitral regurgitation and pulmonary edema commonly occurs. Due to these concerns, moderate or greater aortic regurgitation has always been a contraindication to LVAD support. Current strategies to address aortic regurgitation include AV closure, AV repair, AV replacement, but there are currently sparse data on short- and long-term outcomes that influence decisions for current management of aortic regurgitation in LVAD patients. Significant aortic regurgitation can also result from progression of minor aortic insufficiency with time on device support. In this case no clear recommendations exist for how to proceed. Surgical procedures like aortic valve replacement or left ventricle outflow tract closure could be considered while balancing the high risk of complications. Percutaneous procedures, such

* Corresponding Author's Email: andrea.montalto@libero.it.

transcatheter aortic valve replacement or AV closure with an occlusion device, have been reported with good immediate results, but mid- and long-term outcomes should be further investigated. In this chapter we describe the biggest considerations related to aortic valve pathology during LVAD support and illustrate the different surgical approaches for managing this physiology.

Keywords: left ventricle assist device, aortic regurgitation, aortic repair, ramp test

INTRODUCTION

Mechanical ventricular assistance systems are increasingly acquiring a pivotal role in the treatment of heart failure refractory to medical therapy. The technological evolution has led to the development of remarkably reliable left ventricle assist device (LVAD), also suitable for use as destination therapy in those who are not candidates for heart transplantation. The implantation of these devices is recommended in selected patients when advanced ventricular dysfunction not responsive to medical therapy is diagnosed (class IIa, level of evidence B) [1, 2]. The purposes for implanting these mechanical supports include: DT = Destination therapy; BTT = Bridge to Transplant; BTC = Bridge to Candidacy. LVADs are frequently indicated as destination therapy for patients not suitable for heart transplantation because various comorbidities contraindicate their inclusion in the transplant list. The bridge to transplant strategy is appropriately applied in those whose clinical conditions deteriorate rapidly despite maximum medical therapy, and an organ is not expected to be available quickly for transplantation. Bridge to candidacy is the strategy employed for acutely ill patients not yet screened for transplantation or when transplantation is temporarily contraindicated but the clinical conditions are likely to improve after LVAD therapy. Rapid technological advances have led to the development of reliable and high quality systems. The improvement in blood compatibility has resulted in lower thromboembolic risks and improving survival rates, 86% and 79% at 1 and 2 years respectively [3], has led to an increase in the number of patients offered LVADs for DT. The percentage of all patients receiving LVADs for DT out of all those who receive LVADs is as high as 50% based on data from the INTERMACS registry [4]. The longer of survival time of patients with LVAD, the increased number of patients implanted for DT, and the shortage of organ donors have greatly increased the number of LVAD patients and the duration of support significantly, thus raising the incidence of time-related complications. Development of valve disease, particularly aortic valve insufficiency (AI), should be carefully monitored for when long time support is expected. Three main aspects need to be considered:

1) Medical and surgical strategies when de novo AI occur in LVAD patients.
2) Assessment of aortic regurgitation at the time of implantation.
3) Timing and strategies for treatment of aortic valve disease when LVAD implantation is planned.

De Novo Aortic Regurgitation

Aortic valve degeneration during ventricular assist device (VAD) support is a well-documented complication that occurs 15 to 52% of patients. The development of aortic regurgitation results in reduced efficiency of the device due to volume and pressure overload of the left ventricle. A consequence of this overload is an increase in ventricular diastolic pressures, enhanced pulmonary circulation pressures, and pulmonary edema [5, 6]. A recent analysis conducted on data from the INTERMACS registry showed that 50% of patients with continuous flow left ventricular assist devices (CF-LVADs) developed aortic regurgitation within two years post-implantation. By stratifying the analysis according to the preoperative AI severity, 11% of patients without AI before implantation developed moderate AI at one year and 55% of patients with moderate AI at the time of implantation developed severe AI at six months. The mechanism of de novo aortic regurgitation appears multifactorial, although controversy remains [4]. From a strictly hemodynamic point of view, the position of the outflow cannula in the ascending aorta creates essential modifications in the dynamics of the aortic flow and the physiology of the aortic valve [7, 8, 9, 10]. The persistent increase in left ventricular (LV) afterload combined with reduction in LV filling pressure, cause permanent closure of the valve and persistent stretching of the perivalvar tissues [11, 12, 13]. The synergistic effect of the continuous apposition of the leaflets with the turbulent retrograde flow induces pathological changes affecting the aortic valve leaflets and the aortic wall resulting in valve degeneration with consequent stenosis and/or insufficiency. Since the development of AI is time-related, the duration of support with mechanical systems and the use of VAD as destination therapy, are important risk factors. In two important studies, advanced age (> 60 years), low body surface area (BSA), moderate preoperative AI, peripheral vascular disease, and ischemic cardiomyopathy were identified as risk factors for the development of AI. Several additional studies supported the claim above that the loss of pulsatility and the loss of the physiological opening and closing cycle of the aortic valve during support with LVAD is particularly harmful to the normal physiology of the aortic valve [14, 15, 16, 17, 18]. Many studies have clearly shown that patients in whom it was possible to preserve pulsatility and therefore, the physiological opening and closing cycle of the aortic valve, had a reduced incidence of AI. This is not always possible, and is dependent on the diameter of the left ventricle, the degree of mitral regurgitation, and the residual function of the left ventricle. Maintaining pulsatility in patients with severe impairment of ventricular function can only occur at high ventricular filling pressures, which can result in elevated left atrial pressure and pulmonary venous pressure resulting in pulmonary edema and respiratory distress. Eventually this can lead to right ventricular dysfunction. Therefore, hemodynamic optimization, including opening and closing of the aortic valve, must be balanced with the risk of late development of aortic regurgitation and right ventricular failure.

Hemodynamic Effect

The development of AI represents a severe complication in patients with LVAD as it leads to the formation of a circulatory loop between the device, the left ventricle, and the device again. The ultimate result is severe inefficiency of the ventricular support with consequent inadequate ventricular unloading, reduction of the effective antegrade flow, and compromised distal organ perfusion. Ineffective LV unloading leads to an increase in the end-diastolic volume of the left ventricle oftentimes causing worsening mitral valve insufficiency and the symptoms of heart failure [19]. At the same time, the ineffective unloading causes an increase in the afterload of the right ventricle. This could be detrimental to right ventricular function, especially in patients with preoperative right ventricular failure. While important in all patients, this requies special consideration in those who underwent LVAD implantation as a bridge to candidacy. The high ventricular filling pressures lead to development or worsening pulmonary hypertension as a consequence of increased pulmonary vascular resistance, thus compromising the eligibility for heart transplantation.

Lorem ipsum dolor sit amet, consectetuer adipiscing elit. Maecenas porttitor congue massa. Fusce posuere, magna sed pulvinar ultricies, purus lectus malesuada libero, sit amet commodo magna eros quis urna.

Nunc viverra imperdiet enim. Fusce est. Vivamus a tellus.

Pellentesque habitant morbi tristique senectus et netus et malesuada fames ac turpis egestas. Proin pharetra nonummy pede. Mauris et orci.

Treatment Strategies for De Novo AI

Since the pathophysiological problems related to the development of AI in patients implanted with LVAD can be extremely detrimental, preventive measures should be applied to reduce the occurrence of AI. As previously mentioned, a factor that increases the incidence of aortic valve complications is represented by the absence of pulsatility and the lack of the standard opening and closing cycle of the aortic valve. Therefore, numerous authors recommend that a series of ramp tests be performed before the patient is discharged [20]. These tests conducted under echocardiographic guidance should aim to reduce the pump speed until a transaortic gradient is achieved that guarantees opening of the aortic valve. Attention should be paid to optimize the revolution per minutes (RPM) by balancing adequate unloading of the left ventricle, central positioning of the septum, and minimizing mitral regurgitation. Another critical element in preventing AI development is reduction of afterload. Although there is no unanimous consensus in identifying an association between increased after-load and development of AI, Patil et al. suggest that monitoring and controlling blood pressure plays an essential role in preventing the development of AI [21]. The ISHLT guidelines recommend maintaining an average systemic pressure of 80 mm Hg (class II b, level of evidence C). It should be noted that severe AI does not necessarily result in heart failure and high filling pressures. In LVAD patients with severe but asymptomatic moderate-grade AI, there are no recommendations on timing for intervention or modality of treatment. Management should focus on optimizing the speed of the device, on managing the afterload, and and maintaining euvolemia to prevent progression of aortic insufficiency. It is advisable to monitor these patients closely following the pro-beta natriuretic peptide level and hemodynamics during right heart cardiac catheterization. Patients with significant AI and with symptoms of heart failure, treatment is aimed at reducing vascular congestion while at the same time treating valve insufficiency. Medical treatment via diuretics and vasodilator, aimed at reducing congestion and control blood pressure is always the first step to improve symptoms. Ramp testing under echocardiographic guidance is the next non-invasive step in managing symptomatic patients. Those who do not respond to RPM optimization under echocardiographic guidance should undergo right heart catheterization [22] with concomitant echocardiographic direction. An initial increase in RPM could be trialed with the aim of increasing cardiac output and improving organ perfusion. However, it should not be underestimated that an increase in RPM can result in a worsening aortic valve insufficiency. This approach can only be considered as a short-term palliative strategy. If medical therapy and adjustments to the pump are unsuccessful, invasive procedures should be considered and candidates for a heart transplant could be inserted in an emergent transplant list. There are no absolute recommendations for the most appropriate surgical procedure for these patients. Surgical options include:

1) Implantation of an aortic patch [24, 25]
2) Replacing the native aortic valve with a biological valve
3) Partial closure of the aortic valve
4) Transcatheter aortic valve replacement (TAVR)
5) Implantation of an aortic valve occluder

Complete closure of the LV outflow tract completely eliminates the risk of AI but can lead to a disastrous scenario if a device malfunction occurs. If heart function recovery is expected to occur, the closure of the aortic valve is absolutely contraindicated [26]. In this case, valve replacement or repair could be considered. The surgical approaches that require a sternotomy carry higher risks than less invasive options, including possible ventricular damage and risk of hemorrhage, and are burdened by an up to 18% short-term mortality and up to 7% late mortality [27, 28]. The percutaneous approach in patients with contraindications to surgery reduces the risk related to general anesthesia, extracorporeal circulation, and the effect of anticoagulation. Percutaneous treatments include implantation of an occlusion device, which blocks the ventricular outflow tract, or implantation of a transcatheter aortic valve prosthesis (TAVR). Implantation of an occlusion device reduces AI from severe to mild without changing LVAD parameters. However, this procedure is not without complications. In fact, cases complicated by device migration [29] have been described. Long-term consequences of aortic valve occlusion by implanting an occluder have not yet been well studied. In our experience, we reported the strategy carried out in a patient implanted with Heartmate II (Chicago, IL, USA) and admitted with severe signs of heart failure related to the late development of AI. The patient, not eligible for a heart transplant, was considered unsuitable for percutaneous valve implantation because an aortic root diameter larger than 40 mm was estimated. The only alternative was the occlusion of the aortic valve by implanting an oversized occluder [30]. The postoperative echocardiographic evaluation displayed an aortic regurgitation decreased from severe to trivial (Figure 1).

The chest tomography conducted after seven days demonstrated the device was well positioned (Figure 2).

The second option, TAVR, has shown an excellent efficacy in the treatment of AI in patients implanted with LVAD. The advantage of this procedure is that, unlike the occlusion of the AV, the patient is not entirely dependent on mechanical support. If a device malfunction or thrombosis occurs, transaortic flow through the valve prosthesis is maintained by the residual left ventricular function. Problems associated with this procedure include the risk of perivalvular leaks and the difficulties of anchoring the prosthesis in good position. Unbehaun et al. described a procedure of transcatheter valve prosthesis implantation, preceded by implantation of a bare metal stent in the aortic root, in order to prepare a land zone for the valve prosthesis to mitigate this latter issue [31].

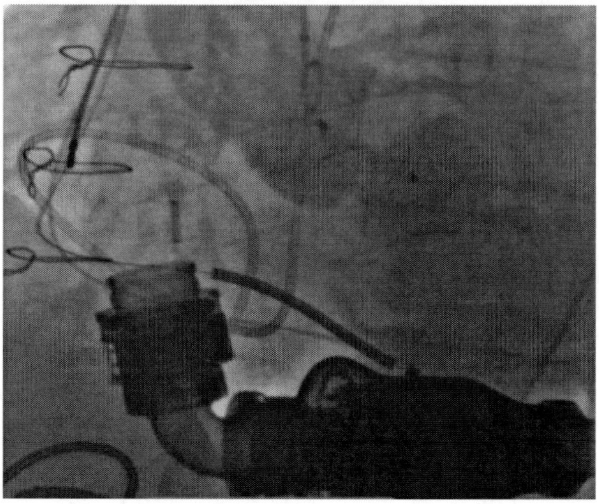

Figure 1. Placement of the Amplatzer patent foramen ovale multi-fenestrated 35-mm device (St Jude Medical, Saint Paul, MN) on the aortic valve with fluoroscopy.

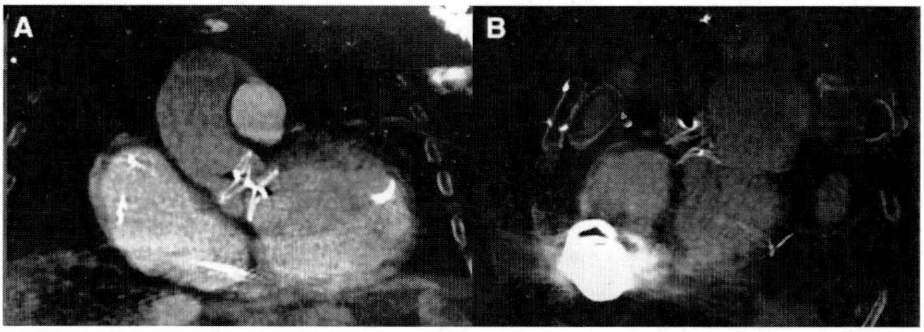

Figure 2. Computed tomographic images of the device after implantation. (A) Coronal view. (B) Axial view.

Assessment and Indication for Treatment of Aortic Regurgitation at the Time of LVAD Implantation

An exhaustive functional and morphological evaluation of the aortic valve should be part of the screening process in patients evaluated for LVAD implantation. It is essential that the AV is assessed under physiological conditions to avoid underestimating the degree of AI when the patient is already under general anesthesia. AI before the LVAD implantation is defined and quantified in the same way as for any other non-VAD patient, namely by pre-operative transthoracic echocardiography followed by transesophageal echocardiography immediately before the surgical procedure and when cardiopulmonary bypass (CPB) is instituted. Because LVAD candidates often have high ventricular filling pressures, a condition can lead to underestimating the AI grade, a further estimate is made after extracorporeal circulation is initiated when the left ventricle has been drained through a vent in the pulmonary vein. This situation reproduces the physiology of the support with LVAD and allows a better definition of the degree of aortic regurgitation. Because the severity of aortic insufficiency progresses in at least 25% of cases and the known negative hemodynamic effect and the clinical consequences that the development of AI entails, it is recommended to proceed with the treatment of moderate or greater aortic regurgitation and the support time is expected to be more than one year [22, 26]. According to data from the INTERMACS registry, 3% of patients underwent a combined aortic valve procedure at the time of LVAD implantation [32]. In a retrospective study of 281 patients, Pal et al., reported a 4% prevalence of moderate or severe AI before LVAD implantation [33]. Patients with moderate AI and risk factors predisposing to AI development during LVAD support (family history, sex, age > 60 years, low body surface area, ischemic cardiomyopathy) should be considered for an aortic valve procedure at the time of implantation of the LVAD. This indication is particularly valid when prolonged support is assumed or when the patient is a candidate for DT. Based on the ISHLT guidelines, patients with aortic valve stenosis of any degree associated with moderate insufficiency must be considered for valve replacement surgery by using a biological prosthesis (class I level of evidence C). Patients with severe stenosis should have SVA regardless of the degree of aortic regurgitation (class II level of evidence C) [26].

STRATEGIES FOR AV REPAIR AT TIME OF LVAD IMPLANTATION

The choice of the surgical procedure for AV repair should be based on the patient's surgical risk, the AI mechanism, the valve and aortic root anatomy, and the support duration. There is currently no worldwide consensus about the most effective and appropriate procedure [22]. In an INTERMACS study conducted on 5344 patients with a CF-LVAD, the most common procedure performed on a malfunctioning aortic valve during LVAD implantation was valve closure (2.3%). Valve replacement was performed in 1.6% of cases. A technique for repairing the valve in which a stich is used to approximate aranzio nodules has been described by Park et al. (Figure 3).

This method is possible when the valve flaps are not overly thin or fragile. The advantage of this technique is to allow blood to be ejected through the aortic valve. The durability of this approach over time remains to be evaluated. Many studies have shown that adverse events and survival rates were similar between patients with and without closure of the AV at the time of VAD implantation [34, 35, 36, 37]. Jorde et al. reported a recurrence rate of 2.3% at one year for mean AI, 2.3% for severe, moderate AI, 2.3% for severe AI and a two-year AI freedom of 66% after the Park stitch was used [20]. The effectiveness and duration of the stitch seem to be most beneficial in DT patients or in patients with risk factors for AI, with a 69% reduction in the risk of developing AI when compared with patients without AV stitch. The analysis conducted by Robertson et al. on INTERMACS databases, revealed a moderate to severe AI progression of 18% at 12 months after aortic valve repair in conjunction with the LVAD implant [35] (Figure 4).

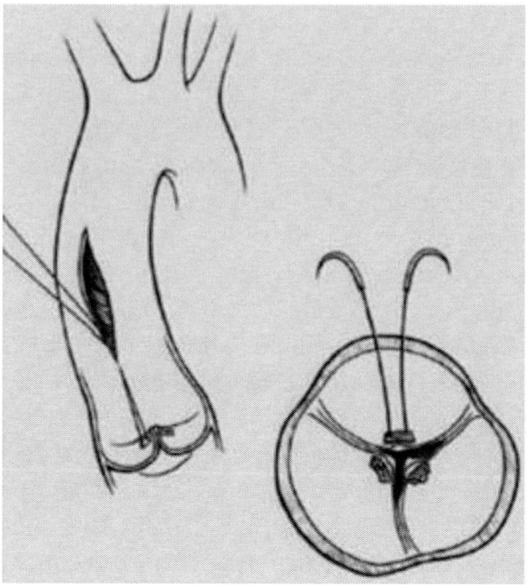

Figure 3. Park stitch: pledgeted 4-0 Prolene sutures are applied to approximate the 3 nodules of Arantius to create a coaptation stitch. Reproduced from Park et al. with permission from Elsevier.

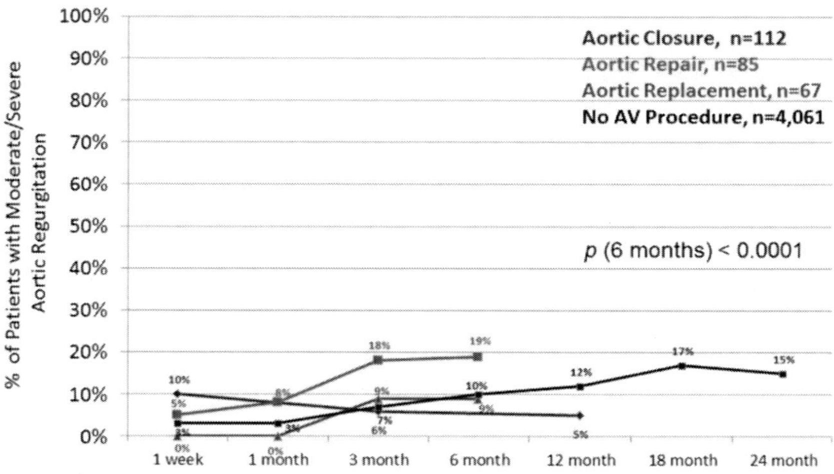

Figure 4. Post-operative recurrence of moderate to severe aortic insufficiency by type of AV procedure performed.

One method to mitigate this risk is by partial closure of the AV with the modified Park technique consisting of additional 5-0 prolene mattress sutures on each side placed between the central point and the commissures to strengthen and reduce the tension on the central point. This technique can be used in cases of degenerated AV with important prolapse or when the aortic leaflets are very fragile. While this allows blood to pass through the AV, the risk of stenosis is greater (Figure 5). A comparison of this technique to the single central point and its durability has yet to be conducted.

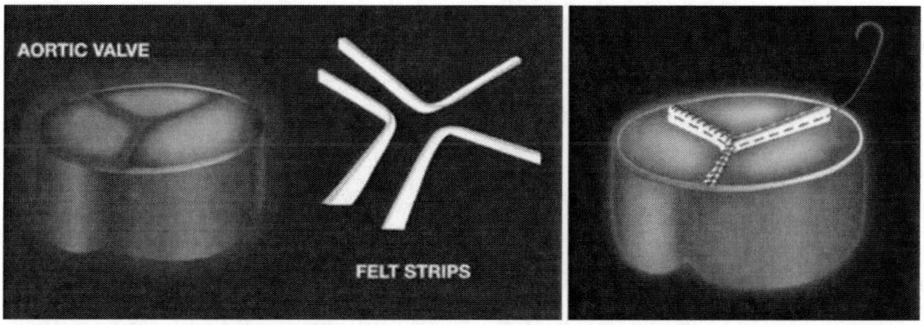

Note: evolved technique, described by Adamson, which incorporates three felt strips rather than individual pledges to expedite closure of the valve.

Figure 5. Native aortic valve closure technique.

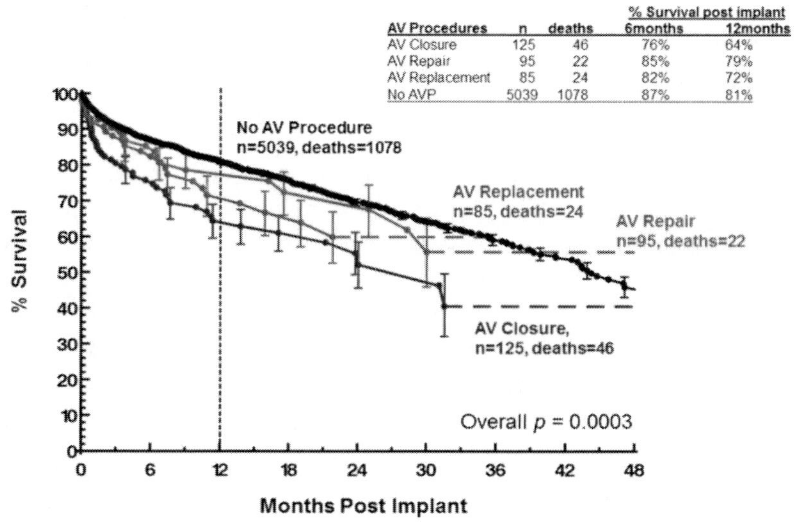

Figure 6. Survival by type of AV procedure performed.

Another treatment strategy is the complete closure of the left ventricle-aorta junction. Two main techniques have been described: 1) direct closure of the native AV with the use of felt strips along the free edge of the flaps; 2) positioning a circular patch of Dacron, Gore-Tex, autologous or heterologous pericardium directly on the native annulus or to the prosthesis ring if already implanted [27]. Total closure of the AV is associated with a low incidence of AI recurrence. However, this technique leaves the patient totally dependent on the device and events such as pump thrombosis can have devastating results. Moreover, this technique is contraindicated if recovery of myocardial function is expected [22]. Two important studies that analyzed the outcome after AV procedures provide mixed results [35, 38]. Using the data of the Heartmate 2, pivotal trials for patients with BTT and DT indications, John et al. found that patients with concomitant AV procedures (n = 80 patients, divided into AV repair [n = 18], closure [n = 32], and replacement [n = 30]) were sicker and had higher early mortality and right ventricular failure rates. In that study, 30-day mortality was lowest for AV closure (6.3%), followed by AV replacement (13%), and finally AV repair (18%). Survival rates at 1 and 2 years were also lower after AV closure than after AV repair or replacement (84.1% vs 70.9% for closure, 75% vs 57% for repair, and 64% vs 43% for replacement, respectively; P <0.001) [38]. In an INTERMACS database analysis (n = 305 patients, divided into AV repair [n = 125], closure [n = 95], and replacement [n = 85]), Robertson et al. reported increased mortality associated with complete over-sewing of the valve, with most deaths occurring early after the procedure [35] (Figure 6).

One-year survival was lower after AV closure compared with AV repair or replacement (81% for patients who did not undergo an AV procedure, 79% for patients who underwent an AV repair, 72% for patients with an AV replacement, and 64% for those with AV closure (P 1⁄4 0.003)). Even if it is unclear whether the deaths were related to the AV closure, complete over sewing has become less popular. This technique is now mainly used when a mechanical valve is already in place to avoid a redo AV replacement with the use of a bioprosthesis.

An additional option for treatment of AI is aortic valve replacement with a biological prosthesis. This procedure is indicated when the aortic valve is calcified or stenotic or when a partial closure does not provide satisfying results. Its potential benefits must be weighed against the risks of an extended clamping time. The duration and superiority of valve replacement when compared with AV over-sewing are unknown. In the INTERMACS analysis, one year after AV replacement at the time of LVAD implantation, survival was 72%, and non-recurrence of AI was observed [35]. Many authors encourage valve replacement with bioprosthesis, especially in stable and long-term supported patients, such as DT. However, the fusion of the cusps, fibrosis, subvalvular thrombosis and obstruction have been reported early after LVAD implantation [39, 40]. Furthermore, abnormal loading conditions cause an increased probability of prosthtesis dysfunction. If a biological prosthesis has been implanted for more than five years or has signs of deterioration, it is advisable to over-sew the valve [22]. In addition with the increase in availability of the transcatheter valve, in the future, it is conceivable that the recommendation will be to use TAVR for the de novo treatment of AI in patients implanted with LVAD. Many reports, albeit with a limited number of patients, have demonstrated the feasibility of TAVR in the case of AI in patients supported with LVAD, both in cases of native AV and in degenerated bioprosthetic valves [41, 42, 43]. The use of mechanical prostheses in an aortic position is highly discouraged given the high thromboembolic risk. If a mechanical valve was already in place, the recommended choice is to replace the mechanical valve with a bioprosthesis or to over-sew the valve with a patch.

CONCLUSION

The presence of acute valvular heart disease in patients with end-stage heart failure presenting for CF-LVAD consideration is frequent. Previously, there has been a lack of understanding and consensus on the adverse impact of VHD on patients receiving LVAD therapy. Recent evidence demonstrates more consistent findings of an adverse impact of valvular pathologies on the hemodynamic benefit of CF- LVAD support, leading surgeons and cardiologists to advocate for more aggressive surgical correction. This is particularly true for AI. Safe and straightforward surgical approaches, such as partial central AV closure, are being used with satisfactory results.

REFERENCES

[1] Yancy CW, Jessup M, Bozkurt B, et al. 2013 ACCF/AHA guideline for the management of heart failure: a report of the American College of Cardiology Foundation/American Heart Association Task Force on Practice Guidelines. *J Am Coll Cardiol* 2013;62:e147-239.

[2] Ezekowitz JA, O'Meara E, McDonald MA, et al. 2017 comprehensive update of the Canadian Cardiovascular Society guidelines for the management of heart failure. *Can J Cardiol* 2017;33:1342-433.

[3] Mehra MR, Uriel N, Naka Y, et al. A fully magnetically levitated left ventricular assist devicedfinal report. *N Engl J Med* 2019;380: 1618-27.

[4] Kirklin JK, Pagani FD, Kormos RL, et al. Eighth annual INTERMACS report: special focus on framing the impact of adverse events. *J Heart Lung Transplant* 2017;36:1080-6.

[5] Cowger J. Aortic regurgitation during continuous-flow left ventricular assist device support: an insufficient understanding of an insufficient lesion. *J Heart Lung Transplant* 2016;35:973-5.

[6] Soleimani B, Haouzi A, Manoskey A, et al. Development of aortic insufficiency in patients supported with continuous flow left ventricular assist devices. *ASAIO J* 2012;58:326-9.

[7] Saito T, Wassilew K, Gorodetski B, et al. Aortic valve pathology in patients supported by continuous-flow left ventricular assist device. *Circ J* 2016;80:1371-7.

[8] Ambardekar AV, Hunter KS, Babu AN, et al. Changes in aortic wall structure, composition, and stiffness with continuous-flow left ventricular assist devices: a pilot study. C*irc Heart Fail* 2015;8:944-52.

[9] Gallen TB, Lau WT, Mehta AR. Complete aortic valve fusion after Heartmate II left ventricular assist device support. *J Cardiothorac Vasc Anesth* 2012;26:1060-2.

[10] Hata H, Fujita T, Ishibashi-Ueda H, Nakatani T, Kobayashi J. Pathological analysis of the aortic valve after long-term left ventricular assist device support. *Eur J Cardiothorac Surg* 2014;46:193-7.

[11] Stephens EH, Han J, Trawick EA, et al. Left-ventricular assist device impact on aortic valve mechanics, proteomics and ultrastructure. *Ann Thorac Surg* 2018;105:572-80.

[12] Ushijima T, Tanoue Y, Ide T, et al. Disuse atrophy of the aortic valve after left ventricular assist device implantation. *Ann Thorac Surg* 2016;101:742-4.

[13] van Rijswijk JW, Vink A, Martina JR, et al. Pathology of aortic valve remodeling after continuous-flow left ventricular assist device support. *J Heart Lung Transplant* 2017;36:113-6.

[14] Truby LK, Garan AR, Givens RC, et al. Aortic insufficiency during contemporary left ventricular assist device support: analysis of the INTERMACS Registry. *JACC Heart Fail* 2018;6:951-60.

[15] Aggarwal A, Raghuvir R, Eryazici P, et al. The development of aortic insufficiency in continuous-flow left ventricular assist device supported patients. *Ann Thorac Surg* 2013;95:493-8.

[16] Imamura T, Kinugawa K, Nitta D, et al. Advantage of pulsatility in left ventricular reverse remodeling and aortic insufficiency prevention during left ventricular assist device treatment. *Circ J* 2015;79:1994-9.

[17] Imamura T, Kinugawa K, Nitta D, Hatano M, Ono M. Opening of aortic valve during exercise is key to preventing development of aortic insufficiency during ventricular assist device treatment. *ASAIO J* 2015;61:514-9.

[18] Saeed D, Westenfeld R, Maxhera B, et al. Prevalence of de novo aortic valve insufficiency in patients after Heartware VAD implantation with an intermittent low-speed algorithm. *ASAIO J* 2016;62:565-70.

[19] Cowger JA, Aaronson KD, Romano MA, Haft J, Pagani FD. Consequences of aortic insufficiency during long-term axial continuous-flow left ventricular assist device support. *J Heart Lung Transplant* 2014;33:1233-40.

[20] Jorde UP, Uriel N, Nahumi N, et al. Prevalence, significance, and management of aortic insufficiency in continuous flow left ventricular assist device recipients. *Circ Heart Fail* 2014;7:310-9.

[21] Patil NP, Mohite PN, Sabashnikov A, et al. Does postoperative blood pressure influence development of aortic regurgitation following continuous-flow left ventricular assist device implantation? *Eur J Cardiothorac Surg* 2016;49:788-94.

[22] Cowger J, Rao V, Massey T, et al. Comprehensive review and suggested strategies for the detection and management of aortic insufficiency in patients with a continuous-flow left ventricular assist device. *J Heart Lung Transplant* 2015;34:149-57.

[23] Sayer G, Sarswat N, Kim GH, et al. The hemodynamic effects of aortic insufficiency in patients supported with continuous-flow left ventricular assist devices. *J Card Fail* 2017;23:545-51.

[24] Park SJ, Liao KK, Segurola R, Madhu KP, Miller LW: Management of aortic insufficiency in patients with left ventricular assist devices: a simple coaptation stitch method (Park's stitch). *J Thorac Cardiovasc Surg* 127: 264–266, 2004.

[25] Rao V, Slater JP, Edwards NM, Naka Y, Oz MC: Surgical management of valvular disease in patients requiring left ventricular assist device support. *Ann Thorac Surg* 71: 1448–1453, 2001.

[26] Feldman D, Pamboukian SV, Teuteberg JJ, et al; International Society for Heart and Lung Transplantation: The 2013 International Society for Heart and Lung Transplantation Guidelines for mechanical circulatory support: executive summary. *J Heart Lung Transplant* 32: 157–187, 2013.

[27] Adamson RM, Dembitsky WP, Baradarian S, et al: Aortic valve closure associated with HeartMate left ventricular device support: technical considerations and long-term results. *J Heart Lung Transplant* 30: 576–582, 2011.

[28] Parikh KS, Mehrotra AK, Russo MJ, et al: Percutaneous transcatheter aortic valve closure successfully treats left ventricular assist device-associated aortic insufficiency and improves cardiac hemodynamics. *JACC Cardiovasc Interv* 6: 84–89, 2013.

[29] Kevin Phan, Joshua M. Haswell, Joshua Xu, Yusuf Assem, Stephanie L. Mick, Samir R. Kapadia, Anson Cheung, Frederick S. Ling, Tristan D. Yan, and Vakhtang Tchantchaleishvili Percutaneous Transcatheter Interventions for Aortic Insufficiency in Continuous-Flow Left Ventricular Assist Device Patients: A Systematic Review and Meta-Analysis. *ASAIO Journal* 2017; 63:117–122.

[30] Francesca Nicolo, Andrea Montalto, Carmine Musto, Marina Comisso, Antonio Lio, and Francesco Musumeci. Percutaneous Aortic Valve Closure in Patient With Left Ventricular Assist Device and Dilated Aortic Annulus Francesca. *Ann Thorac Surg* 2020;109:e25-7.

[31] Axel Unbehaun, Christoph Klein, Semih Buz, Alexander Meyer, Isaac Wamala, Evgenij Potapov, Felix Schoenrath, Volkmar Falk, and Joerg Kempfert. A Novel Technique for Transcatheter Aortic Valve Replacement in Pure Aortic Regurgitation. *Ann Thorac Surg* 2019;107:e177–9.

[32] Truby LK, Garan AR, Givens RC, et al. Aortic insufficiency during contemporary left ventricular assist device support: analysis of the INTERMACS Registry. *JACC Heart Fail* 2018;6:951-60.

[33] Pal JD, Klodell CT, John R, et al. Low operative mortality with implantation of a continuous-flow left ventricular assist device and impact of concurrent cardiac procedures. *Circulation* 2009;120:S215-9.

[34] Fukuhara S, Ikegami H, Polanco AR, et al. Concomitant repair for mild aortic insufficiency and continuous-flow left ventricular assist devices. *Eur J Cardiothorac Surg* 2017;52:1062-8.

[35] Robertson JO, Naftel DC, Myers SL, et al. Concomitant aortic valve procedures in patients undergoing implantation of continuous-flow left ventricular assist devices: an INTERMACS database analysis. *J Heart Lung Transplant* 2015;34:797-805.

[36] Maoz-Metzl D, Morsy M, Khalife WI, Lick SD. Park's stitch for a bicuspid aortic valve in a patient on LVAD support. *J Card Surg* 2014;29:843-5.

[37] Fukuhara S, Takeda K, Chiuzan C, et al. Concomitant aortic valve repair with continuous-flow left ventricular assist devices: results and implications. *J Thorac Cardiovasc Surg* 2016;151:201-210.e201-2.

[38] John R, Naka Y, Park SJ, et al. Impact of concurrent surgical valve procedures in patients receiving continuous-flow devices. *J Thorac Cardiovasc Surg* 2014;147:581-9 [discussion: 589].

[39] Dranishnikov N, Stepanenko A, Potapov EV, et al. Simultaneous aortic valve replacement in left ventricular assist device recipients: single-center experience. *Int J Artif Organs* 2012;35:489-94.

[40] Doi A, Marasco SF, McGiffin DC. Is a bioprosthetic valve in the aortic position desirable with a continuous flow LVAD? *J Card Surg* 2015;30: 466-8.

[41] Yehya A, Rajagopal V, Meduri C, et al. Short-term results with trans- catheter aortic valve replacement for treatment of left ventricular assist device patients with symptomatic aortic insufficiency. *J Heart Lung Transplant* 2019.

[42] Baum C, Seiffert M, Treede H, Reichenspurner H, Deuse T. Concomitant transcatheter aortic valve and left ventricular assist device implantation. *ASAIO J* 2013;59:90-2.

[43] Phan K, Haswell JM, Xu J, et al. Percutaneous transcatheter interventions for aortic insufficiency in continuous-flow left ventricular assist device patients: a systematic review and meta-analysis. *ASAIO J* 2017;63:117-22.

In: Perspectives in Aortic Valve Disease
Editor: Giovanni Concistrè
ISBN: 978-1-53618-769-4

Chapter 11

MULTIDISCIPLINARY APPROACH TO THE TREATMENT OF AORTIC VALVE DISEASE: THE ROLE OF THE HEART TEAM

Giovanni Concistrè**, MD
Ospedale del Cuore "G. Pasquinucci",
Fondazione Toscana Gabriele Monasterio, Massa, Italy

ABSTRACT

Multidisciplinary decision making is becoming increasingly important in health care with ever growing therapeutic options available in complex cases. This is also true for cardiovascular medicine, where the introduction of percutaneous coronary intervention caused a revolution in the treatment of coronary artery disease. Currently, with the development of transcatheter procedures to repair or replace heart valves, the treatment of valvular heart disease is subject to a similar transition. Especially the treatment of severe aortic stenosis in high- and intermediate-surgical-risk patients has changed significantly, with the emergence of the transcatheter aortic valve replace- ment (TAVR) as an accepted treatment.

In order to oversee the extensive set of diagnostic and therapeutic options it is suggested that decision making is performed in a multidisciplinary team, i.e., a Heart Team. This is a summary of the changes that have taken place and continue to take place in the treatment of aortic valve disease. Furthermore, an overview is provided of the advantages and limitations of shared decision making.

Three possible models of decision making in the treatment of patients with severe aortic stenosis are discussed in detail. Subsequently, surgical risk scores, the assessment of frailty in possible TAVR candidates and the necessity of Heart Team reimbursement are discussed.

Keywords: aortic valve, valvular disease, aortic valve prosthesis, aortic valve replacement, aortic valve, transapical, percutaneous, heart team

* Corresponding Author's Email: gioconci@libero.it.

Introduction

With an increasing number of therapeutic options, multidisciplinary decision making (MDM) has become increasingly important for the evaluation of options in medicine, especially in patients with complex diseases. MDM has proven value in disciplines such as cancer treatment, where comprehensive decision making in so-called tumor boards resulted in a change of diagnostic or therapeutic strategies and improved outcomes [1, 2].

Heart Teams, as multidisciplinary teams in cardiovascular disease are usually named, have played a crucial role in decision making. The European Society of Cardiology recommends the consultation of a heart team in the management of valvular heart disease [3], heart failure [4], and myocardial revascularization [5]. A heart team usually consists of cardiologists, cardiac surgeons, interventionists, imaging specialists, anesthetists and midlevel providers. In some cases, the expert opinion of a general practitioner, geriatrician or intensive care specialist can be of additional value.

The evolution of the heart team concept started with a focus on coronary artery disease (CAD). Initially, the options for treatment of CAD were optimal medical therapy and coronary artery bypass grafting (CABG).

The introduction of percutaneous coronary intervention (PCI) revolutionized the treatment of CAD and became an alternative treatment option to CABG. Some studies showed, however, that patients who would benefit most of CABG actually received PCI treatment due to the less invasive nature of PCI [6]. This resulted in a call for standardized preoperative assessment of patients [7].

The invasive treatment of heart valve diseases is undergoing a similar revolution with the introduction of transcatheter heart valve repair and replacement. Of special significance is the rise of the transcatheter aortic valve replacement (TAVR), which is now a first-choice option in patients with severe aortic stenosis (AS) who are considered extreme, high risk or intermediate risk for surgical aortic valve replacement [3]. Furthermore, transcatheter options for mitral and tricuspid valve disease have been developed or are in development and might become increasingly viable as an alternative treatment option. This raises the question whether there is a similar risk of inappropriate use of treatments in heart valve disease now and in the future.

The purpose of this chapter is to describe the innovations in therapeutic options for aortic valve disease and discuss the rationale for involvement of a Heart Team in decision making. Furthermore, patient categories to be discussed with MDM, the use of preoperative surgical risk scores, professionals to be involved in decision making and the limitations and other advantages of shared decision making in valvular heart disease will be discussed.

Developments in Aortic Valve Surgery

The burden of aortic valve disease, especially in elderly people, is an important public-health issue. Studies have shown a prevalence of AS of 0.4% in the general population, but up to 2.8% in people of 75 years or older [8], while a meta-analysis showed a prevalence of severe AS ranging from 1.2% to 6.1% in elderly populations [9]. Patients with severe AS, if left untreated, have a limited life expectancy [10]. The most utilized therapeutic options in severe AS are surgical aortic valve replacement (SAVR) and, more recently, transcatheter aortic valve replacement (TAVR). The potential risk of an unfavorable outcome after surgery in high-risk patients meant that many patients were not referred to SAVR [11]. However, TAVR is now an effective option in inoperable patients, with proven superiority over medical therapy [12] and non-inferior to SAVR in high-risk patients [13, 14]. Recently, TAVR as a treatment option for patients with intermediate surgical risk was demonstrated to be non-inferior to SAVR and was approved as well [15, 16]. TAVR as therapy for low-surgical risk patients is currently under investigation in randomized trials and shows promising first results in nonrandomized studies [17].

Recent trends illustrate a sharp increase in the number of TAVRs procedures, while the number of SAVR procedures remains relatively unchanged, resulting in a more than 2-fold increase in the total number of aortic valve replacements in Germany (Figure 1) [18, 19-21]. This is not the same in every country though, which is attributable to different reimbursement strategies [22]. Although TAVR is less invasive compared to SAVR, the procedure is of course not without risks. TAVR associated risks include: post-procedural aortic regurgitation (mostly paravalvular) [23], necessity for new permanent pacemaker implantation [23], complications associated with vascular access [14, 16], and neurological complications [12, 24-40].

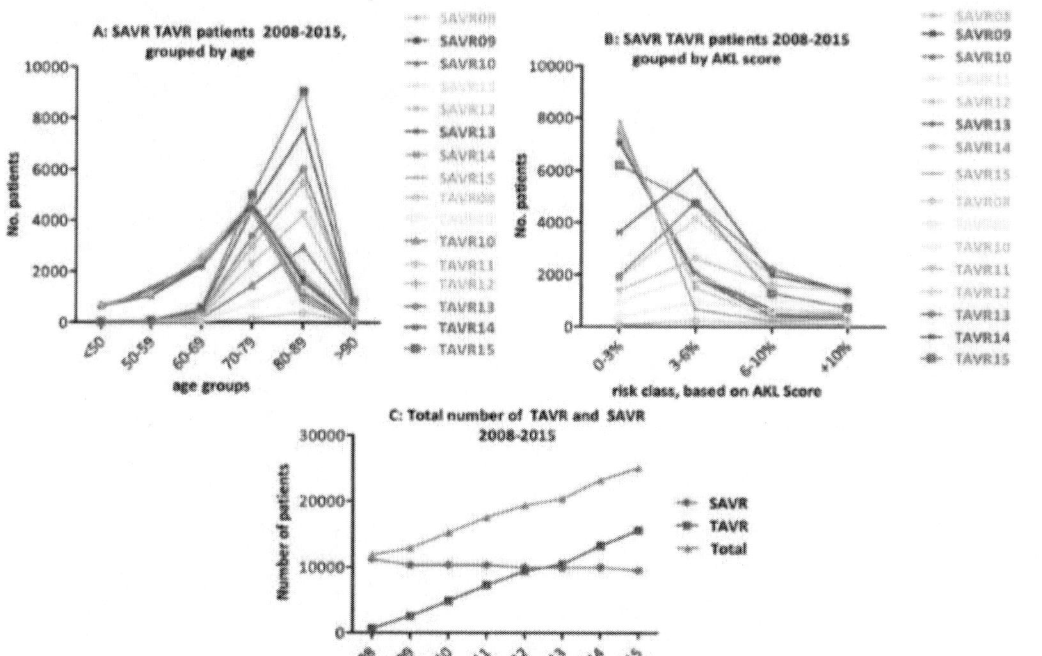

Figure 1. Number of TAVR and SAVR procedures from 2008 to 2015 in Germany. (A) Total number of SAVR and TAVR procedures performed in Germany from 2008 to 2015 grouped by age category per year. (B) Total number of SAVR and TAVR procedures from 2008 to 2015 grouped according to risk scores (AKL: aortenklappen score) per year. (C) Total number of SAVR, TAVR and combined number of AVRs from 2008 to 2015. Adapted from Sektorenübergreifende Qualität in Gesundheitswesen (2008 – 2014) and Institut für Qualitätssicherung und Transparenz im Gesundheitswesen (2015) (18–21).

Advantages of a Multidisciplinary Approach in Aortic Valve Disease

On the face of it, decision making in a multidisciplinary team like a Heart Team has important advantages over solitary decision making. Figure 2 represents the conceptual strengths and weaknesses of the Heart Team model. First, medicine is becoming increasingly complex with various therapeutic options to be considered in older patients with more comorbidities. The combined expertise of a Heart Team provides the basis for a more balanced appraisal of a specific case. This is specifically important if the availability of clear supportive evidence (e.g., risk scores) is limited.

Secondly, use of expensive therapeutic options is likely to be restricted in patients where the benefits of treatment are questionable. Additionally, if an invasive treatment is deemed not to be beneficial for patients, extensive and detailed non-invasive care can be organized immediately. At the same time, underutilization of therapeutic options can be avoided. Furthermore, an open minded, multidisciplinary approach minimizes disagreements between individual clinicians.

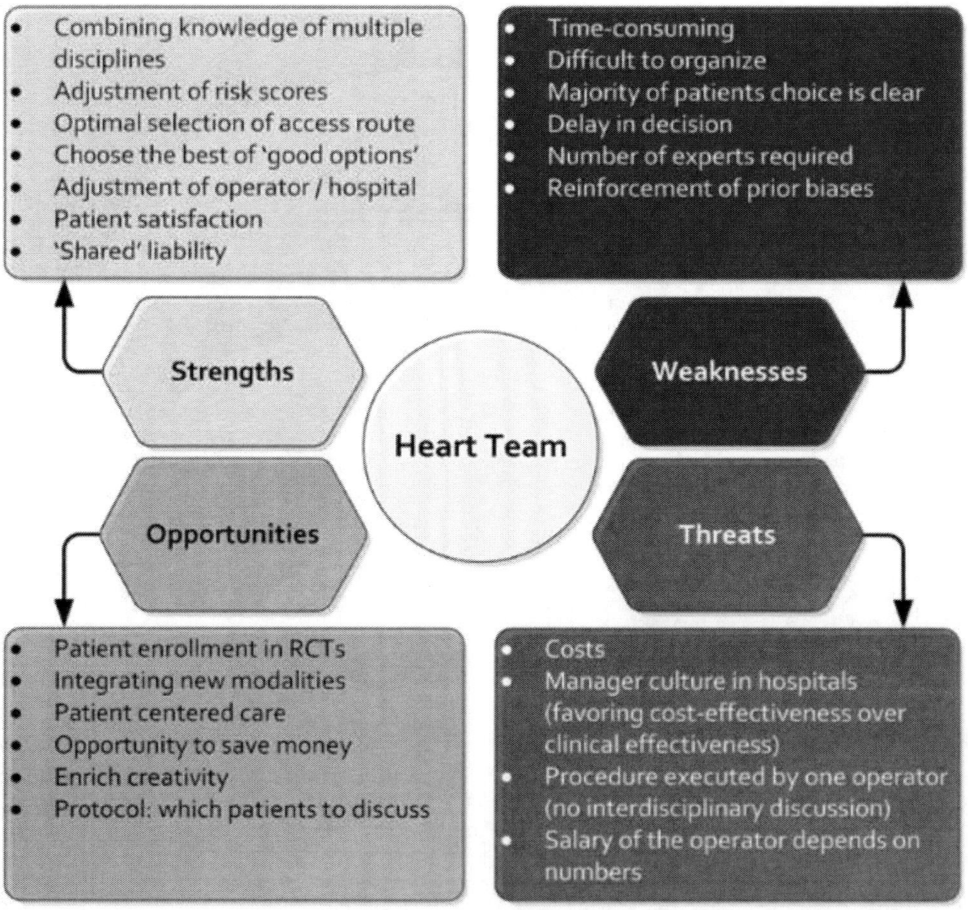

Figure 2. The Heart Team illustrated according to the Strengths, Weaknesses, Opportunities, and Threats model (SWOT).

Another advantage of the Heart Team is that the pre-operative diagnostic work-up will become more standardized, since a protocolized and complete pre-operative assessment is a requirement to have a successful multidisciplinary meeting. Finally, an open discussion about therapeutic options in complex patients creates an environment for clinicians to discuss and expand their knowledge ("Every day is a school day").

Moreover, complex cases sometimes require creative solutions which are not always supported by protocols and guidelines. The Heart Team offers a platform for "creative solutions," and an opportunity to share responsibility for these treatments. Finally, these discussions can deliver an important contribution to the education of medical students and clinical residents in one of the most difficult and rapidly evolving subjects of medicine.

Although evidence of the benefit of Heart Teams is limited, one report has shown that in-hospital mortality and 1-year mortality in patients admitted to the hospital for heart failure was significantly lower if they were discussed in a Heart Team, compared to patients not discussed in a Heart Team [41].

THE HEART TEAM IN VALVULAR HEART DISEASE

Although decision making in a Heart Team is a key element in the treatment of patients with heart valve diseases, the referral pathways, organization and the exact constitution of the Heart Valve Teams are not standardized. Figure 3 shows three possible models of decision making in patients with severe aortic stenosis. Each model comes with specific advan- tages and disadvantages that will be summarized below.

The first flowchart (Figure 3A) represents a model where every patient, after the diagnosis of severe AS by a cardiologist, is referred to the Heart Team. The Heart Team will assess the case and carefully consider the practical options: optimal medical therapy (OMT), TAVR, and SAVR. Advantages of this model are: complete and careful consideration of every case, minimal risk of a possible conflict of interest, learning opportu- nity for decision making in all patients with AS. Disadvantages, however, are: time-consuming and expensive, lack of profes- sional frailty and/or mental health assessment (by e.g., a geria- trician). Two studies reviewed this model and report OMT in 6 – 7% of the patients, while the remaining patients either received TAVR (12 – 43%) or SAVR (51 – 82%) [42, 43].

In Model 3B (Figure 3B), patients with possible AS are seen by a cardiologist of a Heart Valve Clinic who can then refer them directly to a cardiac surgeon, interventional cardiologist or to the Heart Team. The cardiac surgeon or interventional cardiologist can decide on SAVR/TAVR or can decide to discuss the patient in the Heart Team. Advantages of this model are: "fast-track" for patients who are clear SAVR and TAVR candidates (e.g., young patients with low surgical risk as a SAVR candidate), preselection of patients to be discussed in the Heart Team. Disadvantages include: only a select group of patients are discussed by the Heart Team, potentially leading to a higher probability of disagreement. As a future perspective, a similar fast-track could possibly be proposed for patients who are clear TAVR or SAVR candidates. A local protocol defines which patients are directly referred for treatment and which ones will be discussed in the Heart team.

Model 3C (Figure 3C) is a model of a Heart Valve Center as has been proposed before where the goal is to center all specific knowledge on aortic stenosis [44, 45].

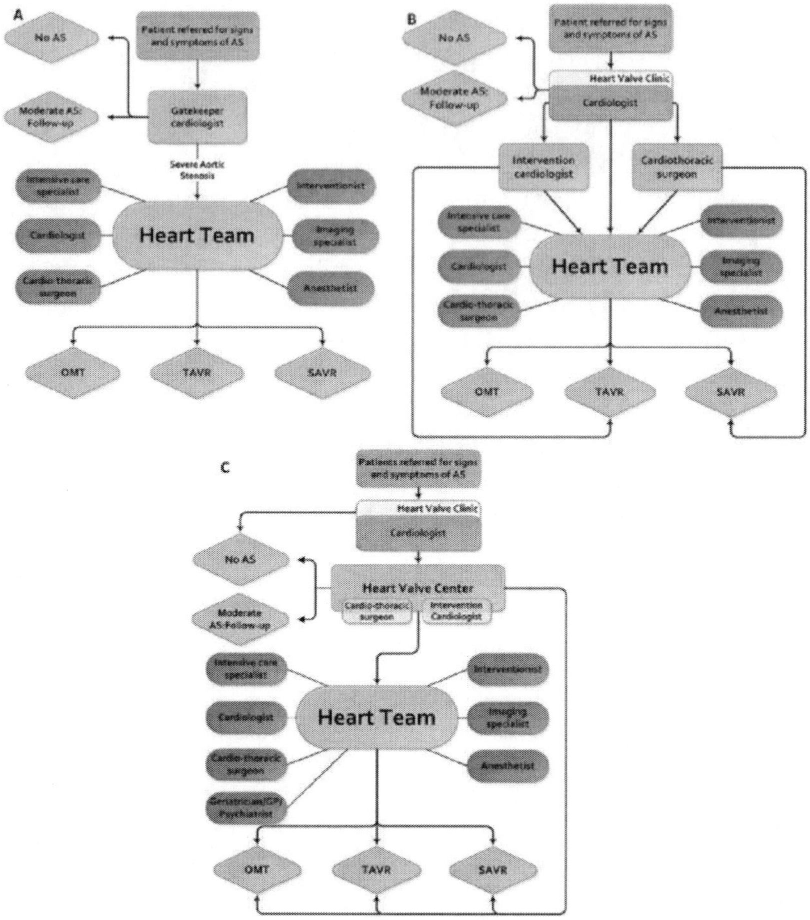

Figure 3. Three different models of implementation of a Heart Team. (A) Model where a cardiologist acts as gatekeeper and every patient with severe AS is discussed in a Heart Team. (B) A cardiologist from a Heart Valve Clinic assesses the possibility of AS, and can refer to the Heart Team or directly to a cardiothoracic surgeon or intervention cardiologist, who can then refer the patient for TAVR/SAVR or also refer the patient to a Heart Team meeting. (C) A cardiologist from the Heart Valve Clinic refers patients with severe AS to a dedicated Heart Valve Center. An interventional cardiologist and cardiac surgeon assess the patient's AS treatment options. If there are/remain doubts about surgical aspects and/or the mental health and frailty of a patient, a patient can be discussed by the Heart Team with the aid of other specialists. AS, aortic stenosis; GP, general practitioner; SAVR, surgical aortic valve replacement; TAVR, transcatheter aortic valve replacement; OMT, optimal medical therapy.

A referred patient by a Heart Valve Clinic is seen by both a cardiologist and a cardiac surgeon of the Heart Valve Center. They can then decide that a patient needs further discussion in a Heart Team and, possibly, that extra diagnostic research has to be done. The patient can also directly be referred to SAVR, TAVR, or OMT. The advantages are: both cardiologist and cardiothor- acic surgeon see the patient, minimizing a potential conflict of interest, possible fast-track, and the creation of a specialized center in aortic stenosis. The disadvantages are: time-consuming (with limited human resources) and expensive.

A recent evaluation of 250 different TAVR centers reported that a Heart Team is consulted in 97% of the centers and that both a cardiac surgeon and a cardiologist are often present (95.6% and 96.8% respectively); however, the involvement of other specialists is not common. Furthermore, at least one surgical risk score for clinical evaluation of the patient is used in nearly all centers. Interestingly, frailty is only tested in 44% of the cases, with over 20 different standards being used [46].

Traditional surgical risk scores are often used to distinguish between possible SAVR and TAVR candidates. The European Society of Cardiology/European Association of Cardio-Thoracic Surgery guideline on the management of valvular heart disease recommends surgical risk stratification performed primarily by a Heart Team with the aid of the logistic EuroSCORE and STS score [3]. A trial comparing the EuroSCORE with a score based on age, creatinine and ejection fraction in cardiac surgery patients showed similar accuracy, highlighting the need for more accurate pre-operative risk scores [47]. Furthermore, these scores do not take aspects such as frailty and mental health status into consideration. Other scores, such as the OBSERVANT-score [48] FRANCE-2 score [49] the SURTAVI risk stratification model [50] and the German Aortic Valve Score [51] have been developed to specifically assess mortality risk in patients undergoing TAVR (and SAVR), but have shown limited additional accuracy in predicting 30-day mortality in comparison with EuroSCORE and STS score in different datasets [52, 53].

The impact of pre-procedural frailty on post-operative outcome after TAVR has been the subject of interest in TAVR research. Frailty is a state of decreased physiologic reserve, resulting in vulnerability when a stressor is applied. Since the number of high-risk patients increases with age, the number of frail patients gradually increases as well. As mentioned earlier, many different scores to assess frailty are used. Criteria that have been used to assess frailty include but are not limited to: gait speed, grip strength, activities of daily living (using the Katz index), and serum albumin. These criteria have shown to be a predictor of decreased long-term survival after TAVR, similarly quality of life (QoL) did not significantly increase after TAVR in the frail patient subgroup [54, 55]. A recent review confirms the association between frailty and decreased survival after TAVR but recognizes the lack of a uniform definition of frailty and a standard protocol to assess frailty in possible TAVR candidates [56]. Efforts are made, though, to find prognostic scores to assess frailty, specifically for patients with severe AS. A recent multicenter comparison of multiple frailty indices has clearly shown that an EFT score (chair standing, mini-mental assessment score, albumin and hemoglobin outperformed all other indices) [57]. However, with the lack of these clear boundaries, it would be recommended to consult an expert on this subject, for example a geriatrician. Another option would be to consult a general practitioner, who is often familiar with the physical and mental capabilities and daily activities of the specific TAVR candidate.

Another aspect to be taken into consideration is how and when to involve the patient in the treatment decisions. This could be done when the patient is referred to the cardiologist, or a patient could be informed about the therapeutic options after the Heart Team meeting. It is clear that patient preference and decision will ultimately be crucial in deciding which alternative therapeutic approach is to be undertaken.

Finally, although MDM has some clear advantages over solitary decision making, it is time-consuming and as it might be difficult to gather the Heart Team participants, meetings can become less efficient. Thus, it is important to promote Heart Team meetings by scheduling them in the agendas of specialists, but also by reimbursing Heart Team meetings or the treatments that are discussed in Heart Team meetings. In the Netherlands, for instance, Heart Team meetings are reimbursed by health insurances. In many countries, TAVR procedures are only reimbursed if they are discussed in a Heart Team [22].

Conclusion

With an increasing number of therapeutic options available in the management of valvular heart disease, multidisciplinary decision making is becoming increasingly important. Not only because of the complexity of treatment options in older patients with significant comorbidities, but also due to the fact that predictive risk scores have limited accuracy. The role of the Heart Team is crucial, since it can comprehensively discuss the accuracy of surgical risk scores, additional unaccounted for comorbidities, frailty, perform a risk-benefit analysis and include other factors that are not necessarily caught in standard procedures or protocols. Nevertheless, there is an urgent need for more accurate risk scores, incorporating frailty and other non-traditional risk factors, specifically for patients with severe AS undergoing TAVR. Although this review focused mainly on the role of the Heart Team in the treatment of severe AS, similar challenges lie ahead for the multiple therapeutic options being developed for the treatment of mitral and tricuspid regurgitation.

References

[1] Van Hagen, P., Spaander, M. C. W., Van Der Gaast, A., et al. Impact of a multidisciplinary tumour board meeting for upper-GI malig- nancies on clinical decision making: a prospective cohort study. *Int. J. Clin. Oncol.,* 2013; 18(2):214 - 219.

[2] Kesson, E. M., Allardice, G. M., George, W. D., Burns, H. J. G., Morrison, D. S. Effects of multidisciplinary team working on breast cancer survival: retrospective, comparative, interventional cohort study of 13 722 women. *BMJ,* 2012; 344:e2718: 1 - 9.

[3] Vahanian, A., Alfieri, O., Andreotti, F. et al. Guidelines on the management of valvular heart disease (version 2012). The joint task force on the management of valvular heart disease of the European Society of Cardiology (ESC) and the European Association for Cardio-Thoracic Surgery (EACTS). *Eur. Heart J.,* 2012; 33(19):2451 - 2496.

[4] Ponikowski, P., Voors, A. A., Anker, S. D. et al. ESC guidelines for the diagnosis and treatment of acute and chronic heart failure. The task force for the diagnosis and treatment of acute and chronic heart failure of the European Society of Cardiology (ESC) developed with the special contribution of the Heart Failure Association (HFA) of the ESC. *Eur. Heart J.,* 2016; 37(27):2129 - 2200.

[5] Windecker, S., Kolh, P., Alfonso, F. et al. ESC/EACTS guidelines on myocardial revascularization. The task force on myocardial revas- cularization of the European Society of Cardiology (ESC) and the European Association for Cardio-Thoracic Surgery (EACTS) developed with the special contribution of the European Association of Percutaneous Cardiovascular Interventions (EAPCI). *Eur. Heart J.,* 2014; 35(37):2541 - 2619.

[6] Hannan, E. L., Racz, M. J., Gold, J. et al. Adherence of catheterization laboratory cardiologists to American College of Cardiology/American Heart Association guidelines for percutaneous coronary interventions and coronary artery bypass graft surgery. What happens in actual practice? *Circulation,* 2010; 121(2):267 - 275.

[7] Head, S. J., Kaul, S., Mack, M. J. et al. The rationale for heart team decision-making for patients with stable, complex coronary artery disease. *Eur. Heart J.,* 2013; 34(32):2510 - 2518.

[8] Nkomo, V. T., Gardin, J. M., Skelton, T. N., Gottdiener, J. S., Scott, C. G., Enriquez-Sarano, M. Burden of valvular heart diseases: a popula- tion-based study. *Lancet,* 2006; 368(9540):1005 - 1011.

[9] Osnabrugge, R. L. J., Mylotte, D., Head, S. J. et al. Aortic stenosis in the elderly. *J. Am. Coll. Cardiol.*, 2013; 62(11):1002 - 1012.

[10] Clark, M. A., Arnold, S. V., Duhay, F. G. et al. Five-year clinical and economic outcomes among patients with medically managed severe aortic stenosis. *Results Med. Claims Anal.,* 2012; 5(5):697 - 704.

[11] Iung, B., Cachier, A., Baron, G. et al. Decision-making in elderly patients with severe aortic stenosis: why are so many denied surgery? *Eur. Heart J.,* 2005; 26(24):2714 - 2720.

[12] Leon, M. B., Smith, C. R., Mack, M. et al. Transcatheter aortic-valve implantation for aortic stenosis in patients who cannot undergo surgery. *N Engl. J. Med.,* 2010; 363(17):1597 - 1607.

[13] Smith, C. R., Leon, M. B., Mack, M. J. et al. Transcatheter versus surgical aortic-valve replacement in high-risk patients. *New Engl. J. Med.,* 2011; 364(23):2187 - 2198.

[14] Adams, D. H., Popma, J. J., Reardon, M. J. et al. Transcatheter aortic- valve replacement with a self-expanding prosthesis. *N Engl. J. Med.,* 2014; 370(19):1790 - 1798.

[15] Leon, M. B., Smith, C. R., Mack, M. J. et al. Transcatheter or surgical aortic-valve replacement in intermediate-risk patients. *New Engl. J. Med.,* 2016; 374(17):1609 - 1620.

[16] Reardon, M. J., Van Mieghem, N. M., Popma, J. J. et al. Surgical or transcatheter aortic-valve replacement in intermediate-risk patients. *N Engl. J. Med.,* 2017; 376(14): 1321 - 1331.

[17] Frerker, C., Bestehorn, K., Schlüter, M. et al. In-hospital mortality in propensity-score matched low-risk patients undergoing routine iso- lated surgical or transfemoral transcatheter aortic valve replacement in 2014 in Germany. *Clin. Res. Cardiol.,* 2017; 106(8):610 - 617.

[18] Institut für Qualitätssicherungund Transparenzim Gesundheitswesen (IQTIG) Ergebnisse/QS-Verfahren. Aorten klappenchirurgie, isoliert (Konvetionell chirurgisch), Bundesauswertung 2015. https://iqtig. org/downloads/ergebnisse/qidb/2015/2016-0525/ QIDB_2015_ DIREKT_PDF/QIDB_2015_direkte_Leistungsbereiche/BuAw_2015_ DIREKT/bu_Gesamt_HCH-AORT-CHIR_2015.pdf. 2016.

[19] Institut für Qualitätssicherungund Transparenzim Gesundheitswesen (IQTIG)/Ergebnisse – QS-Verfahren. Aorten klappenchirurgie, isoliert Kathetergestützt, Bundesauswertung 2015. https://iqtig.org/down loads/ergebnisse/ qidb/2015/2016-0525/ QIDB_2015_DIREKT_PDF/ QIDB_2015_direkte_Leistungsbereiche/BuAw_2015_DIREKT/bu_ Gesamt_HCH-AORT-KATH_2015.pdf. Accessed June 29, 2017.

[20] Sektorenübergreifende Qualität im Gesundheitswesen (SQG)/Ergebnisse – Leistungsbereiche – 2009 – 2014. Aorten klappenchirurgie, isoliert – kathetergestützt. https://sqg.de/front_con tent.php?idart=107.

[21] Sektorenübergreifende Qualität im Gesundheitswesen (SQG)/Ergebnisse – Leistungsbereiche – 2009 – 2014. Aorten klappenchirurgie, isoliert – konventionell. https://sqg.de/front_content. php?idart=106.

[22] Mylotte, D., Osnabrugge, R. L. J., Windecker, S. et al. Transcatheter aortic valve replacement in Europe. *J. Am. Coll. Cardiol.,* 2013; 62 (3):210 - 219.

[23] Holmes, D. R., Nishimura, R. A., Grover, F. L. et al. Annual outcomes with transcatheter valve therapy. *Ann. Thorac Surg.,* 2016; 101 (2):789 - 800.

[24] Nguyen, T. C., Terwelp, M. D., Thourani, V. H. et al. Clinical trends in surgical, minimally invasive and transcatheter aortic valve repla- cement. *Eur. J. Cardio-Thoracic Surg.*, 2017; 51(6):1086 - 1092.

[25] Suri, R. M., Vanoverschelde, J., Grigioni, F. et al. Association between early surgical intervention vs. watchful waiting and outcomes for mitral regurgitation due to flail mitral valve leaflets. *JAMA,* 2013; 310(6):609 - 616.

[26] Kang, D.-H., Kim, J. H., Rim, J. H. et al. Comparison of early surgery versus conventional treatment in asymptomatic severe mitral regurgitation. *Circulation,* 2009; 119(6):797 - 804.

[27] Swaans, M. J., Bakker, A. L. M., Alipour, A. et al. Survival of transcath- eter mitral valve repair compared with surgical and conservative treatment in high-surgical-risk patients. *J. Am. Coll. Cardiol.,* 2014; 7 (8):875 - 881.

[28] Alozie, A., Paranskaya, L., Westphal, B. et al. Clinical outcomes of conventional surgery versus MitraClip® therapy for moderate to severe symptomatic mitral valve regurgitation in the elderly population: an institutional experience. *BMC Cardiovasc. Disord.*, 2017; 17(1):85.

[29] Takagi, H., Ando, T., Umemoto, T., Group, A. A review of compara- tive studies of MitraClip versus surgical repair for mitral regur- gitation. *Int. J. Cardiol.,* 2017; 228:289 - 294.

[30] Deuschl, F., Schofer, N., Lubos, E., Blankenberg, S., Schafer, U. Critical evaluation of the MitraClip system in the management of mitral regurgitation. *Vasc. Health Risk Manag.,* 2016; 12:1 - 8.

[31] Grover, F. L., Vemulapalli, S., Carroll, J. D. et al. 2016 Annual report of the Society of Thoracic Surgeons/American College of Cardiology transcatheter valve therapy registry. *Ann. Thorac Surg.,* 2017; 103 (3):1021 - 1035.

[32] Regueiro, A., Granada, J. F., Dagenais, F., Rodés-Cabau, J. Transcatheter mitral valve replacement. *J. Am. Coll. Cardiol.,* 2017; 69(17):2175 - 2192.

[33] Singh, J. P., Evans, J. C., Levy, D. et al. Prevalence and clinical deter- minants of mitral, tricuspid, and aortic regurgitation (the Framingham heart study). *Am. J. Cardiol.,* 1999; 83(6):897 - 902.

[34] Topilsky, Y., Nkomo, V. T., Vatury, O. et al. Clinical outcome of isolated tricuspid regurgitation. *JACC Cardiovasc. Imaging*, 2014; 7(12):1185 - 1194.

[35] Nath, J., Foster, E., Heidenreich, P. A. Impact of tricuspid regurgita- tion on long-term survival. *J. Am. Coll. Cardiol.*, 2004; 43(3):405 - 409.

[36] Bevan, P. J. W., Haydock, D. A., Kang, N. Long-term survival after isolated tricuspid valve replacement. *Heart, Lung and Circ.,* 2014; 23(8):697 - 702.

[37] De Meester, P., Van De Bruaene, A., Voigt, J.-U., Herijgers, P., Budts, W. Outcome and determinants of prognosis in patients under- going isolated tricuspid valve surgery: retrospective single center analysis. *Int. J. Cardiol.,* 2014; 175(2):333 - 339.

[38] Raikhelkar, J., Lin, H.-M., Neckman, D., Afonso, A., Scurlock, C. Isolated tricuspid valve surgery: predictors of adverse outcome and survival. *Heart, Lung and Circ.,* 2013; 22(3):211 - 220.

[39] Vassileva, C. M., Shabosky, J., Boley, T., Markwell, S., Hazelrigg, S. Tricuspid valve surgery: the past 10 years from the Nationwide Inpatient Sample (NIS) database. *J. Thorac Cardiovasc. Surg.,* 2012; 143(5):1043 - 1049.

[40] Fender, E. A., Nishimura, R. A., Holmes, D. R. Percutaneous therapies for tricuspid regurgitation. *Expert Rev. Med. Dev.,* 2017; 14(1):37 - 48.

[41] Masters, J., Morton, G., Anton, I. et al. Specialist intervention is associated with improved patient outcomes in patients with decompensated heart failure: evaluation of the impact of a multi- disciplinary inpatient heart failure team. *Open Heart,* 2017; 4(1): e000547.

[42] Van Mieghem, N. M., Dumonteil, N. Chieffo, A. et al. Current decision making and short-term outcome in patients with degen- erative aortic stenosis: the Pooled-RotterdAm-Milano-Toulouse In Collaboration Aortic Stenosis survey. *EuroIntervention,* 2016; 11(11): e1305 - e1313.

[43] Thyregod, H. G. H., Holmberg, F., Gerds, T. A. et al. Heart team ther- apeutic decision-making and treatment in severe aortic valve stenosis. *Scand. Cardiovasc. J.,* 2016; 50(3):146 - 153.

[44] Lancellotti, P., Rosenhek, R., Pibarot, P. Heart valve clinic: rationale and organization. *Can. J. Cardiol.,* 2014; 30(9):1104 - 1107.

[45] Chambers, J. B., Prendergast, B., Iung, B. et al. Standards defining a 'Heart Valve Centre': ESC working group on valvular heart dis- ease and European Association for Cardiothoracic Surgery view- point. *Eur. Heart J.,* 2017; 38(28):2177 - 2183.

[46] Cerrato, E., Nombela-Franco, L., Nazif, T. M. et al. Evaluation of current practices in transcatheter aortic valve implantation: the WRITTEN (WoRldwIde TAVI ExperieNce) survey. *Int. J. Cardiol.,* 2017; 228:640 - 647.

[47] Ranucci, M., Castelvecchio, S., Conte, M. et al. The easier, the better: age, creatinine, ejection fraction score for operative mortality risk stratification in a series of 29,659 patients undergoing elective cardiac surgery. *J. Thorac Cardiovasc. Surg.,* 2011; 142(3):581 - 586.

[48] Capodanno, D., Barbanti, M., Tamburino, C. et al. A simple risk tool (the OBSERVANT score) for prediction of 30-day mortality after transcatheter aortic valve replacement. *Am. J. Cardiol.,* 2014; 113 (11):1851 - 1858.

[49] Iung, B., Laouénan, C., Himbert, D. et al. Predictive factors of early mortality after transcatheter aortic valve implantation: individual risk assessment using a simple score. *Heart,* 2014; 100(13):1016 - 1023.

[50] Van Mieghem, N. M., Head, S. J., Van Der Boon, R. M. A. et al. The SURTAVI model: proposal for a pragmatic risk stratification for patients with severe aortic stenosis. *EuroIntervention,* 2012; 8 (2):258 - 266.

[51] Kötting, J., Schiller, W., Beckmann, A. et al. German aortic valve score: a new scoring system for prediction of mortality related to aortic valve procedures in adults. *Eur. J. Cardio-Thoracic Surg.,* 2013; 43(5):971 - 977.

[52] Halkin, A., Steinvil, A., Witberg, G. et al. Mortality prediction fol- lowing transcatheter aortic valve replacement: A quantitative comparison of risk scores derived from populations treated with either surgical or percutaneous aortic valve replacement. The

Israeli TAVR Registry Risk Model Accuracy Assessment (IRRMA) study. *Int. J. Cardiol.,* 2016; 215:227 - 231.

[53] Zbroński, K., Huczek, Z., Puchta, D. et al. Outcome prediction following transcatheter aortic valve implantation: multiple risk scores comparison. *Cardiol. J.,* 2016; 23(2): 169 - 177.

[54] Green, P., Woglom, A. E., Genereux, P. et al. The impact of frailty status on survival after transcatheter aortic valve replacement in older adults with severe aortic stenosis. *J. Am. Coll. Cardiol.,* 2012; 5 (9):974 - 981.

[55] Okoh, A. K., Chauhan, D., Kang, N. et al. The impact of frailty status on clinical and functional outcomes after transcatheter aortic valve replacement in nonagenarians with severe aortic stenosis. *Catheter Cardiovasc. Interv.,* 2017. doi: 10.1002/ccd.27083. [Epub ahead of print] PubMed PMID: 28463403.

[56] Thongprayoon, C., Cheungpasitporn, W., Kashani, K. The impact of frailty on mortality after transcatheter aortic valve replacement. *Ann. Transl. Med.,* 2017; 5(6):144.

[57] Afilalo, J., Lauck, S., Kim, D. H. et al. Frailty in older adults undergoing aortic valve replacement. *J. Am. Coll. Cardiol.,* 2017; 70(6): 689 - 700.

In: Perspectives in Aortic Valve Disease
Editor: Giovanni Concistrè

ISBN: 978-1-53618-769-4

Chapter 12

PHARMACOLOGICAL TREATMENT OF AORTIC VALVE DISEASE

Giovanni Concistrè**, MD
Ospedale del Cuore "G. Pasquinucci,"
Fondazione Toscana Gabriele Monasterio, Massa, Italy

ABSTRACT

Major advances in the diagnostic, evaluation, and particularly surgical treatment of aortic valve disease have redefined the role of medical treatment. Calcific aortic valve disease (CAVD) is the most common valvular disorder in the elderly, with the incidence of 3% in general population of Western countries. Surgical aortic valve replacement and transcatheter aortic valve implantation are the only available treatments when the disease become severe and symptoms occur. Indeed, no approved pharmacological approach is available for CAVD patients. In this review, we describe the current literature evidence on possible future therapeutic targets for this debilitating and fatal disease such as PCSK9, P2Y2 receptor, cadherin 11, and DDP-4.

In acute AR, aortic valve replacement (AVR) is the only life-saving treatment. Medical treatment may improve the hemodynamic state temporarily before surgery. Rationale of medical treatment in chronic AR is based on the natural history and pathophysiology of the disease. The primary goal is to optimize the time of the AVR. If there is any symptom and/or left ventricular (LV) dysfunction, early AVR is required. Vasodilators should only be considered as a short-term treatment before surgery if there is evidence of severe heart failure or as a long-term treatment if AVR is contraindicated because of cardiac or noncardiac factors. In asymptomatic patients with severe chronic AR and normal LV function (even if the left ventricle is moderately dilated), vasodilators may prolong the compensated phase of chronic AR, although proof of their efficacy in delaying AVR is limited. Nifedipine is the best evidence-based treatment in this indication. ACE inhibitors are particularly useful for hypertensive patients with AR. ↑-Adrenoceptor antagonists (↑-blockers) may be indicated to slow the rate of aortic dilatation and delay the need for surgery in patients with AR associated with aortic root

* Corresponding Author's Email: gioconci@libero.it.

disease. Furthermore, they may improve cardiac performance by reducing cardiac volume and LV mass in patients with impaired LV function after AVR for AR.

Keywords: calcific aortic valve disease, aortic valve stenosis, aortic valve regurgitation, pharmacological treatment

Introduction

Although surgery plays a central role in the management of patients with aortic stenosis (AS) and aortic regurgitation (AR), medical treatment remains necessary for two reasons. First, with the increasingly aging population with symptomatic degenerative valve disease, in whom surgery may be too risky, medical treatment may be the only reasonable alternative. Second, some medical therapies have demonstrated their potential to beneficially alter the natural course of AR, resulting in a delay or even reduction in the need for surgery. The objective of this chapter will be to define the role of pharmacotherapy in AR, emphasizing the role of vasodilators, and to analyse the current evidence regarding existing and future pharmacological therapeutic targets for CAVD [1-11].

Novel Pharmacological Targets for Calcific Aortic Valve Disease

Lipid-Lowering Approaches

Failure of Statins

Recently, genetic association and predisposition to high levels of plasma lipids were shown to correlate with presence of aortic valve calcification (AVC), in the Cohorts for Heart and Aging Research in Genetic Epidemiology study, and with AS, in the Malmö Diet and Cancer Study [12]. In the last two decades, several observational studies suggested that lipid-lowering therapy with statins might influence AS progression and its sequelae [13–15]. However, the results from four randomized clinical trials, aimed to investigate the effect of statins on AS progression, showed no difference between statin treatments and placebo, thus demonstrating the absence of AS reduction [16–19].

Parolari et al. [13] performed a meta-analysis to clarify the role of statins and their effect on the incidence of hard endpoints and on the possibility to delay AS progression. In patients affected by non-rheumatic AS, the authors showed that statin treatment does not affect the occurrence of major events, at 4 years of follow-up, and does not reduce the rate of AS progression over time. Partially, the ineffectiveness of statins in these clinical trials might be explained by the advanced stage of the disease. Hence, it has been proposed that lipid-lowering therapy should be initiated in early stage of CAVD in order to prevent AS. However, in the SEAS trail, that assessed patients with mild-to-moderate AS (n = 1.873), simvastatin treatment did not reduce cardiovascular events associated with CAVD [17]. In follow-up, patients were divided in subgroups according to severity of CAVD. The results showed that statin therapy had not effect on CAVD progression, independently of AS severity at baseline [20]. Nevertheless, in one study evaluating 1.641 patients with AVSc, the authors found that statin treatment led to significant reduction in mortality and slowed AS progression, while no significant evidence was noted with angiotensin-converting enzyme inhibitors [21].

Otto et al. [22] described the similarities between AVSc and atherosclerotic lesion of the arterial wall. AVSc, as well as atherosclerosis, are both multifactorial processes associated with various pathological pathways as inflammation, oxidative stress, and matrix remodeling [23, 24]. In addition, lipid deposition, macrophage and T-cell infiltration, and basement membrane disruption have been found in both pathological processes [22]. These two pathological conditions also share similar risk factors, such as hypertension, smoking habits, and male gender. Dyslipidemia, in particular, high levels of low-density lipoprotein cholesterol (LDL), is also known as a risk factor for AS. However, only 40% of patients with AS have concomitant atherosclerosis, and at the same time in the general population affected by atherosclerosis, only a part will developed AS [25, 26]. In addition, only 2% of subjects with AVSc will progress to AS per year [27].

The relationship between circulating oxidized LDL (ox-LDL) levels and fibrocalcific remodeling of valvular tissue in AS has been previously reported [28]. Moreover, lipoprotein-associated phospholipase A2 (Lp-PLA2) is highly expressed in the calcific aortic valve and plays a crucial role in the mineralization process of valve interstitial cells (VICs) [29].

This being said, the hypothesis to use lipid-lowering therapy such as statins at AVSc stage has been put aside since AVSc is still considered a normal echocardiography finding and too many patients will have to be treated to "only" save a small proportion of them who will develop AS and thus requiting aortic valve replacement when AS will reach the severe stage.

Hence, until AVSc will not be recognized as a pathological condition and, more important, until reliable biomarkers (such as bio-humoral or imaging) that will identify AVSc patients with high-risk to develop AS, the use of lipid-lowering therapy will not be sustainable in this particular context.

Lipoprotein(a) Reduction

Lipoprotein(a) [Lp(a)] [30] is an LDL-like particle synthesized by the liver, in which apolipoprotein B100 (apoB100) is covalently bound with apolipoprotein(a) [31–33]. Lp(a) exerts its atherogenic properties through multiple mechanisms: inhibition of the fibrinolytic pathway, interaction with extracellular matrix components such as glycoproteins, binding to macrophage scavenger receptors, accumulation in the vessel wall, and expansion of atherosclerotic plaques [34, 35]. Elevated Lp(a) levels are associated with increased cardiovascular risk, independently of LDL levels [31, 32]. Interestingly, a systematic review, including 36 prospective studies for a total of 126.634 in- dividuals, demonstrated a continuous and independent association of Lp(a) levels with risk of coronary heart disease (CHD) and stroke [36]. In addition, a large population study, including 2.047 patients with either non-fatal myocardial infarction or coronary death and 3.969 controls, showed that the continuous association between Lp(a) levels and CHD risk was independent of traditional cardiovascular risk factors [37]. Hence, elevated levels of Lp(a) are considered an independent risk factor for atherosclerotic disease. A significant association between Lp(a) and CAVD was previously reported [38]. Rogers et al. [39] suggested that Lp(a) plays a key role in the development of CAVD. The mineralization mechanism of the aortic valve mediated by Lp(a) is still controversial. Some authors showed that Lp-PLA2 is highly expressed in mineralized aortic valves, it uses oxidized phospholipids, carried by Lp(a) as substrates to produce lysophosphatidylcholine (LPC), present in AVC [29]. In addition, autotaxin (ATX), a lysophospholipase D enzyme [40], uses LPC as a substrate producing lysophosphatidic acid, which in turn promotes inflammation and mineralization of the aortic valve blocking antagonist of lysophosphatidic receptors 1–3 (LPARs) [39]. Thus, ATX, transported in the aortic valve by Lp(a) and also secreted by VICs, could represent a novel therapeutic target in CAVD.

In 1995, Gotoh et al. [41] found a strong association of Lp(a) with prevalent CAVD, measuring Lp(a) serum concentrations and investigating their relationship to the presence of echocardiographic AVSc. This result was confirmed in a cross-sectional analysis of 129 Dutch individuals with family history of hypercholesterolemia: the results point out that higher Lp(a) levels are associated with calcification of aortic valve [33]. Furthermore, in a prospective Mendelian randomization study including more than 17′500 patients, high Lp(a) levels were associated with an increased risk for CAVD [42]. Recently, in a prospective study in 454 cases of AS incidence in a 20- year follow-up, elevated Lp(a) levels (> 90 mg/dL) predicted a 3-fold increased risk of AS, suggesting that Lp(a) levels are associated not only with presence but also with progression of CAVD [43]. Moreover, the role of Lp(a) in AS development was established with a genome-wide-association analysis of 3 cohorts, including Multi-Ethnic Study of Atherosclerosis (MESA), in which LPA gene variant (rs10455872) was associated with CAVD in both whites and black subjects [44]. Indeed, nowadays, elevated plasma Lp(a) levels are considered as a new risk factor for CAVD. However, screening for Lp(a) and Lp(a) lowering therapy is recommended only in certain patient populations, such as intermediate-to-high-risk patients, patients with premature cardiovascular disease (CVD), or patients with familial hypercholesterolemia [45]. In the Aortic Stenosis Progression Observation: Measuring Effects of Rosuvastatin (ASTRONOMER) trial, elevated oxidized phospholipids and Lp(a) plasma concentrations were independently associated with an increased risk of CAVD progression and this association was more evident in younger patients, providing a strong rationale to test Lp(a)-lowering and/or oxidized phospholipids lowering therapies for reducing CAVD progression [46]. The statins effect on Lp(a) is controversial. It has been shown that different statins (atorvastatin, pravastatin, rosuvastatin and simvastatin/ezetimibe) could stimulate the increment of Lp(a) levels up to twenty percent [30]. The fact that the beneficial LDL lowering effect of statins is balanced by the Lp(a) levels increment could be an explanation of statin failure in AS treatment. Thus, randomized trials including patients at an earlier stage of CAVD treated with the new classes of lipid-lowering therapies are warranted. The second generation of antisense oligonucleotides (ASOs) that inhibit apo(a) mRNA translation [47] was acknowledged as a new potent selective Lp(a) inhibitor with the ability to reduce the risk for CVD and AS in patients with high Lp(a) concentrations [48]. In this randomized, double-blind, placebo-controlled, phase 1 study, 47 volunteers received ISIS-APO(a)RX as a single dose, multi-dose or placebo. Lp(a) plasma levels decreased dose-dependently of 39.6% in the 100mg group, 59.0% in the 200 mg group and 77.8% in the 300 mg group. Similar results were obtained also for oxidized phospholipids associated with apoB100 and apo(a) [47]. In addition, Lp(a) can be significantly lowered by 20–40% with ASOs targeting apoB100 [49], monoclonal antibodies to proprotein convertase subtilisin/kexin type 9 (PCSK9) [50] and cholesterol ester transfer protein inhibitors. However, clinical trials to assess clinical outcomes in patients with elevated Lp(a) levels affected by CAVD are in progress and the results are not available yet. Nicotinic acid (niacin) is known to have beneficial effects on very low-density lipoprotein (VLDL), LDL, and to significantly lower plasma Lp(a) concentrations [51], probably due to an inhibitory effect on LPA transcription [52]. In addition, findings from several studies showed an association of niacin therapy with increment of HDL levels [53]. Of note, there is a relationship between low HDL levels and fast CAVD progression [54]. Indeed, apolipoprotein A–I mimetic peptide, that has been shown to elevate transiently circulating HDL cholesterol in mice and rabbits, prevented mineralization of aortic valve and even pro- moted AS regression [55, 56]. Interestingly, infusion of recombinant apolipoprotein A–I Milano in rabbits had positive effects on morphology and histopathology of stenotic aortic valve, with significant reduction of valve thickening, inflammation, and calcification [57]. Recently, a large clinical trial investigated the effect of statin therapy alone or in combination with extended-release niacin (ERN) in patients with CVD but without high levels of LDL at baseline [58, 59]. In this study, a favourable effect of ERN on apolipoproteins and in particular on Lp(a) was shown. However, these positive changes did not influence CV events occurrence. The pilot randomized trial Early Aortic Valve Lipoprotein (a) Lowering (EAVaLL) (NCT02109614) was designed to evaluate whether lowering Lp(a) at an early stage of CAVD could affect the disease progression. A cohort of 238 participants with elevated Lp(a) and AVSc or mild AS is currently been enrolled and randomized to receive ERN or placebo for 2 years. The primary outcome of the study is the assessment of calcium score progression evaluated by cardiac computed tomography. The secondary outcome is the evaluation of mean change in Lp(a) levels between treatment arms, while other outcomes include: a) rates of CAVD progression by echocardiography; b) drug compliance; and c) side effects and adverse events. The results of this important study will help us to clarify our knowledge about the pharmacological effect of niacin on CAVD progression. Nevertheless, it is important to take into account that niacin has several side effects, such as gastrointestinal and musculoskeletal disorders or even increased risk of diabetes [53]. In light of these recent trials and studies, we believe that in the future guidelines patients affected by AS should be screened for Lp(a) levels and should be treated if high Lp(a) is found.

PCSK9 Inhibition

PCSK9 is a hepatic convertase that binds and internalizes LDL receptors into lysosomes and stimulates their degradation [60]. Cohen and colleagues [61] identified, in a large cohort of subjects (n = 12.887), that variants in PCSK9 locus are associated with different LDL plasma levels and risk of CHD, including myocardial infarction and cardiovascular mortality. In particular, nonsense mutations or a specific sequence variation, resulting in a loss-of-function (LOF), in the PCSK9 locus were associated respectively with 28 and 15% reduction in LDL and with 88 and 47% reduction in CHD risk [61]. Inclisiran is a fully chemically stabilized duplex RNA targeting 3′ UTR of PCSK9 mRNA [62]. Participants receiving either single- or multiple-dose of inclisiran vs placebo experienced a significant reduction in LDL levels in both groups, reaching the peak reduction of ~50% in the single-dose and ~60% in the multiple-dose at day 84. Interestingly, this reduction persisted for up to 180 days after receiving the first dose [62]. Alirocumab and evolocumab, two monoclonal antibodies that inhibit PCSK9, have been implemented for the treatment of patients with elevated LDL and who have not sufficiently responded to or cannot tolerate statins. These drugs, in addition to radically lowering LDL (up to 70%), are also able to lower plasma Lp(a) (up to 30%) [63]. The Lp (a) reduction obtained by inhibiting PCSK9 was surprising since Lp(a) has not been considered to be catabolized through LDL receptors [64]. Both antibodies are associated with a significant reduction in CV events [45]. The FOURIER trial, published on March 2017, is a randomized, double-blind, placebo-controlled, multinational clinical trial in which 27′564 patients, receiving statin therapy, underwent randomization to receive subcutaneous injections of evolocumab (140 mg; 2 weeks or 420 mg; 1 month) or placebo. Overall, LDL levels were reduced by 59% from baseline compared to placebo and this therapy resulted in a significant reduction in the risk of cardiovascular death, myocardial infarction, stroke, coronary revascularization, or hospitalization for unstable angina by 15% and the risk of cardiovascular death, myocardial infarction, or stroke by 20% [65]. In a cohort of Danish individuals (n = 103′083) a LOF mutation of PCSK9 (R46 L) was associated not only with lower levels of LDL but also with lower levels of Lp(a) and with reduced risk of AS and myocardial infarction. These results suggest that individuals with AS could benefit from a therapy with PCSK9 inhibitors [66]. Interestingly, in a small cross-sectional study, PCSK9 levels correlated with the presence but not with the severity of CAVD [67]. Therefore, a randomized control trial (NCT03051360) is now underway to investigate the effects of PCSK9 inhibitors vs placebo on AS progression (Table 3). Final data collection and estimated study completion date are expected by early 2020. Currently, on debate is in which way PCSK9 influences Lp(a) levels. It has been shown a correlation between chronic inflammatory infiltrates, osteochondrogenic metaplasia, and neovascularization of aortic valve [68, 69]. A dense inflammatory infiltrate within the valve tissue was associated with the remodeling process and the peak transaortic gradient [68]. Thanks to fluorodeoxyglucose–positron emission tomography/computed tomography, a method that provides information about valvular metabolic activity, it has been shown that early manifestation of aortic valve lesion (i.e., AVSc) was associated with inflammation [2]. Indeed, early and advanced aortic valve lesions are both characterized by the presence of inflammation [70]. Notably, inflammation induces PCSK9 overexpression that leads to increasing LDL levels as a result of an accelerated LDL receptor degradation [71, 72]. In addition, circulating PCSK9 positively correlated with C reactive protein (CRP) [73], and, at the same time, CRP was found in the fibrosa of stenotic aortic valve. Thus, the presence of CRP in AS might activate the classical complement system [74]. In summary, since PCSK9 seems directly linked to inflammation, PCSK9 inhibitors may have also therapeutic benefits in patients with early/asymptomatic manifestation of CAVD.

Aortic Valve Adverse Remodeling Therapeutic Targets

Purinergic Receptor 2Y2 Activation

Considering that bone mineralization is the result of a balance between deposit and absorption of minerals, it is reasonable to think that, during disease progression involving the mineralization (CAVD or calcified atherosclerotic plaques) it is possible to shift the balance of this process towards calcium removal [75]. Interestingly, Miller et al. [76], using a "genetic switch" in Reversa mice, showed that reducing plasma lipid levels in hypercholesterolemic mice with early CAVD normalized oxidative stress, reduced pro-osteogenic signaling, and halted the pro- gression of AS. These observations suggested that AVC could be re- versible.

VICs are the main cellular components involved in AVC. The role of the purinergic receptor 2Y2 (P2Y2R) in the mineralization process of VICs has been reported [77]. In particular, P2Y2R agonists promoted the membrane translocation of carbonic anhydrase XII (CAXII) that led to a regression of the mineralization of the aortic valve [75]. CAXII is an enzyme catalyzing the formation of bicarbonate and protons from water and carbon dioxide and thus plays an important role in pH homeostasis [78]. Using in vitro and in vivo models, Bouchareb et al. [75] showed that the membrane translocation of CAXII mediated by P2Y2R, in VICs, acidified the extracellular space and promoted the regression of CAVD. Thus, a new class of compounds able to modulate this pathway may open novel research opportunities in the field of medical treatment for CAVD. However, we need to be careful since the AS model used was a hypercholesterolemic mouse model. It is important to note that this animal model develops a significant hemodynamic obstruction of the aortic valve mimicking AS, but with low calcification. Indeed, in this model, the lesion is rich in lipids that create flow obstruction, while the main process observed in AS patients is the calcification of the leaflets.

Phosphate Inorganic Transporter 1 Inhibition

Expression of phosphate-related genes and proteins as sodium-phosphate co-transporter 1 (PiT-1), ectonucleotide pyrophosphatase/phosphodiesterase 1 (ENPP1), alkaline phosphatase (ALP), and oteopontin (OPN) was associated with lysophosphatidylcholine (LPC) induced mineralization in VICs [29]. Interestingly, high phosphate concentrations as well as Ox-LDL, involved in inflammation, stimulate PiT- 1 expression, inducing calcification in human VICs [79, 80]. Treatment with sodium phosphonoformate hexahydrate, a PiT-1 inhibitor, effectively reduced in vitro calcification of VICs [81]. Based on this result, Seya et al. [81], evaluated the effects of an evocarpine derivative, called 1-methyl-2-undecyl-4(1 H)-quinolone (MUQ), on high phosphate induced calcification on human VICs. The authors suggested that MUQ, due to ability to decrease PiT-1 gene expression and protein levels, inhibits high phosphate-induced VICs calcification. Nevertheless, further studies aimed to clarify the molecular mechanism of MUQ calcification inhibitory effects are needed.

Peroxisome Proliferator-Activated Receptor-Gamma Activation

Activation of peroxisome proliferator-activated receptor-gamma (PPARγ) by thiazolidinedione (TZD) mediates positive effects on me- tabolism regulation, inflammation, apoptosis, and cardiovascular cal- cification [82], usually prescribed for type II diabetes treatment [83]. In particular, pioglitazone, a member of the TZD class, attenuates AVC progression in hypercholesterolemic rabbits via down-regulation of receptor for advanced glycation end products (RAGE) [84]. Recently, effectiveness of pioglitazone in slowing CAVD progression has also been shown in a study conducted on hypercholesterolemic mice [85]. Indeed, pioglitazone avoided lipid deposition, attenuated apoptosis, re- duced AVC, and improved mobility of valve leaflets [85]. Despite these positive findings, clinical use of TZD for CAVD patients is limited due to safety concerns. Adverse effects such as reduction of bone density in postmenopausal women [86] or increase risk for cardiovascular disease [87, 88] hindered the application of this therapy.

Dipeptidyl Peptidase 4 Inhibition

Dipeptidyl peptidase 4 (DPP-4) enzyme inactivates the glucagon- like peptide 1 (GLP-1). Thus, DDP-4 inhibitors, preventing GLP-1 inactivation, increase GLP-1 concentration that, in turn, improves the glycaemic control in type 2 diabetes patients [89]. Clinical studies showed that DPP-4 inhibitors decreased atherosclerosis incidence, inflammation [90], improved heart failure, and cognitive functions [91, 92]. The favourable effects of DDP-4 inhibitors attenuated the high glucose-induced cellular alteration such as proliferation, migration, apoptosis, and calcification via extracellular signal-regulated kinase 1/2 pathway [93]. Recently, it was suggested that DPP-4 inhibitors could serve as a potential therapeutic target to prevent CAVD progression as well [94]. Indeed, inhibition of DDP-4 activity resulted in osteogenic differentiation block in human VICs, in reduced AVC in a mouse model, and it led to improvement of echocardiographic characteristics of aortic leaflets features in a rabbit model [94]. Hence, future clinical studies are warranted to evaluate the efficacy of DDP-4 inhibitors on CAVD development and progression.

5-Hydroxytryptamine Receptor 2B Inhibition

Transforming growth factor-beta1 (TGF-β1) is highly expressed in calcified aortic valves, promotes the activation of VICs, and induces myofibroblastic differentiation that leads to CAVD [95, 96]. It has been shown that an interaction exists between serotonin 5-hydro- xytryptamine receptor 2B (5-HT2B) and TGF- β1 pathway in CAVD. Indeed, serotonin stimulates the up-regulation of TGF- β1 in aortic VICs [97]. In addition, 5-HT2B agonists were found to increase the risk of valve diseases due to stimulation of VICs proliferation within the aortic valve [98]. Based on this, Hutcheson et al. [99] hypothesized that 5-HT2B antagonism may have protective effects on myofibroblastic differentiation and calcific nodule formation. The main results of this study suggested that 5-HT2B antagonism blocked tyrosine-protein kinase SRC phosphorylation, preventing the activation of non-canonical TGF-β1 signaling and myofibroblastic differentiation of VICs. Hence, the inhibition of 5-HT2B might be a potential target for CAVD pre- vention [99].

Cadherin 11 Inhibition

Cadherin 11, a cell-cell adhesion protein, can be considered another possible target for CAVD treatment since fibroblastic differentiation, induced by TGF-β1 activation, promotes a strong upregulation of cadherin 11. Of note, rise in cadherin 11 expression has been associated with calcific nodule formation of aortic VICs, in vitro [100]. Indeed, Bowen et al. [101] demonstrated that cadherin 11 knock out adult mice were protected from AVC. These results strongly support cadherin 11 as an important regulator of calcium nodule tissue homeostasis. Interestingly, it was reported that VICs from Notch1+/−mice over-express cadherin 11 [102]. In another study conducted on the same mouse model, it was demonstrated a protective effect of SYN0012 (a cadherin 11-blocking antibody) on AS development, including leaflet thickening and stiffening, by the block of pathological phenotype ob- served in Notch1+/−mice [103]. In human, Notch1 haploinsufficiency resulted in early developmental defects of the aortic valve and later an increment in calcium deposition, leading to severe CAVD with 100% penetrance [104]. Specifically, it has been shown that Notch1 repressed the activity of runt related transcription factor 2 (Runx2), a pivotal transcriptional regulator of osteoblast cell fate [104]. It is worth mentioning that a specific antibody against cadherin 11 is under evaluation in phase I clinical trials for rheumatoid arthritis [103]. Hopefully, after the safety results, new clinical trials evaluating if cadherin 11 block will affect CAVD progression will be performed.

Cathepsin S Inhibition

The pathophysiological changes in stenotic aortic valves include accumulation and degradation of extracellular matrix (ECM). Elastin, a ubiquitous ECM protein, is a crucial factor in this process, as demonstrated in elastin insufficient mice, in which progressive aortic valve malformation and subsequently valve diseases were observed [105]. Interestingly, Helske et al. [106] suggested a potential involvement of elastolytic cysteine proteases (such as cathepsin S, K, and V) in ad- verse ECM remodelling. In the study, stenotic valves, collected at the time of valve replacement, showed increased mRNA expression and activity of cathepsin S, K, and V compared to control valves [106]. The involvement of cathepsin S in CAVD was confirmed in animal models by Aikawa et al. [107]. The authors demonstrated, in hypercholesterolemic mice with Chronic Renal Disease, that aortic valve calcification is completely abolished in cathepsin S deficient mice [107]. These results indicate that the preservation of elastin integrity, for example with a selective inhibition of cathepsin S, may also represent a novel therapeutic strategy in the prevention of CAVD.

Multi-Omic Approach

The recent advances in omics technologies and network medicine allow a better understanding of the CAVD complexity from onset, progression, and treatment [108]. Recently, Schlotter et al. [109] presented the first "spatiotemporal multi-omics" mapping proteome and transcriptome of human CAVD. Differences at transcriptional and protein level were identified among non-diseased, fibrotic, and calcific stages of CAVD. Authors suggest that pathological process involved in CAVD may act in parallel to promote valvular fibrosis and calcification. Thanks to their experimental approach, the authors highlighted that structural matrix proteins, such as proline-arginine-rich end leucine-rich repeat protein (PRELP) and procollagen C-endopeptidase enhancer 2 (PCOLCE2), as well as secreted proteins, such as clusterin (CLU) and high-temperature requirement A serine peptidase 1 (HTRA1), con- tributed to the calcification propensity [109]. Hence, the identified molecular pathways and the associated proteins could represent novel therapeutic targets to halt CAVD progression.

Conclusion

It is worth mentioning that angiotensin-converting-enzyme inhibitors (ACEi) and angiotensin-receptor blockers (ARBs) use in patients with AS and hypertension are extensively reported in the literature and actually, represent the first treatment of choice even if clinical studies reported contradictory results [110]. Like statin trials, positive outcomes have been described mainly by retrospective studies. Thus, without prospective placebo-controlled, random double-blind studies, it is uncertain whether any of these therapies will any favourable effects [110]. In conclusion, nowadays there is no effective pharmacological treatment for the patients with overt CAVD. It is worth mentioning that after symptoms manifestation, CAVD mortality occurs within 5 years without aortic valve replacement [111]. Conservative surgical intervention is the standard therapeutic approach in non-high risk CAVD patients, improving significantly symptoms and survival [112]. Recently, TAVI was shown to be effective in elderly high-risk patients, being less invasive; however, the treatment of AS patients with low to intermediate operative risk with this new technique it is still uncertain [113]. That being sad, all current transcatheter heart valves are bioprosthesis, hence the durability of these valves remain questionable, particularly in younger patients [114]. Thanks to the new multiomic approach, we will be able to considerably advance our knowledge of molecular and cellular pathways involved in this multifactorial disease, allowing us to unravel new targets to be exploited in CAVD pharmacological therapies and appropriated follow up. Finally, to tackle CAVD effectively, we believe that it will be important: 1) to identify and treat patients in the early stage of the disease to halt CAVD progression; 2) to focus the attention not only on risk factors known to affect the atherosclerotic disease but also on direct pathological mechanisms involved in CAVD; and 3) to intensify the effort to design new studies focused on "direct therapy" of CAVD, such as P2Y2 receptor, cadherin 11 and DDP-4.

RATIONAL FOR MEDICAL TREATMENT IN AORTIC AORTIC REGURGITATION

Vasodilators

Acute AR

Sodium nitroprusside may help to temporarily manage the symptoms of acute AR before surgery by decreasing the signs of heart failure. The drug may transiently augment forward flow and reduce LV end-diastolic pressure [1].

Chronic AR

AR volume varies as the product of the regurgitant orifice area (which remains constant) [17] by the square root of the pressure gradient across the aortic orifice in diastole and by the duration of diastole. AR may vary if any one of the determinants of regurgitant volume changes. Therefore, bradycardia and diastolic hypertension should be avoided. Most vasodilator therapies reduce both the aortic diastolic pressure and LV diastolic pressure, resulting in little change in the mean transaortic pressure gradient [18]. All this suggests that if pharmacologic treatment is to be effective in the management of AR, another parameter, indepen- dent of changes in regurgitant volume, may be involved. In fact, the first response of the left ventricle to volume overload of chronic AR is to increase end-diastolic volume, with a concomitant increase in chamber compliance (to avoid an increase in filling pressures) and development of LV hypertrophy. As a result of this ventricular remodeling, forward stroke volume and LVEF tend to remain within the normal range. LV preload reserve is also maintained. However, LV dilatation associated with increased systolic wall stress induces an increase in LV afterload. Effects of continued preload and afterload reduction induced by vasodilator therapy differ with treatment type and duration [18] (Figure 1). With short-term treatment, reduced fiber shortening is associated with a decrease in preload that is countered by a reduction in afterload, to maintain a stable stroke volume. With long-term treatment, regression of hypertrophy is associated with a reduction in ventricular volume and wall stress. The diastolic pressure-volume curve shifts leftward, resulting in an improvement of preload reserve and a relatively preserved stroke volume [18]. Moreover, preload and afterload are interrelated: because peak systolic stress is substantially elevated in AR [19] afterload reduction enables such a volume-overload ventricle to perform more work merely by moving the workload relation to a more favorable and efficient operative load [18]. Thus, the primary goal of vasodilator therapy should focus on correction of this excessive afterload, which is predominant in AR. Therefore, vasodilators are particu- larly useful in patients with systolic hypertension [20, 21]. This reduction in afterload enables an increase in LVEF despite a decrease in preload. Other goals of this treatment are the reduction of venous congestion signs and the restoration of preload reserve.

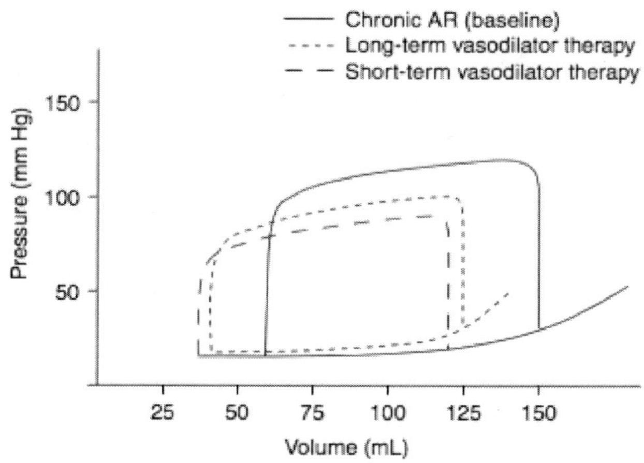

Figure 1. Effects of combined preload and afterload reduction induced by vasodilator therapy differ with treatment type and duration (reproduced from Levine and Gaasch [18], with permission from the American College of Cardiology Foundation). AR = aortic regurgitation.

Short-Term Effects of Vasodilators

Among vasodilators used as short-term treatment of AR, intra-venous sodium nitroprusside allows for rapid decrease of AR by a rapid decrease of arterial pressure, LV end-diastolic pressure and volume, and by concomitant increase in the LVEF and cardiac index [22, 23]. In these studies, patients with high filling pressures, reduced LVEF, and elevated systolic pressures were the most likely to benefit from this drug. Similar results were obtained with intravenous hydralazine [24]. Despite an increase in cardiac index and a decrease in end- diastolic pressure after a single oral dose of nifedipine [25] the drug failed to significantly reduce LV end-diastolic volume [26]. Banaszewski et al. [27] compared single treatments with nifedipine and captopril. Nifedipine significantly reduced systemic vascular resistance compared with captopril, whereas captopril reduced pulmonary capillary wedge more than nifedipine.

Long-Term Effects of Vasodilators

The results of long-term therapy with vasodilators are more impressive than those after single dose administration. Five trials with hydralazine have been published [29-33]. In the largest randomized, double-blind, placebo-controlled trial with hydralazine (average dose 216 mg/day given to 45 asymptomatic patients), Greenberg et al. [31] found a significant reduction in LV volumes (end-diastolic and end-systolic) and a small improvement of LVEF in hydralazine recipients. ACE inhibitors may increase LV emptying, resulting in a favorable systolic unloading effect [21]. However, only a few small studies have evaluated the use of ACE inhibitors in chronic AR, with equivocal results, possibly because plasma renin activity is not increased in this setting [20]. Whereas Wisenbaugh et al. [36] found no change in LV volume or LVEF in 23 patients given captopril 25 mg/day for 6 months, Schön [37] found a significant decrease in LV volume and increase in LVEF in 12 patients given quinapril 10–20 mg/day for 12 months. Banaszewski et al., [27] comparing 3 years' treatment with captopril or nifedipine, found no change in LV end-systolic diameter or LVEF in either group, even though LV end-diastolic diameter was more reduced in captopril recipients. Moreover, several investigators have reported the effectiveness of ACE inhibitors in reducing not only LV volume overload but also LV hypertrophy [32, 36, 37]. Schön [37] demonstrated a 35% reduction in LV mass and a complete reversal of LV hypertrophy with quinapril 10-20 mg/day. Lin et al., [32] in a large randomized, double-blind trial comparing enalapril and hydralazine, found a significant reduction in LV volume and mass at 1 year in the enalapril group. Because of the physiological role of the cardiac renin-angiotensin system in normal growth of the left ventricle, the benefits of ACE inhibition are particularly interesting in reducing LV hypertrophy in growing children with LV overload [35, 38]. Calcium channel antagonists have also been used in chronic AR. After one year nifedipine 20mg twice daily reduced systolic and diastolic blood pressure, and produced an important reduction in LV volume and mass and a large increase in the LVEF in a randomized trial [34]. Nifedipine was superior to hydralazine in this trial; [34] reduction in LV volume and increase in LVEF at 1 year was greater with nifedipine, and there was a reduction in LV mass. In 16 patients with chronic asymptomatic AR given 3 months' treatment with oral felodipine 10 mg/day (after initial IV infusion of 0.3mg), Sondergaard et al. [28] found a pronounced decrease in systemic vascular resistance, in regurgitant fraction, in LV mass, and an increased forward cardiac output index. The short duration of the study (3 months) may explain the absence of effect on LV volumes and LVEF. Few studies have demonstrated a potential for pharmacologic treatment to delay the need for surgery by prolonging the asymptomatic period while preserving LVEF. Scognamiglio et al. [39] demonstrated that long-term use of nifedipine can achieve that goal. In this study, 143 asymptomatic patients with isolated severe AR and a normal LVEF were randomized to receive either nifedipine 20mg twice daily ($n = 69$) or digoxin 0.25 mg/day ($n = 74$). The cause of AR was rheumatic heart disease in 61% of patients. Digoxin was chosen instead of placebo, even though its beneficial effect on AR was only based on a previously published 1-month trial [40]. The rate of progression to AVR was significantly lower in the nifedipine group at all evaluation times after the first year. No AVR occurred in the first two years in the nifedipine group. At the end of the 6-year follow-up, a mean of 34 α 6% of the patients in the digoxin group had undergone AVR, compared with only 15 α 3% in the nifedipine group ($p < 0.001$). The rate of AVR in the digoxin group (5.8% per year) was similar to that previously reported for patients receiving no medical therapy [5, 41]. Compared with the digoxin group, patients in the nifedipine group had lower LV end-diastolic and end-systolic volume indices and a higher LVEF. In all nifedipine recipients, the LVEF returned to normal values after AVR, whereas it remained abnormal in four patients (20%) treated with digoxin. This study supports the as- sumption that nifedipine is effective in delaying the need for surgery. It also suggests that use of vasodilators requires a careful follow-up to avoid masking of progressive myocardial dysfunction that would not recover despite AVR. To summarize, in chronic AR, an ACE inhibitor may be the most appropriate drug for patients with hypertension and/or LV dilatation, whereas nifedipine appears to be the best 'evidence- based' treatment for asymptomatic patients with severe AR and no LV dysfunction [20].

Limitations

Most of the studies analyzing the effects of vasodilators in AR included only a limited number of patients. It then appears particularly difficult to extrapolate the data for general practice. The proper way to test whether nifedipine is the best treatment to delay surgery would be to test nifedipine against another potentially effective medication rather than digoxin, for which efficacy has not been documented in AR, or a placebo. Furthermore, long-term hydralazine therapy is often poorly tolerated [18]. Another limitation of these trials is that most of the drugs were not titrated against blood pressure. Finally, surrogate endpoints (LV volume, LV mass) rather than clinical outcomes were measured in these studies. In that way, the study by Scognamiglio et al. [39] represented a major advance in measuring surrogate endpoints and clinical outcomes.

↑-ADRENOCEPTOR ANTAGONISTS

↑-Adrenoceptor antagonists (↑-blockers) are not recommended in patients with AR because they block compensatory tachycardia. In patients with disease of the aortic root, such as in Marfan disease, progressive enlargement of the aortic root is associated with AR and dissection. In such patients, the primary goal of a pharmacologic treatment is to limit aortic dilatation and avoid occurrence of aortic dissection. The only treatment proven to be effective is a prophylactic ↑-adrenergic blockade that reduces the progression of the aneurysmal dilatation [9]. In fact, Shores et al., [9] in a randomized trial in 70 patients with Marfan syndrome, found significantly lower aortic-root dimensions and a better survival rate in the propanolol group than in the control group. Recommended ↑-adrenoceptor antagonists are propanolol (mean dosage 212 α 68 mg/day) or atenolol (100 mg/day) [9, 10]. Although likely, this beneficial effect of ↑-adrenoceptor antagonists in patients with Marfan syndrome has not been proven in patients with bicuspid valve or dilatation of the ascending aorta not associated with Marfan syndrome. ↑-Adrenoceptor antagonist therapy may also be useful in patients with impaired LV function after AVR for AR. In these patients, ↑-adrenoceptor antagonist therapy is postulated to improve cardiac performance by reducing cardiac volume and mass [42]. Treatment with different ↑-adrenoceptor antagonists (atenolol 50 mg/day, carvedilol 10 mg/day, or bisoprolol 5mg/day) was associated with benefit in a retrospective study [42].

Other Treatment in AR and Systemic Prevention of Endocarditis

In acute severe AR, while the patient is being prepared for surgery, treatment with an intravenous inotropic agent (dopamine and/or dobutamine) may be necessary [1]. Selection of the agent and dosage should be based on arterial pressure. Atrial fibrillation and/or bradyarrhythmia are usually poorly tolerated and should be treated promptly. In this setting, anticoagulant therapy should be initiated. Rhythm disturbances should be prevented, if necessary, by using antiarrhythmic agents. Finally, endocarditis is still a serious concern in patients with AR. In the Euro Heart Survey, the etiology of AR was endocarditis in 7.5% of patients [8]. The risk of endocarditis in patients with AR is considered moderately low [1]. However, this risk increases after AVR with prosthetic replacement or after Bentall surgery. Therefore, prevention of endocarditis, with antibacterials before procedures expected to produce bacteremia, is always recommended in patients with AR [1, 6]. Moreover, a careful dental evaluation and, if necessary, a complete dental treatment should be undertaken before AVR whenever possible.

Evidence-Based Management of AR: Place of Medical Therapy

Early surgery is recommended, especially in patients with acute AR caused by aortic root dissection. Sodium nitroprusside and sometimes inotropic agents (such as dopamine and/or dobutamine) may help to improve the hemodynamic state temporarily before surgery [1]. Symptomatic patients with chronic AR and those with LV dysfunction should undergo AVR rather than medical therapy [1]. However, vasodilators remain the drugs of choice for the relief of symptoms in patients with chronic AR who are considered unsuitable for AVR because of extra-cardiac comorbidity. Short-term vasodilator therapy may also be indicated in symptomatic patients (NYHA functional class III or IV) with severe heart failure or LV dysfunction to improve their hemodynamic status before AVR [1, 20]. Vasodilators can be used in asymptomatic patients with severe AR and normal LVEF (55%) if there is a moderate LV enlargement (end-systolic diameter <50–55mm or <25 mm/m^2 body surface area and LV end-diastolic diameter <70–75mm) [1, 6]. In this indication, nifedipine has been proved effective in delaying the need for AVR [39]. Vasodilators should not be used in asymptomatic patients with only mild to moderate AR, unless the patients are hypertensive [6]. ACE inhibitors are effective and well tolerated in such patients. ACE inhibitors are also recommended in patients with persistent LV dysfunction after AVR [1]. The class I recommendations for vasodilators in chronic AR are presented in Table 1.

In patients with aortic root dilatation >55mm, surgery should be undertaken, irrespective of the degree of AR or LV dysfunction [6]. This threshold may be lower (>50mm) for patients with bicuspid valve or Marfan syndrome, in particular if a valve-sparing surgery is possible or if there is a rapid increase in aortic diameter [6]. ↑- Adrenergic blockade reduces the progression of the aneurysmal dilatation in Marfan syndrome [9] and should be continued after surgery [42].

Table 1. Class I recommendations for vasodilator therapy for chronic aortic regurgitation (AR)

Long-term therapy in patients with severe AR who have symptoms and/or LV dysfunction when surgery is not recommended because of additional cardiac or noncardiac factors
Long-term therapy in asymptomatic patients with severe AR who have LV dilatation but normal systolic function
Long-term therapy in asymptomatic patients with hypertension and any degree of AR
Long-term ACE inhibitor therapy in patients with persistent LV systolic dysfunction after AVR
Short-term therapy to improve the hemodynamic profile of patients with severe heart failure symptoms and severe LV dysfunction before proceeding with AVR

AVR = aortic valve replacement; **LV** = left ventricular.

American College of Cardiology/American Heart Association guidelines (reproduced from Bonow et al.)

FUTURE PROSPECTS

Recent data suggest that primary myocardial fibrosis in AR may result from abnormal strain on myocardial fibroblasts, i.e., the extra strain induces production of extra-cellular matrix rich in non-collagen component [43]. Growing understanding of the molecular transduction pathways underlying the myocardial fibroblast response to AR may lead to new pharmacologic therapies in AR, such as metalloproteinase inhibitors.

CONCLUSION

The role of medical treatment in AR has to be defined against surgery. In acute AR, surgery is the only life-saving treatment and medical treatment may improve the hemodynamic state temporarily before surgery. In patients with AR associated with aortic root disease, ↑-adrenoceptor antagonists may slow the rate of aortic dilatation and delay the need for surgery. Chronic AR associated with any symptom and/or LV dysfunction requires AVR. In these patients, vasodilators should only be considered as a short-term treatment before surgery if there is evidence of severe heart failure or as a long-term treatment if surgery is contra-indicated because of cardiac or noncardiac factors. In asymptomatic patients with severe chronic AR and normal LV function, the goal of vasodilator therapy is to prolong the compensated phase of chronic AR, although proof of their efficacy in delaying AVR is limited. Nifedipine is the best evidence-based treatment in this indication. However, vasodilator therapy should not be used in asymptomatic patients with mild to moderate AR unless the patients are hypertensive. ACE inhibitors are particularly indicated in this setting and in children. ↑-Adrenoceptor antagonists are indicated in patients with persistent LV dysfunction after AVR for AR. New insight into the pathophysiology of AR may lead to new medications, such as metalloproteinase inhibitors.

REFERENCES

[1] Leopold, J. A., Cellular mechanisms of aortic valve calcification, *Circ. Cardiovasc. Interv.* 5 (4) (2012) 605–614 Epub 2012/08/17.

[2] Abdelbaky, A., E. Corsini, A. L. Figueroa, S. Subramanian, S. Fontanez, H. Emami, et al., Early aortic valve inflammation precedes calcification: a longitudinal FDG-PET/CT study, *Atherosclerosis* 238 (2) (2015) 165–172 Epub 2014/12/20.

[3] Mathieu, P., Y. Bosse, G.S. Huggins, A. Della Corte, P. Pibarot, H. I. Michelena, et al., The pathology and pathobiology of bicuspid aortic valve: state of the art and novel research perspectives, *J. Pathol. Clin. Res.* 1 (4) (2015) 195–206 Epub 2016/ 08/09.

[4] Otto, C. M., I. G. Burwash, M. E. Legget, B. I. Munt, M. Fujioka, N. L. Healy, et al., Prospective study of asymptomatic valvular aortic stenosis. Clinical, echocardiographic, and exercise predictors of outcome, *Circulation* 95 (9) (1997) 2262–2270 Epub 1997/05/06.

[5] Freeman, R. V., C. M. Otto, Spectrum of calcific aortic valve disease: pathogenesis, disease progression, and treatment strategies, *Circulation* 111 (24) (2005) 3316–3326 Epub 2005/06/22.

[6] Nkomo, V. T., J. M. Gardin, T. N. Skelton, J. S. Gottdiener, C. G. Scott, M. Enriquez-Sarano, Burden of valvular heart diseases: a population-based study, *Lancet* 368 (9540) (2006) 1005–1011 Epub 2006/09/19.

[7] Eveborn, G. W., H. Schirmer, G. Heggelund, P. Lunde, K. Rasmussen, The evolving epidemiology of valvular aortic stenosis. *The Tromso Study, Heart* 99 (6) (2013) 396–400 Epub 2012/09/04.

[8] Hadar, H., D. Meiraz, Thickenedrenalfascia–asignofretroperitonealpathology, *J. Comput. Tomogr.* 5 (2) (1981) 193–198 Epub 1981/06/01.

[9] Lindman, B. R., M. A. Clavel, P. Mathieu, B. Iung, P. Lancellotti, C. M. Otto, et al., Calcific aortic stenosis, *Nat. Rev. Dis. Primers* 2 (2016) 16006 Epub 2016/05/18.

[10] Tsimikas, S., Lipoprotein(a): novel target and emergence of novel therapies to lower cardiovascular disease risk, *Curr. Opin. Endocrinol. Diabetes Obes.* 23 (2) (2016) 157–164 Epub 2016/01/31.

[11] Hutcheson, J. D., E. Aikawa, W. D. Merryman, Potential drug targets for calcific aortic valve disease, *Nat. Rev. Cardiol.* 11 (4) (2014) 218–231 Epub 2014/01/22.

[12] Smith, J. G., K. Luk, C. A. Schulz, J. C. Engert, R. Do, G. Hindy, et al., Association of low-density lipoprotein cholesterol-related genetic variants with aortic valve cal- cium and incident aortic stenosis, *Jama* 312 (17) (2014) 1764–1771 Epub 2014/10/27.

[13] Parolari, A., E. Tremoli, L. Cavallotti, M. Trezzi, S. Kassem, C. Loardi, et al., Do statins improve outcomes and delay the progression of non-rheumatic calcific aortic stenosis? *Heart* 97 (7) (2011) 523–529 Epub 2011/01/29.

[14] Rajamannan, N. M., M. Subramaniam, F. Caira, S. R. Stock, T. C. Spelsberg, Atorvastatin inhibits hypercholesterolemia-induced calcification in the aortic valves

via the Lrp5 receptor pathway, *Circulation* 112 (Suppl. 9) (2005) I229–34 Epub 2005/09/15.

[15] Novaro, G. M., I. Y. Tiong, G. L. Pearce, M. S. Lauer, D. L. Sprecher, B. P. Griffin, Effect of hydroxymethylglutaryl coenzyme a reductase inhibitors on the progression of calcific aortic stenosis, *Circulation* 104 (18) (2001) 2205–2209 Epub 2001/10/31.

[16] Dichtl, W., H. F. Alber, G. M. Feuchtner, F. Hintringer, M. Reinthaler, T. Bartel, et al., Prognosis and risk factors in patients with asymptomatic aortic stenosis and their modulation by atorvastatin (20 mg), *Am. J. Cardiol.* 102 (6) (2008) 743–748 Epub 2008/09/09.

[17] Rossebo, A. B., T. R. Pedersen, K. Boman, P. Brudi, J. B. Chambers, K. Egstrup, et al., Intensive lipid lowering with simvastatin and ezetimibe in aortic stenosis, *N. Engl. J. Med.* 359 (13) (2008) 1343–1356 Epub 2008/09/04.

[18] Cowell, S. J., D. E. Newby, R. J. Prescott, P. Bloomfield, J. Reid, D. B. Northridge, et al., A randomized trial of intensive lipid-lowering therapy in calcific aortic stenosis, *N. Engl. J. Med.* 352 (23) (2005) 2389–2397 Epub 2005/06/10.

[19] Chan, K. L., K. Teo, J. G. Dumesnil, A. Ni, J. Tam, Effect of Lipid lowering with rosuvastatin on progression of aortic stenosis: results of the aortic stenosis progression observation: measuring effects of rosuvastatin (ASTRONOMER) trial, *Circulation* 121 (2) (2010) 306–314 Epub 2010/01/06.

[20] Gerdts, E., A. B. Rossebo, T. R. Pedersen, K. Boman, P. Brudi, J. B. Chambers, et al., Impact of baseline severity of aortic valve stenosis on effect of intensive lipid lowering therapy (from the SEAS study), *Am. J. Cardiol.* 106 (11) (2010) 1634–1639 Epub 2010/11/26.

[21] Ardehali, R., N. J. Leeper, A. M. Wilson, P. A. Heidenreich, The effect of angiotensin-converting enzyme inhibitors and statins on the progression of aortic sclerosis and mortality, *J. Heart Valve Dis.* 21 (3) (2012) 337–343 Epub 2012/07/20.

[22] Otto, C. M., J. Kuusisto, D. D. Reichenbach, A. M. Gown, K. D. O'Brien, Characterization of the early lesion of' degenerative' valvular aortic stenosis. Histological and immunohistochemical studies, *Circulation* 90 (2) (1994) 844–853 Epub 1994/08/01.

[23] Stewart, B. F., D. Siscovick, B. K. Lind, J. M. Gardin, J. S. Gottdiener, V. E. Smith, et al., Clinical factors associated with calcific aortic valve disease. Cardiovascular Health Study, *J. Am. Coll. Cardiol.* 29 (3) (1997) 630–634 Epub 1997/03/01.

[24] Parolari, A., C. Loardi, L. Mussoni, L. Cavallotti, M. Camera, P. Biglioli, et al., Nonrheumatic calcific aortic stenosis: an overview from basic science to pharmacological prevention, *Eur. J. Cardiothorac. Surg.* 35 (3) (2009) 493–504 Epub 2009/01/24.

[25] Novaro, G. M., B. P. Griffin, Calcific aortic stenosis: another face of atherosclerosis? *Cleve. Clin. J. Med.* 70 (5) (2003) 471–477 Epub 2003/06/05.

[26] Otto, C. M., K. D. O'Brien, Why is there discordance between calcific aortic stenosis and coronary artery disease? *Heart* 85 (6) (2001) 601–602 Epub 2001/05/23.

[27] Nsaibia, M. J., M. C. Boulanger, R. Bouchareb, G. Mkannez, K. Le Quang, F. Hadji, et al., OxLDL-derived lysophosphatidic acid promotes the progression of aortic valve stenosis through a LPAR1-RhoA-NF-kappaB pathway, *Cardiovasc. Res.* 113 (11) (2017) 1351–1363 Epub 2017/05/05.

[28] Leopold, J. A., Cellular mechanisms of aortic valve calcification, *Circ. Cardiovasc. Interv.* 5 (4) (2012) 605–614 Epub 2012/08/17.

[29] Abdelbaky, A., E. Corsini, A. L. Figueroa, S. Subramanian, S. Fontanez, H. Emami, et al., Early aortic valve inflammation precedes calcification: a longitudinal FDG-PET/CT study, *Atherosclerosis* 238 (2) (2015) 165–172 Epub 2014/12/20.

[30] Mathieu, P., Y. Bosse, G. S. Huggins, A. Della Corte, P. Pibarot, H. I. Michelena, et al., The pathology and pathobiology of bicuspid aortic valve: state of the art and novel research perspectives, *J. Pathol. Clin. Res.* 1 (4) (2015) 195–206 Epub 2016/ 08/09.

[31] Otto, C. M., I. G. Burwash, M. E. Legget, B. I. Munt, M. Fujioka, N. L. Healy, et al., Prospective study of asymptomatic valvular aortic stenosis. Clinical, echocardiographic, and exercise predictors of outcome, *Circulation* 95 (9) (1997) 2262–2270 Epub 1997/05/06.

[32] Freeman, R. V., C. M. Otto, Spectrum of calcific aortic valve disease: pathogenesis, disease progression, and treatment strategies, *Circulation* 111 (24) (2005) 3316–3326 Epub 2005/06/22.

[33] Nkomo, V. T., J. M. Gardin, T. N. Skelton, J. S. Gottdiener, C. G. Scott, M. Enriquez-Sarano, Burden of valvular heart diseases: a population-based study, *Lancet* 368 (9540) (2006) 1005–1011 Epub 2006/09/19.

[34] Eveborn, G. W., H. Schirmer, G. Heggelund, P. Lunde, K. Rasmussen, The evolving epidemiology of valvular aortic stenosis. *The Tromso Study, Heart* 99 (6) (2013) 396–400 Epub 2012/09/04.

[35] Hadar, H., D. Meiraz, Thickenedrenalfascia–asignofretroperitonealpathology, *J. Comput. Tomogr.* 5 (2) (1981) 193–198 Epub 1981/06/01.

[36] Lindman, B. R., M. A. Clavel, P. Mathieu, B. Iung, P. Lancellotti, C. M. Otto, et al., Calcific aortic stenosis, *Nat. Rev. Dis. Primers* 2 (2016) 16006 Epub 2016/05/18.

[37] Tsimikas, S., Lipoprotein(a): novel target and emergence of novel therapies to lower cardiovascular disease risk, *Curr. Opin. Endocrinol. Diabetes Obes.* 23 (2) (2016) 157–164 Epub 2016/01/31.

[38] Hutcheson, J. D., E. Aikawa, W. D. Merryman, Potential drug targets for calcific aortic valve disease, *Nat. Rev. Cardiol.* 11 (4) (2014) 218–231 Epub 2014/01/22.

[39] Smith, J. G., K. Luk, C. A. Schulz, J. C. Engert, R. Do, G. Hindy, et al., Association of low-density lipoprotein cholesterol-related genetic variants with aortic valve cal- cium and incident aortic stenosis, *Jama* 312 (17) (2014) 1764–1771 Epub 2014/10/27.

[40] Parolari, A., E. Tremoli, L. Cavallotti, M. Trezzi, S. Kassem, C. Loardi, et al., Do statins improve outcomes and delay the progression of non-rheumatic calcific aortic stenosis? *Heart* 97 (7) (2011) 523–529 Epub 2011/01/29.

[41] Rajamannan, N. M., M. Subramaniam, F. Caira, S. R. Stock, T. C. Spelsberg, Atorvastatin inhibits hypercholesterolemia-induced calcification in the aortic valves via the Lrp5 receptor pathway, *Circulation* 112 (Suppl. 9) (2005) I229–34 Epub 2005/09/15.

[42] Novaro, G. M., I. Y. Tiong, G. L. Pearce, M. S. Lauer, D. L. Sprecher, B. P. Griffin, Effect of hydroxymethylglutaryl coenzyme a reductase inhibitors on the progression of calcific aortic stenosis, *Circulation* 104 (18) (2001) 2205–2209 Epub 2001/10/31.

[43] Dichtl, W., H. F. Alber, G. M. Feuchtner, F. Hintringer, M. Reinthaler, T. Bartel, et al., Prognosis and risk factors in patients with asymptomatic aortic stenosis and their

modulation by atorvastatin (20 mg), *Am. J. Cardiol.* 102 (6) (2008) 743–748 Epub 2008/09/09.

[44] Rossebo, A. B., T. R. Pedersen, K. Boman, P. Brudi, J. B. Chambers, K. Egstrup, et al., Intensive lipid lowering with simvastatin and ezetimibe in aortic stenosis, *N. Engl. J. Med.* 359 (13) (2008) 1343–1356 Epub 2008/09/04.

[45] Cowell, S. J., D. E. Newby, R. J. Prescott, P. Bloomfield, J. Reid, D. B. Northridge, et al., A randomized trial of intensive lipid-lowering therapy in calcific aortic stenosis, *N. Engl. J. Med.* 352 (23) (2005) 2389–2397 Epub 2005/06/10.

[46] Chan, K. L., K. Teo, J. G. Dumesnil, A. Ni, J. Tam, Effect of Lipid lowering with rosuvastatin on progression of aortic stenosis: results of the aortic stenosis progression observation: measuring effects of rosuvastatin (ASTRONOMER) trial, *Circulation* 121 (2) (2010) 306–314 Epub 2010/01/06.

[47] Gerdts, E., A. B. Rossebo, T. R. Pedersen, K. Boman, P. Brudi, J. B. Chambers, et al., Impact of baseline severity of aortic valve stenosis on effect of intensive lipid lowering therapy (from the SEAS study), *Am. J. Cardiol.* 106 (11) (2010) 1634–1639 Epub 2010/11/26.

[48] Ardehali, R., N. J. Leeper, A. M. Wilson, P. A. Heidenreich, The effect of angiotensin-converting enzyme inhibitors and statins on the progression of aortic sclerosis and mortality, *J. Heart Valve Dis.* 21 (3) (2012) 337–343 Epub 2012/07/20.

[49] Otto, C. M., J. Kuusisto, D. D. Reichenbach, A. M. Gown, K. D. O'Brien, Characterization of the early lesion of' degenerative' valvular aortic stenosis. Histological and immunohistochemical studies, *Circulation* 90 (2) (1994) 844–853 Epub 1994/08/01.

[50] Stewart, B. F., D. Siscovick, B. K. Lind, J. M. Gardin, J. S. Gottdiener, V. E. Smith, et al., Clinical factors associated with calcific aortic valve disease. Cardiovascular Health Study, *J. Am. Coll. Cardiol.* 29 (3) (1997) 630–634 Epub 1997/03/01.

[51] Parolari, A., C. Loardi, L. Mussoni, L. Cavallotti, M. Camera, P. Biglioli, et al., Nonrheumatic calcific aortic stenosis: an overview from basic science to pharmacological prevention, *Eur. J. Cardiothorac. Surg.* 35 (3) (2009) 493–504 Epub 2009/01/24.

[52] Novaro, G. M., B. P. Griffin, Calcific aortic stenosis: another face of atherosclerosis? *Cleve. Clin. J. Med.* 70 (5) (2003) 471–477 Epub 2003/06/05.

[53] Otto, C. M., K. D. O'Brien, Why is there discordance between calcific aortic stenosis and coronary artery disease? *Heart* 85 (6) (2001) 601–602 Epub 2001/05/23.

[54] Nsaibia, M. J., M. C. Boulanger, R. Bouchareb, G. Mkannez, K. Le Quang, F. Hadji, et al., OxLDL-derived lysophosphatidic acid promotes the progression of aortic valve stenosis through a LPAR1-RhoA-NF-kappaB pathway, *Cardiovasc. Res.* 113 (11) (2017) 1351–1363 Epub 2017/05/05.

[55] Leopold, J. A., Cellular mechanisms of aortic valve calcification, *Circ. Cardiovasc. Interv.* 5 (4) (2012) 605–614 Epub 2012/08/17.

[56] Abdelbaky, A., E. Corsini, A. L. Figueroa, S. Subramanian, S. Fontanez, H. Emami, et al., Early aortic valve inflammation precedes calcification: a longitudinal FDG-PET/CT study, *Atherosclerosis* 238 (2) (2015) 165–172 Epub 2014/12/20.

[57] Mathieu, P., Y. Bosse, G. S. Huggins, A. Della Corte, P. Pibarot, H. I. Michelena, et al., The pathology and pathobiology of bicuspid aortic valve: state of the art and novel research perspectives, *J. Pathol. Clin. Res.* 1 (4) (2015) 195–206 Epub 2016/ 08/09.

[58] Otto, C. M., I. G. Burwash, M. E. Legget, B. I. Munt, M. Fujioka, N. L. Healy, et al., Prospective study of asymptomatic valvular aortic stenosis. Clinical, echocardiographic, and exercise predictors of outcome, *Circulation* 95 (9) (1997) 2262–2270 Epub 1997/05/06.

[59] Freeman, R. V., C. M. Otto, Spectrum of calcific aortic valve disease: pathogenesis, disease progression, and treatment strategies, *Circulation* 111 (24) (2005) 3316–3326 Epub 2005/06/22.

[60] Nkomo, V. T., J. M. Gardin, T.N. Skelton, J. S. Gottdiener, C. G. Scott, M. Enriquez-Sarano, Burden of valvular heart diseases: a population-based study, *Lancet* 368 (9540) (2006) 1005–1011 Epub 2006/09/19.

[61] Eveborn, G. W., H. Schirmer, G. Heggelund, P. Lunde, K. Rasmussen, The evolving epidemiology of valvular aortic stenosis. *The Tromso Study, Heart* 99 (6) (2013) 396–400 Epub 2012/09/04.

[62] Hadar, H., D. Meiraz, Thickened renal fascia–asignofretroperitonealpathology, *J. Comput. Tomogr.* 5 (2) (1981) 193–198 Epub 1981/06/01.

[63] Lindman, B. R., M. A. Clavel, P. Mathieu, B. Iung, P. Lancellotti, C. M. Otto, et al., Calcific aortic stenosis, *Nat. Rev. Dis. Primers* 2 (2016) 16006 Epub 2016/05/18.

[64] Tsimikas, S., Lipoprotein(a): novel target and emergence of novel therapies to lower cardiovascular disease risk, *Curr. Opin. Endocrinol. Diabetes Obes.* 23 (2) (2016) 157–164 Epub 2016/01/31.

[65] Hutcheson, J. D., E. Aikawa, W. D. Merryman, Potential drug targets for calcific aortic valve disease, *Nat. Rev. Cardiol.* 11 (4) (2014) 218–231 Epub 2014/01/22.

[66] Smith, J. G., K. Luk, C. A. Schulz, J. C. Engert, R. Do, G. Hindy, et al., Association of low-density lipoprotein cholesterol-related genetic variants with aortic valve cal- cium and incident aortic stenosis, *Jama* 312 (17) (2014) 1764–1771 Epub 2014/10/27.

[67] Parolari, A., E. Tremoli, L. Cavallotti, M. Trezzi, S. Kassem, C. Loardi, et al., Do statins improve outcomes and delay the progression of non-rheumatic calcific aortic stenosis? *Heart* 97 (7) (2011) 523–529 Epub 2011/01/29.

[68] Rajamannan, N. M., M. Subramaniam, F. Caira, S. R. Stock, T. C. Spelsberg, Atorvastatin inhibits hypercholesterolemia-induced calcification in the aortic valves via the Lrp5 receptor pathway, *Circulation* 112 (Suppl. 9) (2005) I229–34 Epub 2005/09/15.

[69] Novaro, G. M., I. Y. Tiong, G. L. Pearce, M. S. Lauer, D. L. Sprecher, B. P. Griffin, Effect of hydroxymethylglutaryl coenzyme a reductase inhibitors on the progression of calcific aortic stenosis, *Circulation* 104 (18) (2001) 2205–2209 Epub 2001/10/31.

[70] Dichtl, W., H. F. Alber, G. M. Feuchtner, F. Hintringer, M. Reinthaler, T. Bartel, et al., Prognosis and risk factors in patients with asymptomatic aortic stenosis and their modulation by atorvastatin (20 mg), *Am. J. Cardiol.* 102 (6) (2008) 743–748 Epub 2008/09/09.

[71] Rossebo, A. B., T. R. Pedersen, K. Boman, P. Brudi, J. B. Chambers, K. Egstrup, et al., Intensive lipid lowering with simvastatin and ezetimibe in aortic stenosis, *N. Engl. J. Med.* 359 (13) (2008) 1343–1356 Epub 2008/09/04.

[72] Cowell, S. J., D. E. Newby, R. J. Prescott, P. Bloomfield, J. Reid, D. B. Northridge, et al., A randomized trial of intensive lipid-lowering therapy in calcific aortic stenosis, *N. Engl. J. Med.* 352 (23) (2005) 2389–2397 Epub 2005/06/10.

[73] Chan, K. L., K. Teo, J. G. Dumesnil, A. Ni, J. Tam, Effect of Lipid lowering with rosuvastatin on progression of aortic stenosis: results of the aortic stenosis progression observation: measuring effects of rosuvastatin (ASTRONOMER) trial, *Circulation* 121 (2) (2010) 306–314 Epub 2010/01/06.

[74] Gerdts, E., A. B. Rossebo, T. R. Pedersen, K. Boman, P. Brudi, J. B. Chambers, et al., Impact of baseline severity of aortic valve stenosis on effect of intensive lipid lowering therapy (from the SEAS study), *Am. J. Cardiol.* 106 (11) (2010) 1634–1639 Epub 2010/11/26.

[75] Ardehali, R., N. J. Leeper, A. M. Wilson, P. A. Heidenreich, The effect of angiotensin-converting enzyme inhibitors and statins on the progression of aortic sclerosis and mortality, *J. Heart Valve Dis.* 21 (3) (2012) 337–343 Epub 2012/07/20.

[76] Otto, C. M., J. Kuusisto, D. D. Reichenbach, A. M. Gown, K. D. O'Brien, Characterization of the early lesion of' degenerative' valvular aortic stenosis. Histological and immunohistochemical studies, *Circulation* 90 (2) (1994) 844–853 Epub 1994/08/01.

[77] Stewart, B. F., D. Siscovick, B. K. Lind, J. M. Gardin, J. S. Gottdiener, V. E. Smith, et al., Clinical factors associated with calcific aortic valve disease. Cardiovascular Health Study, *J. Am. Coll. Cardiol*. 29 (3) (1997) 630–634 Epub 1997/03/01.

[78] Parolari, A., C. Loardi, L. Mussoni, L. Cavallotti, M. Camera, P. Biglioli, et al., Nonrheumatic calcific aortic stenosis: an overview from basic science to pharmacological prevention, *Eur. J. Cardiothorac. Surg.* 35 (3) (2009) 493–504 Epub 2009/01/24.

[79] Novaro, G. M., B. P. Griffin, Calcific aortic stenosis: another face of atherosclerosis? *Cleve. Clin. J. Med.* 70 (5) (2003) 471–477 Epub 2003/06/05.

[80] Otto, C. M., K. D. O'Brien, Why is there discordance between calcific aortic stenosis and coronary artery disease? *Heart* 85 (6) (2001) 601–602 Epub 2001/05/23.

[81] Nsaibia, M. J., M. C. Boulanger, R. Bouchareb, G. Mkannez, K. Le Quang, F. Hadji, et al., OxLDL-derived lysophosphatidic acid promotes the progression of aortic valve stenosis through a LPAR1-RhoA-NF-kappaB pathway, *Cardiovasc. Res.* 113 (11) (2017) 1351–1363 Epub 2017/05/05.

[82] Leopold, J. A., Cellular mechanisms of aortic valve calcification, *Circ. Cardiovasc. Interv.* 5 (4) (2012) 605–614 Epub 2012/08/17.

[83] Abdelbaky, A., E. Corsini, A. L. Figueroa, S. Subramanian, S. Fontanez, H. Emami, et al., Early aortic valve inflammation precedes calcification: a longitudinal FDG-PET/CT study, *Atherosclerosis* 238 (2) (2015) 165–172 Epub 2014/12/20.

[84] Mathieu, P., Y. Bosse, G. S. Huggins, A. Della Corte, P. Pibarot, H. I. Michelena, et al., The pathology and pathobiology of bicuspid aortic valve: state of the art and novel research perspectives, *J. Pathol. Clin. Res.* 1 (4) (2015) 195–206 Epub 2016/ 08/09.

[85] Otto, C. M., I. G. Burwash, M. E. Legget, B. I. Munt, M. Fujioka, N. L. Healy, et al., Prospective study of asymptomatic valvular aortic stenosis. Clinical, echocardiographic, and exercise predictors of outcome, *Circulation* 95 (9) (1997) 2262–2270 Epub 1997/05/06.

[86] Freeman, R. V., C. M. Otto, Spectrum of calcific aortic valve disease: pathogenesis, disease progression, and treatment strategies, *Circulation* 111 (24) (2005) 3316–3326 Epub 2005/06/22.

[87] Nkomo, V. T., J. M. Gardin, T. N. Skelton, J. S. Gottdiener, C .G. Scott, M. Enriquez-Sarano, Burden of valvular heart diseases: a population-based study, *Lancet* 368 (9540) (2006) 1005–1011 Epub 2006/09/19.

[88] Eveborn, G. W., H. Schirmer, G. Heggelund, P. Lunde, K. Rasmussen, The evolving epidemiology of valvular aortic stenosis. *The Tromso Study, Heart* 99 (6) (2013) 396–400 Epub 2012/09/04.

[89] Hadar, H., D. Meiraz, Thickenedr enalfascia–asignofretroperitonealpathology, *J. Comput. Tomogr.* 5 (2) (1981) 193–198 Epub 1981/06/01.

[90] Lindman, B. R., M. A. Clavel, P. Mathieu, B. Iung, P. Lancellotti, C. M. Otto, et al., Calcific aortic stenosis, *Nat. Rev. Dis. Primers* 2 (2016) 16006 Epub 2016/05/18.

[91] Tsimikas, S., Lipoprotein(a): novel target and emergence of novel therapies to lower cardiovascular disease risk, *Curr. Opin. Endocrinol. Diabetes Obes.* 23 (2) (2016) 157–164 Epub 2016/01/31.

[92] Hutcheso, J. D., E. Aikawa, W. D. Merryman, Potential drug targets for calcific aortic valve disease, *Nat. Rev. Cardiol.* 11 (4) (2014) 218–231 Epub 2014/01/22.

[93] Smith, J. G., K. Luk, C. A. Schulz, J. C. Engert, R. Do, G. Hindy, et al., Association of low-density lipoprotein cholesterol-related genetic variants with aortic valve cal- cium and incident aortic stenosis, *Jama* 312 (17) (2014) 1764–1771 Epub 2014/10/27.

[94] Parolari, A., E. Tremoli, L. Cavallotti, M. Trezzi, S. Kassem, C. Loardi, et al., Do statins improve outcomes and delay the progression of non-rheumatic calcific aortic stenosis? *Heart* 97 (7) (2011) 523–529 Epub 2011/01/29.

[95] Rajamannan, N. M., M. Subramaniam, F. Caira, S. R. Stock, T. C. Spelsberg, Atorvastatin inhibits hypercholesterolemia-induced calcification in the aortic valves via the Lrp5 receptor pathway, *Circulation* 112 (Suppl. 9) (2005) I229–34 Epub 2005/09/15.

[96] Novaro, G. M., I. Y. Tiong, G. L. Pearce, M. S. Lauer, D. L. Sprecher, B. P. Griffin, Effect of hydroxymethylglutaryl coenzyme a reductase inhibitors on the progression of calcific aortic stenosis, *Circulation* 104 (18) (2001) 2205–2209 Epub 2001/10/31.

[97] Dichtl, W., H. F. Alber, G. M. Feuchtner, F. Hintringer, M. Reinthaler, T. Bartel, et al., Prognosis and risk factors in patients with asymptomatic aortic stenosis and their modulation by atorvastatin (20 mg), *Am. J. Cardiol.* 102 (6) (2008) 743–748 Epub 2008/09/09.

[98] Rossebo, A. B., T. R. Pedersen, K. Boman, P. Brudi, J. B. Chambers, K. Egstrup, et al., Intensive lipid lowering with simvastatin and ezetimibe in aortic stenosis, *N. Engl. J. Med.* 359 (13) (2008) 1343–1356 Epub 2008/09/04.

[99] Cowell, S. J., D. E. Newby, R. J. Prescott, P. Bloomfield, J. Reid, D. B. Northridge, et al., A randomized trial of intensive lipid-lowering therapy in calcific aortic stenosis, *N. Engl. J. Med.* 352 (23) (2005) 2389–2397 Epub 2005/06/10.

[100] Chan, K. L., K. Teo, J. G. Dumesnil, A. Ni, J. Tam, Effect of Lipid lowering with rosuvastatin on progression of aortic stenosis: results of the aortic stenosis progression observation: measuring effects of rosuvastatin (ASTRONOMER) trial, *Circulation* 121 (2) (2010) 306–314 Epub 2010/01/06.

[101] Gerdts, E., A. B. Rossebo, T. R. Pedersen, K. Boman, P. Brudi, J. B. Chambers, et al., Impact of baseline severity of aortic valve stenosis on effect of intensive lipid lowering therapy (from the SEAS study), *Am. J. Cardiol.* 106 (11) (2010) 1634–1639 Epub 2010/11/26.

[102] Ardehali, R., N. J. Leeper, A. M. Wilson, P. A. Heidenreich, The effect of angiotensin-converting enzyme inhibitors and statins on the progression of aortic sclerosis and mortality, *J. Heart Valve Dis.* 21 (3) (2012) 337–343 Epub 2012/07/20.

[103] Otto, C. M., J. Kuusisto, D. D. Reichenbach, A. M. Gown, K. D. O'Brien, Characterization of the early lesion of' degenerative' valvular aortic stenosis. Histological and immunohistochemical studies, *Circulation* 90 (2) (1994) 844–853 Epub 1994/08/01.

[104] Stewart, B. F., D. Siscovick, B. K. Lind, J. M. Gardin, J. S. Gottdiener, V. E. Smith, et al., Clinical factors associated with calcific aortic valve disease. Cardiovascular Health Study, *J. Am. Coll. Cardiol.* 29 (3) (1997) 630–634 Epub 1997/03/01.

[105] Parolari, A., C. Loardi, L. Mussoni, L. Cavallotti, M. Camera, P. Biglioli, et al., Nonrheumatic calcific aortic stenosis: an overview from basic science to pharmacological prevention, *Eur. J. Cardiothorac. Surg.* 35 (3) (2009) 493–504 Epub 2009/01/24.

[106] Novaro, G. M., B. P. Griffin, Calcific aortic stenosis: another face of atherosclerosis? *Cleve. Clin. J. Med.* 70 (5) (2003) 471–477 Epub 2003/06/05.

[107] Otto, C. M., K. D. O'Brien, Why is there discordance between calcific aortic stenosis and coronary artery disease? *Heart* 85 (6) (2001) 601–602 Epub 2001/05/23.

[108] Nsaibia, M. J., M. C. Boulanger, R. Bouchareb, G. Mkannez, K. Le Quang, F. Hadji, et al., OxLDL-derived lysophosphatidic acid promotes the progression of aortic valve stenosis through a LPAR1-RhoA-NF-kappaB pathway, *Cardiovasc. Res.* 113 (11) (2017) 1351–1363 Epub 2017/05/05.

[109] Leopold, J. A., Cellular mechanisms of aortic valve calcification, *Circ. Cardiovasc. Interv.* 5 (4) (2012) 605–614 Epub 2012/08/17.

[110] Abdelbaky, A., E. Corsini, A. L. Figueroa, S. Subramanian, S. Fontanez, H. Emami, et al., Early aortic valve inflammation precedes calcification: a longitudinal FDG-PET/CT study, *Atherosclerosis* 238 (2) (2015) 165–172 Epub 2014/12/20.

[111] Mathieu, P., Y. Bosse, G. S. Huggins, A. Della Corte, P. Pibarot, H. I. Michelena, et al., The pathology and pathobiology of bicuspid aortic valve: state of the art and novel research perspectives, *J. Pathol. Clin. Res.* 1 (4) (2015) 195–206 Epub 2016/ 08/09.

[112] Otto, C. M., I. G. Burwash, M. E. Legget, B. I. Munt, M. Fujioka, N. L. Healy, et al., Prospective study of asymptomatic valvular aortic stenosis. Clinical, echocardiographic, and exercise predictors of outcome, *Circulation* 95 (9) (1997) 2262–2270 Epub 1997/05/06.

[113] Freeman, R. V., C. M. Otto, Spectrum of calcific aortic valve disease: pathogenesis, disease progression, and treatment strategies, *Circulation* 111 (24) (2005) 3316–3326 Epub 2005/06/22.

[114] Nkomo, V. T., J. M. Gardin, T. N. Skelton, J. S. Gottdiener, C. G. Scott, M. Enriquez-Sarano, Burden of valvular heart diseases: a population-based study, *Lancet* 368 (9540) (2006) 1005–1011 Epub 2006/09/19.

[115] Eveborn, G. W., H. Schirmer, G. Heggelund, P. Lunde, K. Rasmussen, The evolving epidemiology of valvular aortic stenosis. *The Tromso Study, Heart* 99 (6) (2013) 396–400 Epub 2012/09/04.

[116] Hadar, H., D. Meiraz, Thickened renalfascia–asignofretroperitonealpathology, *J. Comput. Tomogr.* 5 (2) (1981) 193–198 Epub 1981/06/01.

[117] Lindman, B. R., M. A. Clavel, P. Mathieu, B. Iung, P. Lancellotti, C. M. Otto, et al., Calcific aortic stenosis, *Nat. Rev. Dis. Primers* 2 (2016) 16006 Epub 2016/05/18.

In: Perspectives in Aortic Valve Disease
Editor: Giovanni Concistrè
ISBN: 978-1-53618-769-4

Chapter 13

SURGICAL TREATMENT OF AORTIC VALVE DISEASE: INDICATIONS, RISK STRATIFICATION AND OUTCOMES

Rafik Margaryan**, MD, PhD
Ospedale del Cuore "G. Pasquinucci,"
Fondazione Toscana Gabriele Monasterio, Massa, Italy

ABSTRACT

Aortic stenosis (AS) is the most common valve disease requiring surgical intervention in high income countries [1]. Calcification of the aortic cusps is the most common cause of aortic stenosis [1]. Valve replacement is the only durable treatment for this lesion and, unlike aortic insufficiency, which can be managed by means of valve repair in selected patients(see chapter 19, 20), aortic stenosis resulting from calcification of the cusps almost always requires valve replacement, and in recent years also sutureless trans-cathter valve implantation. A comprehensive review of transcatheter aortic valve implantation is well coverd [2], and this technique will be reviewed and discussed deeply in chapter 21. In this chapter we will mainly focus on aortic valve replacement (aortic valve repair will be discussed in chapters 19 and 20).

Interes in severe aortic stenosis treatment still remainsof many researchers and clinicians (see Figure 2). Since the replacement of aortic valve is only known treatment, nowadays different approaches are applied to it: surgical (radical, real replacement) and catheter bases techniques(implantation, not replacement). However when to do it is important. For a note there is a recent randomized trial [3] who has addressed that question beautifully.

Keywords: aortic stenosis, surgical aortic valve replacement, transfemoral aortic valve implantation, outcomes

* Corresponding Author's Email: margaryan@ftgm.it.

INTRODUCTION

In 1947, Smithy and Parker at the University of South Carolina in Charleston first reported an experimental study of aortic valvotomy [4]. During the early 1950s, Bailey and coauthors in Philadelphia used closed methods either a dilator introduced transventricularly or a digital approach through a 'poncho' sewn onto the ascending aorta in clinical attempts to relieve severe aortic stenosis [5, 6]. Success in some patients was obtained by them and by Ellis and Kirklin. [7] In 1951 developed a ball valve prosthesis for rapid insertion into the descending thoracic aorta [8].

An effective approach to surgical treatment of aortic valve disease in adults began with the advent of clinical cardiopulmonary bypass in 1954 and 1955. At first, aortic valvotomy and removal of calcific deposits were all that could be acchieved [9, 10]. Then Bahnson and colleagues and, independently, Hufnagel and Conrad developed a single-leaflet prosthesis that was commercialized [11, 12]. Generally, the leaflets were used to partially replace the aortic valve, but three leaflets could be used together for total aortic valve replacement. Probably the first single-unit prosthesis for total aortic valve replacement was the polytetrafluroethylene (PTFE) sleeve prosthesis developed and first used by McGoon at the Mayo Clinic in 1961. Introduction of the ball valve prosthesis by Harken and colleagues and Starr and colleagues in 1960 and reported in 1963 established aortic valve surgery on a firm basis [13, 14]. Many types of prosthetic valves have subsequently developed. In 1956, Murray demonstrated that the aortic valve could be used as an allograft valve transplant in the descending thoracic aorta in patients with aortic regurgitation, [15] and Kerwin and colleagues reported 6-year follow-up [16]. The first orthotopic insertions of an allograft valve using the double-suture-line technique were performed in 1962 by Barratt-Boyes and separately by Ross using a single-sutureline technique described by Duran and Gunning [17, 18]. In 1967, Ross and colleagues introduced the pulmonary autograft for aortic valve replacement [19]. In 1965, Binet and colleagues in Paris implanted porcine xenograft aortic valves, sterilized and preserved in a special formaldehyde solution, directly into the aortic root [20]. Stent-mounted bioprostheses are manufactured to provide a standard device that is easily implanted and provides reproducible results in the aortic position. Glutaraldehyde preserved stent-mounted porcine valves were introduced by Carpentier and colleagues in Paris in 1967 [21]. David and colleagues revived the concept of direct insertion of nonstented porcine xenografts into the aortic root [22]. This valve was manufactured on a limited trial basis by Hancock Laboratory and by St. Jude Medical as the Toronto SPV (stentless porcine valve). In April 2002, Professor Alan Cribier at the University of Rouen, France, performed the first percutaneous aortic valve implantation for aortic stenosis in a 62-year-old man who was not a candidate for surgery [23]. Cribier used the antegrade transseptal approach through the femoral vein. Frirst transapical approach was used by Lange et al. [24] in 2007 with successful implantation of suturles Corevalve (Medtronic Inc). First suturless aortic valve Shrestha et al. [25] have describe first implantation of Perceval suturless valve implatation in human. All the timeline related to surgical treatment of aortic valve is designed in Figure 1.

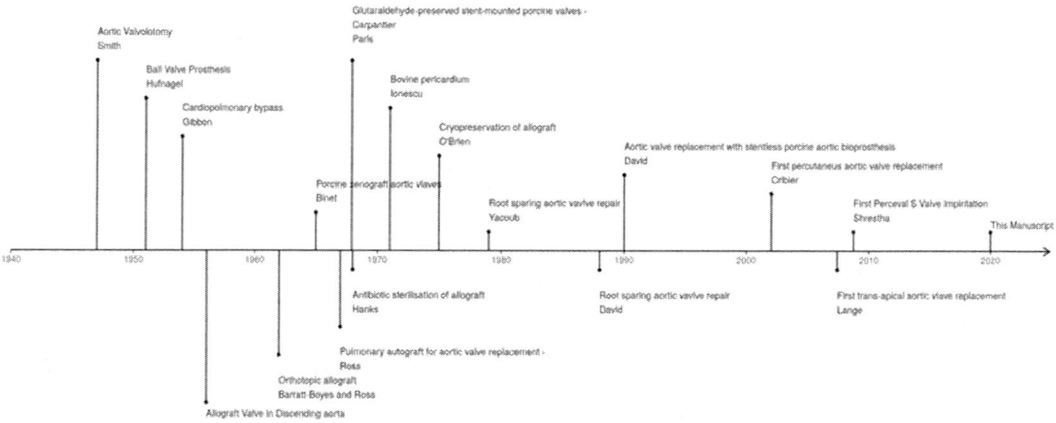

Figure 1. Timeline related to Aortic Valve Procedures.

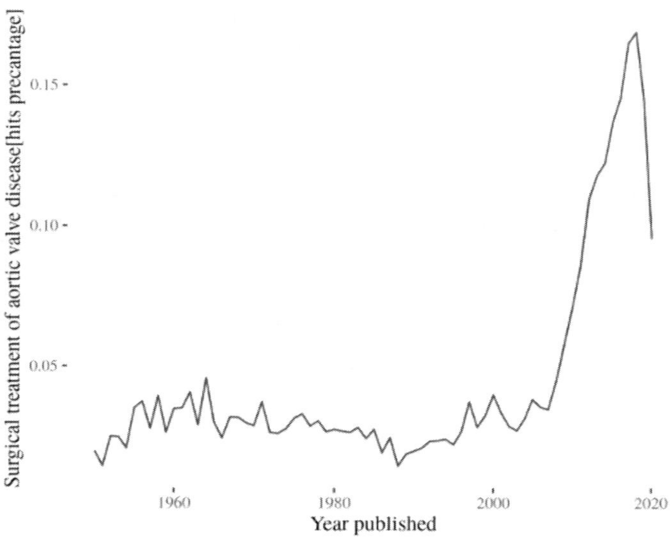

Figure 2. Hits percentage of 'Surgical Treatment of Aortic Valve Disease' term in European PUBMED.

INDICATIONS

Early therapy should be strongly recommended in all symptomatic patients with severe aortic stenosis because of their bad prognosis [26, 27]. Watchfull waiting for asyntomatic patients seem to harm more the one has expected, early surgical aortic valve replacement resulted in a significantly lower risk of operative mortality or death from cardiovascular causes during the follow-up period than conservative care among asymptomatic patients with very severe aortic stenosis [3]. Patients with severe comorbidities indicating a survival of < 1 year and patients in whom severe comorbidities or their general condition at an advanced age make it unlikely that the intervention will improve quality of life or survival [27]. In all other patients surgery should be recommended in particular circumstances, such as impaired left ventricular function, abnormal exercise test, or the presence of left ventricular hypertrophy in the absence of systemic hypertension [26, 27]. Aortic valve surgery is recommended in asymptomatic patients with aortic insufficiency and left ventricular ejection fraction ≤50%, and in patients with normal systolic function, but an enlarged left ventricle (end-diastolic diameter ≥35 mm/m2, end-systolic diameter ≥25 mm/m2 [26, 27]). Patients with ascending aortic aneurysm and aortic insufficiency should undergo surgery when the diameter of the aorta is ≥55 mm, and at an earlier stage when associated with particular conditions, such as BAV or genetic aneurysms. Patients with low-flow, low-gradient aortic stenosis and reduced ejection fraction in whom the depressed ejection fraction is predominantly caused by excessive afterload, LV function usually improves after intervention [28, 29]. Intervention is definitely advised when severe aortic stenosis is confirmed at increasing flow, 10 while patients who are classified as having pseudosevere aortic stenosis at increasing flow should receive conventional treatment for heart failure [28, 30]. Although the outcome of patients without flow reserve is compromised by a higher operative mortality, SAVR (as well as TAVI) has also been shown to improve ejection fraction and clinical status in such patients [31, 32]. Patients with low-flow, low-gradient aortic stenosis and preserved ejection fraction are the most challenging subgroup. Data on their natural history and outcome after surgical or catheter intervention remain controversial [33–35]. In concomitatn aneruismatic dilatation of thoracic aorta surgery is recommended when the aortic root reaches 45 mm as measured by CT scanning or MRI in patients with Loeys–Dietz syndrome, at a diameter of 50 mm in patients with Marfan syndrome or familial aneurysms, or at a smaller diameter in patients with a family history of aortic dissection [26, 27]. There are no specific guidelines for choosing thype of prosthesis. However, in our istitution there is patient/case based method and generally meccanical valve is recommended for patients ≤ 60 years old, above that boundery the biological vavlves are preffered. Stutureless vlaves, sience these are fairly new to our practice is preffered ≥ 75 years old [36].

RISK STRATIFICATION

Risk stratification applies to any sort of intervention and is required for weighing the risk of intervention against the expected natural history of aortic valve desease as a basis for decision making. Most experience relates to surgery and TAVI. The EuroSCORE I (http://www.euroscore.org/calc.html) overestimates operative mortality and its calibration of risk is poor and it is was mainly build for conventional surgery. Consequently, it should no longer be used to guide decision making not for conventiona nor for minimally invasive surgery. The EuroSCORE II and the Society of Thoracic Surgeons (STS) score (http://riskcalc.sts.org/stswebriskcalc/#/) more accurately discriminate high- and low-risk surgical patients and show better calibration to predict postoperative outcome after valvular surgery in conventional [37, 38] and minimally invasive surgery [39]. Scores have major limitations for practical use by insufficiently considering disease severity and not including major risk factors such as frailty, porcelain aorta, chest radiation etc. While EuroSCORE I markedly overestimates 30-day mortality and should therefore be replaced by the better performing EuroSCORE II in this regard as it has been used in many TAVI studies/registries and may still be useful to identify the subgroups of patients for decision between intervention modalities and to predict 1-year mortality. However, it seems that there is necessity to update some scores (EuroSCORE II) as STS is updated continously. A very simple score (age, creatinine and ejection fractio, ACEF [40]) and its subsequent update offer very simple but practically very useful scoring system. We have evaluated its' performance in MICS with sodisfying results for its simplicity. Both scores have shown variable results in predicting the outcomes of intervention in TAVI but are useful for identifying low-risk patients for surgery. New scores have been developed to estimate the risk of 30-day mortality in patients undergoing TAVI, with better accuracy and discrimination, albeit with numerous limitations [41, 42]. Experience with risk stratification is being accumulated for other interventional procedures, such as mitral edge-to-edge repair. It remains essential not to rely on a single risk score figure when assessing patients or to determine unconditionally the indication and type of intervention. Patient's life expectancy, expected quality of life and patient preference should be considered, as well as local resources. The futility of interventions in patients unlikely to benefit from the treatment has to be taken into consideration, particularly for TAVI and mitral edge-to-edge repair [43]. The role of the Heart Team is essential to take all of these data into account and adopt a final decision on the best treatment strategy. Finally, the patient and family should be thoroughly informed and assisted in their decision on the best treatment option [44].

OUTCOMES

For past seven decades the defenitive treatment for severe aortic stenosis has been surgical replacement (SAVR). Trans-catheter based procedure technically are not replacements (native valve remains in situ). There are numerous article are published every year (see the Figure 2). Today, tran-catheter alternative has been devoloped in order to face high risk patients. There no long term reports for the SAVR versus TAVI, however there are sufficient for different risk groups and terms. In this chapter we will discuss only surgical ortic valve replacement resutls.

There is a subdivision of outcome in aortica valve disease: early and long term reuslts.

Early or Peri-Operative Mortatlity

Early mortality after SAVR is most commonly related to acute cardiac failure, neurologic complications, hemorrhage, and infection. The Society of Thoracic Surgeons (STS) National Database reports a 3.2% 30-day mortality for isolated SAVR [45]. When adding CABG, mortality rises to 5.6% [46]. Although, in the past, isolated reoperative SAVR increased the risk of early mortality [47], it does not appear to do so in the current era [47]. Early mortality has improved with time and continues to do so. In the 1990s early mortality for isolated SAVR was approximately 4.3% compared with the more contemporary 3.2% [45]. Similarly, the early mortality of combined SAVR and CABG improved significantly with time from 8.0% to 5.6% [46]. Double valve surgery, including an SAVR and either mitral valve or tricuspid valve replacement, raises the operative mortality to 11% to 14% [48]. Triple valve surgery, including SAVR, mitral valve replacement, and tricuspid valve replacement, raises the operative mortality rate to higher than 15%. [48] Risk factors for early mortality include increasing age, higher New York Heart Association (NYHA) functional class, LVH, left ventricular enlargement, presence of aortic regurgitation, renal dysfunction, severe chronic obstructive pulmonary disease (COPD), multiple reoperations, and concomitant CABG or heart valve surgery [49–52]. In minimally invasive approaches early and perioperative mortality seems significantly lower [53], although a fairly recent clnical trial failed to show a significat diffrence [54].

Early Complications

Neurologic Complications

The joint Society of Thoracic Surgeons/American Association for Thoracic Surgery (STS/AATS) panel subclassified cerebral embolic events into transient ischemic attacks (TIAs), which are fully reversible neurologic events lasting less than 24 hours; reversible ischemic neurologic deficit, which are fully reversible neurologic events lasting between 24 hours and 3 weeks; and strokes, which are nonreversible neurologic deficits lasting longer than 3 weeks [27]. The rate of stroke for isolated SAVR, according to the STS database, is 1.5% [45]. In high-risk (STS predicted risk of mortality >10%) and older patients (>80 years old), the risk of stroke rises to between 2% and 4.4% [55, 56]. The addition of CABG to the SAVR also raises the risk to between 4.9% and 5.8% [57]. Risk factors for early postoperative stroke include low LVEF (<40%), ascending aortic calcification, older than 70 years, female sex, diabetes mellitus, bypass time greater than 120 minutes, a history of stroke, carotid artery disease, and walking less than 300 meters during a 6-minute walk test [58, 59].

The annual rate of late stroke is 1.3% and 1.4% for bioprosthetic and mechanical valves, respectively. Risk factors for late stroke include female sex, older than 75 years, atrial fibrillation, current or previous smoking, diabetes mellitus, and carotid artery disease [60]. Postoperative strokes (55% to 76%) occur within the first 24 to 48 hours after surgery, but the high-risk period likely lasts for 3 months after surgery [61, 62]. Postoperative stroke is a significant predictor of mortality, raising the mortality rate to 31% for those with early stroke (<24 h) and 14% for those with late stroke (>24 h) compared with the baseline 4.6% mortality rate in one study [63]. Although early strokes seem to be related to the operation, late strokes are more influenced by patient- and disease-related factors [62]. Approximately one third of patients who have undergone cardiac surgery experience postoperative delirium [64]. Preexisting organic mental disorders, significant prior alcohol consumption, advanced age, intracranial cerebral artery disease, and longer cardiopulmonary bypass time are risk factors for postoperative delirium [64]. Suturless valves and catheter based valves have specific complicatione in early stages: itravalvular thrombosi. We have noteced (not published data) that it is majoraly related to valvular oversizing [65].

Heart Block and Permanent Pacemaker Implantation

Atrioventricular node block occurs more frequently after heart valve surgery compared with other types of cardiac surgery, with 3% to 8% of patients requiring permanent pacemaker insertion [66, 67].

It is a unique feature of valve surgery, and it is because of the very close proximity of the conduction system to the aortic valve in the area of the membranous septum. Decalcification must be exercised and shallower needle bites must be taken at the level of the commissure between the non-coronary and right coronary cusps. Heart block may be transient because of edema of the tissues around the con- duction system. However, if a patient remains pacer-dependent 7 to 10 days postoperatively, we recommend a permanent pacemaker insertion. Predictors of complete heart block and permanent pacemaker insertion include preoperative first-degree atrioventricular block or bundle branch block, postoperative cardiac arrest, combined aortic and mitral valve surgery, and infective endocarditis [67]. The type of aortic valve prosthesis used was not an important predictor in one study [67]. In suturless valves, mainly for intraanular position, there is a slighty high percantage of atriventricolar complete blockage, but with time it seems to recover [68]. In our institution we do not have any elevated risk of atrioventricular blockage when it consernec to sutureless valves. However it is very important not to oversize the intraannular suturless valves [65] for two reasons: transvalvular gradient and atrioventricualar conduction worsening.

Long-Term Survival

Late mortality can be divided into valve-related mortality and non–valve-related cardiac mortality. The former includes deaths caused by structural valve deterioration, nonstructural valve dysfunction, valve thromboembolism, bleeding, valve endocarditis, death related to a reoperation on an operated valve, or sudden and unexpected death in a patient with an operated valve. Non–valve-related mortality comprises other cardiac causes of death, such as progressive heart failure in a patient with a well functioning prosthetic valve [27]. The latter makes up 63% of all deaths in patients with mechanical valves and 59% of all deaths in patients with bioprosthetic valves at 15 years [69] Although there does not appear to be a survival difference between patients with bioprosthetic and mechanical aortic valves at 10 years, 24 structural bioprosthetic valve deterioration leads to a survival benefit for patients with mechanical valves at 15 years and over follow-up [69]. In contrast, other research has shown that even at 15, 20, and 25 years, there is no survival difference between patients who receive biopros- thetic versus mechanical valves in the aortic position [70]. Risk factors for late mortality include increasing age, higher NYHA functional class, LVH, left ventricular enlargement, left ventricular dysfunction, increased left atrial size, functional mitral regurgitation, atrial fibrilla- tion, ventricular arrhythmia, renal dysfunction, diabetes mellitus, peripheral arterial disease, female gender, smoking, severe COPD, multiple cardiac reoperations, and concomitant CABG or heart valve surgery [49–52, 71] There are no long term result on suturless aortic valves, however our group and others [72] has demostrated neat imporvement in early and mid term follow-up [36, 73].

Late Complications

Thromboembolism, Anticoagulation, and Bleeding Complications

Beyond the 3-month period after surgery when the risk of thromboembolism and bleeding is highest, the risk of thromboembolism is approximately constant. The overall linearized rate of thromboembolism for mechanical aortic valves is quoted as 2 per 100 patient-years and approximately half of that for bioprosthetic aortic valves, according to one report [74]. In another report, the rates of thromboembolism are similar among various mechanical valves, ranging between 1.16% and 1.33%, with one report quoting a lower rate for the On-X bileaflet mechanical valve (On-X Life Technologies Inc., Austin, TX) at 0.6% per year [75]. The rates are also comparable among different stented bioprosthetic valves, ranging between 0.78% and 1.22% per year [76].

However, the rate is much lower for allografts with a median of 0.23% per year [76]. Bleeding rates from anticoagulation appear to be independent of the prosthesis and range from 1% to 2% per year in a recent report [76]. Fluctuations in the interna- tional normalized ratio (INR) seem to be an important risk factor for both thromboembolic and bleeding events [77, 78].

Therefore, close monitoring of the INR to minimize fluctuations may be important to prevent these complications [78]. New point-of-care home testing may aid in achieving this goal. 58 Anticoagulation with a minimum target INR of 2.0 to 3.0 for low-risk patients and valves with low thrombogenicity (bileaflet valves) is recom- mended for mechanical SAVR. 59-61 However, interim results from the first limb of the Prospective Randomized On-X Anticoagulation Clinical Trial (PROACT) suggest that INR may be safely maintained between 1.5 and 2.0 with lower risk of bleeding and without a significant increase in thromboembolism. 62 The target INR should be 2.5 to 3.5 for patients at high risk for thromboembo- lism or who receive mechanical valves with high throm- bogenicity (disc valves). For bioprosthetic SAVR, the bulk of the evidence favors no anticoagulation in patients at low risk for thromboembolism because antiplatelet therapy suffices in this patient population [79–84]. The recommendations are shifting from anticoagulation in the first 3 months followed by antiplatelet therapy thereafter in low-risk patients to only antiplatelet therapy right after surgery [27, 85, 86]. Patients at high risk for thromboembolism should have a different consideration and anticoagulation may be warranted in this group. Prosthesis thrombosis is a serious but rare complica- tion of SAVR that occurs in less than 0.2% of cases per year [87]. It is more common in mechanical valves. Although often ineffective, thrombolysis may be attempted in patients with heart failure caused by valve dysfunction and who are considered too high risk for surgery. Surgi cal thrombectomy or re-replacement of the prosthetic valve is usually required and is associated with a high mortality rate of 10% to 15% [87].

Prosthetic Valve Endocarditis

Prosthetic valve endocarditis (PVE) is a serious complica- tion of SAVR and is divided into early PVE if it occurs less than 60 days post implantation and late PVE if it occurs more than 60 days post implantation. The rate of PVE is approximately 0.5% to 1% per year, with a slightly higher rate in the first 6 to 12 months compared to less than 12 months [88, 89]. Early PVE is usually a result of perioperative seeding of the prosthetic valve either intraoperatively or from wound infections or indwelling intravascular catheters postoperatively. Late PVE usually results from noncardiac sources of bacteremia or some- times from insidious infections with less virulent organ- isms introduced perioperatively. The microbiological profile of early PVE includes Staphylococcus aureus, S. epidermidis, gram-negative bacteria, and fungal infections. For late PVE, the microbiological profile resembles that of native endocarditis and includes Streptococcus and Staphylococcus species. Patients presenting with fever after an SAVR should be thoroughly investigated for PVE. Serial blood cultures and transthoracic or transesophageal echocardiography are important components of the diagnostic workup. Surgical indications for the management of PVE include early PVE, valve dysfunction including dehiscence or paravalvular leak, associated heart failure, presence of new conduction defect, abscess, aneurysm or fistula, persistent bacteremia despite maximum and appropriate medical therapy, vegetations larger than 10 mm in size, systemic embolization, all fungal infections, and virulent strains of S. aureus, Serratia marcescens, and Pseudomonas aeruginosa. The timing of surgery has been an area of debate. Sterilization of the valve is ideal before reoperation and is more likely if the vegetation is limited to the leaflets without annular involvement. Strokes from septic emboli are a common occurrence in patients with PVE, and differentiating ischemic stroke from hemorrhagic stroke is important because the former does not adversely affect outcome after reoperation whereas the latter does [90]. Computed tomography is an important modality in patients with neurologic signs or symptoms of stroke. The outcome following PVE is poor. Early PVE is associated with 30% to 80% mortality, whereas late PVE is associated with 20% to 40% mortality [91].

Structural Valve Deterioration and Freedom from Reoperation

In the quest for the ideal valve, new valves are constantly being introduced to the market after testing and short- term clinical trials, making the choice between different valves for SAVR a challenge. Thirdgeneration bileaflet mechanical valves have high structural integrity, and SVD is not observed or reported in several large series totaling more than 50,000 patient-years of follow-up [92–95]. The durability of these valves is excellent, resulting in a freedom from reoperation of approximately 94% at 10 years [95] and in one report up to 98% at 25 years after surgery [92, 96].

Glutaraldehyde-treated biological valves are subject to degenerative changes and calcification with time. Thera- pies to mitigate these processes help to slow down SVD and include using compounds such as surfactants, alpha oleic acid, and ethanol. The use of bioprosthetic valves has increased dramatically over the past couple of decades, increasing from 42% in 1996 to 82% in 2011 [97]. Although the risk of thromboembolism and anticoagulation-related bleeding events is lower in bioprosthetic valves, the concern about higher rates of SVD and perhaps higher rates of PVE remains [96].

Surgeons must therefore balance between the risks and benefits of various valve choices. There is no convincing evidence to suggest that various second-generation pericardial and porcine bioprosthe- ses differ in longevity; therefore, choice of the valve should depend on surgeon comfort and institutional preferences. Age is an important contributing factor to SVD in patients with bioprosthetic valves. Younger patients seem to have an accelerated rate of SVD probably as a result of a combination of factors, such as calcium metab- olism and hemodynamics. In all series, patients older than 70 years have a greater than 90% freedom from reoperation at 15 to 25 years. This rate falls slowly in patients 60 to 70 years old, and precipitously in patients younger than 60 years [98–101]. Actuarial freedom from reoperation in these studies probably overestimates the rate of SVD compared with actual freedom. In a recent report, the reoperation rate was 4% at 25 years after biopros- thetic SAVR, with 2.6% due to SVD [102]. Paravalvular Leak and Hemolysis The continuous suture technique of aortic valve implantation was traditionally thought to be a risk factor for paravalvular leak compared with an interrupted suture technique. However, recent reports show no difference in the rate of paravalvular leak between the two suture techniques [103, 104]. In the absence of infection, important paravalvular leak in mechanical or bioprosthetic aortic valves is uncommon, although minor leaks may occur. A contemporary report quotes a 0.01% annual rate [92]. If a paravalvular leak occurs, it can usually be detected in the first few months after surgery. There may be an anatomic predisposition in the area extending from the right and noncoronary commissure to one third the dis- tance along the right coronary cusp in one direction and two thirds the distance along the noncoronary cusp in the other direction [105]. Minor hemolysis may be managed conservatively, whereas clinically significant hemolysis requires surgical intervention.

Symptomatic Relief

Most surviving patients experience significant functional improvement after an SAVR, with 70% to 90% of patients in NYHA functional classes II through IV becoming class I. Even 10 years after surgery, 90% of patients remain in NYHA class I or II.

Left Ventricular Remodeling

Increased left ventricular mass (LVM) is a common occurrence later in patients with aortic valve disease, either through concentric LVH in AS or through left ventricular dilation and eccentric hypertrophy in aortic regurgitation. Increased LVM is a strong negative prognostic factor in aortic valve disease [106]. SAVR relieves the left ventricular pressure and volume overload in AS and aortic regurgitation, allowing the left ventricular myocardium to remodel and the LVM to regress. Left ventricular remodeling occurs in the first 18 months after surgery but can last up to 5 years [107]. However, in patients with decreased left ventricular contractility, signifying late-stage aortic valve disease, or reduced exercise capacity preoperatively, remodeling may fail to occur [108]. Myocardial gene expression of microRNA- 133a (miR-133a) is currently being explored as a poten- tial predictor of left ventricular remodeling in patients with AS, with several reports demonstrating promising results [109]. Further research may clarify the role of miR-133a in SAVR decision making, especially in asymp- tomatic patients with signs of LVH. The presence of prosthesis-patient mismatch may also hinder LVM regression, as discussed in the next subsection.

Prosthesis-Patient Mismatch

The theoretical goal of an SAVR is to reduce the pressure and volume overload on the left ventricle. Although transprosthetic gradients postoperatively should be minimal to allow left ventricular remodeling, high gradi- ents are occasionally seen despite an appropriately func- tioning valve. The persistence of left ventricular outflow obstruction postoperatively is termed prosthesis-patient mismatch (PPM) [110]. The parameter that most consis- tently correlates with postoperative transprosthetic gra- dients is the effective orifice area (EOA) indexed to the patient's body surface area or, indexed effective orifice area (IEOA) [111]. The EOA is measured by echocardiogra- phy using the continuity equation or by cardiac catheter- ization using the Gorlin formula. An IEOA of 0.65 to 0.85 cm 2/m 2 is generally defined as moderate PPM, and less than 0.65 cm 2 /m 2 is defined as severe PPM. The prevalence of moderate PPM ranges from 20% to 70% and severe PPM ranges from 2% to 11% [110]. The signifi- cance of PPM is a controversial topic and may depend on the definition of PPM used in various studies. Some studies have shown that PPM does not influence mid- term and long-term survival or left ventricular mass at mid-term follow-up [50, 112]. In contrast, other groups have shown that PPM after SAVR is associated with less improvement in functional status, less regression of LVH, higher risk of congestive heart failure, and increased long-term mortality [113, 114]. Patients with left ventricular dysfunction, including low-gradient AS, and younger patients (<60 years) who may be more active are particu- larly susceptible to PPM [113, 115]. Several options exist if a surgeon anticipates PPM in a large patient with a small aortic annulus. In young active patients or patients with left ventricular dysfunction (ejection fraction <50%) choosing prosthetic valves with larger IEOAs according to manufacturer-available user-friendly charts is one option. Aortic root enlargement is another method to allow for the implantation of larger prosthetic valve sizes. However, in older and sedentary patients, the extra risk in performing aortic root enlargement may not be worth the benefit of the extra valve size, and a certain amount of PPM may need to be accepted [116].

REFERENCES

[1] Iung B, Baron G, Butchart EG, Delahaye F, Gohlke-Bärwolf C, Levang OW, et al. A prospective survey of patients with valvular heart disease in Europe: The Euro Heart Survey on Valvular Heart Disease. *European Heart Journal* [Internet]. 2003 Jul [cited 2020 Feb 24];24(13):1231–43. Available from: https://academic.oup.com/eurheartj/article/24/13/1231/397045.

[2] Rodés-Cabau J. Transcatheter aortic valve implantation: Current and future approaches. *Nature Reviews Cardiology* [Internet]. 2012 Jan [cited 2020 Feb 25];9(1): 15–29. Available from: https://www.nature.com/articles/nrcardio.2011.164.

[3] Kang DH, Park SJ, Lee SA, Lee S, Kim DH, Kim HK, et al. Early Surgery or Conservative Care for Asymptomatic Aortic Stenosis. *New England Journal of Medicine* [Internet]. 2020 Jan [cited 2020 Feb 3];382(2):111–9. Available from: https://doi.org/10.1056/NEJMoa1912846.

[4] Smithy HG, Parker EF. Experimental aortic valvulotomy; a preliminary report. *Surgery, Gynecology & Obstetrics*. 1947 Apr;84(4-A):625–8.

[5] Bailey CP, Glover RP, O'neill TJE, Redondo Ramirez HP. Experiences with the experimental surgical relief of aortic stenosis; a preliminary report. *The Journal of Thoracic Surgery*. 1950 Oct;20(4):516–41.

[6] Bailey CP, Redondo Ramirez HP, Larzelere HB. Surgical treatment of aortic stenosis. *Journal of the American Medical Association*. 1952 Dec;150(17):1647–52.

[7] Ellis FH, Kirklin JW. Aortic stenosis. *The Surgical Clinics of North America*. 1955 Aug;Mayo Clinic No.:1029–34.

[8] Hufnagel CA. *Aortic plastic valvular prosthesis*. Bulletin Georgetown University Medical Center. 1951 Mar;4(5):128–30.

[9] Hurley PJ, Lowe JB, Barratt-Boyes BG. Débridement-valvotomy for aortic stenosis in adults. A follow-up of 76 patients. *Thorax*. 1967 Jul;22(4):314–9.

[10] Kirklin JW, Mankin HT. Open operation in the treatment of calcific aortic stenosis. *Circulation*. 1960 Apr;21:578–86.

[11] Bahnson HT, Spencer FC, Busse EF, Davis FW. Cusp Replacement and Coronary Artery Perfusion in Open Operations on the Aortic Valve. *Annals of Surgery*. 1960 Sep;152(3):494–503.

[12] Hufnagel CA, Conrad PW. The direct approach for the correction of aortic insufficiency. *JAMA*. 1961 Oct;178:275–9.

[13] Harken DE, Soroff HS, Taylor WJ, Lefemine AA, Gupta SK, Lunzer S. Partial and complete prostheses in aortic insufficiency. *The Journal of Thoracic and Cardiovascular Surgery*. 1960 Dec;40:744–62.

[14] Starr Albert, Edwards M. Lowell, Mccord Colin W., Griswold Herbert E. Aortic Replacement. Circulation [Internet]. 1963 Apr [cited 2020 Apr 16];27(4):779–83. Available from: https://www.ahajournals.org/doi/10.1161/01.CIR.27.4.779.

[15] Murray G. Homologous aortic-valve-segment transplants as surgical treatment for aortic and mitral insufficiency. *Angiology*. 1956 Oct;7(5):466–71.

[16] Kerwin AJ, Lenkei SC, Wilson DR. Aortic-valve homograft in the treatment of aortic insufficiency. Report of nine cases, with one followed for six years. *The New England Journal of Medicine*. 1962 Apr;266:852–7.

[17] Duran CG, Gunning AJ. A method for placing a total homologous aortic valve in the subcoronary position. *Lancet* (London, England). 1962 Sep;2(7254):488–9.

[18] Segal J, Harvey WP, Hufnagel C. A clinical study of one hundred cases of severe aortic insufficiency. *The American Journal of Medicine*. 1956 Aug;21(2):200–10.

[19] Ross DN. Replacement of aortic and mitral valves with a pulmonary autograft. *Lancet* (London, England). 1967 Nov;2(7523):956–8.

[20] Binet JP, Duran CG, Carpenter A, Langlois J. Heterologous aortic valve transplantation. *Lancet* (London, England). 1965 Dec;2(7425):1275.

[21] Carpentier A, Lemaigre G, Robert L, Carpentier S, Dubost C. Biological factors affecting long-term results of valvular heterografts. *The Journal of Thoracic and Cardiovascular Surgery*. 1969 Oct;58(4):467–83.

[22] David TE, Pollick C, Bos J. Aortic valve replacement with stentless porcine aortic bioprosthesis. *The Journal of Thoracic and Cardiovascular Surgery*. 1990 Jan;99(1): 113–8.

[23] Cribier A, Eltchaninoff H, Bash A, Borenstein N, Tron C, Bauer F, et al. Percutaneous transcatheter implantation of an aortic valve prosthesis for calcific aortic stenosis: First human case description. *Circulation*. 2002 Dec;106(24):3006–8.

[24] Lange R, Schreiber C, Götz W, Hettich I, Will A, Libera P, et al. First successful transapical aortic valve implantation with the Corevalve Revalving system: A case report. *The Heart Surgery Forum*. 2007;10(6):E478–479.

[25] Shrestha M, Khaladj N, Bara C, Hoeffler K, Hagl C, Haverich A. A staged approach towards interventional aortic valve implantation with a sutureless valve: Initial human implants. *The Thoracic and Cardiovascular Surgeon*. 2008 Oct;56(7):398–400.

[26] Nishimura RA, Otto CM, Bonow RO, Carabello BA, Erwin JP, Fleisher LA, et al. 2017 AHA/ACC Focused Update of the 2014 AHA/ACC Guideline for the Management of Patients With Valvular Heart Disease: A Report of the American College of Cardiology/American Heart Association Task Force on Clinical Practice Guidelines. *Circulation*. 2017;135(25):e1159–95.

[27] 2017 ESC/EACTS Guidelines for the management of valvular heart disease. *European Heart Journal* [Internet]. 2017 Sep [cited 2020 Apr 22];38(36):2739–91. Available from: https://academic.oup.com/eurheartj/article/38/36/2739/4095039.

[28] Monin J-L, Quéré J-P, Monchi M, Petit H, Baleynaud S, Chauvel C, et al. Low-gradient aortic stenosis: Operative risk stratification and predictors for long-term outcome: A multicenter study using dobutamine stress hemodynamics. *Circulation.* 2003 Jul;108(3).

[29] Thourani VH, Kodali S, Makkar RR, Herrmann HC, Williams M, Babaliaros V, et al. Transcatheter aortic valve replacement versus surgical valve replacement in intermediate-risk patients: A propensity score analysis. *The Lancet* [Internet]. 2016 May [cited 2020 Apr 29];387(10034):2218–25. Available from: https://www.thelancet.com/journals/lancet/article/PIIS0140-6736(16)30073-3/abstract.

[30] Fougères E, Tribouilloy C, Monchi M, Petit-Eisenmann H, Baleynaud S, Pasquet A, et al. Outcomes of pseudo-severe aortic stenosis under conservative treatment. *European Heart Journal.* 2012 Oct;33(19):2426–33.

[31] Levy F, Laurent M, Monin JL, Maillet JM, Pasquet A, Le Tourneau T, et al. Aortic valve replacement for low-flow/low-gradient aortic stenosis operative risk stratification and long-term outcome: A European multicenter study. *Journal of the American College of Cardiology.* 2008 Apr;51(15):1466–72.

[32] Tribouilloy C, Lévy F, Rusinaru D, Guéret P, Petit-Eisenmann H, Baleynaud S, et al. Outcome after aortic valve replacement for low-flow/low-gradient aortic stenosis without contractile reserve on dobutamine stress echocardiography. *Journal of the American College of Cardiology.* 2009 May;53(20):1865–73.

[33] Clavel M-A, Dumesnil JG, Capoulade R, Mathieu P, Sénéchal M, Pibarot P. Outcome of patients with aortic stenosis, small valve area, and low-flow, low-gradient despite preserved left ventricular ejection fraction. *Journal of the American College of Cardiology.* 2012 Oct;60(14):1259–67.

[34] Tribouilloy C, Rusinaru D, Maréchaux S, Castel A-L, Debry N, Maizel J, et al. Low-gradient, low-flow severe aortic stenosis with preserved left ventricular ejection fraction: Characteristics, outcome, and implications for surgery. *Journal of the American College of Cardiology.* 2015 Jan;65(1):55–66.

[35] Jander N, Minners J, Holme I, Gerdts E, Boman K, Brudi P, et al. Outcome of patients with low-gradient "severe" aortic stenosis and preserved ejection fraction. *Circulation.* 2011 Mar;123(8):887–95.

[36] Concistrè G, Chiaramonti F, Bianchi G, Cerillo A, Murzi M, Margaryan R, et al. Aortic Valve Replacement With Perceval Bioprosthesis: Single-Center Experience With 617 Implants. *The Annals of Thoracic Surgery* [Internet]. 2018 Jan [cited 2020 May 12];105(1):40–6. Available from: https://www.annalsthoracicsurgery.org/article/S0003-4975(17)30832-9/abstract.

[37] Osnabrugge RL, Speir AM, Head SJ, Fonner CE, Fonner E, Kappetein AP, et al. Performance of EuroSCORE II in a large US database: Implications for transcatheter aortic valve implantation. *European Journal of Cardio-Thoracic Surgery: Official Journal of the European Association for Cardio-Thoracic Surgery.* 2014 Sep;46(3): 400–408; discussion 408.

[38] Barili F, Pacini D, Capo A, Rasovic O, Grossi C, Alamanni F, et al. Does EuroSCORE II perform better than its original versions? A multicentre validation study. *European Heart Journal.* 2013 Jan;34(1):22–9.

[39] Margaryan R, Moscarelli M, Gasbarri T, Bianchi G, Kallushi E, Giuseppe Cerillo A, et al. EuroSCORE performance in minimally invasive cardiac surgery: Discrimination ability and external calibration. *Innovations.* 2017;12(4):282–6.

[40] Margaryan R, Bianchi G, Concistre G, Gasbarri T, Kallushi E, Farneti P, et al. *Three Risk Scores For Mortality Prediction in Minimally Invasive Cardiac Surgery.* medRxiv [Internet]. 2020 Jun [cited 2020 Jun 10];2020.06.03.20120949. Available from: https://www.medrxiv.org/content/10.1101/2020.06.03.20120949v1.

[41] Iung B, Laouénan C, Himbert D, Eltchaninoff H, Chevreul K, Donzeau-Gouge P, et al. Predictive factors of early mortality after transcatheter aortic valve implantation: Individual risk assessment using a simple score. *Heart* (British Cardiac Society). 2014 Jul;100(13):1016–23.

[42] Edwards FH, Cohen DJ, O'Brien SM, Peterson ED, Mack MJ, Shahian DM, et al. Development and Validation of a Risk Prediction Model for In-Hospital Mortality After Transcatheter Aortic Valve Replacement. *JAMA cardiology.* 2016;1(1):46–52.

[43] Arnold SV, Reynolds MR, Lei Y, Magnuson EA, Kirtane AJ, Kodali SK, et al. Predictors of poor outcomes after transcatheter aortic valve replacement: Results from the PARTNER (Placement of Aortic Transcatheter Valve) trial. *Circulation.* 2014 Jun;129(25):2682–90.

[44] Puri R, Iung B, Cohen DJ, Rodés-Cabau J. TAVI or No TAVI: Identifying patients unlikely to benefit from transcatheter aortic valve implantation. *European Heart Journal.* 2016 Jul;37(28):2217–25.

[45] O'Brien SM, Shahian DM, Filardo G, Ferraris VA, Haan CK, Rich JB, et al. The Society of Thoracic Surgeons 2008 cardiac surgery risk models: Part 2–isolated valve surgery. *The Annals of Thoracic Surgery.* 2009 Jul;88(1 Suppl):S23–42.

[46] Shahian DM, O'Brien SM, Filardo G, Ferraris VA, Haan CK, Rich JB, et al. The Society of Thoracic Surgeons 2008 cardiac surgery risk models: Part 3–valve plus coronary artery bypass grafting surgery. *The Annals of Thoracic Surgery.* 2009 Jul;88(1 Suppl):S43–62.

[47] LaPar DJ, Yang Z, Stukenborg GJ, Peeler BB, Kern JA, Kron IL, et al. Outcomes of reoperative aortic valve replacement after previous sternotomy. *The Journal of Thoracic and Cardiovascular Surgery.* 2010 Feb;139(2):263–72.

[48] Rankin JS, Hammill BG, Ferguson TB, Glower DD, O'Brien SM, DeLong ER, et al. Determinants of operative mortality in valvular heart surgery. *The Journal of Thoracic and Cardiovascular Surgery.* 2006 Mar;131(3):547–57.

[49] Beach JM, Mihaljevic T, Rajeswaran J, Marwick T, Edwards ST, Nowicki ER, et al. Ventricular hypertrophy and left atrial dilatation persist and are associated with reduced survival after valve replacement for aortic stenosis. *The Journal of Thoracic and Cardiovascular Surgery.* 2014 Jan;147(1):362–369.e8.

[50] Blackstone EH, Cosgrove DM, Jamieson WRE, Birkmeyer NJ, Lemmer JH, Miller DC, et al. Prosthesis size and long-term survival after aortic valve replacement. *The Journal of Thoracic and Cardiovascular Surgery.* 2003 Sep;126(3):783–96.

[51] Di Eusanio M, Fortuna D, De Palma R, Dell'Amore A, Lamarra M, Contini GA, et al. Aortic valve replacement: Results and predictors of mortality from a contemporary

series of 2256 patients. *The Journal of Thoracic and Cardiovascular Surgery*. 2011 Apr;141(4):940–7.

[52] Mihaljevic T, Nowicki ER, Rajeswaran J, Blackstone EH, Lagazzi L, Thomas J, et al. Survival after valve replacement for aortic stenosis: Implications for decision making. *The Journal of Thoracic and Cardiovascular Surgery*. 2008 Jun;135(6):1270–1278; discussion 1278–9.

[53] Mkalaluh S, Szczechowicz M, Dib B, Sabashnikov A, Szabo G, Karck M, et al. Early and long-term results of minimally invasive mitral valve surgery through a right mini-thoracotomy approach: A retrospective propensity-score matched analysis. *PeerJ*. 2018;6:e4810.

[54] Speziale G, Nasso G, Esposito G, Conte M, Greco E, Fattouch K, et al. Results of mitral valve repair for Barlow disease (bileaflet prolapse) via right minithoracotomy versus conventional median sternotomy: A randomized trial. *The Journal of Thoracic and Cardiovascular Surgery*. 2011 Jul;142(1):77–83.

[55] ElBardissi AW, Shekar P, Couper GS, Cohn LH. Minimally invasive aortic valve replacement in octogenarian, high-risk, transcatheter aortic valve implantation candidates. *The Journal of Thoracic and Cardiovascular Surgery*. 2011 Feb;141 (2):328–35.

[56] Thourani VH, Ailawadi G, Szeto WY, Dewey TM, Guyton RA, Mack MJ, et al. Outcomes of surgical aortic valve replacement in high-risk patients: A multiinstitutional study. *The Annals of Thoracic Surgery*. 2011 Jan;91(1):49–55; discussion 55–6.

[57] Alexander KP, Anstrom KJ, Muhlbaier LH, Grosswald RD, Smith PK, Jones RH, et al. Outcomes of cardiac surgery in patients > or = 80 years: Results from the National Cardiovascular Network. *Journal of the American College of Cardiology*. 2000 Mar;35(3):731–8.

[58] Chikwe J, Croft LB, Goldstone AB, Castillo JG, Rahmanian PB, Adams DH, et al. Comparison of the results of aortic valve replacement with or without concomitant coronary artery bypass grafting in patients with left ventricular ejection fraction < or =30% versus patients with ejection fraction >30%. *The American Journal of Cardiology*. 2009 Dec;104(12):1717–21.

[59] Arenaza DP de, Pepper J, Lees B, Rubinstein F, Nugara F, Roughton M, et al. Preoperative 6-minute walk test adds prognostic information to Euroscore in patients undergoing aortic valve replacement. *Heart* (British Cardiac Society). 2010 Jan;96(2):113–7.

[60] Gulbins H, Florath I, Ennker J. Cerebrovascular events after stentless aortic valve replacement during a 9-year follow-up period. *The Annals of Thoracic Surgery*. 2008 Sep;86(3):769–73.

[61] Al-Atassi T, Lam K, Forgie M, Boodhwani M, Rubens F, Hendry P, et al. Cerebral microembolization after bioprosthetic aortic valve replacement: Comparison of warfarin plus aspirin versus aspirin only. *Circulation*. 2012 Sep;126(11 Suppl 1):S239–244.

[62] Miller DC, Blackstone EH, Mack MJ, Svensson LG, Kodali SK, Kapadia S, et al. Transcatheter (TAVR) versus surgical (AVR) aortic valve replacement: Occurrence, hazard, risk factors, and consequences of neurologic events in the PARTNER trial. *The Journal of Thoracic and Cardiovascular Surgery*. 2012 Apr;143(4):832–843.e13.

[63] Filsoufi F, Rahmanian PB, Castillo JG, Bronster D, Adams DH. Incidence, imaging analysis, and early and late outcomes of stroke after cardiac valve operation. *The American Journal of Cardiology*. 2008 May;101(10):1472–8.

[64] Guenther U, Theuerkauf N, Frommann I, Brimmers K, Malik R, Stori S, et al. Predisposing and precipitating factors of delirium after cardiac surgery: A prospective observational cohort study. *Annals of Surgery*. 2013 Jun;257(6):1160–7.

[65] Cerillo AG, Amoretti F, Mariani M, Cigala E, Murzi M, Gasbarri T, et al. Increased Gradients After Aortic Valve Replacement With the Perceval Valve: The Role of Oversizing. *The Annals of Thoracic Surgery*. 2018;106(1):121–8.

[66] Baraki H, Al Ahmad A, Jeng-Singh S, Saito S, Schmitto JD, Fleischer B, et al. Pacemaker dependency after isolated aortic valve replacement: Do conductance disorders recover over time? *Interactive Cardiovascular and Thoracic Surgery*. 2013 Apr;16(4):476–81.

[67] Huynh H, Dalloul G, Ghanbari H, Burke P, David M, Daccarett M, et al. Permanent pacemaker implantation following aortic valve replacement: Current prevalence and clinical predictors. *Pacing and clinical electrophysiology*: PACE. 2009 Dec;32(12): 1520–5.

[68] Vogt F, Moscarelli M, Nicoletti A, Gregorini R, Pollari F, Kalisnik JM, et al. Sutureless Aortic Valve and Pacemaker Rate: From Surgical Tricks to Clinical Outcomes. *The Annals of Thoracic Surgery*. 2019;108(1):99–105.

[69] Hammermeister K, Sethi GK, Henderson WG, Grover FL, Oprian C, Rahimtoola SH. Outcomes 15 years after valve replacement with a mechanical versus a bioprosthetic valve: Final report of the Veterans Affairs randomized trial. *Journal of the American College of Cardiology*. 2000 Oct;36(4):1152–8.

[70] Ruel M, Chan V, Bédard P, Kulik A, Ressler L, Lam BK, et al. Very long-term survival implications of heart valve replacement with tissue versus mechanical prostheses in adults <60 years of age. *Circulation*. 2007 Sep;116(11 Suppl):I294–300.

[71] Casaclang-Verzosa G, Malouf JF, Scott CG, Juracan EM, Nishimura RA, Pellikka PA. Does left atrial size predict mortality in asymptomatic patients with severe aortic stenosis? *Echocardiography* (Mount Kisco, NY). 2010 Feb;27(2):105–9.

[72] Schlömicher M, Bechtel M, Taghiyev Z, Naraghi H, Haldenwang PL, Moustafine V, et al. Intermediate Outcomes after Rapid Deployment Aortic Valve Replacement in Multiple Valve Surgery. *The Thoracic and Cardiovascular Surgeon*. 2019 Apr;

[73] Concistrè G, Bianchi G, Chiaramonti F, Margaryan R, Marchi F, Kallushi E, et al. Minimally Invasive Sutureless Aortic Valve Replacement is Associated With Improved Outcomes in Patients With Left Ventricular Dysfunction. *Innovations* (Philadelphia, Pa). 2019 Oct;14(5):445–52.

[74] Edmunds LH. Thrombotic and bleeding complications of prosthetic heart valves. *The Annals of Thoracic Surgery*. 1987 Oct;44(4):430–45.

[75] Chambers JB, Pomar JL, Mestres CA, Palatianos GM. Clinical event rates with the On-X bileaflet mechanical heart valve: A multicenter experience with follow-up to 12 years. *The Journal of Thoracic and Cardiovascular Surgery*. 2013 Feb;145(2):420–4.

[76] Grunkemeier GL, Li HH, Naftel DC, Starr A, Rahimtoola SH. Long-term performance of heart valve prostheses. *Current Problems in Cardiology*. 2000 Feb;25(2):73–154.

[77] Bourguignon T, Bergöend E, Mirza A, Ayegnon G, Neville P, Aupart MR, et al. Risk factors for valve-related complications after mechanical heart valve replacement in 505

patients with long-term follow up. *The Journal of Heart Valve Disease*. 2011 Nov;20(6):673–80.

[78] Rhie S, Choi JY, Jang IS, Kim JW, Lee CE, Park HO. Relationship between the Occurrence of Thromboembolism and INR Measurement Interval in Low Intensity Anticoagulation after Aortic Mechanical Valve Replacement. *The Korean Journal of Thoracic and Cardiovascular Surgery*. 2011 Jun;44(3):220–4.

[79] Sundt TM, Zehr KJ, Dearani JA, Daly RC, Mullany CJ, McGregor CGA, et al. Is early anticoagulation with warfarin necessary after bioprosthetic aortic valve replacement? *The Journal of Thoracic and Cardiovascular Surgery*. 2005 May;129(5):1024–31.

[80] Aramendi JI, Mestres C-A, Mestres C-A, Martinez-León J, Campos V, Muñoz G, et al. Triflusal versus oral anticoagulation for primary prevention of thromboembolism after bioprosthetic valve replacement (trac): Prospective, randomized, co-operative trial. *European Journal of Cardio-Thoracic Surgery: Official Journal of the European Association for Cardio-Thoracic Surgery*. 2005 May;27(5):854–60.

[81] Colli A, Mestres CA, Castella M, Gherli T. Comparing warfarin to aspirin (WoA) after aortic valve replacement with the St. Jude Medical Epic heart valve bioprosthesis: Results of the WoA Epic pilot trial. *The Journal of Heart Valve Disease*. 2007 Nov;16(6):667–71.

[82] ElBardissi AW, DiBardino DJ, Chen FY, Yamashita MH, Cohn LH. Is early antithrombotic therapy necessary in patients with bioprosthetic aortic valves in normal sinus rhythm? *The Journal of Thoracic and Cardiovascular Surgery*. 2010 May;139 (5):1137–45.

[83] Gherli T, Colli A, Fragnito C, Nicolini F, Borrello B, Saccani S, et al. Comparing warfarin with aspirin after biological aortic valve replacement: A prospective study. *Circulation*. 2004 Aug;110(5):496–500.

[84] Colli A, Verhoye J-P, Heijmen R, Antunes M, ACTION Investigators. Low-dose acetyl salicylic acid versus oral anticoagulation after bioprosthetic aortic valve replacement. Final report of the ACTION registry. *International Journal of Cardiology*. 2013 Sep;168(2):1229–36.

[85] Bonow RO, Carabello BA, Chatterjee K, Leon AC de, Faxon DP, Freed MD, et al. 2008 focused update incorporated into the ACC/AHA 2006 guidelines for the management of patients with valvular heart disease: A report of the American College of Cardiology/American Heart Association Task Force on Practice Guidelines (Writing Committee to revise the 1998 guidelines for the management of patients with valvular heart disease). Endorsed by the Society of Cardiovascular Anesthesiologists, Society for Cardiovascular Angiography and Interventions, and Society of Thoracic Surgeons. *Journal of the American College of Cardiology*. 2008 Sep;52(13):e1–142.

[86] Whitlock RP, Sun JC, Fremes SE, Rubens FD, Teoh KH. Antithrombotic and thrombolytic therapy for valvular disease: Antithrombotic Therapy and Prevention of Thrombosis, 9th ed: American College of Chest Physicians Evidence-Based Clinical Practice Guidelines. *Chest*. 2012 Feb;141(2 Suppl):e576S–600S.

[87] Lengyel M, Vandor L. The role of thrombolysis in the management of left-sided prosthetic valve thrombosis: A study of 85 cases diagnosed by transesophageal echocardiography. *The Journal of Heart Valve Disease*. 2001 Sep;10(5):636–49.

[88] Gordon SM, Serkey JM, Longworth DL, Lytle BW, Cosgrove DM. Early onset prosthetic valve endocarditis: The Cleveland Clinic experience 1992-1997. *The Annals of Thoracic Surgery*. 2000 May;69(5):1388–92.

[89] Wang A, Athan E, Pappas PA, Fowler VG, Olaison L, Paré C, et al. Contemporary clinical profile and outcome of prosthetic valve endocarditis. *JAMA*. 2007 Mar;297(12):1354–61.

[90] Prendergast BD, Tornos P. Surgery for infective endocarditis: Who and when? *Circulation*. 2010 Mar;121(9):1141–52.

[91] David TE, Ivanov J, Armstrong S, Feindel CM, Cohen G. Late results of heart valve replacement with the Hancock II bioprosthesis. *The Journal of Thoracic and Cardiovascular Surgery*. 2001 Feb;121(2):268–77.

[92] Emery RW, Krogh CC, Arom KV, Emery AM, Benyo-Albrecht K, Joyce LD, et al. The St. Jude Medical cardiac valve prosthesis: A 25-year experience with single valve replacement. *The Annals of Thoracic Surgery*. 2005 Mar;79(3):776–782; discussion 782–3.

[93] Ikonomidis JS, Kratz JM, Crumbley AJ, Stroud MR, Bradley SM, Sade RM, et al. Twenty-year experience with the St Jude Medical mechanical valve prosthesis. *The Journal of Thoracic and Cardiovascular Surgery*. 2003 Dec;126(6):2022–31.

[94] Khan SS, Trento A, DeRobertis M, Kass RM, Sandhu M, Czer LS, et al. Twenty-year comparison of tissue and mechanical valve replacement. *The Journal of Thoracic and Cardiovascular Surgery*. 2001 Aug;122(2):257–69.

[95] Bouhout I, Stevens L-M, Mazine A, Poirier N, Cartier R, Demers P, et al. Long-term outcomes after elective isolated mechanical aortic valve replacement in young adults. *The Journal of Thoracic and Cardiovascular Surgery*. 2014 Oct;148(4):1341–1346.e1.

[96] Brennan JM, Edwards FH, Zhao Y, O'Brien S, Booth ME, Dokholyan RS, et al. Long-term safety and effectiveness of mechanical versus biologic aortic valve prostheses in older patients: Results from the Society of Thoracic Surgeons Adult Cardiac Surgery National Database. *Circulation*. 2013 Apr;127(16):1647–55.

[97] Brown JM, O'Brien SM, Wu C, Sikora JAH, Griffith BP, Gammie JS. Isolated aortic valve replacement in North America comprising 108,687 patients in 10 years: Changes in risks, valve types, and outcomes in the Society of Thoracic Surgeons National Database. *The Journal of Thoracic and Cardiovascular Surgery*. 2009 Jan;137(1):82–90.

[98] McClure RS, Narayanasamy N, Wiegerinck E, Lipsitz S, Maloney A, Byrne JG, et al. Late outcomes for aortic valve replacement with the Carpentier-Edwards pericardial bioprosthesis: Up to 17-year follow-up in 1,000 patients. *The Annals of Thoracic Surgery*. 2010 May;89(5):1410–6.

[99] Mykén PSU, Bech-Hansen O. A 20-year experience of 1712 patients with the Biocor porcine bioprosthesis. *The Journal of Thoracic and Cardiovascular Surgery*. 2009 Jan;137(1):76–81.

[100] Valfrè C, Ius P, Minniti G, Salvador L, Bottio T, Cesari F, et al. The fate of Hancock II porcine valve recipients 25 years after implant. *European Journal of Cardio-Thoracic Surgery: Official Journal of the European Association for Cardio-Thoracic Surgery*. 2010 Aug;38(2):141–6.

[101] Yankah CA, Pasic M, Musci M, Stein J, Detschades C, Siniawski H, et al. Aortic valve replacement with the Mitroflow pericardial bioprosthesis: Durability results up to 21 years. *The Journal of Thoracic and Cardiovascular Surgery*. 2008 Sep;136(3):688–96.

[102] Forcillo J, Pellerin M, Perrault LP, Cartier R, Bouchard D, Demers P, et al. Carpentier-Edwards Pericardial Valve in the Aortic Position: 25-Years Experience. *The Annals of Thoracic Surgery* [Internet]. 2013 Aug [cited 2020 May 10];96(2):486–93. Available from: https://www.annalsthoracicsurgery.org/article/S0003-4975(13)00609-7/abstract.

[103] Choi JB, Kim JH, Park HK, Kim KH, Kim MH, Kuh JH, et al. Aortic valve replacement using continuous suture technique in patients with aortic valve disease. *The Korean Journal of Thoracic and Cardiovascular Surgery*. 2013 Aug;46(4):249–55.

[104] Watanabe G, Ushijima T, Tomita S, Yamaguchi S, Koshida Y, Iino K. Revival of continuous suture technique in aortic valve replacement in patient with aortic valve stenosis: A novel modified technique. *Innovations* (Philadelphia, Pa). 2011 Sep;6(5):311–5.

[105] De Cicco G, Lorusso R, Colli A, Nicolini F, Fragnito C, Grimaldi T, et al. Aortic valve periprosthetic leakage: Anatomic observations and surgical results. *The Annals of Thoracic Surgery*. 2005 May;79(5):1480–5.

[106] Haider AW, Larson MG, Benjamin EJ, Levy D. Increased left ventricular mass and hypertrophy are associated with increased risk for sudden death. *Journal of the American College of Cardiology*. 1998 Nov;32(5):1454–9.

[107] Kühl HP, Franke A, Puschmann D, Schöndube FA, Hoffmann R, Hanrath P. Regression of left ventricular mass one year after aortic valve replacement for pure severe aortic stenosis. *The American Journal of Cardiology*. 2002 Feb;89(4):408–13.

[108] Bonow RO, Borer JS, Rosing DR, Henry WL, Pearlman AS, McIntosh CL, et al. Preoperative exercise capacity in symptomatic patients with aortic regurgitation as a predictor of postoperative left ventricular function and long-term prognosis. *Circulation*. 1980 Dec;62(6):1280–90.

[109] García R, Villar AV, Cobo M, Llano M, Martín-Durán R, Hurlé MA, et al. Circulating levels of miR-133a predict the regression potential of left ventricular hypertrophy after valve replacement surgery in patients with aortic stenosis. *Journal of the American Heart Association*. 2013 Aug;2(4):e000211.

[110] Pibarot P, Dumesnil JG. Prosthesis-patient mismatch: Definition, clinical impact, and prevention. *Heart* (British Cardiac Society). 2006 Aug;92(8):1022–9.

[111] Pibarot P, Dumesnil JG, Cartier PC, Métras J, Lemieux MD. Patient-prosthesis mismatch can be predicted at the time of operation. *The Annals of Thoracic Surgery*. 2001 May;71(5 Suppl):S265–268.

[112] Hanayama N, Christakis GT, Mallidi HR, Joyner CD, Fremes SE, Morgan CD, et al. Patient prosthesis mismatch is rare after aortic valve replacement: Valve size may be irrelevant. *The Annals of Thoracic Surgery*. 2002 Jun;73(6):1822–1829; discussion 1829.

[113] Blais C, Dumesnil JG, Baillot R, Simard S, Doyle D, Pibarot P. Impact of valve prosthesis-patient mismatch on short-term mortality after aortic valve replacement. *Circulation*. 2003 Aug;108(8):983–8.

[114] Tasca G, Brunelli F, Cirillo M, DallaTomba M, Mhagna Z, Troise G, et al. Impact of valve prosthesis-patient mismatch on left ventricular mass regression following aortic valve replacement. *The Annals of Thoracic Surgery*. 2005 Feb;79(2):505–10.

[115] Price J, Lapierre H, Ressler L, Lam B-K, Mesana TG, Ruel M. Prosthesis-patient mismatch is less frequent and more clinically indolent in patients operated for aortic insufficiency. *The Journal of Thoracic and Cardiovascular Surgery*. 2009 Sep;138(3):639–45.

[116] Kulik A, Al-Saigh M, Chan V, Masters RG, Bédard P, Lam B-K, et al. Enlargement of the small aortic root during aortic valve replacement: Is there a benefit? *The Annals of Thoracic Surgery*. 2008 Jan;85(1):94–100.

In: Perspectives in Aortic Valve Disease
Editor: Giovanni Concistrè
ISBN: 978-1-53618-769-4

Chapter 14

SURGICAL APPROACH: CONVENTIONAL AND MINIMALLY INVASIVE TREATMENTS

Giovanni Concistrè*, MD and Marco Solinas, MD
Ospedale del Cuore "G. Pasquinucci,"
Fondazione Toscana Gabriele Monasterio, Massa, Italy

ABSTRACT

Treatment of aortic valve disease is rapidly evolving. Aortic valve replacement (AVR) via a full sternotomy is well tolerated and has demonstrated excellent long-term event-free survival and quality of life. At the same time the use of minimally invasive surgical approaches, after decades of scepticism, is increasing in the attempt to further reduce postoperative morbidity and to improve patient satisfaction. However, not all cardiac surgeons offer minimal access approach aortic valve replacement. In 1993, the first mini-AVR was performed through a right thoracotomy. Subsequently, a variety of incisions, including partial lower and transverse sternotomy as well as a parasternal approach, have been adopted. Nowadays, the right anterior minithoracotomy, ministernotomy and in the recent times endoscopic right axillar minithoracotomy are the predominant approaches for the mini-AVR. At present, there are no guidelines to either recommend or discourage surgeons from using minimally invasive approaches in aortic valve surgery because of the lack of definitive prospective randomized studies.

Keywords: aortic valve, valvular disease, aortic valve prosthesis, aortic valve replacement, conventional aortic valve replacement, minimally invasive aortic valve replacement

INTRODUCTION

Aortic valve replacement can be performed through a median sternotomy with standard or limited skin incision, through an upper midline sternotomy extending to the right third or fourth intercostal space, or through a right thoracotomy in the second or third intercostal

* Corresponding Author's Email: gioconci@libero.it.

space. Although median sternotomy remains the surgical approach most used, less invasive surgery represents the treatment of choice for AVR in many Centers.

CONVENTIONAL TREATMENT

Cardiopulmonary Bypass and Myocardial Protection

AVR is performed with a venous cannula in the right atrium for venous return and distal ascending aorta is cannulated for systemic perfusion. A cannula for antegrade cardioplegia is inserted in the ascending aorta and a preshaped catheter is inserted in the coronary sinus through the right atrium for retrograde cardioplegia in selected cases. Left ventricular venting is performed through the right superior pulmonary vein. Once all cannulae are in place, an activated clotting time (ACT) of >400 seconds is necessary before cardiopulmonary bypass (CPB) is initiated. Attention should be given at this time to proper venous drainage and absence of LV distension. The plane between the aorta and the pulmonary artery is divided for secure and proper positioning of the aortic cross-clamp. We use mild systemic hypothermia (34°C). Normothermic blood cardioplegia is used with antegrade induction followed by intermittent retrograde perfusion, in selected cases. When the procedure is prolonged and the aortic root open, additional protection can be obtained with intermittent antegrade direct cardioplegia administration into the coronary ostia every 15 minutes. In more complex procedures, we use single dose of cold crystalloid cardioplegia (Custodiol), dosed according to patient's body weight.

Exposure of the Aortic Valve

We performe the aortotomy anteriorly approximately 2 cm above the commissures In cases of stented prosthesis implantation, extending the incision obliquely into the non-coronary sinus allows easier passage of a large valve prosthesis. This incision can be extended into the aortic annulus or further into the anterior mitral leaflet in cases requiring aortic root enlargement. Commissural sutures are pulled outward to improve valve and root exposure.

Valve Excision, Debridement, and Sizing

Valve leaflets excision is started at the commissures. Using scissors, the aortic valve leaflets are resected en bloc at their hinge point. Further debridement is carefully performed using two surgical forceps or a rongeur. The aim is to remove all calcium at the level of the annulus in order to suture the prosthesis into pliable tissues, which reduces the risk of paravalvular leaks. Care should be taken to avoid disruption of the annulus in cases of generous debridement, as well as preventing calcium fragments from falling into the left ventricle, as these may embolize systemically or into the coronary ostia. The annulus is then sized and an appropriate prosthesis chosen. Patient body surface area (BSA) and valve effective orifice area (EOA) characteristics should be considered to avoid patient-prosthesis mismatch (PPM). In addition, the importance of implanting a large stented bioprosthesis at first operation is increasingly important should a valve-in-valve procedure be considered.

Valve Implantation

Stented Prosthesis

Pledgeted Ticron 2-0 U-stitches are used to secure the prosthesis to the annulus. Typically, four or five pledgeted sutures are needed per sinus. The sutures should be strong enough but not include too much annular tissue to avoid crowding the space beneath the prosthesis, which may cause turbulence and favor pannus formation. Attention should be given when placing the sutures at the level of the right and non-coronary cusp commissure to avoid injury to the conduction tissue. These sutures should follow the crown shape of the annulus instead of a straight line in the subcommissural triangle. Pledgets can be placed on the aortic side or ventricular side. We prefer placing them on the ventricular side because it allows a larger prosthetic valve in a supra-aortic position. However, when implanting mechanical prostheses, pledgets are placed on the aortic side to ensure proper placement of the prosthesis and avoid losing any pledgets in the ventricular cavity. Once all sutures are placed in the sewing ring, the prosthesis is lowered onto the annulus. Care should be taken not to force the prosthesis to avoid aortic tearing or prosthesis deformation. After the prosthesis is tied in place, the coronary ostia should be visible. In case of doubt about potential paravalvular leaks, a small right-angle clamp is used to probe the spaces between the sutures.

In patients with a small aortic annulus, annular enlargement should be considered. To do this, the aortotomy is extended toward the nadir of the non-coronary sinus. Depending on the targeted degree of annular enlargement, the incision can be continued into the aortic annulus, or further into the anterior leaflet of the mitral valve. Once the incision has been prolonged, the space is filled with a diamond-shaped patch of Dacron or bovine pericardium, sutured first to the anterior leaflet of the mitral valve. When both limbs of the suture have passed beyond the native aortic annulus, the prosthesis is sutured into place as previously described. The non-coronary sinus is then sutured to the interposition graft, before the aortotomy is fully closed. Extending the incision into the anterior leaflet of the mitral valve allows the placing of a prosthesis one or two sizes larger than the original measurement.

Homograft Prosthesis

Stentless AVR can be performed using the total root or the subcoronary techniques. Total root replacement minimizes leaflet distortion and ensures an even distribution of stresses on the leaflets. A continuous running suture or interrupted single 4-0 polypropylene sutures are used to suture the prosthesis to the aortic annulus. Suturing is started at the commissure between the right and left coronary sinuses. The prosthesis is placed in its anatomical position. However, because the angle between the pig coronary ostia is significantly narrower than in humans, the xenograft buttons should be ligated and the patient coronaries alternately positioned within the sinus wall.

Alternatively, the stentless root can be placed in a subcoronary position. First, the sinuses of Valsalva from the xenograft root are resected, leaving 2–3 mm of sinus wall at the attachment of the leaflets. Three 4-0 polypropylene sutures are then placed at each commissure, and through the stentless root. The stentless root is lowered and the proximal suture line is performed at the level of the aortic annulus. The second suture line is then performed following the crown shape of the xenograft onto the native sinus wall, ensuring coronary ostial permeability.

Stentless Prosthesis

A transverse aortotomy should be performed high above the commissures, in order to provide good vision over the sinuses as well as sufficient space for stentless commissure attachment to the aortic wall. Three reference "stay" sutures placed slightly above the commissures are helpful. Particular attention must be paid to the aortic root anatomy, and a correct sizing is critical. Symmetric implantation may be difficult with a wide and deep noncoronary (NC) sinus and particularly in the case of bicuspid aortic valve (BAV), when the commissure landmark is missing. We therefore discourage use of a stentless valve in a BAV root anatomy. There is also a potential risk of regurgitation over time, due to presumed coexistent aortic disease and potentially later aortic dilatation in these patients. The use of stentless prosthesis should therefore be avoided in patients with BAV and in those with moderate dilatation of the ascending aorta. The fundamental importance of accurate sizing and prosthesis selection must be emphasized. The probe should tightly fit the aortic annulus (Figure 2A). The prosthetic valve corresponding to the probe is already upsized by the manufacturer, to one size more or 2 mm larger than the annular diameter. When in doubt with determining the correct valve size, one should consider that oversizing the stentless valve may result in S-shaped leaflet folding with functional stenosis and high gradients. Another source of dysfunction can be the presence or likelihood of future root and/or sinotubular junction dilatation, which have the potential to cause regurgitation. This means that both oversizing and undersizing have the potential to cause prosthesis failure. In general, if one size is too small and the larger one fits the annulus with some resistance, the larger one should be implanted. Three equidistant, intercommissural sutures (polypropylene 4-0, using a small semicircular needle) are then placed in the supra-annular position at the nadir of each sinus, at 2–3 mm above the native annulus. Each of these sutures must be placed at the corresponding part of the tissue valve cusps, using the pericardial strip available at the basis of the stentless valve (Figure 2B). Placement of sutures below or through the annulus must be avoided. At the level of the commissures, the sutures are passed out of the aorta and tied together (Figure 2C-E). At the end of the suturing process, the sutureless bioprosthesis becomes somewhat fixed in the aortic root and the exposition may be more difficult, potentially making suturing difficult, especially in cases with small valve sizes. It is important to avoid too small suture bites, to prevent dehiscence. Care must be taken to avoid any laceration of the valve leaflets with a needle tip and also to prevent any damage of the assembly suture of the valve. Some surgeons have suggested to start suturing at the right coronary sinus, followed by the left coronary sinus, and finally the NC sinus, but in fact, any order can be followed (Figure 2F). There is large individual variability in root anatomy, and the NC sinus often presents wider and deeper than the symmetric prosthesis. Therefore, the suture line can be longer, and consequently, relatively less valve tissue might be available for a longer distance between commissures, resulting in bites that create folding or tension. In fact, most reported failures and thrombosis were thought to be associated with the NC cusp. In the NC sinus, the suturing plane should be intentionally elevated by 1–2 mm, but care must be taken to follow the annular line (and not to create a straight line). It was also suggested to begin suturing the NC sinus by applying only the first 2–3 stitches on each side, in order to assure tension-free seating of the prosthesis on a nonwrinkled aortic sinus under perfect exposure, and then to continue with the right and left sinus, and finally complete the NC sinus suture line. In our opinion, the key is to perform correct and tension-free sutures comfortably, regardless of the sequence. We have made it routine to check for folding and leaks with a small instrument (nerve hook). Additional stitches to correct for folding or suspected leaks can be made through the prosthesis and with the knot tied outside the aorta.

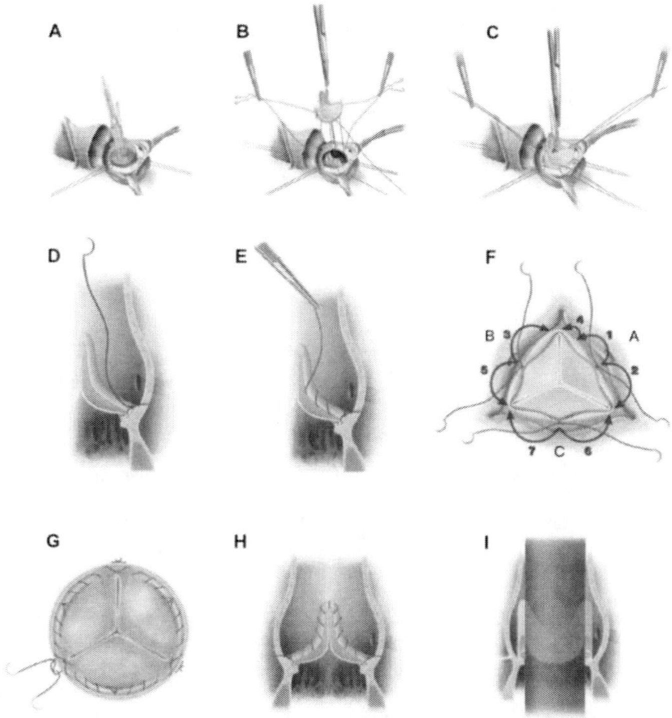

Notes: (A) Transverse aortotomy, 3 string sutures at the level of the commissures and sizing. (B) The first three stitches are passed at the nadir of each sinus and through the pericardial rim of the tissue valve. (C) The valve is parachuted down into the aortic anulus. (D) The first stitch is demonstrated at the nadir of the sinus. (E) The continuous suture is performed in direction of the commissure. (F) This picture demonstrates the sequence of suturing the tissue valve. Starting below the right coronary artery and moving to both commissures (1, 2, and 4) then below the left coronary artery (3 and 5) and finally suturing the non-coronary leaflet at the end (6 and 7). A, right-coronary cusp; B, left-coronary cusp; C, non-coronary cusp. (G) Tying of the sutures is performed outside the aorta at the level of the three commissures. (H) Final view of the supraanular, subcoronary continuous suture line from inside the aorta. (I) Final view from outside the aorta with demonstration of a maximized central and homogeneous flow through the valve.

Reprinted from Stanger O, Tevaerarai H, Carrel T. The Freedom SOLO bovine pericardial stentless valve. Res Rep Clin Cardiol. 2014;5:1-13.

Figure 1. Implantation technique of the Freedom SOLO stentless valve.

Sutureless and Rapid Deployment Prostheses

We describe these two new technologies in Chapter 18.

Ross Procedure

- Pulmonary autograft harvesting

Once the decision to replace the aortic valve has been confirmed, a transverse incision is made on the main pulmonary artery (PA) 5 mm proximal to the origin of the right PA. The pulmonary valve is inspected and will be used only if it has a normal-appearing trileaflet configuration with no major fenestrations. The PA is transected and freed from the aortic root down to the right ventricular muscle. Using a right-angle clamp through the pulmonary valve, the right ventricle is poked approximately 5 mm below the nadir of the non-facing cusp. The pulmonary root is then carefully harvested, leaving no more than 5 mm of infundibular muscle under the insertion line of the leaflets. By staying close to the leaflets, injury to the first septal artery is greatly minimized. After harvesting the pulmonary autograft, the infundibular muscle is trimmed leaving 2 mm below the insertion of the cusps and cut 2–3 mm above the level of the STJ to avoid exposing the PA to systemic pressures.

- Pulmonary autograft implantation

As with stentless roots, both total root replacement and subcoronary implantation techniques can be used. We favor the total root technique. The autograft is implanted in a sub-annular position using single interrupted 4-0 polypropylene sutures, while ensuring symmetrical spatial distribution of the commissures. Distal autograft anastomosis to native aorta or Dacron graft is performed using 5-0 polypropylene sutures. The coronary buttons are reimplanted in their corresponding sinuses using 6-0 polypropylene sutures. If the aortic annulus is more than 2 mm larger than the pulmonary annulus, an extra-aortic ring annuloplasty is performed to educe the size of the native aortic annulus. The coronary ostia are anastomosed to their respective sinuses. Following surgery, strict blood pressure control is immediately instituted and maintained for the first 6–12 months to allow adaptive remodeling of the autograft. Maximum target sys- tolic blood pressure should be 100–110 mmHg.

- Pulmonary homograft implantation

The largest pulmonary homograft available is always used to replace the pulmonary root (28–30 mm), irrespective of the original pulmonary annulus diameter. Proximal and distal implantation is made with a standard running suture. Care is taken to avoid purse-stringing the distal suture line between the pulmonary homograft and the main PA.

Aortotomy Closure and De-airing

The aorta is closed using a running 4-0 polypropylene suture. Before unclamping the aorta, de-airing maneuvers are performed. The left ventricular vent is stopped, Valsalva maneuvers are initiated, and root suction is started while manually shaking the heart to dislodge air bubbles from the left-sided chambers. The cross-clamp is then removed. If residual air is observed on transesophageal echocardiography, suction on the aortic root is continued until it can no longer be observed.

MINIMALLY INVASIVE TREATMENT

Principles and Advantages

The main principle of minimally invasive surgery (MIS) AVR surgery is to perform a safe and effective aortic valve procedure, without an increase in complication rates. The key to this goal is a well-planned approach that will lead to good exposure of the aortic valve. Speed of the procedure should not be the primary concern of the surgeon, particularly early in his/her experience. The increased operative times associated with MIS are not clinically relevant in the majority of patients requiring isolated AVR surgery. Although a definite learning curve exists for MIS AVR surgery, it is less than for many other cardiac operations (e.g., MIS mitral valve surgery, complex aortic procedures, high-risk reoperative surgery). In addition, improvements in low- and high-fidelity surgical models, increased surgical mentoring, and establishment of peer-to-peer MIS learning centers should help mitigate the learning curve effect for future cardiac surgeons. Several lines of evidence justify the performance of MIS AVR surgery. As stated above, several studies have demonstrated clinical benefits associated with this operation. A meta-analysis of 4667 patients demonstrated a statistically significant reduction in ventilation time, blood loss, ICU stay, supraventricular arrhythmia rate, hospital stay, and early mortality rate in patients undergoing MIS AVR procedures [1]. However, myocardial ischemic and CPB times were longer in the MIS group, with an average of 9 and 11 minutes, respectively. A large retrospective study from Leipzig also suggested improved long-term survival in propensity-matched MIS AVR patients, although the mechanism behind this observation is unclear [2]. Several other reasons may justify the performance of MIS AVR surgery.

- Some studies have demonstrated additional clinical benefits other than those listed above, including decreased transfusion rates, decreased pain, decreased sternal infection rate, better quality of life, and shortened return to work times.
- The history of cardiovascular interventional medicine demonstrates that patients prefer less invasive procedures. Increased acceptance by patients and their family members may result in better psychological preparation for their cardiac operation, as well as increased motivation for a faster postoperative recovery.
- The decreased surgical exposure (particularly of the right atrium and ventricle) leads to decreased postoperative adhesions and easier re-entry in the case of future reoperation.
- The additional technical skills that surgeons acquire during MIS AVR surgery are similar to those required for many other types of less invasive cardiovascular interventions, which are likely to increase in number in the future.

- Establishment of a successful MIS program may result in increased patient referrals and increased recognition from referring cardiologists and surgical peers.

Preoperative Assessment and Preparation

Preoperative assessment for patients undergoing a MIS AVR procedure is similar to that for all patients undergoing AVR surgery including transthoracic echocardiography (TTE), chest X-ray (CXR), routine blood work, and cardiac catheterization for patients. Thoracic computed tomography (CT) scan without contrast medium injection is a routine preoperative screening facility in our department before AVR to choose the appropriate surgical approach for the patient. In the last 3 years, we prefer CT scan with contrast to better evaluate the characteristics of the native valve and to measure the aortic annulus. Generally, relative dextraposition of the ascending aorta (at least 50% of the calliper beyond the right parasternal line in the right part of the thorax at the level of the pulmonary trunk bifurcation) and moderate profoundness of the aortic root (not >10 cm from skin to the aortic valve annulus) provide optimal surgical exposure for the right minithoracotomy. Otherwise, the patient is eligible for upper ministernotomy or full midline sternotomy. However, thanks to technical feasibility of sutureless and rapid deployment valves implantation, these criteria are of relative importance now. Exclusion criteria for right anterior minithoracotomy approach were severe thorax deformities, right pleural cavity adhesions, severe COPD complicated by emphysema, or technical impossibility for peripheral percutaneous venous cannulation.

Anesthesia

A single lumen endotracheal tube is sufficient for both of the most common MIS AVR approaches (i.e., ministernotomy and right anterior minithoracotomy). If the lung interferes with exposure during the minithoracotomy approach, then a moist sponge placed in the right pleura will suce. Endocavitary wires for temporary pacemaker are inserted in internal jugular vein. Some surgeons request that the anesthesiologist insert a percutaneous retrograde cardioplegia catheter in the coronary sinus prior to starting the procedure, but we find this to be unnecessary and cumbersome. We prefer antegrade cardioplegia via the aortic root or coronary ostia. Patients can be extubated according to institutional protocol.

Ministernotomy: Surgical Technique

A skin incision 6–8 cm in length is made starting 1–2 cm above the sternal manubrium junction and extending 5–7 cm toward the xiphoid. The incision is continued from the skin down to the sternum with electrocautery. The sternal saw is used to divide the sternum midline from the sternal notch to the level of the third intercostal space. Division of the sternum is then either continued as a "J" or "T" to the third intercostal space. Four pericardial stay sutures are placed at the four "corners" of the incision, then pulled up with force in order to bring the mediastinal structures closer to the skin. We prefer percutaneous cannulation of the femoral vein under echocardiographic guidance (Figure 2).

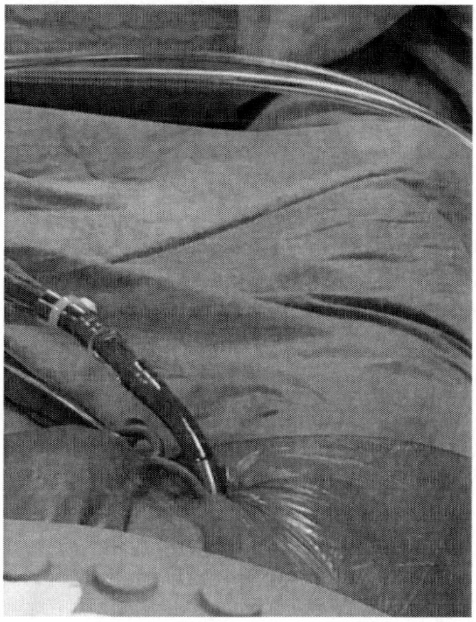

Figure 2. Percutaneous femoral vein cannulation.

A Finochietto retractor is inserted and pericardial stay sutures are placed. Percutaneous femoral venous cannulation has the advantage of completely eliminating the cannula from the surgical field, but risks the complications of peripheral cannulation (i.e., injury to the deep venous structures or local groin complications). Once CPB has been initiated, venous drainage is assisted with vacuum pressure. In our experience, the total negative pressure is maintained at no greater than -40 mmHg. Aortic cannulation is performed in the standard manner.

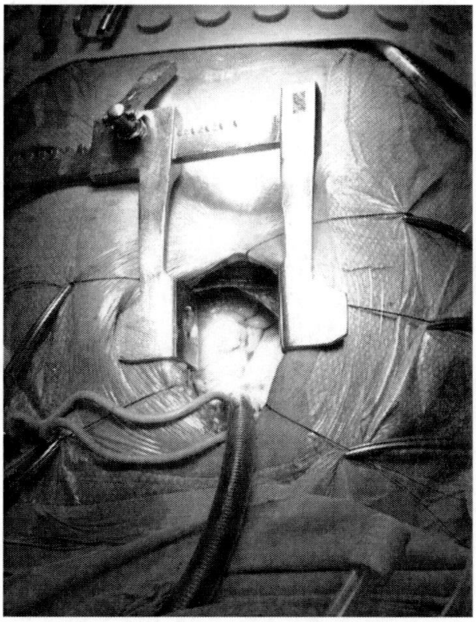

Figure 3. Ascending aorta cannulation.

Since vacuum-assisted cardiopulmonary bypass was established, a left ventricular vent was placed through the right superior pulmonary vein. A needle vent is used for administering antegrade cardioplegia, as well as to assist in de-airing the heart at the conclusion of the case. We do not use retrograde cardioplegia because of difficulties in positioning the catheter via the MIS approach, as well as obscuring of the operative field from blood that runs out of the coronary ostia. The ascending aorta was clamped with the Cygnet cross-clamp (Novare Surgical Systems, Cupertino, California). We prefer to administer normothermic blood cardioplegia or cold crystalloid solution (Custodiol Koehler Chemie, Alsbach-Haenlein, Germany).

Transverse aortotomy was performed approximately 2 cm above the commissures and aortic valve was inspected. The aortic valve leaflets were totally excised and the aortic annulus decalcified. Three stay sutures may be placed at the top of each commissure in order to improve valve exposure. Annular non-everting pledgeted mattress sutures are placed in a standard fashion, with the pledgets on the ventricular side of the annulus for the bioprosthesis or on the aorta side of the annulus for the mechanical prosthesis. The valve prosthesis is lowered into place. Once the valve sutures have been tied, the coronary ostia are checked to ensure patency. The space between the annulus and the sewing ring is also probed circumferentially, in order to assess for a possible paravalvular leak. The use of sutureless aortic valves and automatic knotting devices may simplify these stages of the procedure. The aortotomy is closed with a single layer using a 4-0 polypropylene suture. Prior to removal of the aortic cross-clamp, de-airing techniques are performed. The heart is filled with venous blood, the left ventricle is compressed and the lungs are inflated with sustained positive pressure. In addition, manual compression over the left ventricular apex may be applied externally. The left ventricular vent is stopped prior to these maneuvers, and the needle vent is applied to high suction immediately prior to opening of the cross-clamp. The left ventricular vent is applied to gentle suction following cross-clamp removal. Once the aortic cross clamp is removed, intracavitary air is assessed by transesophageal echocardiography (TEE). Chest tube should be placed when the right ventricle while it is completely decompressed, prior to coming off CPB. When TEE confirms adequate de-airing of the left ventricle, the patient is weaned from CPB in a standard fashion. Once surgical hemostasis has been confirmed, protamine is administered. The sternum is closed with sternal wires. The skin and subcutaneous tissue are closed using a standard technique.

Right Anterior Minitoracothomy: Surgical Technique

RAMT was performed through an incision (5-6 cm) in the second intercostal space. In patients with associated mitral and tricuspid procedures, third intercostal space anterior minithoracotomy was preferred. The soft tissue retractor are used to open the working field. A Finochietto retractor is inserted and pericardial stay sutures are placed. Some surgeons prefer detache third rib. Direct aortic cannulation was performed using low-profile cannulas. Venous drainage was achieved with a variety of percutaneous venous cannulas inserted through the femoral vein into the venae cavae. The correct placement of the venous cannula was obtained using the Seldinger technique under transoesophageal echocardiographic guidance. Vacuum-assisted venous drainage can facilitate venous return. Since vacuum-assisted cardiopulmonary bypass was established, a left ventricular vent was placed through the right superior pulmonary vein, and the patients were cooled down to 34 or 35°C. The ascending aorta was clamped with the Cygnet cross-clamp (Novare Surgical Systems, Cupertino, California).

Antegrade cardioplegic solution was given into the aortic root or selectively into the coronary ostia using normothermic blood cardioplegia or cold crystalloid solution. In all cases of RAMT, the surgical field was flooded with carbon dioxide at a flow of 0.5–1.0 l/min. The procedures of decalcification and prosthesis implantation are the same as for ministernotomy and full sternotomy. At the end of RAMT procedure, we prefer juxtaposed the second (or third, in case of mutliple procedures) intercostal space with non-absorbable stitches. The skin and subcutaneous tissue are closed using a standard technique (Figure 4).

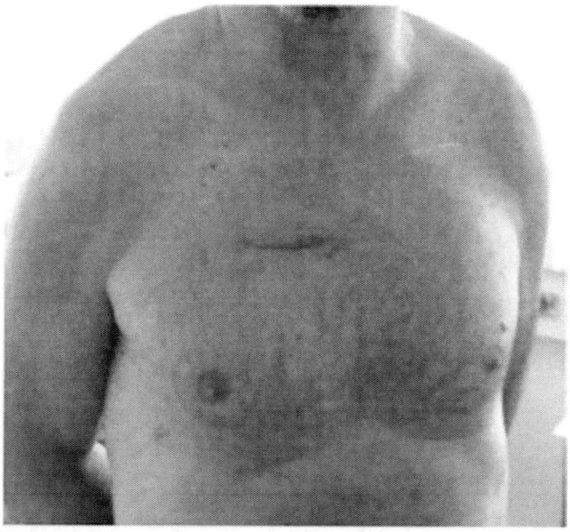

Figure 4. Final result of RAMT approach.

OUTCOMES IN MINIMALLY INVASIVE AORTIC SURGERY

The evidence to date shows that MIS AVR can be performed safely and effectively and is associated with several clinical advantages. Potential drawbacks of MIS AVR, however, include increased operative, bypass, and cross-clamp times, particularly during the early portion of the surgeon's experience. Multiple studies have compared outcomes of conventional versus MIS AVR in a prospective and retrospective fashion. Doll et al. [3] retrospectively compared 175 patients who underwent MIS AVR to 258 patients who underwent conventional AVR via full sternotomy. Patients who underwent MIS AVR had decreased morbidity and mortality, lower incidence of respiratory failure, shorter ICU and hospital length of stay, and less transfusion requirements at the expense of slightly longer cross-clamp time (5 minutes) and operating room time (14 minutes), but no significant difference in CPB time. Patient selection bias limits the interpretation of such retrospective studies, but subsequent small, randomized controlled trials have largely confirmed their results. A large, single-center study by Tabata et al. [4] involving 1005 patients showed excellent short-term and long-term outcomes for MIS AVR out to 11 years postoperatively. Of note, this study also included 130 patients (13%) who underwent reoperative AVR and 62 patients (6%) who had concomitant ascending aortic surgery, highlighting the potential for this technique in more complex procedures. The authors achieved excellent results with a median length of stay of 6 days, operative mortality rate of 1.9%, and reoperation for bleeding rate of 2.4%. In addition, pneumonia was observed in only 1.3% of patients and deep sternal wound infection in 0.5%. Also notable was a significant decrease in CPB time, incidence of bleeding, and operative mortality over time, confirming the presence of a learning curve associated with this approach. Bakir et al. [5] also reviewed their results of 506 patients who underwent MIS AVR compared to conventional AVR and found that the MIS patients had shorter cross-clamp and CPB times, less blood loss, and shorter hospital stay. Similarly, Glauber et al. [6] used propensity matching to compare their results of 192 MIS AVR patients (using a right anterior minithoracotomy approach) to patients undergoing conventional AVR. The MIS patients had a lower incidence of atrial fibrillation and blood transfusions, shorter ventilation duration, shorter length of stay, and no difference in mortality. A recent large propensity-matched study by Merk et al. [2] compared 479 MIS AVR patients to matched controls. MIS patients had better medium-term survival compared to matched conventional AVR patients (5-year survival 89.3 ± 2.4% vs 77.7 ± 4.7%) with a hazards ratio of 0.47 on Cox-regression analysis. The study also demonstrated less bleeding in MIS patients while cross-clamp times were slightly longer (3 minutes), similar to the results of previous studies. Few randomized controlled trials examining MIS AVR compared to conventional approach exist to date. However, Bonacchi et al. [7] randomized a total of 80 patients to the two techniques and demonstrated no significant differences in CPB or cross-clamp times between groups but longer total operating time in the MIS patients. MIS patients also had fewer transfusions, shorter ventilation times, decreased pain at 1 hour and 12 hours postoperatively, and better lung function 5 days postoperatively. Machler et al. [8] randomized 120 patients to MIS or conventional AVR and showed no difference in cross-clamp, CPB, or operating times. However, MIS AVR patients had shorter ventilation times, less blood loss, and less analgesic use. A meta-analysis by Murtuza et al. from 2008 [1] showed marginal benefits in perioperative mortality (odds ratio, OR, 0.72 [range: 0.51–1.0], $p = 0.05$), but statistically significant shorter ICU and lengths of hospital stay, decreased ventilation duration, and decreased transfusion requirements, at the potential expense of longer cross-clamp, CPB, and total operating times in MIS AVR patients.

In conclusion, MIS AVR surgery is associated with an improved survival, cosmetic result and decreased bleeding, pain, and ICU/hospital length of stay, but it is associated with longer cross-clamp and CPB times. In the last years, new technologies (Sutureless and Rapid Deployments) have limited significantly ACC and CPB times (We discusse this aspect in Chapter 18). Although MIS AVR can be performed safely, a learning curve exists and surgeons should be aware of potential pitfalls in both patient selection and operative techniques.

References

[1] Murtuza B, Pepper JR, Stanbridge RD, et al. Minimal access aortic valve replacement: is it worth it? *Ann Thorac Surg*. 2008; 85: 1121–31.

[2] Merk DR, Lehmann S, Holzhey DM, et al. Minimal invasive aortic valve replacement surgery is associated with improved survival: a propensity-matched comparison. *Eur J Cardiothorac Surg*. 2015; 47(1): 11–17.

[3] Doll N, Borger MA, Hain J, et al. Minimal access aortic valve replacement: effects on morbidity and resource utilization. *Ann Thorac Surg*. 2002; 74(4): S1318–22.

[4] Tabata M, Umakanthan R, Cohn LH, et al. Early and late outcomes of 1000 minimally invasive aortic valve operations. *Eur J Cardiothorac Surg*. 2008; 33: 537–41.

[5] Bakir I, Casselman FP, Wellens F, et al. Minimally invasive versus standard approach aortic valve replacement: A study in 506 patients. *Ann Thorac Surg*. 2006; 81: 1599–604.

[6] Glauber M, Miceli A, Gilmanov D, et al. Right anterior minithoracotomy versus conventional aortic valve replacement: A propensity score matched study. *J Thorac Cardiovasc Surg*. 2013; 145: 1222–6.

[7] Bonacchi M, Prifti E, Giunti G, et al. Does ministernotomy improve postoperative outcome in aortic valve operation? A prospective randomized study. *Ann Thorac Surg*. 2002; 73: 460–5.

[8] Machler HE, Bergmann P, Anelli-Monti M, et al. Minimally invasive versus conventional aortic valve operations: aprospective study in 120 patients. *Ann Thorac Surg*. 1999; 67: 1001–5.

In: Perspectives in Aortic Valve Disease
Editor: Giovanni Concistrè
ISBN: 978-1-53618-769-4

Chapter 15

TOTALLY ENDOSCOPIC AORTIC VALVE REPLACEMENT (EAVR)

Tommaso Hinna Danesi*, MD
Department of Cardiac Surgery, Osp. San Bortolo, Vicenza, Italia

ABSTRACT

In the last 15 years minimally invasive approach in cardiac surgery (MICS) become a strong reality involving valvular and revascularization surgery. A variety of different surgical approaches are described as minimally invasive, but may be be substantially different one from another.

The trend of wound's reduction requires the application of the thoracoscope in order to perform surgery under indirect vision; this is the era of endoscopic minimally invasive cardiac surgery (Endoscopic MICS) or cardiac endoscopy.

Performing surgery using videoscopy and long shaft instruments requires specific skills and a wide expertise in other endoscopic surgeries such as mitral valve one should be a pivotal startup.

All aspects of cardiac surgery are involved in this innovative procedure, including the anesthesiological and cardio-pulmonary bypass setups.

Keywords: MICS, minimally invasive cardiac surgery, endoscopic cardiac surgery, cardiac endoscopy, aortic valve replacement

INTRODUCTION

Over the past 15 years, minimally invasive cardiac surgery (MICS) has been increasingly adopted especially with mitral valve surgery. Minimally invasive approach for the aortic valve was often represented by mini-sternotomy.

* Corresponding Author's Email: tommasohinnadanesi@gmail.com.

The MICS growth was driven by the desire to translate the benefits observed in other surgery specialties, such as decreased pain, reduced surgical trauma, faster recovery and meeting the patient's needs to cardiac surgery.

The complexity of performing operations through a small incision, a reduced operating field with no dedicated technologies, rudimentary minimally invasive instruments and the compelling need of avoiding longer cross clamp time mitigated the initial enthusiasm.

However, innovation in perfusion techniques and devices, the devolpement of dedicated surgical instruments and the availability of fast implanting bioprosthesis has made the way to establish endoscopic MICS the standard of care in high volume centers in the current era.

MICS over a long period has undergone several changes with regard to techniques and philosophy making it easier and reproducible, with surgical results comparable to the conventional surgical approach.

In this chapter aortic valve replacement in an endoscopic fashion will be explored referring to a surgery performed in a totally endoscopic under indirect vision where the use of a thoracoscope is mandatory.

Minimally Invasive Concept

MICS and Endoscopic MICS

Figure 1 shows a right anterior thoracotomy (RAT) in which the divarication of the ribs provides a large operative field and surgery can be performed under direct vision.

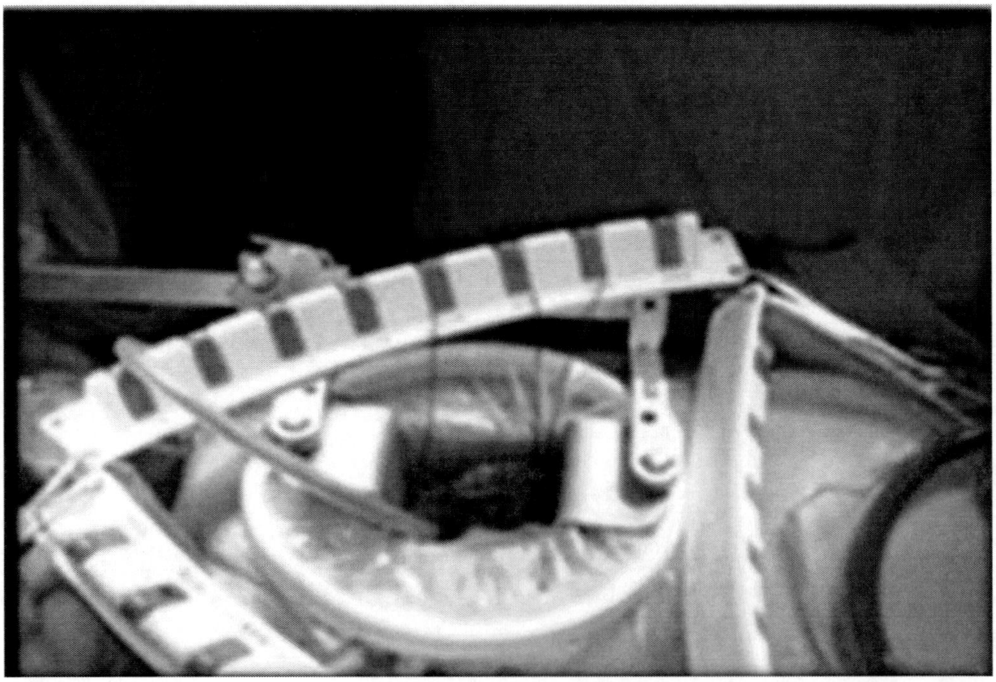

Figure 1. RAT in direct vision.

There are several interpretations of minimally invasive concepts as shown in Figures 1, 2, 3.

Figures 2 and 3 show a minimally invasive RAT (MRAT). Both approaches are intended as minimally invasive but there are several differences. First of all in MRAT the thoracoscope is mandatory to perform surgery, otherwise the reduction of the skin incision does not allow to preserve the natural stereo-vision of the operator and often the aortic valve should not be directly visualized.

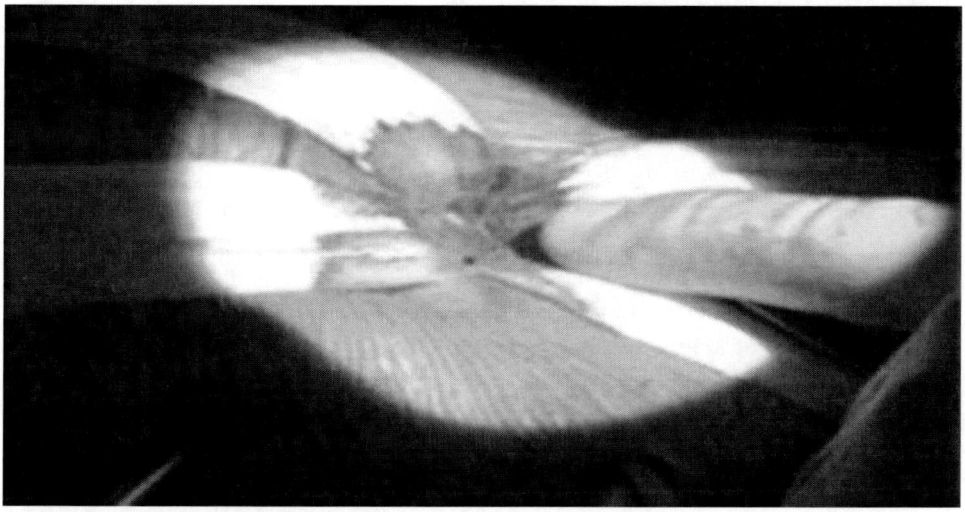

Figure 2. MRAT in thoracoscopic vision.

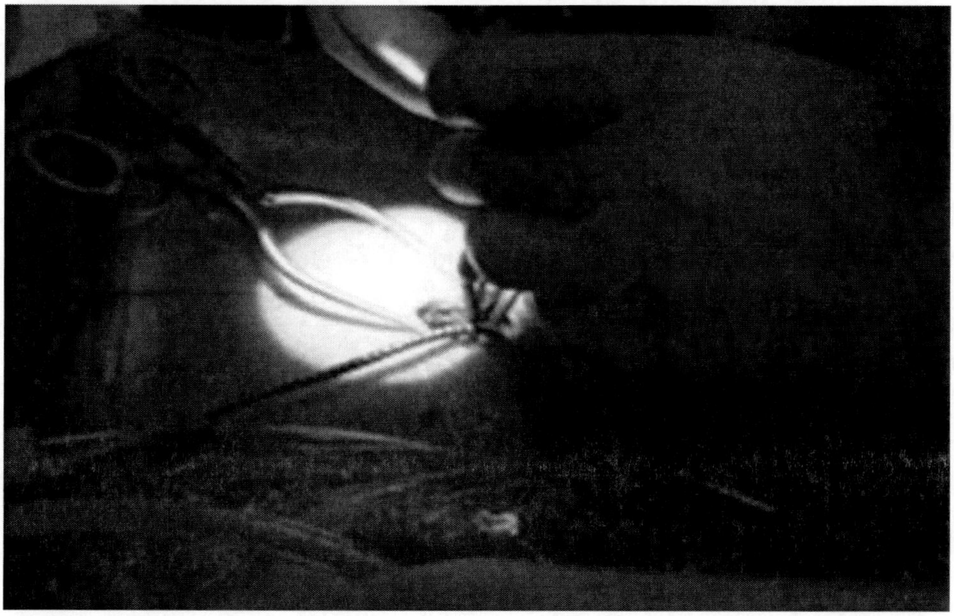

Figure 3. MRAT in thoracoscopic vision.

The chapter will discuss only surgery performed trough MRAT in which the small skin incision serves only to introduce the endoscopic surgical instruments, the plegia/root venting line and the prosthetic valve.

This access is done without any rib spreading just wit the aid of soft tissue retractor and any sacrifice of right mammary artery or cutting rib. The use of thoracoscope wit indirect vision, the miniaturized skin incision, no rib spreading, dislocation or cutting and no right mammary artery sacrifice are fundamental characteristics of endoscopic aortic valve MICS.

Rib spreading leads to postoperative pain ignoring one of the principles of endoscopic MICS which is pain avoidance.

General Considerations

From the Society of Thoracic Surgery database (STS database), a minimally invasive valve surgery is defined as the one not performed with a full sternotomy and with a CPB support [1]. According to Chitwood et al., [2] MICS should not be defined in term of a specific procedure, but rather a philosophy that requires an operation-specific strategy. Each minimally invasive strategy introduces alternatives for CPB cannulation (central or peripheral), aortic occlusion (endovascular or external trasnthoracic i.e., in mitral valve surgery) and cardioplegia delivery (antegrade, atrial retrograde or transjugular retrograde) [2-3]. The concept of avoiding a full sternotomy translates into a wide range of surgical procedures in which a partial sternotomy and a full length right thoracotomy are both considered minimally invasive surgery.

Preoperative assessment of aortic patient candidates to MICS surgery is still debated, i.e., several centers consider a full aortic CT scan mandatory to assess the feasibility of fem-fem cannulation. While in mitralic patients in which 60 t0 70% of mitral valve pathology is due to degenerative disease and the average age of them is quite low a preoperative CT scan could be considered useful to detect ascending aorta calcification affecting aortic cross clamp as well as prediction of peripheral cannulation-related complications [4] in aortic population a preoperative CT scan should be routinely performed.

Anesthesiological setup is not very different from conventional cardiac surgery. Although double lumen endo-tracheal intubation is widespread this often is not mandatory. A retrospective study on 96 patients from Kim et al., who underwent MICS procedure using a single lumen tube or double lumen tube did not show any difference in ICU stay of failure in fast track protocols [5].

Double lumen tube should be considered for patients with previous sternotomy and is mandatory in redo patient with a previous right thoracotomy or a right lung procedure i.e., pleurodesis or chest tube insertion.

Central venous cannulation can be achieved through either the right or the left internal jugular veins. the right subclavian vein should be generally spread because is proximal to the insertion site of the Chitwood clamp which is placed in the 1st or the 2nd intercostal space (ICS).

The right internal jugular vein may be also necessary for double venous CPB drainage in case of elevated BMI patients or in redo cases.

Cannulation techniques for MICS have constantly evolved over the past few years; until 2010 cannulation strategies evolved in our experience to favor peripheral femoral cannulation over central ascending aorta one. [6] Percutaneous or surgical dual stages bicaval venous drainage over a percutaneous adjunctive neck access and direct external aortic cross clamp with Chitwood clamp.

Currently, the most common aortic valve minimally invasive approach is PortAccess through RAT or MRAT, depending on the center preference or experience (direct or indirect vision). Because our large experience with endoscopic Mitral Valve surgery and this endoscopic approach is more attractive for both patients and surgeons we translate our knowledge in the setting of aortic surgery.

Patient Selection and Preoperative Assessment for EAVR

In an experienced MICS center used to completely thoracoscopic surgery no Patient selection is needed. The endoscopic indirect vision surgery is not affected by the position of the aorta (several Centers needs a more than 50% of dextroposition of the aorta respect the right margin-sternal line) [7].

The habitus of the Patient do not affect the surgical access because once the thoracoscope is positioned in the right way every mediastinal structure is easily accessible.

Moving to a full video guided surgical procedure, no specific preoperative assessment is needed. For medical and legal reasons a CT scan or Echo Color Doppler of groin's vascular axis can be made. It can be reasonable considering that aortic population is older than mitral one and may present some vascular comorbidities such as aortopathy or lower limb atherosclerosis precluding a safe aortic cross clamp or retrograde perfusion.

Once the endoscopic skills are well acquired a Patient undergoing to EAVR could follow the same path of other standard surgery candidates.

Operating Theatre Setup and Patient Positioning

EAVR does not need any specific setup except for the videocoloumn and the CO" insufflator connected to the thoracoscope trocar. [8]

The patient must lay supine with an elevation of 30 to 40° of the right hemithorax. It can be useful the use of an inflating pillet that can be deflated in case of need to convert the procedure into a full sternotomy.

Surgical Access

In endoscopic aortic valve replacement surgery (EAVR), the choice of the skin incision and the ICS in the MRAT is crucial, in order to achieve a comfortable surgical procedure.Usually the 2nd ICS is entered through a prepectoral skin incision performed above the 3rd rib extended for 2 to 4 cm laterally from the midclavicular line. This is the "Working

Port." The incision over the 3rd rib easily allow to access the 3rd ICS in case the 2nd results too high for a short ascending aorta.

The incorrect ICS or a very medial MRAT can result in an uncomfortable setup and may lead to a more invasive needs such as rib dislocation, cutting or right mammary artery sacrifice to improve the rib spreading and the operating field. If the chosen ICS is too high the approaching angle, may be very uncomfortable making difficult any maneuver on the aortic valve. There are not differences preparing men and women.

It is preferable to enter the ICS more laterally in order to achieve a better divarication of the ribs which are more fix close to the sternum.

A soft tissue retractor is needed, it allows to gently increase the working port. Other two 5 mm incisions are needed: one in the 2nd or 1 st ICS laterally to the midclavicular line to introduce the aortic clamp and one in the 3rd i.s. at the level of the anterior axillary line to introduce the ventricular vent-line. These are the "Mini-Ports."

Cardiopulmonary Bypass

The small Working Port doesn't allow direct aortic and right atrial cannulation may be difficult and can steal lot of space of operating field. The CPB is instituted through femoral vessels. Is mandatory to check the position of the venous guidewire into the superior vena cava with TEE to avoid any atriocaval junction injury or malpositioning of the cannula resulting in an inappropriate venous drainage.

The usage of the vacuum assisted venous drainage is mandatory. The vacuum should not exceed -60 mmHg into the venous reservoir to avoid RBCs damage [9].

In large Patients (BSA > 1.9 m2) an additional venous drainage cannula can be considered. Usually a 14 fr. cannula inserted into the right internal jugular vein is enough [10].

Aortic Cross Clamping, Cardioplegia and Ventricular Venting

Aortic cross clamp is obtained using a Chitwood clamp, other clamps can be used too i.e., Cygnet and Glauber MIS clamps. Once the CPB has been instituted is mandatory to obtain a gentle dissection of the transverse sinus to allow the aortic cross clamp as distal as possible and avoiding any injury of the right branch of the pulmonary artery that may result in an emergency conversion to full sternotomy.

As for mitral valve endoscopic surgery a root needle is putted in place and the cardioplegia is delivered. Custodiol or Bretschneider cardioplegic solutions may be a valid option giving lot of time free from adjunctive doses. If aortic regurgitation is present the first shot may be delivered into the root and then the dose completed directly into the coronary ostia.

Unfortunately the Working Port is too small to allow the positioning of a retroplegia catheter, if desired additional neckline such as Propledge (Edwards Lifescience, Irvine CA) can be used.

The left ventricle is vented as usual through the superior right pulmonary vein and the sump is passed through the 5 mm mini-port inte the 3rd I.S. Putting in place the purse string and the tourniquet at this time may steel some operating field space making the Working Port uncomfortable. If desired a percutaneous ventline can be used (Endovent by Edwards Lifescience, Irvine, CA).

Aortic Valve Access in Endoscopic Surgery

The 30° thoracoscope is essential and provides a magnified surgical view and allows to navigate the mediastinum accessing alla cardiac structures involved in the operation; sometimes the visualization results better than in standard surgery i.e., pulmonary veins and Sondergaard groove.

Many attention must be paid to the aortotomy, in general concepts we must consider that median structures toward the pulmonary artery are very difficult to reach from a right sided access.

A good strategy should be to remove accurately the pleuro-pericardial fat, identify the phrenic nerve to avoid any injury and then open the pericardium. This maneuver should be attempted once the patient is on CPB in order to avoid any right atrium injury.

Once the pericardium has been opened our goal is to pull the target structures towards us reducing the distance. Pericardial retraction stitches should be placed in order to achieve this goal. Usually three stitches are enough to expose the aorta and the Sondergaard groove.

The aortotomy should be made considering the prosthetic valve chosen; a 3 to 3.5 cm high aortotomy should be mad in case of sutureless valve implantation meanwhile a standard J stick or italic S incision can be performed for standard stented or rapid deployment valves.

Surgical Technique

Aortotomy

Aortotomy is made the right on possible avoiding any extension or tear towards the pulmonary artery. This zone is very difficult to manage once the aorta has been declamped in case of bleeding.

Three to four suspension stitches can be placed in order to maximize the exposition of the aortic valve.

One stitch should be placed on the distal part of the ascending aorta and secured to the pericardium avoiding any interference with the operating field by the distal stump of the aorta. Other two or three stitches can be placed in order to open wide the aortic root and achieve a better exposition of the aortic valve; we have to consider that just one Surgeon can act into the operating field.

Aortic Valve Replacement (AVR)

The aortic valve is normally excised and the annulus decalcified. The technique for AVR implantation depends on the chosen prosthesis. If a standard biological or mechanical prosthesis is chosen a standard technique of implantation can be adopted (2-0 polyester suture with subannular pledgets); in case of Rapid deployment valve implantation three 2-0 polyester suture are required. Considering the small working space check with the thoracoscope the correct position of the three tourniquets required for the implantation of these kind of bioprosthesis; in some cases (discrepancy between non coronary sinus and right/left coronary sinuses) we used to secure rapid deployment valves with at least six 2-0 polyester stitches. This technique increase the safety of a correct valve positioning considering that the Working Port do not allow rude manipulation of the bioprosthesis such as hard pushing into the annulus and allows or hard pulling of the stitches that may lead to an annular damage.

If a sutureless bioprosthesis is chosen the thoracoscope allows to easily check the correct positioning of the valve. Once the bioprosthesis has been released as a tip we suggest to introduce the thoracoscope into the ventricle to check its correct positioning.

Aortorrhaphy

Start from the medial part of the aortotomy paying attention to that zone.

Deairing

EAVR does not allow an efficient deiaring as well as in standard sternotomic surgery, but continuous CO_2 inflation during the procedure significantly reduces gaseous emboli.

Electrodes

The small Working Port does not allow to easily reach a safe landing zone for the pacing wire. This must be placed when the heart is empty because once the heart has been filled is no longer possible to expose the right ventricle. If desired consider an endocavitary temporary pacing.

Drainages

Two small 24 fr flexible silastic drains are enough to maintain an efficient drainage of the chest. They can be passed through the miniports used to place te ventline and the clamp or the thoracoscope.

Conclusion

In conclusion EAVR is a safe, reproducible and appealing technique. Many attention must be paid at the beginning in order to avoid failure which may leads to a minimally invasive program stop. A large experience in minimally-invasive and endoscopic mitral valve surgery may represent a must do to approach a safe EAVR.

A strong standardization of the procedure plays a key role in a successful Endoscopic Cardiac Surgery Program.

References

[1] Durham NC. Executive Summary. *STS National Database* 2003.

[2] Chitwood WR Jr, Gulielmos V. *What is minimally invasive cardiac surgery?* CTSnet.org. Accessed June 22, 2010.

[3] Felger JE, Nifong LW, Chitwood WR Jr. The evolution of and early experience with robot-assisted mitral valve surgery. *Surg. Laparosc. Endosc. Percutan. Tech.* 2002;12:58-63.

[4] Enriquez-Sarano M, Akins CW, Vahanian A. Mitral regurgitation. *Lancet* 2009;373:1382-94.

[5] Kim HY, Baek SH, Je HG, Kim TK, Kim HJ, Ahn JH, Park SJ. Comparison of the single-lumen endotracheal tube and double-lumen endobronchial tube used in minimally invasive cardiac surgery for the fast track protocol. *J. Thorac. Dis.* 2016;8(5):778-83.

[6] Chan EY1, Lumbao DM, Iribarne A, Easterwood R, Yang JY, Cheema FH, Smith CR, Argenziano M. Evolution of cannulation techniques for minimally invasive cardiac surgery: a 10-year journey. *Innovations* (Phila) 2012;7(1):9-14.

[7] A. Miceli, M. Murzi, D. Gilmanov, R. Fuga,' M. Ferrarini, M. Solinas, et al. Minimally invasive aortic valve replacement using right minithoracotomy is associated with better outcomes than ministernotomy. *J. Thorac. Cardiovasc. Surg.*, 148 (2014), pp. 133-137.

[8] Svensson LG1, D'Agostino RS "J" incision minimal-access valve operations. *Ann. Thorac. Surg.* 1998 Sep;66(3):1110-2.

[9] Colangelo N1, Torracca L, Lapenna E, Moriggia S, Crescenzi G, Alfieri O. Vacuum-assisted venous drainage in extrathoracic cardiopulmonary bypass management during minimally invasive cardiac surgery. *Perfusion.* 2006 Nov;21(6):361-5.

[10] UpToDate: *Obesity in adults: Prevalence, screening and evaluation.* Retrieved on 7/18/17 from https://www.uptodate.com/contents/obesity-in-adults-prevalence-screening-and evaluation?source=search_result&search=bmi&selectedTitle=1~150.

In: Perspectives in Aortic Valve Disease
Editor: Giovanni Concistrè
ISBN: 978-1-53618-769-4

Chapter 16

REDO SURGERY FOR AORTIC VALVE: DEMOGRAPHICS AND OPERATIVE OPTIONS

Antonio Miceli[1,*], MD, PhD and Mattia Glauber[1], MD
[1]Minimally Invasive Cardiac Surgery Department,
Istituto Clinico Sant'Ambrogio,
Gruppo Ospedaliero San Donato, Milan, Italy

ABSTRACT

Redo aortic valve surgery (RVAD) is a challenging procedure and associated with higher intraoperative and postoperative risks compared to first operation. It is technically more demanding than primary operation, because of adhesions and scars around the heart, the risk of iatrogenic injury to cardiovascular structures and the presence of cardiac and non-cardiac morbidities related to aging. These surgical difficulties determine prolonged operative times, which increase the risk of bleeding, transfusion-related morbidity and organ failures [1, 2]. According to EuroSCORE II, patients undergoing redo surgery have 2-fold increased risk of death compared to those undergoing isolated surgery [3].

Historically, mortality rate is high and ranges from 5% to 17% [4-7]. Nevertheless, advancements in cardiac surgery, myocardial protection and alternative surgical strategies have dramatically reduced operative complications, making redo surgery for aortic valve almost safe as primary cardiac surgery, reaching an overall mortality of 4 - 6% [8-10]. An analysis of STS database has shown that compared to primary AVR, RAVR was associated with higher operative mortality (4.6% vs. 2.2%), post-operative stroke (1.9 vs 1.4%), pacemaker requirement (11% vs. 4.3%) and vascular complications (0.06% vs. 0.01%) [11].

Keywords: aortic valve disease, reintervention, conventional aortic surgery, minimally invasive surgery

[*] Corresponding Author's Email: antoniomiceli79@alice.it.

Introduction

The number of patients undergoing repeat surgery is increasing because of aging, improved durability of newer generation tissue valves, and patient's preference for biological valve to avoid long-life anticoagulation. According to Society of Thoracic Surgeons (STS) national database report, the use of bioprostheses increased from 42% in 1996 to 78.4% in 2006 [12].

In addition, the introduction of valve in valve transcatheter aortic valve implantation, as alternative strategy for the treatment of failed bioprostheses, will further increase this percentage. It has been estimated that after AVR, 10% of patients receiving biological valve will require a reoperation within 10 years. After 15 years, this percentage rises up to 30%. As consequence, reoperation for bioprosthetic valve degeneration represents the most common indication for repeated aortic valve replacement [13]. Nevertheless, The incidence of reoperation for mechanical valve is low and amounts < 0.3% per patient-year [14]. Paravalvular leaks, pannus formation and acute thrombosis are the most frequent causes of mechanical valve replacement.

Other indications are prosthetic valve endocarditis, failed valve repair, paravalvular leak. An observational, nationwide, population-based cohort study on 26, 580 patients undergoing aortic valve replacement reports that the overall incidence of prosthetic valve endocarditis (PVE) after AVR is 0.57% per person-year. The risk of PVE is highest during the first year after AVR with 1% per person year; then, the yearly rate of PVE is halved and remains stable during years [15].

Despite not frequent, paravalvular leak (PVL) is the most common nonstructural valve after valve replacement. The annual incidence annual incidence of paravalvular leak ranges between 0.1% and 1.0% per year after aortic valve replacement, whereas the cumulative incidence of PVL recurrence after AVR is was 3%, 14%, and 32%% at 1, 5, and 10 years, respectively. Interestingly, the number of previous surgeries is a predictor PVL recurrence [16].

Last indication for redo AVR is failure of aortic valve repair. Aortic valve repair is a procedure that should not be done in low volume institution on an episodic basis. In this regard, it is difficult to estimate the incidence.

In experienced center, freedom from reoperation can reach 96% after almost 20 years, whereas for bicuspid aortic valve repair freedom from reoperation after 10 years is 90% [17, 18].

In addition to traditional risk factors of EurosCORE II, preoperative intraaortic ballon pump, number of redo operations and previous CABG surgery have been associated with higher risk of in-hospital mortality.

A preoperative score card was created for the preoperative estimation of in-hospital mortality in redo cardiac procedures [19]. Table 1 shows preoperative variables associated with a score point.

The sum of the score for each individual risk factor gives a total score, which assigns a percentage of risk. Six risk categories of in-hospital mortality were identified: 1. Score 0 - 6 mortality risk 0 - 5%; score 6.5 - 10.5 mortality risk 5 - 10%; score 10.5 - 12 mortality risk 10 - 15%; score 12.5 - 14 mortality risk 15 - 20%; score 14.5 - 19 mortality risk 20-40%; > 19 mortality risk >40%) [19].

Table 1. Score for preoperative prediction of in hospital mortality risk [19]

Risk factor	Score
Age (years):	
<60	0
60-69	2
70-79	5
≥80	6
Current procedure:	
Isolated aortic valve or isolated mitral valve	0
Isolated CABG	1
Not isolated CABG, isolated aortic valve, or isolated mitral valve	5
Previous CABG	2
Number of previous sternotomies	
1	0
2	1
3	5
Peripheral vascular disease	2
Renal failure (creatinine>176 µmol/L)	2.5
One or more of the following: Urgent/emergent procedure within 24 h MI within 21 days, Active endocarditis IABP placement	6

CABG = coronary artery bypass grafting; IABP = intraaortic balloon pump; MI = myocardial infarction. According to ref Launcelott et al. [19].

SURGICAL APPROACH

Resternotomy

Median resternotomy is the most common and standard approach for the treatment of redo aortic valve surgery, as it gives full access to whole of the heart. However, in reoperative patients, repeating sternotomy may increase surgical risk because of the risk of iatrogenic injury of the right ventricular, ascending aorta, innominate vein and grafts. The incidence of hemorrage after resternotomy is between 2% and 6% per patient reoperation [20]. Preoperative computed tomography scanning is mandatory to evaluate the relationship among these structures and sternum and identify patients at risk of injury during reentry. If pericardium was closed to previous during the primary procedure, median sternotomy is quite safe, although we recommend having cardiopulmonary machine ready to start in case of catastrophic events. Conversely, if the mediastinal contents are closely attached to the sternum, an alternative strategy is to perform resternotomy once the heart is empty through cardiopulmonary bypass (CPB) machine, cannulating the femoral vessels. In presence of advanced peripheral vessel disease, axillary cannulation may be useful to reduce the risk of stroke and vessels injuries. When major hemorrhage occurs on sternal reentry for right ventricular or aortic injury, sternotomy should be abandoned and chest reapproximated. CPB should be established cooling down the patient for potential circulatory arrest and the remaining sternal division can be completed and injury repaired. After safe re-entry, the patient may be weaned off for further dissection to avoid prolonged cardiopulmonary bypass time. Careful attention should be taken to avoid de-adventializing the aorta, as well as the space between pulmonary artery and aorta, innominate vein and right phrenic nerve during dissection at the level of superior vena cava.

Minimally Invasive Approach

The number of minimally invasive procedures for isolated primary AVR is increasingly performed, as minimally invasive AVR (MIAVR) has shown excellent results in terms of mortality, morbidities and patient's satisfaction. It reduces risk of bleeding, blood transfusion and associated with shorter hospital stay [21]. In the setting of redo surgery, the rational of a minimally invasive approach is to minimize surgical trauma because it does not require extensive dissection, reduce the risk of cardiac structures injuries and consequently less bleeding. However, several concerns have been expressed regarding myocardial protection, prolonged operative times, chambers dearing, as well as retrograde perfusion related to peripheral cannulation. A systematic review and meta-analysis on 441 redo patients concluded that minimally invasive redo AVR is a valid alternative option for patients requiring redo AVR, as it has showed similar efficacy, mortality and morbidity outcomes (renal failure, stroke, pacemaker implantation and myocardial infarction) compared conventional redo AVR [22]. Ministernotomy is the most common minimally invasive approach used for redo AVR and consists in a J partial resternotomy at the 3rd or 4th intercostal space. Mediastinal dissection is limited to the only ascending aorta necessary for aortotomy and aortic clamping. Ministernotomy is our preferred approach for those patients requiring repeated AVR, especially for degenerated biological valve or mechanical valve dysfunction. Nevertheless, the introduction of sutureless valves and our increased experience in right anterior minithoracotomy for primary AVR have facilitated the redo AVR via right minithoracotomy.

In this setting, the computed tomography allows to evaluate the anatomic relationship among the intercostal spaces, ascending aorta, and aortic valve. Patients are suitable for RT only if the following criteria were met: (1) at the level of main pulmonary artery, the ascending aorta is rightward (more than one half located on the right in respect to the right sternal border) (2) the distance from the ascending aorta to the sternum is between 2cm-10cm and (3) good valve exposure with α angle (angle between the midline and the inclination of ascending aorta) $\geq 45°$ (Figure 1). We describe our surgical approach. Minimally invasive RT AVR is performed through a 5 to 7cm skin incision placed at the level of the second intercostal space without rib resection.

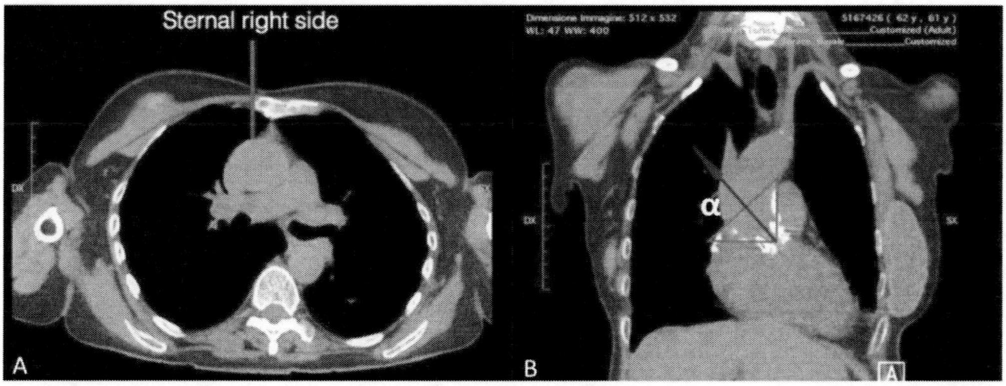

Figure 1. Evaluation of anatomic relationship among the intercostal spaces, ascending aorta, and aortic valve with CT-scan.

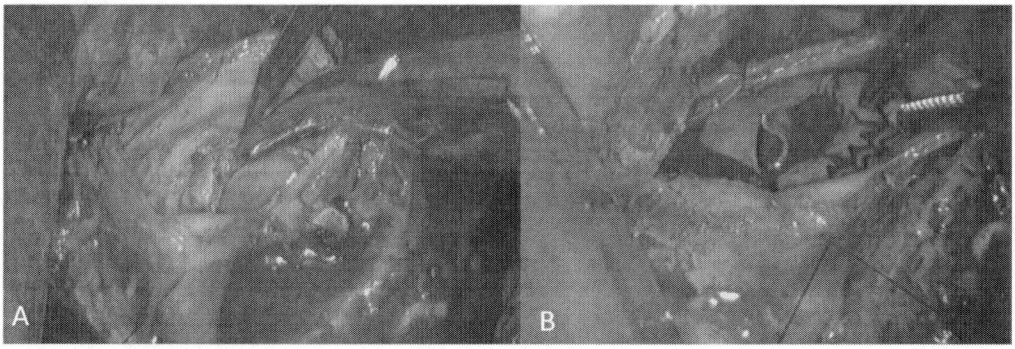

Figure 2. Transverse aortotomy.

The right internal thoracic artery is excluded and vacuum-assisted cardiopulmonary bypass (between -30mm Hg -40mm Hg) is established though femoral vessels. Mediastinal dissection is limited to the ascending aorta for aortic clamping. After clamping, antegrade crystalloid cardioplegic solution is given into the aortic root or selectively into the coronary ostia in presence of severe regurgitation for cusp fractures. This approach is used also in patients with patent LIMA-LAD graft without the need of cooling the patients. In case of significant blood flow out the coronary ostium and obscured surgical field, the pump flow is turned down temporarily and a pediatric vent is used through the aortic annulus for better visualization.

A transverse aortotomy is usually performed 2 - 3cm above the sinotubular junction (Figure 2).

Once the prosthesis is removed, the aortic annulus is inspected and the excess of pannus or fibrotic tissue is removed to favor annular, taking care to avoid annular defects. After sizing, 3 guiding 4 - 0 Prolene sutures are placed at the nadir point of each valve sinuses for accurate alignment of the inflow portion of the prosthesis into the aortic annulus. Often, nadir points are not evident, as the previous prosthesis has altered annulus geometry. To manage this problem, we recreate 3 nadirs that are positioned at approximately 120 degrees. Landmarks are right and left coronary artery and previous commissures. To achieve this result, the surgeon may use instruments such as a sizer with 120-degree markings to recreate a normal nadir. Then the valve is collapsed using a specific device system and connected to the guiding sutures through 3 bottom holes placed on the midpart of the inflow ring. The valve is released into the aortic annulus and once coaptation of the 3 leaflets has been checked, a balloon was inserted into the sutureless valve and expanded with warm saline solution for 30 seconds at a pressure of 4 mmBar. Finally, the 3 guiding sutures were removed; the valve is again checked for the correct position, and the aortotomy is closed using 4-0 or 5-0 running sutures.

Valve in Valve for Failed Aortic Bioprosthesis

The operative surgical risk and the non-inferiority of transcatheter AVR (TAVR) compared with conventional AVR in high and intermediate risk patients, have brought medical community to consider the concept of valve in valve TAVR for failed aortic bioprostheses [23-26]. In August 2015, the Food and Drug Administration approved the use of percutaneous valves for patients in need of a second tissue AVR after undergoing previous one. Several studies show that valve in valve TAVR is a safe and clinically effective procedure with similar mortality compared to surgical AVR at least in the short term [27-29]. Nevertheless, valve in valve TAVR requires and extensive preoperative work up and is associated with complications such as coronary obstruction (stentless internally oriented stented bioprosthetic valves) and high gradients with small failed aortic bioprosthes [30]. Moreover, no long-term results are available.

Conclusion

Redo surgery for aortic valve is expected to increase in next years because of aging and patients' preference for biological valve to improve quality of life. Despite the surgical risk is higher than first operation, advancement in cardiac surgery in terms of minimally invasive approaches, myocardial protection and sutureless technology, have improved postoperative outcomes. Valve in Valve TAVR is a safe and effective procedure in high-risk patients; however, the lack of long term durability and the high gradients in small prostheses make this procedure still not indicated in young and low risk patients.

References

[1] Balsam, L. B., Grossi, E. A., Greenhouse, D. G. et al. Reoperative valve surgery in the elderly: predictors of risk and long-term survival. *Ann. Thorac Surg.,* 2010; 90:1195 - 200.

[2] Ranucci, M., Frigiola, A., Menicanti, L. et al. Aortic cross clamp time, new prosthese and outcome in aortic valve replacement. *J. Heart Valve Dis.,* 2012; 21:732 - 9.

[3] Nashef, S. A. M., Roques, F., Sharples, L. D. et al. EuroSCORE II. *Eur. J. Cardiothoracic Surg.*, 2012; 41:734 - 44.

[4] Akins, C. W., Buckley, M. J., Daggett, W. M. et al. Risk of reoperative valve replacement for failed mitral and aortic bioprostheses. *Ann. Thorac. Surgery,* 1998; 65, 1545 - 1551.

[5] Furukawa, H., Tanemoto, K. Redo valve surgery-current status and future perspectives. *Ann. Thorac Cardiovasc. Surg.,* 2014; 20:267 - 275.

[6] Jamieson, W. R., Burr, L. H., Miyagishima, R. T. et al. Reoperation for bioprosthetic aortic structural failure-risk assessment. *Eur. J. Cardiothoracic Surg.,* 2003; 31:43 - 8.

[7] Cohn, L. H. Evolutions of redo cardiac surgery: review of personal experience. *J. Card. Surg.*, 2004: 19:320 - 4.

[8] Onorati, F., Biancari, F., De Feo, M., Mariscalco, G., Messina, A., Santarpino, G., Santini, F., Beghi, C., Nappi, G., Troise, G., Fischlein, T., Passerone, G., Heikkinen, J., Faggian, G. Mid-term results of aortic valve surgery in redo scenarios in the current practice: results from the multicentre European RECORD (REdo Cardiac Operation Research Database) iniziative. *Eur. J. Cardiothorac. Surg.,* 2015 Feb.; 47(2):269 - 80.

[9] Gummert, J. F., Funkat, A., Beckmann, A. et al. Cardiac surgery in Germany during 2007: a report on behalf of the German Society for Thoracic and Cardiovascular Surgery. *Thorac. Cardiovasc. Surg.,* 2008; 56:328 - 36.

[10] Leontyev, S., Borger, M. A., Davierwala, P., Walther, T., Lehmann, S., Kempfert, J. et al. Redo aortic valve surgery: early and late outcomes. *Ann. Thorac. Surg.,* 2011; 91:1120 - 6.

[11] Kaneko, T., Vassileva, C. M., Englum, B. et al. Contemporary outcomes of repeat aortic valve replacement: a Benchmark for transcatheter valve in valve procedures. *Ann. Thorac. Surg.,* 2015; 100:1298 - 1304.

[12] Brown, J. M., O'Brien, S. M., Wu, C. et al. Isolated aortic valve replacement in North America comprising 108,687 patients in 10 years changes in risks, valve types and outcomes in the Society of Thoracic Surgeons National Database. *J. Thoracic Cardiovasc. Sur.,* 2009; 137:82 - 90.

[13] Potter, D. D., Sundt, T. M., 3rd, Zehr, K. J. et al. Operative risk reoperative aortic valve replacement. *J. Thoracic Cardiovasc. Surg.,* 2005; 129:878 - 84.

[14] Emery, R. W., Krogh, C. C., Arom, D. V. et al.: The St. Jude Medical cardiac valve prosthesis: A 25-year experience with single valve replacement. *Ann. Thorac. Surg.,* 2005; 79:776.

[15] Glaser, N., Jackson, V., Holzmann, M. J., Franco-Cereceda, A., Sartipy, U. Prosthetic Valve Endocarditis after Surgical Aortic Valve Replacement. *Circulation,* 2017; 136:329 - 331.

[16] Bouhout, I., Mazine, A., Ghoneim, A., Mill, X., El-Hamamsy, I., Pellerin, M., Cartier, R. et al. Long-term results after surgical treatment of paravalvular leak in the aortic and mitral position. *J. Thorac. Cardiovasc. Surg*., 2016; 151:1260 - 6.

[17] Miceli, A., Lio, A., Glauber, M. The art of repair. *J. Thoracic Cardiovasc. Surg*., 2017; 153:1021 - 2.

[18] Lansac, E., Kercove Aortic valve repair techniques: state of the art. *Eur. J. Cardiothoracic Surg*., 2018: 53; 1101 - 1107.

[19] Launcelott, S., Ouzonian, M., Buth, K. J., Légaré, J. F. Predicting In-Hospital Mortality after Redo Cardiac Operations: Development of a Preoperative Scorecard. *Ann. Thorac. Surg.,* 2012; 94:778 - 84.

[20] Dobell, A. R. C., Jain, A. K. Catastrophic Hemorrhage during Redo Sternotomy. *Ann. Thorac. Surg.,* 1984; 37:273 - 278.

[21] Glauber, M., Ferrarini, M., Miceli, A. Minimally invasive aortic valve surgery: state of art and future direction. *Ann. Cardiothorac. Surg.,* 2015; 4:26 - 32.

[22] Phan, K., Zhou, J. J., Niranjan, N., Di eusanio, M., Yan, T. D. Minimally invasive reoperative aortic valve replacement: a systematic review and meta-analysis. *Ann. Cardiothoracic Surg.,* 2015; 4:15 - 25.

[23] Smith, C. R., Leon, M. B., Mack, M. J. et al. PARTNER Trial Investigators. Transcatheter versus surgical aortic valve replacement in high risk patients. *N Engl. J. Med.,* 2011; 364:2187 - 98.

[24] Adams, D. H., Popma, J. J., Reardon, M. J. Transcatheter aortic valve replacement with a self-expanding prosthesis. *N Engl. J. Med.,* 2014; 37:967 - 78.

[25] Leon, M. B., Smith, C. R., Mack, M. J. et al. Thransccatheter or Surgical aorticac valve replacement in intermediate risk patients. *N Eng. J. Med.,* 2016; 374:1609 - 20.

[26] Reardon, M. J., Van Mieghem, N. M. Popma, J. J. et al. SURTAVI Investigators. Surgical or thranscatheter aortic valve replacement in intermediate risk patients. *N Engl. Med. J.,* 2017; 367;1321 - 31.

[27] Seekek, A. f., Greason, K. L., Sandhu, G. S., Dearani, J. A., Holmes, D. R. Jr., Schaff, H. V. Transcatheter valve in valve vs. Surgical replacement of failing stented aortic biological valves. *Ann. Thorac. Surg.,* 2019; 108:424 - 430.

[28] Takagi, H., Mitta, ando. Meta-analysis of valve in valve transcatheter versus redo surgical aortic valve replacement. *Thorac. Cardiovasc. Surg.,* 2019; 67:243 - 250.

[29] Nalluri, N., Atti, V., Minir, A. B., Karam, B., Patel, N. J., Kumar, V., Vemula, P. et al. Valve in valve transcatheter aortic valve implantation (ViV-TAVI) versus redo—Surgical aortic valve replacement (redo-SAVR): A systematic review and meta-analysis. *J. Int. Cardiol.,* 2018; 31:661 - 671.

[30] Reul, R. M., Ramchandani, K., Readon, M. J. Thranscatheter aortic valve-in-valve procedure inpatients with bioprosthetic structural valve deterioration. *Methodist Debakey Cardiovasc. J.,* 2017; 13:132 - 141.

In: Perspectives in Aortic Valve Disease
Editor: Giovanni Concistrè ISBN: 978-1-53618-769-4

Chapter 17

Aortic Prosthesis: Mechanical and Sutured Biological Valves

Giuseppe Santarpino[1,2,3,*], Giuseppe Filiberto Serraino[3] and Pasquale Mastroroberto[3]

[1]Anthea Hospital, GVM Care and Research, Bari, Italy
[2]Paracelsus Medical University, Nuremberg, Germany
[3]Cardiac Surgery Unit, Department of Experimental and Clinical Medicine, University "Magna Graecia" of Catanzaro, Catanzaro, Italy

Abstract

Within a context of innovation, between transcatheter prostheses, stentless and sutureless prostheses, the use of stented and mechanical prostheses seems to represent a "historical" chapter of cardiac surgery. This chapter provides an overview of the most commonly used prostheses in terms of prevalence, and therefore of importance, also from an economic perspective. Furthermore, new studies on biological designs and materials, as well as new anticoagulant therapy protocols, open new frontiers for the future use of these prostheses (still) in a large proportion of patients suffering from aortic valve disease.

Keywords: mechanical valves, sutured biological valves

Introduction

The progressive rise in the average age of the population has resulted in a growing proportion of elderly patients who may benefit from medical and surgical treatment options that were previously offered only to younger subjects. This applies, for example, to aortic valve replacement for symptomatic severe aortic stenosis, where biological tissue valves are

[*] Corresponding Author's Email: gsantarpino@gvmnet.it.

generally considered the device of choice for older patients. Aortic valve bioprostheses are commonly implanted in the current era (also in younger patients) as they may obviate the need for anticoagulation while providing better hemodynamic performance and a more favorable quality of life. The steady increase in the use of biological valves has prompted the development of several different models of conventional stented bioprostheses.

In this chapter we describe the features of different bioprosthetic valve models. As these devices are well recognized and available on the market worldwide, the ultimate aim is to understand how to select the most appropriate prosthetic model for the individual patient in order to establish the indication for aortic valve replacement with a stented bioprosthesis based on a patient- rather than a prosthesis-oriented approach.

Furthermore, we will describe the new anticoagulation regimes necessary for mechanical prostheses and their hemodynamic characteristics; both factors that can recover space for these prostheses, even in non-young patients.

Finally, we will describe new biological tissues and models that seem to have excellent future prospects based on *in vitro* studies that may represent a hope of reduced risk of structural valve degeneration (SVD) even in young patients who want to make a "biological" choice.

BIOLOGICAL MODELS

The classic classification of stented biological valves divides them into two large families: porcine prostheses and pericardial prostheses. In reality, and in light of the most recent studies on the hemodynamic effects and on the risk of SVD, it is necessary to divide the prostheses - probably more important than the aspect of the origin of the biological tissue - into two other families: those with leaflets mounted inside the stent and those with leaflets mounted outside.

One of the models with externally mounted leaflets is the Livanova Crown PRT. This stented bioprosthesis is a device built on the previous generation of the Mitroflow aortic valve model. The Mitroflow valve design was already shown to provide good hemodynamic performance, especially in patients with small aortic annulus [1, 2]. The valve design consists of a single bovine pericardium layer mounted outside the stent, combined with an advanced tissue treatment - the phospholipid reduction treatment (PRT) - which is intended to bolster durability through mitigation of valve calcification. The Crown PRT bioprosthetic aortic valve can be implanted in either the supra-annular or intra-annular position. Since its market introduction in 1982, the Mitroflow pericardial bioprosthesis demonstrated good long-term performance in both European 1 and north-American 2 multicenter studies. However, Sénage et al., reported a high incidence of structural valve deterioration with the Mitroflow pericardial bioprosthesis [3]. For a deeper understanding of this concept and the difficulty in comparing different models in different patients, we suggest meta-analysis (2017): Fischlein T., et al., Patterns of use and durability for the Mitroflow aortic valve: a systematic review of the literature. J Cardiovasc Surg (Torino) [4-6].

The second model with leaflets mounted outside the stent is the St. Jude Trifecta. The Trifecta valve is a third-generation heart valve that complements the St. Jude Medical Epic and Epic Supra bioprosthetic aortic valves. It is a one-leaflet stented pericardial valve designed for supra-annular placement in the aortic position. The valve is fabricated using a polyester-covered titanium stent. The stent, excluding the sewing cuff, is then covered with porcine pericardial tissue. This covering is designed to provide protection from mechanical wear by allowing only tissue-to-tissue contact during valve function. A silicone insert in the polyester sewing cuff is slightly contoured to conform to the shape of the native annulus. The valve leaflets are fabricated from bovine pericardium. The porcine and bovine pericardium are preserved and crosslinked in glutaraldehyde. Glutaraldehyde, formaldehyde and ethanol are used in the valve sterilization process. Additionally, the Trifecta valve is processed with LinxTM anti-calcification technology, a patented proprietary anti-calcification treatment that in animal studies has demonstrated resistance to calcification [7-10].

These are the external stent mounted valve (Crown and Trifecta). The following models mounted the leaflets inside the stent:

The Carpentier-Edwards Perimount Magna Ease is a recent stented aortic bioprosthesis developed by Edwards Lifesciences, with a device design based on its two predecessor models (the Perimount and the Perimount Magna aortic valves). The advanced Carpentier-Edwards Perimount Magna ease aortic bioprosthesis adds enhanced implantability to the unsurpassed hemodynamics of the Magna valve platform, setting the new standard for tissue valve performance. In particular, the low valve profile enables easier insertion and aortotomy closure minimizing the risk for coronary obstruction[11-18]. In addition, the presence of suture markers aids in valve orientation and suture placement. The implantation of the Carpentier- Edwards Perimount Magna Ease aortic valve seems to result in improved hemodynamic performance, as suggested by industry-leading effective orifice areas (EOA) and low gradients documented in multiple studies, with hemodynamic stability reported up to 20 years post- implantation. According to the manufacturer, this model is designed for endurance as it is built on the proven performance of Perimount aortic valves, with over 27 years of clinical experience [19, 20]. The Carpentier-Edwards ThermaFix process is the only anti-calcification technology designed to compare both major calcium binding sites. However, no clinical data are available to evaluate the long-term impact of the Edwards Lifesciences tissue treatment in patients.

Medtronic offers three stented aortic bioprostheses, including the Hancock II, the Mosaic and the Mosaic Ultra tissue valve that will be described here. The Mosaic Ultra valve is delivered with a Cinch® implant System that facilitates aortic valve insertion, particularly through a tight sinotubular space (and helps prevent suture "looping" around the stent posts for mitral valve replacement) [21-27]. It is mounted on a flexible stent that reduces tissue stress, making this bioprosthesis especially suited for minimally invasive procedures. Thirteen-year results demonstrate clinical safety and excellent performance. Third-generation tissue technology - aoa® (alpha amino oleic acid) tissue treatment and Physiologic FixationTM - has improved the durability of this valve and helps mitigate valve calcification while preserving leaflet structure, with leaflets that function similarly to native aortic valves. However, again no clinical data are available to evaluate the long-term impact of the aoa® tissue treatment and Physiologic Fixation process in patients. Because tissue valves open physiologically as native valves, they provide excellent forward flow.

Different from the other bioprosthetic valves, the Mosaic Ultra is made from a single porcine aortic valve, using physiological pressure fixation that maintains the natural leaflet form and function. By contrast, aortic valve reconstruction with bovine pericardium is usually performed when using the other three valve models [28-33]. The Mosaic Ultra has a reduced sewing cuff that allows greater flexibility to implant a larger valve size for improved hemodynamics. Its scalloped sewing ring conforms to the aortic annulus for complete supra-annular placement.

Hemodynamic Performance and Durability

It is essential to underline that the two aspects of hemodynamic performance and durability, or structural valve degeneration, are concepts that must be followed simultaneously also because this says the definition of SVD. In fact, according to the new unified definition of SVD, it is not only necessary to consider the cases of SVD that lead to re-intervention but also the cases in which the prosthesis over time has moderate or severe valve insufficiency or if it develops gradients above 20 or 40 mmHg. Therefore, a worsening of hemodynamic performance corresponds "by definition" to a poor durability of the valve. We suggest reading the recent review (2020) on this reflection: New Year's Eve, Søndergaard L. How to Define Durability of Transcatheter and Surgical Bioprosthetic Aortic Valves: Facts and Misconceptions. JACC Cardiovasc Interv.

A number of studies evaluated the hemodynamic performance of stented aortic valves, although hemodynamic data mostly refer to old models with longer follow-up, as only scanty information is available in the literature on the latest generation of these valves.

It is difficult to compare data on the hemodynamic performance of stented pericardial and porcine aortic valves. It has been demonstrated that aortic valve replacement with a pericardial bioprosthesis provides superior hemodynamic performance, resulting in significantly lower transvalvular gradients. However, is there an influence of that on the durability? Andreas et al., compared a porcine prosthesis with a traditional pericardial heart valve with leaflets sutured inside of the stent and found that patients with a porcine bioprosthesis had a higher postoperative transvalvular gradient. Durability comparisons are made between the three types of pericardial aortic valves, given the different structural profile of the Mosaic Ultra porcine bioprosthesis. Again, data are mostly derived from studies conducted with the predecessor models, which include longer follow-up periods. In particular, durability after aortic valve replacement with the Mitroflow and Perimount pericardial bioprostheses has been evaluated, but no long-term follow-up data are available for both the Crown PRT and Magna/Magna Ease valves. Conversely, mid-term data are available for the Trifecta valve [34-40].

In summary, we therefore consider it essential to read and comment on 3 recent studies to be able to give a "to date" answer to the hemodynamic/durability ratio:

First, Wang M. et al., (Ann Thorac Surg. 2017) did a meta-regression of published studies at that time. The aim of this study was to extract published SVD information on the four most widely used aortic bioprosthetic heart valve types (Medtronic and Edwards porcine and Sorin and Edwards pericardial), to compare their durability [41]. They conclude that Sorin pericardial valves have a significantly shorter main time to valve failure than the other three valve types. There were no significant differences in main time to valve failure among the Edwards pericardial valves and the Hancock and Edwards porcine valves.

This analysis, together with other more recently published data, indicate that the importance of the classification of biological prostheses in two large families based on the tissue of origin (porcine valve or bovine pericardium) has less importance than it seemed in terms of degeneration risk [42-44].

Second, an intersting paper from Biancari F. et al., (Ann Thorac Surg. 2020) [45]. This is a comparative analysis of the outcome of the Trifecta and Perimount Magna Ease bioprostheses from the FinnValve registry, a Finnish nationwide database including patients with aortic stenosis who underwent aortic valve replacement with a bioprosthesis. They conclude that the Trifecta aortic bioprosthesis is associated with a higher occurrence of repeat aortic valve replacement for structural valve failure compared to the Perimount Magna Ease bioprosthesis. These results are of clinical significance because the early degeneration of the Trifecta bioprosthesis was observed in an advanced age cohort and such a risk could be higher in younger patients. These findings highlight the importance of a vigilant assessment of the long-term outcome of surgical aortic valve replacement bioprostheses.

The pathological basis underlying Biancari's clinical results can be found in the third important and recent paper (Vriesendorp M. D. et al., Interact Cardiovasc Thorac Surg. 2020) [46-48]. In this elegant paper an *in vitro* methodology for the assessment of long-term mechanical durability of prosthetic tissue valves was conducted using accelerated wear testing. Valves were cycled between 10 and 20 Hz for 600 million cycles, which corresponds to 15 years of simulated use.

These authors conclude that externally mounted leaflet valves showed superior hydrodynamic performance but inferior mechanical durability versus internally mounted leaflet valves after 600 million cycles of testing. The primary failures were because of significant mechanical abrasion at the commissural region, which may warrant close monitoring of externally mounted leaflet valves over the course of long-term follow-up.

In summary, up to now 2020, we can speculate that the most important factor to influence SVD is the "design." Hemodynamics, gradients, patient-prosthesis mismatch, porcine or bovine valves appear to have a low impact on the destiny of the valve [49-52].

In this direction we can say that a new prosthetic model with stent characteristics mounted inside, in bovine pericardium with good immediate hemodynamic data, gave very encouraging results in its trial for marketing (PERIGON trial) with data at one year. Following these hypotheses, the results on durability should also be very encouraging from a distance (See: Robert J. M. et al., Eur J Cardiothorac Surg. 2017) [53].

In conclusions, part of the above-described types of stented aortic valves have only recently been introduced into the market, which makes direct comparisons challenging. Second and third-generation prosthetic valves were considered and, hence, comparative analysis is of limited value. The data derived from the different studies also pose interpretation issues, either because of the small sample size or because each cardiac surgery center usually performs aortic valve replacement predominantly with the same prosthesis model, which further limits interstudy comparisons. However, early structural valve deterioration of the "external mounted stent valves" has also been reported. These observations call for a cautious use of these prosthetic valves.

The assessment of hemodynamic performance is commonly performed through measurement of EOA and mean pressure gradients, and these two indicators allow for comparisons between the different prosthesis models. Also the cited guidelines to define SVD used these parameters. However, in the context of the competing transcatheter approach and an increased focus on quality of life, it would be more appropriate to consider additional functional parameters that may provide an estimate of the impact on the myocardium and not merely on left ventricular mass. Such information could be obtained through echocardiographic parameters for myocardial tissue characterization (e.g., tissue Doppler imaging) that enable assessment of left ventricular diastolic function after correction of aortic stenosis.

Despite the advances in stent structure and anti-calcification technology, contemporary aortic bioprostheses suffer from the same disadvantages of the early models, including the risk of degenerative bioprosthetic stenosis or regurgitation and the need for suture lines. Future research should aim at developing faster and easier suturing techniques, so as to compete with sutureless devices and achieve shorter implantation and ischemic times - the Cinch® Implant System on the Mosaic Ultra valve partially meets this need. In addition, further refinement in the field of biomaterials should be pursued to obtain more ideal autologous prostheses and minimize the risk for immunoreaction and bioprosthetic valve failure.

Indeed, the search for new biomaterials with enhanced biocompatibility and for the production of autologous aortic valves has been going on for many years, but none of these is yet commercially available. However, the enlargement of the prosthetic heart valve market to emerging countries and failure to eradicate several infectious diseases (e.g., rheumatic heart disease in developing areas of the world) are expected to draw interest in the development of more ideal autologous devices. This means that hopefully in the near future, stent and aortic bioprostheses will be biocompatible, less expensive and free from the risk of valve degeneration, will not require anticoagulant medication, and will adapt to patient growth from childhood into adulthood.

Probably the biggest innovation we currently have on the market in terms of new biomaterials is the RESILIA tissue from the Inspiris Edwards prosthesis. RESILIA tissue is made of bovine pericardium that undergoes integrity preservation technology. This technology consists of stable capping that permanently blocks calcium (Ca2+) binding sites, and glycerolization that allows dry storage of the bioprosthesis prior to implant. The RESILIA™ tissue was incorporated within a standard bioprosthesis design and called "Edwards Inspiris." Bartus K. et al., (J Thorac Dis. 2019) have reported their experience (the first ever published) on the first 4 years of implants with very encouraging results, but it is still too early for real results in terms of long-term durability [22].

As for the "innovations" for mechanical valve prostheses in an aortic position, the discussion is much simpler. This is because in recent years, probably due to the small number of patients who need or require a mechanical prosthesis, new products have not been marketed, but the two-disc prostheses have been the same on the market for years.

Mechanical valves remain the most durable option for valve replacement with most new generation valves reporting 0% structural failures with follow-up of >10 years and valve thrombosis risk <1% in both the aortic and mitral positions.

Based on current guidelines in North America and Europe, mechanical valves are recommended in patients <50 years old who can tolerate anticoagulation and should be considered in patients between 50 and 65 years old after a discussion of the risks and benefits.

Moreover, an important innovation was introduced last year for the Sorin Bicarbon mechanical prosthesis. This prosthesis had - on the basis of a 2010 study (Torella M., et al., "LOWERING-IT" Trial. Am Heart J) - approval for a lower INR anticoagulation regimen (1.5-2.5) [54-55]. This value, while maintaining the same degree of protection from thromboembolic complications, ensures a lower risk of bleeding events. The consequence of all this could be a greater use of mechanical prostheses, since the risk of anticoagulant therapy is lower. In fact, we are skeptical in this regard, given that for years there has been an on the mark (On-X) prosthesis that has approved this anticoagulation regimen, but this has not increased the number of patients in whom mechanical prostheses were impanted. Other reasoning could be, in perspective and in a speculative sense, if the new direct anticoagulants can be approved for mechanical prostheses and, therefore, these "would compete again" with biological prostheses even in patients of advanced age.

References

[1] Conte J., et al., 2010 "A North American, prospective, multicenter assessment of the Mitroflow aortic pericardial prosthesis." *Ann Thorac Surg*. 90:144-152.

[2] iSTHMUS investigators. 2011 "The italian study on the Mitroflow postoperative results (ISTHMUS): a 20-year, multicentre evaluation of Mitroflow pericardial bioprosthesis." *Eur J Cardiothorac Surg*. 39:18-26.

[3] Sénage T., et al., 2014 "Early structural valve deterioration of Mitroflow aortic bioprosthesis: mode, incidence, and impact on outcome in a large cohort of patients." *Circulation*. 130:2012-2020.

[4] Pfeiffer S., et al., 2015 "Early Structural valve deterioration of Mitroflow aortic bioprosthesis: mode, incidence, and impact on outcome in a large cohort of patients." *Circulation*. 132:e152.

[5] Gerosa G., et al., 2006 "Small aortic annulus: the hydrodynamic performances of 5 commercially available tissue valves." *J Thorac Cardiovasc Surg*. 131:1058-1064.

[6] Pollari F., et al., 2015 "First experience with the new Sorin Crown PRT bioprosthetic aortic valve: early postoperative outcome and hemodynamic performance in 90 patients." *J Cardiovasc Surg (Torino)*. 56:939-943.

[7] Brennan J. M., et al., 2012 "Early anticoagulation of bioprosthetic aortic valves in older patients: results from the Society of Thoracic Surgeons Adult Cardiac Surgery national database." *J Am Coll Cardiol*. 60:971-977.

[8] Frater R. W., et al., 1997 "Anticalcification, proendothelial, and anti-inflammatory effect of post aldehyde polyol treatment of bioprosthetic material." in: Gabbay S., Wheatley D., editors. *Advances in anticalcific and antidegenerative treatment of heart valve bioprostheses*. First edition. Austin, TX: Silent Partners, Inc.

[9] Chen W., et al., 1994 "Mechanism of efficacy of 2-amino oleic acid for inhibition of calcification of glutaraldehyde-pretreated porcine bioprosthetic heart valves." *Circulation*. 90:323-329.

[10] Vyavahare N., et al., 1997 "Prevention of bioprosthetic heart valve calcification by ethanol preincubation." *Circulation*. 95:479-488.

[11] Vyavahare N., et al., 1998 "Prevention of calcification of glutaraldehyde-crosslinked porcine aortic cusps by ethanol preincubation." *J Biomed Mater Res*. 40:577-585.

[12] Shen M., et al., 2001 "Effect of ethanol and ether in the prevention of calcification of bioprostheses." *Ann Thorac Surg*. 71:S413-S416.

[13] Vyavahare N., et al., 2000 "Prevention of glutaraldehyde-fixed bioprosthetic heart valve calcification by alcohol pretreatment: further mechanistic studies." *J Heart Valve Dis.* 9:561-566.

[14] Dalmau M. J., et al., 2006 "The Carpentier-Edwards Perimount Magna aortic xenograft: a new design with an improved hemodynamic performance." *Interact Cardiovasc Thorac Surg* 5:263-267.

[15] Botzenhardt F., et al., 2005 "Hemodynamic per- formance and incidence of patient-prosthesis mismatch of the complete supraannular Perimount Magna bioprosthesis in the aortic position." *Thorac Cardiovasc Surg.* 63:459-466.

[16] Botzenhardt F., et al., 2005 "Hemodynamic comparison of bioprostheses for complete supra-annular position in patients with small aortic annulus." *J Am Coll Cardiol.* 45:2054-2060.

[17] Totaro P., et al., 2005 "Carpentier-Edwards PERIMOUNT Magna bioprosthesis: a stented valve with stentless performance?" *J Thorac Cardiovasc Surg.* 130:1668-1674.

[18] Dalmau M. J., et al., 2007 "One year hemodynamic performance of the Perimount Magna pericardial xenograft and the Medtronic Mosaic bioprosthesis in the aortic position: a prospective randomized study." *Interact Cardiovasc Thorac Surg.* 130:1668-1674.

[19] Wagner I. M., et al., 2007 "Influence of completely supra-annular placement of bioprostheses on exercise hemodynamics in patients with a small aortic annulus." *J Thorac Cardiovasc Surg.* 133:1234-1241.

[20] Borger M. A., et al., 2007 "Carpentier-Edwards Perimount Magna valve versus Medtronic Hancock II: a matched hemodynamic comparison." *Ann Thorac Surg.* 83:2054-2058.

[21] Banbury M. K., et al., 2002 "Hemodynamic stability during 17 years of the Carpentier-Edwards aortic pericardial bioprosthesis." *Ann Thorac Surg.* 73:1460-1465.

[22] Aupart M. R., et al., 2006 "Perimount pericardial bioprosthesis for aortic calcified stenosis: 18-year experience with 1133 patients." *J Heart Valve Dis.* 15:768-775.

[23] Riess F. C., et al., 2010 "Clinical results of the Medtronic Mosaic porcine bioprosthesis up to 13 years." *Eur J Cardiothorac Surg.* 37:145-153.

[24] Bakhtiary F., et al., 2007 "Opening and closing kinematics of fresh and calcified aortic valve prostheses: an *in vitro* study." *J Thorac Cardiovasc Surg.* 134:657-662.

[25] Chen W., et al., 1994 "Mechanism of efficacy of 2-amino oleic acid for inhibition of calcification of glutaraldehyde-pretreated porcine bioprosthetic heart valves." *Circulation.* 90:323-329.

[26] Girardot M. N., et al., 1995 "Role of glutaraldehyde in calcification of porcine heart valves: comparing cusp and wall." *J Biomed Mater Res.* 29:793-801.

[27] González-Juanatey Jr., et al., 1996 "Hemodynamics of various designs of 19 mm pericardial aortic valve bioprosthesis." *Eur J Cardiothorac Surg.* 10:201-206.

[28] Yankah C. A., et al., 2005 "Seventeen-year clinical results of 1,037 Mitroflow pericardial heart valve prostheses in the aortic position." *J Heart Valve Dis.* 14:172-179.

[29] Tasca G., et al., 2006 "Impact of prosthesis-patient mismatch on cardiac events and midterm mortality after aortic valve replacement in patients with pure aortic stenosis." *Circulation.* 2006:570-576.

[30] García-Bengochea J., et al., 2006 "Left ventricular mass regression after aortic valve replacement with the new Mitroflow 12A pericardial bioprosthesis." *J Heart Valve Dis.* 15:451-452.
[31] Bleiziffer S., et al., 2009 "Hemodynamic characterization of the Sorin Mitroflow pericardial bioprosthesis at rest and exercise." *J Heart Valve Dis.* 18:95-100.
[32] Jamieson W. R., et al., 2010 "Hemodynamic performance of Mitroflow aortic pericardial bioprosthesis - optimizing management for the small aortic annulus." *Thorac Cardiovasc Surg.* 58:69-75.
[33] Hartrumpf M., et al., 2012 "Favorable gradients with the Mitroflow aortic valve prosthesis in everyday surgery." *Thorac Cardiovasc Surg.* 60:326-333.
[34] Asch F. M., et al., 2012 "Mitroflow aortic bioprosthesis 5-year follow-up: North American prospective multicenter study." *Ann Thorac Surg.* 94:1198-1203.
[35] Suri M., et al., 2012 "A prospective, randomized comparison of 3 contemporary bioprosthetic aortic valves: should hemodynamic performance influence device selection?" *J Thorac Cardiovasc Surg.* 144:1387-1395.
[36] Wilbring M., et al., 2013 "Isolated aortic valve replacement in patients with small aortic annulus - a high-risk group on long-term follow-up." *Thorac Cardiovasc Surg.* 61:379-385.
[37] Ugur M., et al., 2014 "Comparison of early hemodynamic performance of 3 aortic valve bioprostheses." *J Thorac Cardiovasc Surg.* 148:1940-1946.
[38] Bleiziffer S., et al., 2007 "Prediction of valve prosthesis-patient mismatch prior to aortic valve replacement: which is the best method?" *Heart.* 93:615-622.
[39] Dalmau M. J., et al., 2001 "Hemodynamic performance of the Medtronic Mosaic and Perimount Magna aortic bioprostheses: five-year results of a prospectively randomized study." *Eur J Cardiothorac Surg.* 39:844-852.
[40] Minardi G., et al., 2014 "Early Doppler-echocardiography evaluation of Carpentier-Edwards Standard and Carpentier-eEdwards Magna aortic prosthetic valve: comparison of hemodynamic performance. *Thorac Cardiovasc Surg.* 9:37.
[41] Suri M., et al., 2012 "Aortic annulus diameter and valve design each determine the valve size implanted election?" *J Thorac Cardiovasc Surg.* 149:163-73.
[42] Von Oppell U. O., et al., 2012 "Aortic annulus diameter and valve design each determine the valve size implanted." *J Heart Valve Dis.* 21:591-598.
[43] Bobiarski J., et al., 2013 "One-year hemodynamic comparison of Perimount Magna with St Jude epic aortic bioprostheses." *Arch Med Sci.* 9:445-451.
[44] Wendt D., et al., 2014 "The new St Jude Trifecta versus Carpentier-edwards Perimount Magna and Magna ease aortic bioprosthesis: is there a hemodynamic superiority?" *J Thorac Cardiovasc Surg.* 147:1553-1560.
[45] Dell'Aquila A. M., et al., 2013 "Clinical and echocardiographic outcomes after implantation of the Trifecta aortic bioprosthesis: an initial single-centre experience." *Interact Cardiovasc Thorac Surg.* 16:112-115.
[46] Bavaria J. E., et al., 2014 "The St Jude Medical Trifecta aortic pericardial valve: results from a global, multicenter, prospective clinical study." *J Thorac Cardiovasc Surg.* 147:590-597.
[47] Permanyer E., et al., 2013 "St. Jude Medical Trifecta TM aortic valve perioperative performance in 200 patients." *Interact Cardiovasc Thorac Surg.* 17:669-672.

[48] Seo H., et al., 2012 "Clinical outcomes and hemodynamics of the 19-mm Perimount Magna bioprosthesis in an aortic position: comparison with the 19-mm Medtronic Mosaic Ultra valve." *Circ J*. 76:102-108.

[49] Flécher E., et al., 2014 "Hemodynamic performance during exercise of the new St. Jude Trifecta aortic bioprosthesis: results from a French multicenter study." *J Am Soc Echocardiogr*. 27:590-597.

[50] Eichinger W. B., et al., 2005 "Exercise hemodynamics of bovine versus porcine bioprostheses: a prospective randomized comparison of the mosaic and Perimount aortic valves." *J Thorac Cardiovasc Surg*. 129:1056-1063.

[51] Eichinger W. B., et al., 2004 "The effective orifice area/patient aortic annulus area ratio: a better way to compare different bioprostheses? A prospective randomized comparison of the Mosaic and Perimount bioprostheses in the aortic position." *J Heart Valve Dis*. 13:388-389.

[52] Pettenazzo E., et al., 2008 "Octanediol treatment of glutalaldehyde fixed bovine pericardium: evidence of anticalcification efficacy in the subcutaneous rat model." *Eur J Cardiothorac Surg*. 34:418-422.

[53] Ganapathi A. M., et al., 2015 "Long-term survival after bovine pericardial versus porcine stented bioprosthetic aortic valve replacement: does valve choice matter?" *Ann Thorac Surg*. 100:550-559.

[54] Kim W. K., et al., 2015 "Trans-femoral valve-in-valve implantation of a St. Jude Medical Portico in a failing trifecta bioprosthesis: a case report." *Clin Res Cardiol*. 104:363-365.

[55] Campisi S., et al., 2014 "Early failures of Trifecta aortic bioprosthesis." *J Thorac Cardiovasc Surg*. 148:133-134.

In: Perspectives in Aortic Valve Disease
Editor: Giovanni Concistrè
ISBN: 978-1-53618-769-4

Chapter 18

NEW GENERATION OF AORTIC BIOPROSTHESIS: SUTURELESS AND RAPID DEPLOYMENT VALVES

Giovanni Concistrè*, MD, Francesca Chiaramonti, PhD, MD and Marco Solinas, MD
Ospedale del Cuore "G. Pasquinucci,"
Fondazione Toscana Gabriele Monasterio, Massa, Italy

ABSTRACT

Over the last decade, the therapeutic options for patients with aortic valve disease have expanded considerably as demonstrated by the exponential growth of catheter-based aortic valve implants, the popularizing of minimally invasive surgical aortic valve replacement (AVR) techniques and the introduction of new valve technologies such as sutureless and rapid deployment (SURD) bioprostheses. SURD technologies reduce operative times and facilitate complex procedure and minimally invasive AVR.

This chapter aimed to explain chercteristics, surgical technique and published results of these two very similar but very different new generation of aortic bioprostheses.

Keywords: aortic valve, valvular disease, aortic valve prosthesis, aortic valve replacement, conventional aortic valve replacement, minimally invasive aortic valve replacement

INTRODUCTION

Historically, aortic valve replacement (AVR) has been the gold standard for patients with aortic stenosis (AS) since the 1960. In the recents years we have observed an increase in the number of elderly patients undergoing aortic valve surgery with high surgical risk profile due to presence of multiple comorbidities. Although much of this growth will likely be transcatheter AVR (TAVI), technologic advances in valve design and materials continue to improve the procedural success and long-term safety and performance of surgical aortic

* Corresponding Author's Email: gioconci@libero.it.

valves. Technologies have been improved to find any solutions to spread the indication of surgery for a broader spectrum of patients with AS. In this setting, the sutureless and the rapid deployment (SURD) bioprostheses can represent a good option. The sutureless concept of aortic valve implantation was developed in the early 60s. However, this approach was abandoned due to frequent valve-related thromboembolic complications and severe paravalvular leakage [1]. More recently, this concept has been reintroduced based on modern experience with TAVI and with the advent of bovine pericardial material for tissue valves. SURD valves are designed to allow faster and easier aortic valve implantation avoiding the need for sutures, reducing the cardiopulmonary bypass (CPB) and the aortic cross clamp (ACC) times. These characteristics make it especially suitable for minimally invasive approaches (MIA) and for patients requiring AVR and concomitant surgery. The rapid deployment aortic bioprosthesis Edwards INTUITY-Elite® valve (Edwards Lifesciences, Irvine, CA, USA) received CE Mark European approval in April 2014 and the sutureless aortic bioprosthesis Perceval (LivaNova, London, United Kingdom) in February 2011. Starting from these dates more than sixty-thousand Perceval and twenty-thousand Intuity valves have been implanted worldwide.

Methods

Sutureless Perceval S Bioprosthesis

Perceval Platform Technology

Perceval is a biological prosthesis composed of bovine pericardium stabilized in a buffered glutaraldehyde solution and assembled on a nitinol stent. This sutureless technique is achieved by the nitinol stent, which has the dual role of valve support and anchoring to the aortic root. A distinctive design built around a super elastic stent with unique features and mechanical behavior. The elastic structure aims at reproducing the stress absorption properties of the native tissue at the valve commissures level. The Perceval stent is able to adapt to the movements of the aorta during the cardiac cycle (Figure 1). Perceval gives patients even broader treatment options for their future. Its exclusive stent design allows even circumferential expansion to accommodate future transcatheter valves. The nitinol stent provides clear visibility under fluoroscopy. The inflow ring can be evenly and circumferentially expanded to accommodate transcatheter aortic valve placement. The sinusoidal struts allow identification of clear landmarks which may help avoid coronary ostia obstruction at annulus level.

Thanks to dedicated accessories (Figure 2), the valve diameter can be reduced prior to implantation, increasing visibility and facilitating more complex procedures.

Perceval is not crimped and it has been shown in literature that the collapsing procedure of Perceval does not affect leaflet integrity (Figure 3).

Pericardial leaflets are not connected to the stent directly but through an intermediate outer layer to minimize the stress transferred to the leaflets (Figure 4).

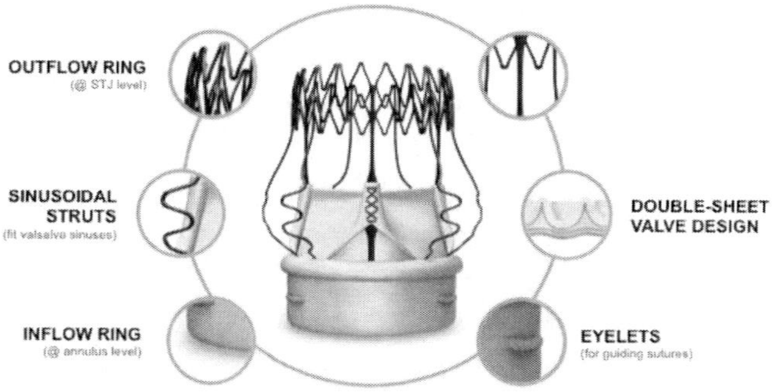

Figure 1. Structural characteristics of sutureless Perceval S bioprosthesis (Reprinted from Livanova website).

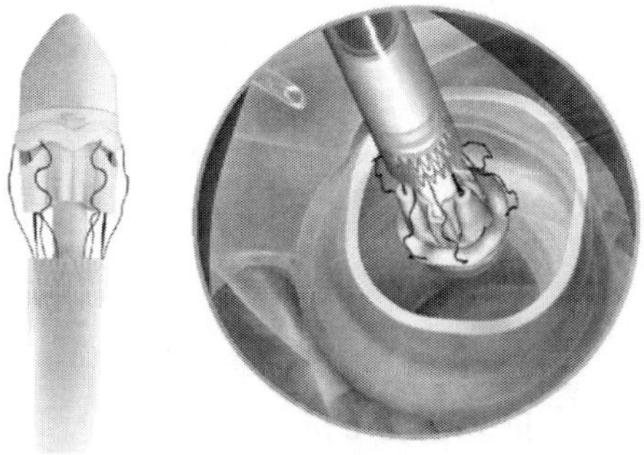

Figure 2. Perceval collapsed in delivery system (Reprinted from Livanova website).

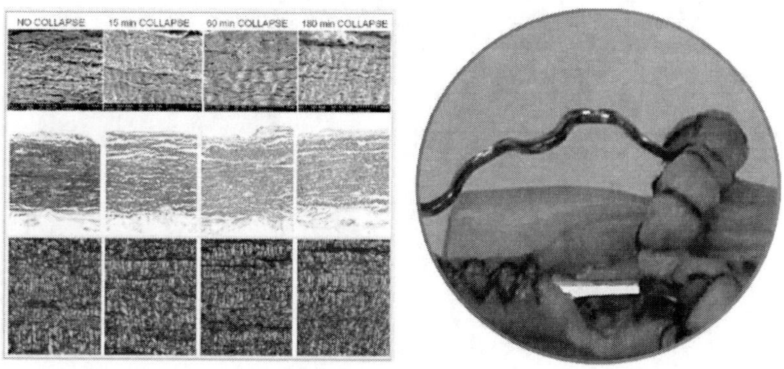

Figure 3. Pre-implantation collapse and ballooning does not affect the structural integrity of the collagen network of the pericardial cusp tissue (Reprinted from Livanova website).

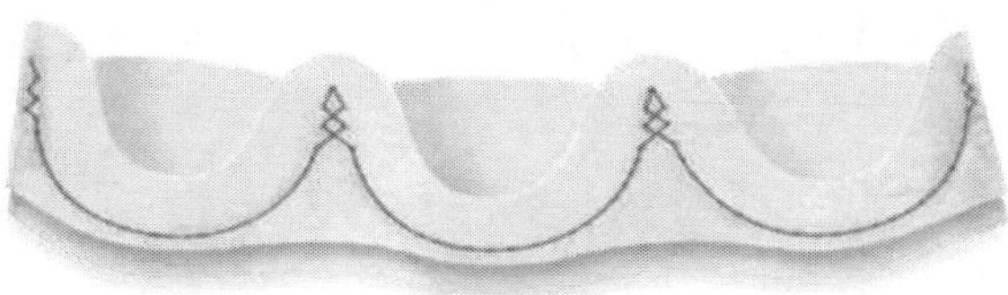

Figure 4. Pericardial characteristic of Perceval prosthesis (Reprinted from Livanova website).

This sutureless aortic valve prosthesis is available in size S, M, L, and XL. Perceval obtained U.S. Food and Drug Administration (FDA) approval in January 2016. We instituted oral anticoagulation therapy with warfarin sodium for 3 months after Perceval implantation reaching an international normalized ratio between 2.0 and 3.0. After 3 months we recommend, when there are no contraindications to suspension, the replacement of warfarin with 100 mg daily of aspirin.

The use of sutureless bioprosthesis is contraindicated in case of acute endocarditis, pure aortic regurgitation, irregular aortic annulus or ascending aorta geometry. The ratio between the diameter of the sinotubular junction and the diameter of the superior annulus should not exceed 1.3 (a ratio >1.3 can prevent a correct fixation of the valve-stent on the aorta). This ratio was routinely determined with echocardiography and also with CT-scan in case of isolated AVR. We performed in all patients undergoing isolated AVR CT-scan to planning minimally invasive approach.

Implantation Technique

A higher aortotomy is required to accommodate the height of the cage and to allow for closure of the aorta. We recommend a transverse aortotomy 3.5 cm above the annulus, or 0.5 cm above the sinotubular junction (STJ), approximating the epiaortic fat pad (Figure 5). Commissural traction sutures for native valve exposure should be removed before Perceval valve deployment because they distort the annulus. If the aortotomy is too low, care must be taken to avoid catching the outflow ring during suture closure because this can displace the valve and potentially cause intimal tears when the heart fills with blood.

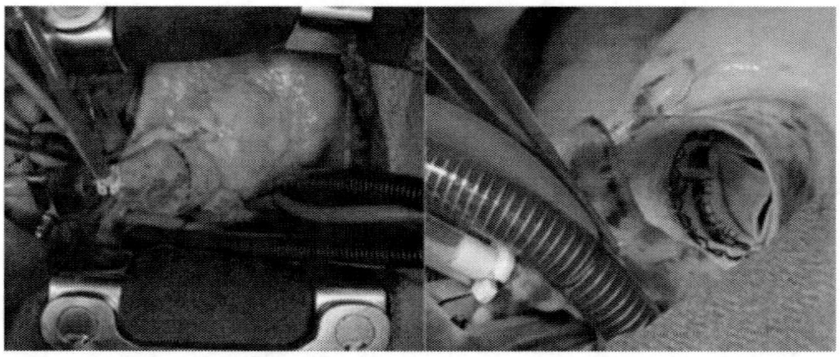

Figure 5. High transverse aortotomy for Perceval implantation outlined in blue marking pen, approximately 3.5 cm above annulus, and then after implantation.

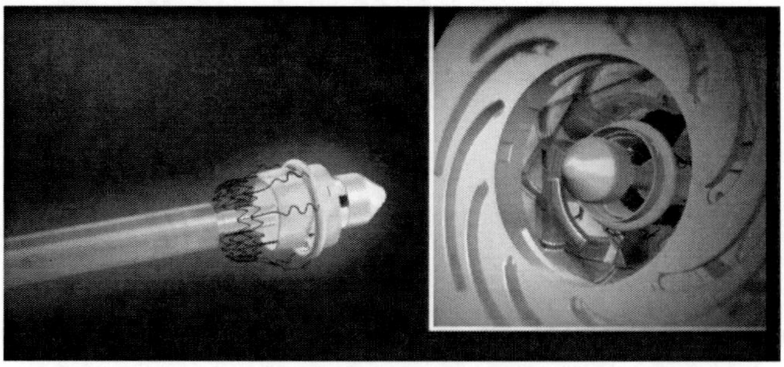

Figure 6. Collapsing device (Reprinted from Livanova website).

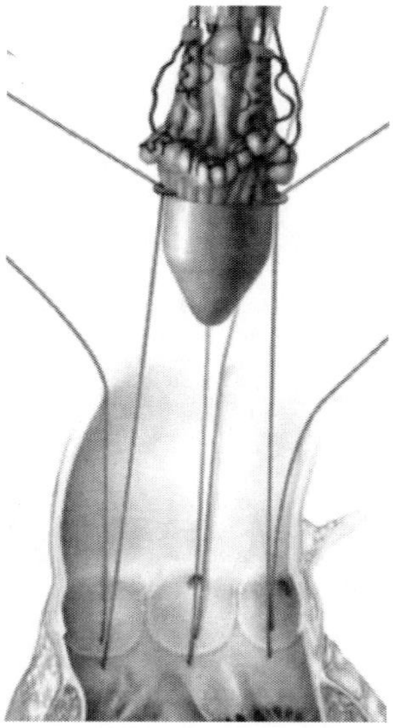

Figure 7. Perceval implantation.

This bioprosthesis can be collapsed through a dedicated device and positioned by means of a delivery system (Figure 6).

Temporary guiding sutures are placed in the annulus at the nadir of each sinus and are then passed though the eyelets of the valve (Figure 7).

During deployment, continuous traction is important to ensure that the valve is positioned at the correct height. Because the non-coronary sinus is lower, the valve holder is tilted toward the operator, thus aligning the valve with the left ventricular outflow tract (LVOT), perpendicular to the annulus. Once the delivery system is in position, the prosthesis is deployed, the guiding sutures are removed and the valve is finally in place; at this point a post-dilation modeling is performed with a dedicated balloon (30 seconds at a pressure of 4 Atmosphere) and the valve flushed with warm saline at 37°C to optimize final sealing. The operator visually confirms positioning, alignment, leaflet symmetry, coaptation, and patency of the coronary ostia (Figure 7). Visible annulus above or below the valve indicates that the height of deployment is incorrect. The commissures will be visible above the valve, but the annulus should not appear. Forceps should be used to open the leaflets to confirm that the annulus is not visible below the inflow ring. Circumferential examination of the prosthesis-tissue interface should detect PVL. This valve is retrievable and replaceable if necessary. When a malposition occurs the Perceval valve can safely be removed even after balloon dilation. The procedure performed is a 'χ-movement' with the aid of anatomical forceps. If the prosthesis does not show any malformation after the procedure, it can be reimplanted in the correct intra-annular position [2].

Sizing

Correct sizing requires particular attention. The transparent sizer must easily traverse the annulus, whereas the white sizer must meet significant resistance or fail to pass (Figure 8).

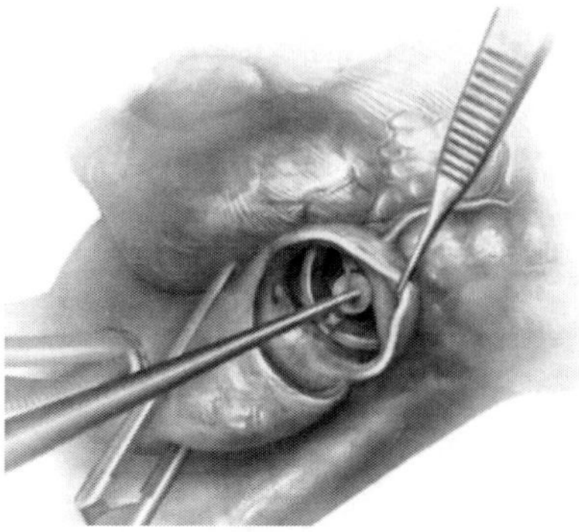

Figure 8. Sizing procedure.

Undersizing causes PVL secondary to inadequate annular sealing, central leak from failure of central leaflet coaptation, or possible late proximal migration. Oversizing is a more common mistake and it is discussed in the next paragraph.

Intraoperative transesophageal echocardiography assessment includes the same parameters as those for evaluating a stented bioprosthesis. Additional evaluation is required, focusing on correct intraannular position, thereby ensuring full cage expansion, appropriate deployment height, presence of leaks, and leak significance. Short-axis views assess deployment of the device (rule out infolding) and circumferential annular apposition. Circumferential deformities warrant additional cross-clamping for visual evaluation, particularly if they are associated with more than mild intravalvular regurgitation, PVL, rocking, or high gradients. Normal Perceval leaflets may appear to open and coapt slightly asymmetrically or display accentuated "leaflet fluttering" because they lack the rigid struts of a typical stented valve. In isolation, these findings are of no concern. Central regurgitation occasionally accompanies the asymmetric coaptation. It should be no greater than mild in severity and typically resolves over time. Long-axis views assess angulation of the valve and aortic root parameters. Although an angulated conventional stented prosthesis does not always entail poor valve implantation, it should raise more concern with the Perceval valve. Visible edges of the device should line up with the virtual parallel lines formed by the LVOT, aortic root, and ascending aorta. The cage should also conform to the aortic root and engage the STJ. The proximal inflow ring will extend below the native valve annulus. If the valve is deployed at the appropriate height, the location of the Perceval and native valves' hinge points should match (within 1 to 2 mm). The known dimensions of the Perceval valve can locate a "virtual hinge point" when shadowing occurs. Create a reference point using distances from the anterior mitral leaflet and STJ to the native hinge point and compare with the virtual hinge point described earlier. Observation of inflow ring impedance of anterior mitral leaflet opening may suggest low deployment, as well as membranous septum compression and risk of atrioventricular conduction block. After valve deployment, isolated trace PVL is rarely concerning. Eccentric PVLs make grading challenging, and jets splaying across the LVOT can be overestimated. Generally, any PVL greater than trace or the presence of multiple jets warrants repeat visual inspection of the valve and potentially further annulus debridement and valve redeployment.

Role of Oversizing

Excessive oversizing of the Perceval valve is associated with increased transprosthetic gradients and should be avoided. Grossly oversized Perceval bioprostheses tend to recoil, causing loss of contact between the prosthesis and the annulus, which results in paravalvular leakage and, possibly, in significant aortic regurgitation. Recoiling has been observed in the clinical setting and in the laboratory [3, 4]. An oversizing of 30% or more in the annular cross-sectional area was associated with a 16-fold increase of the risk of developing increased postoperative gradients [5]. In our experience some typical predictors of prosthesis-patient mismatch, such as the patients' body surface area and the size of the implanted prosthesis, were not related to the outcome, whereas a greater degree of oversizing was associated with increased gradients. This apparent paradox is, in our opinion, well explained by the fact that the full expansion of the valved stent inside the patient aortic annulus could be associated with smoother leaflet kinetics, improved valve opening, and increased effective orifice area (EOA), whereas the stent compression or deformation that follows the implantation of a prosthesis that is too big with respect to the patient annulus could lead to altered kinetics of the leaflets, incomplete valve opening, and increased gradients. In fact, the Perceval valve has an in vitro EOA that is much higher than that of conventional sutured bioprostheses [6, 7]: the in vitro EOA for the S size ranges from 2.07 to 2.2 cm2 [6], and in a study of patients with small annuli, the measured in vivo EOA index was 1.12 ` 0.2 cm2/m2 vs 0.82 ` 0.1 cm2/m2 for small size conventional, sutured valves [8], indicating that the fluid dynamics of valved stents might be superior to those of conventional surgical valves. The observation that the use of transcatheter aortic valves is associated with a higher EOA index and with a reduced incidence of prosthesis-patient mismatch would also support this idea [8]. A secondary finding of our experience is that intraoperative sizing for the Perceval valve, as recommended by the instructions for use, does not reflect the true in vivo measure of the aortic annulus and could be misleading. Surgical obturator-based sizing is a complex process that converts to a number several nonnumeric inputs, including visual assessment, tactile feedback, stiffness of the cardiac tissues, the amount and distribution of calcium, the fragility of the aortic wall or the height of the coronary arteries, and others. Furthermore, the surgical sizers and the sizing strategy both differ significantly between different prostheses, making the sizing process even more complex [9]. In our experience, there was an impressive degree of overlapping between the four prosthetic sizes. Surgical sizing resulted in a mean oversizing of more than 20% and probably led to the implantation of a too big prosthesis in a significant proportion of patients. Other authors have reported difficulties with the Perceval sutureless sizing process. Baert and coworkers [4] recently reported valve recoiling caused by excessive oversizing in 4 patients (2.9% of their Perceval population). They suggested to modify the sizing process and to implant the valve size "Given by the sizer of which the white obturator pass the annulus with friction" [4]. This would certainly reduce the number of grossly oversized prostheses but that the choice between different valve sizes in patients with similar annular dimensions would remain arbitrary. In our opinion, cardiac CT could offer a simple solution to this problem. In fact, cardiac CT has become a very standardized process and is used with an extremely high rate of success in thousands of TAVI patients every year. Given the surprising forgivingness of the Perceval valve, the development of a CT-based sizing reference chart would not be complex: the valve showed good hemodynamic performance in a wide range of conditions and still behaved acceptably in the extreme conditions of virtually no to almost 50% oversizing (Figure 9).

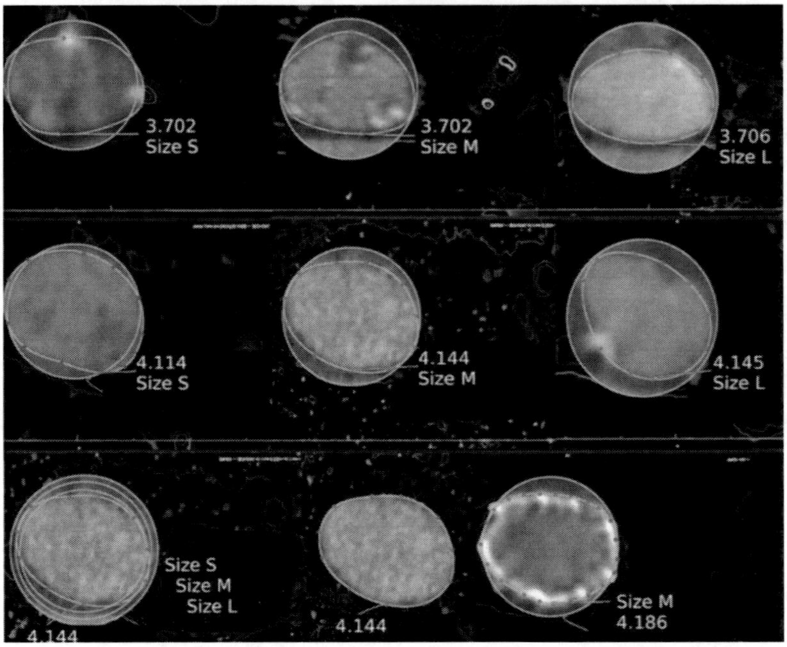

Figure 9. Double oblique axial computed tomography images of the virtual basal ring (VBR) from 6 patients. (Upper row) Three patients with virtually identical aortic annular sizes (3.7 cm^2) who received 3 different prosthesis sizes (small [S], medium [M], and large [L], respectively). The ex vivo area of the implanted prostheses is represented with 3 closed circles for comparison. (Middle row) Three patients with virtually identical aortic annular sizes (4.1 cm^2) who received 3 different prosthesis sizes (S, M, and L, respectively). (Bottom row) The VBR area of this patient (4.14 cm^2, center) is depicted against the ex vivo area of the S, M and L Perceval (LivaNova, Saluggia, Italy) valve (left). The patient received an M valve. The postimplant area of the VBR was 4.18 cm^2, indicating minimal expansion of the aortic annulus after the implantation. The patient underwent valve-in-valve implantation with a 23-mm Sapien 3 valve (Edwards Lifesciences, Irvine, CA) for valve failure 3 years after the original operation.

Results

First clinical results of Perceval bioprosthesis were reported in 2011 by the group of Flameng and colleagues [10]. A larger multicentre experience with Perceval aortic bioprosthesis was reported by Shrestha et al. [11]. Fischlein et al. reported low 1-year event rates in intermediate-risk patients undergoing AVR from a large multicentre cohort study [12]. In our experience up to 2015, 30-day mortality was 1.9% (12/617) and survival was 91.3% at follow-up. Relative to others series, we found similar results in terms of paravalvular leakage and hemodynamic performance. Specifically, we found 3 patients with moderate paravalvular leakage without hemolysis not requiring any treatment. Two patients had incomplete expansion of Perceval valve due to oversizing of bioprosthesis, caused early moderate paravalvular leakage, required reoperations at 2 and 9 postoperative days. The Perceval bioprosthesis selected for implant should match the measured diameter of the aortic annulus. Margaryan et al. analyzed 54 patients underwent Perceval who had preoperative contrast-enhanced multidetector-row computed tomography (MDCT). Echocardiographic measurements showed lower accuracy compared to MDCT measurements. They concluded that possibly for precise aortic annulus measurement, contrast-enhanced MDCT is preferable [13]. According to the 2-year follow-up of the PARTNER trial, paravalvular leakage was more frequent in patients undergoing transcatheter aortic valve implantation (TAVI) and this was associated with increased risk of mid-term mortality, even in those with mild leakage [14]. In our single center series, paravalvular leakage occurred at follow-up in 36 patients, of whom 3 had moderate paravalvular leakage. Although the reduced time needed for implantation is a theoretic potential advantage of this prosthesis, in our experience mean CPB and ACC time were longer than other studies [10-12]. This might certainly be related to surgical approach. In 475 (77%) patients Perceval was implanted in minimally invasive approach. A meta-analytical study showed CPB time of 104.4 minutes for minimal access group underwent AVR versus 94.0 minutes for conventional access group ($p < 0.00001$) [15]. Our experience showed CPB time of 81.7 minutes for minimal access group underwent AVR with Perceval valve. As minimally invasive AVR has shown longer CPB and ACC time than conventional surgery, we strongly believe that sutureless technology might be the solution for less invasive approaches. In our experience ACC and CPB times of minimally invasive AVR with conventional sutured bioprosthesis were 87 and 121 minutes versus 50.5 and 81.7 with Perceval bioprosthesis. The advantages of Perceval implantation in ministernotomy approach have been described by Fischlein et al. with good results [16]. On the other hand, we reported AVR through a right minithoracotomy, which avoids opening the sternum, but requires greater technical skills, and may be a challenging and long procedure even for expert surgeons. The potential advantages of the right minithoracotomy for AVR as well as the potential limitations and drawbacks of this technique have been recently reviewed [17]. Especially when the ribs are not resected or disconnected from the sternum, this procedure may be very challenging because of the limited field and the difficult exposure of some regions of the aortic annulus, this reflected by the longer operative and cross-clamp times reported with this approach. The sutureless prostheses might represent a solution to this problem. Semsroth et al. compared patients underwent AVR with sutured prosthesis through an anterolateral minithoracotomy versus partial upper hemisternotomy. In this study a median cross-clamp time of minithoracotomy group was 93 minutes and a median perfusion time was 137 minutes [18]. In our series, patients underwent AVR with sutureless Perceval bioprosthesis presented a mean cross-clamp time of 52 minutes and a mean perfusion time of 82.3 minutes. Besides the possible facilitation of minimally invasive approach, this prosthesis may also be advantageous for patients needing AVR replacement long with concomitant procedures that prolong CPB and ACC times. In our experience, there were a significant number of patients who had concomitant mitral surgery. The procedures on the mitral valve are always mitral anuloplasty with incomplete ring implantation. Incomplete mitral ring prosthesis allows correct implantation of sutureless bioprosthesis. In concomitant mitral surgery, we performed before mitral anuloplasty and after the Perceval implantation to avoid dislocation of bioprosthesis during the mitral surgery. Mean transvalvular gradient at mid-term follow-up was 11.9 ± 5.4 mmHg. Left ventricular mass decreased from 146.57 g/m2 before surgery to 112.6 g/m2 at follow-up ($P < 0.001$). In our experience the rate of perioperative pacemaker implantation was 5% (30/617). This result is lower than the largest European multicentre experience [19]. Until 2020, we have implanted more than thousand

Perceval in our Center. Vogt et al. identified preoperative presence of right bundle branch block (RBBB) as independent predictors of postoperative conduction disorder [20]. The rate of preoperative RBBB was lower than the study of Vogt (3.6% vs. 7.8%). This could be the reason why the rate of pacemaker implantation is lower in our experience than the other studies. In TRASFORM clinical trial, the rate of permanent pacemaker implantation for the Edwards Intuity was 11.9% [21].

Rapid Deployment Intuity Elite Valve

INTUITY Platform Technology

Starting from 2012 the first-generation of Intuity Valve System (model 8300A; Edwards Lifesciences) was available for surgical AVR. The Edwards Intuity valve system consist is a stented trileaflet bovine pericardial bioprosthesis with a balloon-expandable, cloth-covered stent frame at the inflow aspect and combines the long-term safety and efficacy in terms of hemodynamics results of bioprosthesis Carpentier Edwards Perimount with the simplicity and quickness on implantation of transcatheter valve prosthesis. The pericardial stented aortic valve is based on the design and the proven performance of the PERIMOUNT valve family. A balloon expandable stainless steel cloth-covered frame is incorporated into the inflow aspect of the valve. The valve is implanted with the aid of a delivery system, which incorporates a balloon catheter to expand the frame within the left ventricular outflow tract (LVOT). The expandable frame works in conjunction with the sewing ring to position and stabilize the valve at implant. The system reduces the number of sutures required to secure the valve, while the frame establishes a seal within the LVOT. These new valves are so termed "rapid-deployment valves" because their implantation (rapid-deployment aortic valve replacement [RDAVR]) requires only 3 sutures. Another design improvement of these bioprosthesis is a shaped skirt along the underside of the valve; the skirt acts to mechanically maintain effective orifice area (EOA) in aortic placement and to provide a substrate for fixation and an associated significantly reduced need for suturing. The second generation Intuity Valve System (model 8300AB; Edwards Lifesciences), named INTUITY-Elite® valve (Edwards Lifesciences, Irvine, CA, USA) received CE Mark European approval in April 2014 and presents three minor design modifications made to enhance seating during implantation. First, the number of cloth layers on the frame was reduced and the cloth was shifted down closer to the inflow edge of the annulus frame. With the cloth on the annulus frame moved down, the resulting tissue annulus diameter was reduced by 1 mm. Second, the single, crimped cloth-covered, expandable stainless steel frame was double crimped to further reduce the implant profile. Third, the valve holder is now cusp-mounted instead of commissural-mounted to increase the visibility for the nadir suture markers.

The model 8300AB is a stented trileaflet valve comprised of bovine pericardium treated with the Carpentier-Edwards ThermaFix process. The leaflets are mounted on a flexible cobalt-chromium alloy wireform. The inflow of the valve incorporates the cloth-covered balloon expandable frame. The EDWARDS INTUITY Elite valve system is available in sizes 19, 21, 23, 25, and 27 mm (Table 1).

Table 1. Nominal dimensions (mm) EDWARDS INTUITY Elite Valve

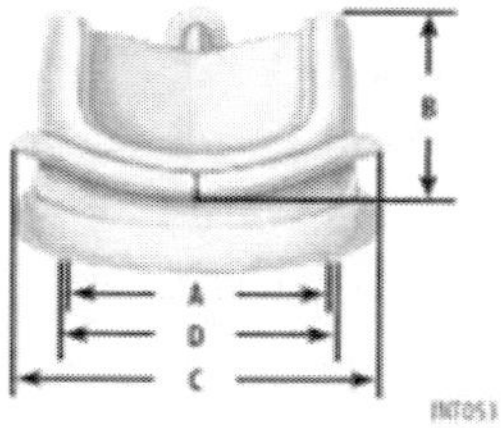

Legend
A. Internal Diameter
B. Profile Height
C. External Sewing Ring Diameter
D. Stent Diameter (wireform)*

Size	19 mm	21 mm	23 mm	25 mm	27 mm
A. Internal Diameter	18	20	22	24	26
B. Profile Height	13	14	15	16	17
C. External Sewing Ring Diameter	24	26	28	30	32
D. Stent Diameter (wireform)*	19	21	23	25	27

*TAD (Tissue Annulus Diameter)

Reprinted from accessdata.fda.gov

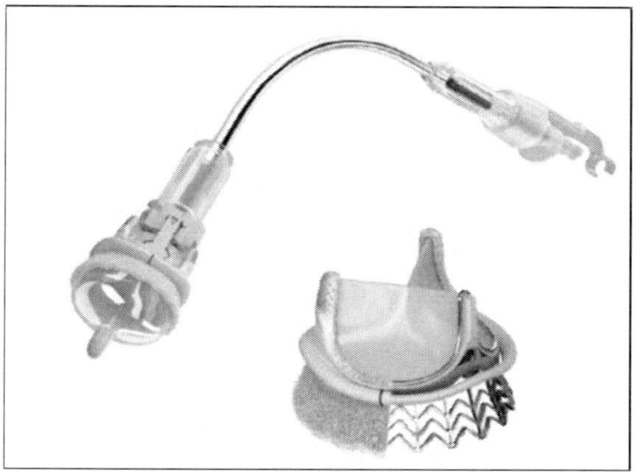

Figure 10. Edwards INTUITY Valve System Elite - Valve Technology and Delivery System. Reprinted from Edwards website.

The valve is packaged and terminally sterilized in glutaraldehyde. Glutaraldehyde is shown to both reduce the antigenicity of tissue xenograft valves and increase tissue stability. The wireform is made of cobalt-chromium alloy. The wireform is covered with a knitted polyester fabric. A thin, cobalt-chromium alloy/polyester film laminate band surrounds the base of the wireform. A silicone sewing ring which is covered with a porous, seamless polytetrafluoroethylene (PTFE) cloth is attached to the wireform. The scalloped sewing ring is designed to conform to the native aortic annulus. The compliant nature of the sewing ring facilitates coaptation between the valve and an often irregular or calcific tissue bed. The sewing ring has three suture markers to aid in valve orientation. A holder is attached to the valve by means of sutures to facilitate handling, deployment, and suturing the valve during the implant procedure. The holder is easily detached by the surgeon. The delivery system includes an integrated balloon catheter and malleable tubular handle shaft through which the catheter extends. The distal end of the handle shaft includes an adapter, which mates with the holder of the valve, and a locking sleeve for rapidly connecting the delivery system to the valve holder. The balloon portion of the delivery system resides within the adapter, and advances distally into position for expanding the frame. A tubular balloon introducer is attached, when removing the valve from a storage jar, and facilitates passage of the balloon through the valve. The malleable handle is made of aluminum and has chromate conversion coating applied over the entire surface of the part. The inflation device is used to pressurize and expand the balloon (Figure 10).

The Edwards Intuity Valve is indicated for the replacement of the diseased, damaged or malfunctioning native or prosthetic aortic valves. The use of this valve system is contraindicated in case of pure aortic regurgitation and in patients with aneurysms of the aortic root or ascending aorta.

Implantation Technique

A standard CPB is established. Most important is the incision of aorta that will allow for coaxial delivery of the Intuity valve; proper angulation of the delivery device is critical to seating the valve perpendicular to the annulus. While a transverse aortotomy may be sufficient in patients with dilated ascending aorta, the aortotomy in patients with normal diameter of ascending aorta should be directed to the non-coronary sinus and extended past the sinotubular junction (STJ) [22], especially in patients with narrow supracoronary aorta (Figure 11).

The native aortic valve leaflets are excised and a total decalcification of the annulus is performed. Debridement of the calcium from the annulus, left ventricular outflow tract (LVOT), and the anterior mitral valve leaflet must be performed beacause the inside of the annulus and LVOT should be smooth to ensure proper seating of the prosthetic valve to achieve a good seal and minimize the risk of paravalvular leaks. Otherwise an excessive debridement may result in annular injury or creates divots, compromise the integrity of the aortic annulus, and it must to be avoided and/or results in paravalvular leak. Three equidistant guiding sutures are placed through the nadir of the aortic annulus and then placed in corresponding positions through the sewing ring of the valve. A simple suture technique is recommended to help confirm seating of the valve. The pledgeted sutures or monofilament sutures are not recommended. The use of pledgets may create leak channels resulting in paravalvular leaks. The use of monofilament sutures and resulting suture tails may damage the leaflets. Simple suture technique is recommended with suture entering just below the annulus and exiting 2-3 mm above the annulus. A suture entry site too low, in order to avoid deep-seating the valve, may lead to conduction disturbance. The exit site should be high enough on the aorta to visualize around the sewing cuff of the seated valve (Figure 12). If one of the sinuses appears relatively large and prolapsed, two sutures can be placed within that sinus to bring the tissue in plane with the valve.

By using the guiding sutures, the valve and attached delivery system are lowered onto the annulus and secured into position under direct vision. It should also be confirmed that any atherosclerotic plaque be debrided from the aortic root and STJ. During parachuting must be maintained counter traction on the sutures. It is importantant to avoid bending the malleable handle greater than 90 degrees and more than three times. Once seated, we must hold the valve in place with the delivery system, and toconfirm the seating position of the valve onto the annulus. The commissure posts should correspond to the remnants of the native valve commissures so as not to obstruct the coronary ostia. Maintaining proper seating of the valve is recommended to prevent valve displacement. After we must secure the valve by snares compressed with hemostats over the sewing ring, ensuring that the snares are placed directly on the sewing ring, not on the valve holder legs as this may result in loose sutures or difficulty in removing the holder/delivery system once the holder sutures are cut. After securing the snares, appropriate valve seating should be confirmed by direct visual inspection. In particular, the valve must be firmly seated in the non-coronary sinus and no gaps should exist between the sewing cuff and native annulus. If adjustment is necessary, the snares may be loosened and the valve repositioned. After that we must verify that the coronary ostia are not obstructed, the commissure posts do not interfere with the aortic wall at the sinotubular junction and there is good apposition between the sewing ring and the annulus (Figure 13).

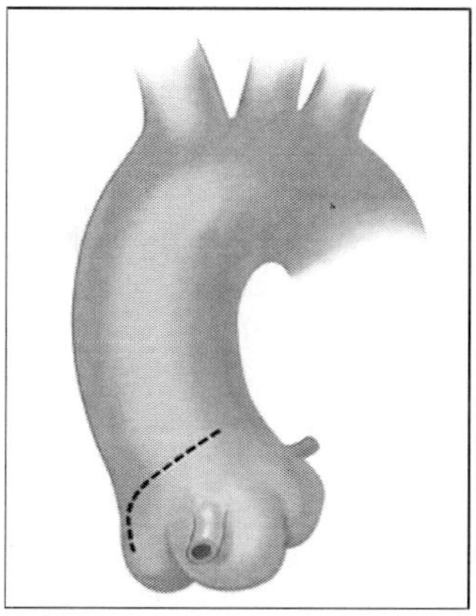

Figure 11. Hockey-stick aortotomy crossing the sinotubular junction into the noncoronary sinus. Reprinted from Step-by-Step Aortic Valve Replacement With a New Rapid Deployment Valve. Accola KD, Chitwood WR Jr, Mumtaz MA, Barnhart GR. Ann Thorac Surg. 2018;105(3):966-971.

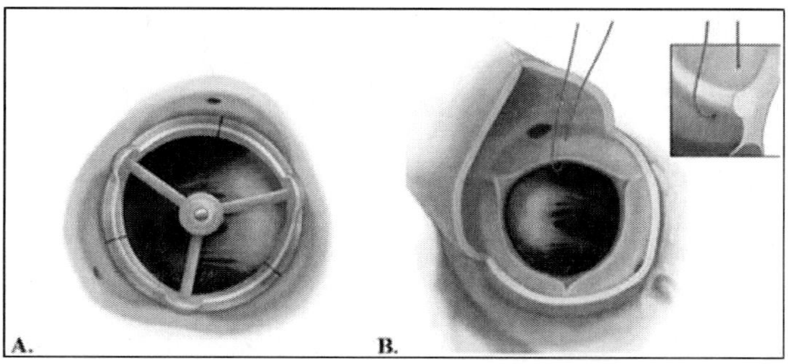

Figure 12. Edwards Intuity Valve System – Placing sutures. (A) Location of sutures correspond to markers on sizer to ensure proper valve seating. (B) Placement of guiding suture at the nadir of the right, left, and noncoronary cusps with exit site well away from annulus (inset). Reprinted from Step-by-Step Aortic Valve Replacement With a New Rapid Deployment Valve. Accola KD, Chitwood WR Jr, Mumtaz MA, Barnhart GR. Ann Thorac Surg. 2018;105(3):966-971.

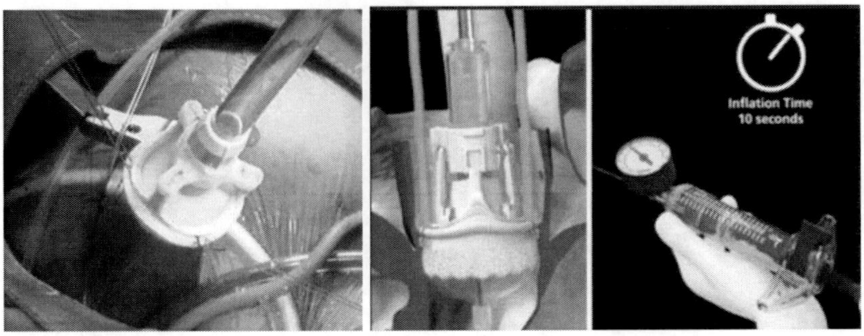

Figure 13. Valve delivery.

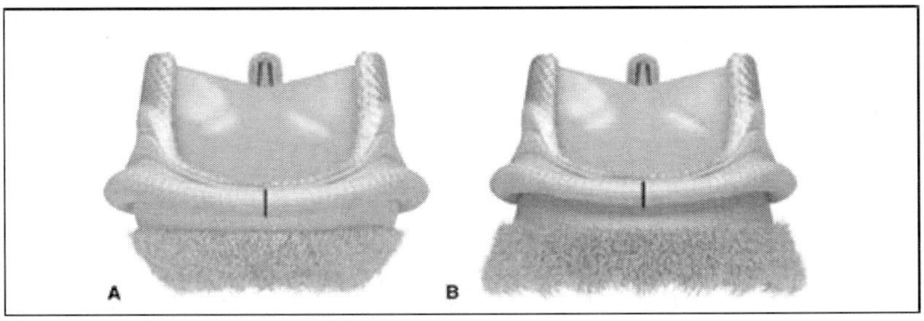

Figure 14. Edwards INTUITY Aortic Valve. A. Valve before deployment B. Valve after deployment. Reprinted from TRANSFORM (Multicenter Experience With Rapid Deployment Edwards INTUITY Valve System for Aortic Valve Replacement) US clinical trial: Performance of a rapid deployment aortic valve. Barnhart GR, Accola KD, Grossi EA, et al. J Thorac Cardiovasc Surg. 2017; 153(2):241-251.e2.

Then we fill the inflation device with sterile physiological saline and remove any air to a final volume of 25 cc . The balloon catheter is advanced distally until the catheter snaps into place and an audible "click" is heard. We must be sure to stabilize the handle while advancing the balloon catheter and that the distal portion of the delivery system is perpendicular to the plane of the valve and apply gentle pressure in a distal direction to maintan proper valve seating during balloon inflation. During balloon inflation pressure must be maintained for 10 seconds to ensure proper frame expansion. The delivery system must be held in position during balloon inflation to ensure that the valve remains seated in the annulus. Inflation of the sealing frame should be performed up to the recommended pressure in a slow and controlled fashion; this slow expansion against the septum may reduce the risk of heart block. Over-inflation may cause excessive frame expansion and may result in annular damage, conduction interference/arrhythmia, or sub-annular tissue damage. Under-inflation may cause insufficient expansion of the frame and may result in paravalvular leak, thrombosis, and/or thromboembolism. If the inflation pressure is not achieved is recommended to completely deflate the balloon by fully retracting the syringe plunger, remove the valve and delivery system beginning with the removal of the snares and sutures and then to use a new valve and delivery system. We must to take attention to not retract the balloon catheter through the valve holder when removing the whole system to avoid possible valve displacement. Once the inflation pressure is achieved and maintained for 10 seconds, we deflate the balloon by unlocking the inflation device, fully retracting the plunger, and locking the plunger in the retracted position. We remove the delivery system and valve holder as a single unit. To tie the sutures first we remove one snare while maintaining valve seating position by applying downward pressure on the sewing ring and then we tie the suture (we repeat the process for the other two or three snares) (Figure 14). The aortotomy is closed using standard surgical techniques. Minimal manipulation of the heart after valve implant is recommended to avoid valve displacement.

Sizing

The sizing is crucial for the good results of the implant of an edwards Intuity bioprosthesis. The final decision to use the EDWARDS INTUITY Elite valve system should be made after the native aortic valve is excised and the annulus is debrided, or decalcified. An assessment of the potential interaction between the EDWARDS INTUITY Elite valve system and surrounding cardiac structures, such as, the aortic annulus, anterior leaflet of the mitral valve, and coronary ostia, should be conducted. Severely calcified LVOT that is not properly debrided may result in balloon rupture during inflation. When choosing a valve, the size, age, and physical condition of the patient in relation to the size of the prosthesis must be taken into consideration to minimize the possibility of obtaining a suboptimal hemodynamic result. A combined intra- and supra-annular sizing technique is recommended for this valve. The practice of using only a supra-annular sizing technique is not recommended, due to the intra-annular and sub-annular aspects of the EDWARDS INTUITY Elite valve.

- Intra-annular sizing: is recommanded to insert the sizer barrel end through the aortotomy and place it into the aortic root and annulus. If a transverse aortotomy is used and the sinotubular junction diameter is estimated to be equal or smaller than the annulus diameter, it is recommended to extend the aortotomy into the non-coronary sinus to facilitate sizer and implant insertion. If extension of the aortotomy is not possible, it is not recommended to use the product as parachuting the valve through a narrow sinotubular junction may result in increased difficulty of valve implant and/or aortic injury. It is suggested to sized the valve choosing the largest diameter barrel end that is a comfortable fit in the annulus. It is important to ensure that the lip of the barrel does not pass through the annulus. The lip of the barrel represents the sewing cuff of the valve, therefore it is intended to rest on the annulus and not go through it. We do not have to implant a valve larger than the size indicated by the barrel end of the sizer as it may result in annular or aortic damage. We do not have to select a valve size based on the sizer that will fit through the sinotubular junction as it may result in paravalvular leak due to the use of an undersized valve.
- Supra-annular sizing : the replica end of the same sizer may be used to verify adequate fit and orientation of the supra-annular section of the valve in the aortic root. Adequate fit includes good seating on the aortic annulus and no interference of the commissure posts of the valve with the aortic wall at the sinotubular junction or with the coronary ostia. We can also use three black orientation markers on the replica end to assess guiding suture placement in the annulus.

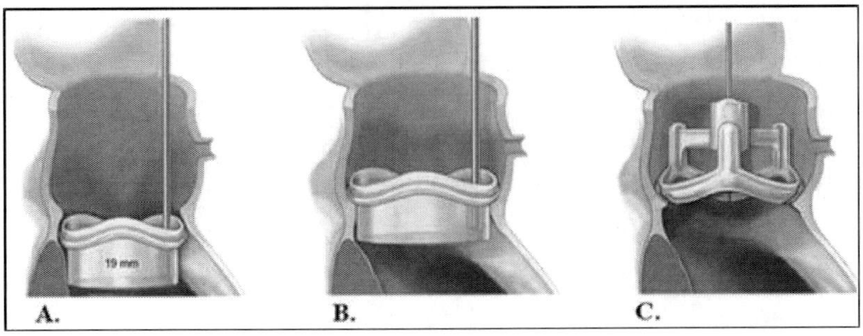

Figure 15. SIZING: (A) Incorrect sizing: Loose fit with flange protruding through the annulus. (B) Correct sizing: Sizer barrel seen intraannular with flange sitting on annulus. (C) Sizer replica end placed in a supra-annular position. Reprinted from Step-by-Step Aortic Valve Replacement With a New Rapid Deployment Valve. Accola KD, Chitwood WR Jr, Mumtaz MA, Barnhart GR. Ann Thorac Surg. 2018;105(3):966-971.

When using either sizer, a barrel sizer that falls through the annulus is too small, and one that requires significant force to push it through the annulus is too big. When using the sizer, the correct size will not allow the flange to comfortably pass into the LVOT. In cases of "in-between" sizes, the smaller size should be chosen without concern for perivalvular leak and with the confidence of improved hemodynamics. The expanded frame width is 2.5 mm larger in diameter than the nominal size of each valve. Oversizing may lead to tearing of the aorta, failure to completely seat the valve within the LVOT, or increased risk of conduction disturbance. If oversizing is clinically required, EIE should not be used (Figure 15).

Intra-operative trans-esophageal echocardiography (TEE) is required to assess bioprosthetic valve function. While trace of paravalvular leak is acceptable, mild or greater paravalvular leak should be addressed in the operating room. Because of stainless steel in its sealing frame, the Intuity valve will have an appearance on TEE similar to that following transcatheter aortic valve replacement. First, the sealing frame will be seen in the LVOT extending on the aorta-mitral curtain. Second, the sealing frame casts an acoustic shadow which can obscure the contralateral side of the valve on mid-esophageal and long-axis views. Therefore, to completely assess for paravalvular regurgitation, two additional TEE views should be performed: mid-esophageal, short-axis and deep trans- gastric.

The indications for anticoagulat/antiplatelets terapy management are the same for any other aortic bioprosthetic valve: some medical professional societies recommend anticoagulant therapy, unless contraindicated, during the first 3 months after bioprosthetic aortic valve implantation. Long-term anticoagulant therapy, unless contraindicated, is recommended for patients who have risk factors for thromboembolism. Long-term low dose aspirin, unless contraindicated, is recommended for all patients.

Results

Edwards Intuity valve system combines the long term proven Magna Ease Perimount aortic valve platform with the stent-based technology. First published article by Borger et al. [23] presented the Edwards Intuity valve as an exciting device that may further change the landscape of aortic valve intervention expecially for the possibility to facilitate the performance of minimally invasive aortic valve surgery and for the possibility to reduced implantation times in higher risk patients or in those requiring concomitant procedures. An impportant advantage connected to facilitating surgical implant of Intuity valve bioprosthesis is the reduction in crossclamp and cardiopulmonary bypass (CPB) times. The CADENCE-MIS trial [24], a prospective, multicentre, randomized trial, that compares outcomes in patients undergoing minimally invasive AVR using the EDWARDS INTUITY Valve System with those undergoing conventional full sternotomy with a commercially available bioprosthetic valve, focusing on early and mid-term outcomes particularly on haemodynamic data, showed a highly significant reduction in myocardial ischemic time (54.0 min and 41.3min, respectively), favoring the Intuity valve despite the more challenging minimally invasive surgical access. These findings were confirmed in two articoles that reported the European (TRITON) and the American (TRANSFORM) trials. Kocher [25] presents the 1-year clinical outcomes and device efficacy of the first 146 subjects receiving an EDWARDS INTUITY Valve in a prospective, multicenter study (Surgical Treatment of Aortic Stenosis With a Next Generation Surgical Aortic Valve [TRITON]). Barnhart and collegues [26] show the one year primary and effectiveness endpoints of 839 underwent AVR using an EDWARDS INTUITY Valve in a prospective, nonrandomized, multicenter (n = 29), single-arm trial (Multicenter Experience With Rapid Deployment Edwards INTUITY Valve System for Aortic Valve Replacement [TRANSFORM]). In both TRITON and TRANSFORM trials was documented a remarkable reduction in crossclamp and cardiopulmonary bypass (CPB) times for both isolated full sternotomic approaches and minimally invasive RDAVR operations when compared with Society of Thoracic Surgeons (STS) National Database values. Even more important, these times were reduced significantly in combined cardiac procedures. Both trials involved the surgeon implanting the Intuity valve for the first time. Thus, without the learning curve effect, crossclamp and CPB times might have been even shorter. These benefits are impressive and suggest a positive impact on hard clinical end points (eg. 30-day mortality). The 30-day mortality in the TRITON and TRANSFORM studies was 1.7% and 0.9%, respectively. This appears to be noticeably low, considering the risk profiles of patients in both studies (mean age, 75/73 years; only 55/62% isolated RDAVR; mean STS score, 3.5/2.5, respectively). The data collected through the clinical trial were confirmed by short-term outcomes of the Assessing Standard oF Care and Clinical Outcomes UsiNg the EDWARDS INTUITY VAlve SysTem in a European multI-center, Active, pOst-market surveillaNce Study (FOUNDATION) registry, representing the largest series of patients receiving the EDWARDS INTUITY valve system in a registry setting. The FOUNDATION registry was a prospective, multicenter, single-arm, postmarket 2-year study designed to determine the safety and effeciveness of the EDWARDS INTUITY rapid-deployment valve system in a broad registry setting across Europe. In this registry we observed a valve-related mortality of 1.4% early and 1.4%/patient-year beyond 30 days, within the range of those reported with this valve in TRITON, CADENCE and TRANSFORM. The Intuity valve system design not only enables quicker and easier aortic valve implantation but also promises improved hemodynamic performance.

With the use of in vitro testing, Capelli and colleagues [27] demonstrated that pledget-armed sutures adversely affect the hemodynamic performance of biologic aortic valves when compared with the stent-based anchoring system of the Intuity system. Moreover low transvalvular gradients of this valve is also related to the shape of expanded stent frame. The stent skirt frame is seated below the annulus in a flared configuration within the left ventricular outflow tract. The stent may limit active constriction of the LVOT during systole which may lead to more laminar blood flow across the prosthesis. In addition, the lack of pledgeted sutures may contribute to more laminar flow across the LVOT/aortic annulus. Both TRITON and TRANSFORM trials confirm these previously postulated advantages with a 1-year mean gradients of 9.0 ± 3.5mm Hg and 10.3 ± 3.8mm Hg and effective orifice areas of 1.7 ± 0.2cm2 and 1.7 ± 0.2cm2, respectively. A noteworthy hemodynamics also was observed on FOUNDATION registry confirming smaller reports with a mean EOA at 1 year of 1.88 +/- 0.6 cm2 and the mean and peak valve gradients of 9.6 +/- 4.6 mm Hg and 17.7+/- 7.3 mm Hg at 1 year. In the TRITON trial, optimal hemodynamic performance was shown for the Intuity valve by the low rate of severe patient–prosthesis mismatch (PPM) from discharge to 3 years (2.4%-3.9%). In FOUNDATION registry was unexpectly observed a 9.76% severe PPM at 1 year, especially given this registry's 43% proportion of small 19- and 21-mm valves. Device sizing is critical; in this series, standard sizing criteria were used, but there was also a deliberate tendency not to oversize. Maybe the high incidence of small valves in this registry reflects the cohort rather than undersizing. In routine clinical practice, PPM is a concern, especially in patients with small valve sizes. Theron and colleagues [28] focused on the small aortic root (only 19-mm and 21-mm Intuity valves) and reported a severe PPM rate as low as 15% in this subset. This is remarkable because severe PPM rates with conventional bioprosthesis SAVR have been approximately 20% according to a meta-analysis by Takagi and colleagues [29]. The anchoring mechanism design of the Intuity valve is based on balloon inflation of a subvalvular stent frame with radial pressure apposition throughout the distal subvalvular outflow tract.

A highly debated aspect is the new early permanent pacemaker implantations (PPI) rate. Theoretically, any pressure below the leaflet attachment zone induces the risk of a cardiac conduction disturbance. With a rapid deployment valve, the implantation mechanical stress is restricted to the leaflet attachment zone and immediately below where the sutures are placed. In both TRITON and TRANSFORM trials, AVR was performed in patients with the higher-risk profile of a combined cardiac operation in 45.9% and 37.5%, respectively. Thus, a higher likelihood for new conduction disturbances existed preoperatively, but the PMI rates reported tend to have increased compared to conventional prostheses. Although European TRITON data showed an early PPI rate of 6.9%, the US TRANSFORM trial revealed a higher early PPI rate (14.0% overall and 6.0% without previous conduction abnormalities). These observed differences in PPIs have to be interpreted with caution: First, the implant technique, although the valve is fixed at the nadir in all 3 sinuses, allows variability as to how deep the valve descends in the outflow tract. If commissural suspension sutures are used for better exposure and traction is exerted during introduction of the valve, the stent frame can be deployed deeper into the conduction sensitive area in the right nonsubcommissural triangle, promoting a higher risk of new conduction disturbances. Second, sizing is critical. Surgeons in the "learning phase" of implantation may tend to oversize the valve to avoid paravalvular leak, which can result in increased radial stress along the subvalvular rim. Third, with this valve, approximately 30% of new conduction disturbances revert within 1 week postoperatively. Generally, in the United States an earlier patient discharge strategy is present than in European centers. Thus, in TRANSFORM more patients may have had pacemakers implanted early to ensure safety at discharge. A watchful waiting strategy should allow more patients to recover from transitory rhythm disturbances and result in a lower PPI rate. As shown by Romano M. A. and collegues [30] patient factors associated with PPI after RDAVR were RBBB, AVB, female gender and larger valve size. In FOUNDATION registry was experienced a pacemaker rate of 6.1%. An interesting observation was conducted by Mogilansky et al. [31] who studied 183 patients undergoing RDAVR. Out of these 38.1% had new left bundle branch block, 2.5% of patients had new right bundle branch block and 9.6% had atrioventricular block III requiring either a pacemaker or defibrillator. Another quality of this valve is a remarkable resistance to prosthetic valve endocarditis (PVE). In the TRITON trial, the early incidence was 0.2% (late 0.2%/per patient-year), and in TRANSFORM there were no early cases or throughout late follow-up. This advatage could be releated to a low paravalvular leak rates that could been associated with subsequent PVE (the exceptionally low PVE rates may be explained by the covered stent smooth surface, which reduces surface roughness that is present with multiple pledgets in the outflow tract). Moreover, the valve can be implanted with almost no contact between the surgeon's gloves and the prosthesis, especially if a knot pusher is used to tie the guiding sutures. Valve thrombosis in TRITON and TRANSFORM patients (n = 1126) was absent at both early and late clinical follow-ups. Underreporting of early subclinical bioprosthesis valve thrombosis (BPVT) in TRITON and TRANSFORM cannot be excluded because subclinical valve thrombosis often is associated with absent or minimal gradient increases. However, in the TRITON trial, the lack of BPVT evidence on high-quality, core laboratory–adjudicated TTE images (N=1126 patients) at 1 year and 5 years and gradient stability suggest that it is unlikely. Nevertheless, a prospective study using 4-dimensional volume-rendered computed tomography scans with different antithrombotic strategies would add valuable information. A very important benefit related to this valve is representing by the possibility to increase minimally invasive AVR as shows in CADENCE-MIS (24% reduction in XCT). Minimally invasive AVR has been shown to improve operative mortality, with a risk ratio of 0.74 for mini-AVR versus full sternotomy [32]. Moreover in all types of cardiac surgery, resternotomy is associated with increased mortality. However, resternotomy after a minimally invasive approach approaches is straightforward because the right ventricle is not adherent to the posterior table of the sternum.

In the past few years, the proportion of patients receiving tissue valves as opposed to mechanical valves has been recently increasing, especially in younger patients in whom the prospect of lifelong anticoagulation therapy is unappealing and fraught with risks. Therefore, it can be expected that there will be an increase in revision aortic valve procedures in the future. If this bioprosthesis facilitates an increase in minimally invasive approaches, then it can be expected that the mortality of repeat surgery may be significantly reduced when the Edwards Intuity valve implantation is used through a minimally invasive approach. One of the main drawbacks, like that seen with transcatheter heart valve systems, is the complication of paravalvular leaks (PVL). The association of PVL with mortality and poor long-term outcomes make a search for standardized treatment options essential. Currently, there is no universally agreed single treatment option. Various transcatheter methods for treating with PVL, such as the use of coils and plugs, have been tried. The ease of access and superior forward flow valve hemodynamics seen with balloon expandable valves used during RDAVR make balloon valvuloplasty a promising treatment option in cases complicated by PVL as shown by Grant J. K. et al. [33] in a case report that explained a case of a patient that received an Edwards Intuity valve and developed a PVL 6 moins after the procedure. In this patient a balloon valvuloplasty with a 25 mm True Balloon was performed with resolution of the PVL that remained stable also at 1 year follow up. The costs of this bioprosthesis is higher compared with standard prostheses, but general economic outcome end points have been documented to be equal or even superior as shown by Moore et al. [34]·

References

[1] Magovern GJ, Cromie HW. Sutureless prosthetic heart valves. *J Thorac Cardiovasc Surg*. 1963;46:726-36.

[2] Santarpino G, Pfeiffer S, Concistrè G, Fischlein T. A supra-annular malposition of the Perceval S sutureless aortic valve: the 'χ-movement' removal technique and subsequent reimplantation. *Interact Cardiovasc Thorac Surg*. 2012 Aug;15(2):280-1.

[3] Di Eusanio M, Saia F, Pellicciari G, et al. In the era of the valve-in-valve: is transcatheter aortic valve implantation in sutureless valves feasible? *Ann Cardiothorac Surg* 2015;4: 214–7.

[4] Baert J, Astarci P, Noirhomme P, de Kerchove L. The risk of oversizing with the Perceval S sutureless bioprosthesis in small aortic annulus. *J Thorac Cardiovasc Surg* 2017;153: 270–2.

[5] Cerillo AG, Amoretti F, Mariani M, et al. Increased gradients after aortic valve replacement with the Perceval valve: the role of oversizing. *Ann Thorac Surg*. 2018 Jul;106(1):121-128. doi: 10.1016/j.athoracsur.2017.12.044. Epub 2018 Feb 2.

[6] Belluschi I, Moriggia S, Giacomini A, et al. Can Perceval sutureless valve reduce the rate of patient- prosthesis mismatch? *Eur J Cardiothorac Surg* 2017;51: 1093–9.

[7] Tasca G, Vismara R, Mangini A, et al. Comparison of the performance of a sutureless bioprosthesis with two pericar- dial stented valves on small annuli: an in vitro study. *Ann Thorac Surg* 2017;103:139–44.

[8] Shalabi A, Spiegelstein D, Sternik L, et al. Sutureless versus stented valve in aortic valve replacement in patients with small annulus. *Ann Thorac Surg* 2016;102:118–22.

[9] Doenst T, Amorim PA, Al-Alam N, Lehmann S, Mukherjee C, Faerber G. Where is the common sense in aortic valve replacement? A review of hemodynamics and sizing of stented tissue valves. *J Thorac Cardiovasc Surg* 2011;142:1180–7.

[10] Flameng W, Herregods MC, Hermans H, Van der Mieren G, Vercalsteren M, Poortmans G, Van Hemelrijck J, Meuris B. Effect of sutureless implantation of the Perceval S aortic valve bioprosthesis on intraoperative and early postoperative outcomes. *J Thorac Cardiovasc Surg*. 2011 Dec;142(6):1453-7.

[11] Shrestha M, Fischlein T, Meuris B, Flameng W, Carrel T, Madonna F, Misfeld M, Folliguet T, Haverich A, Laborde F. European multicentre experience with the sutureless Perceval valve: clinical and haemodynamic outcomes up to 5 years in over 700 patients. *Eur J Cardiothorac Surg*. 2016 Jan;49(1):234-41.

[12] Fischlein T, Meuris B, Hakim-Meibodi K, Misfeld M, Carrel T, Zembala M, Gaggianesi S, Madonna F, Laborde F, Asch F, Haverich A; CAVALIER Trial Investigators. The sutureless aortic valve at 1 year: A large multicenter cohort study. *J Thorac Cardiovasc Surg*. 2016 Jun;151(6):1617-1626.e4.

[13] Margaryan R, Kallushi E, Gilmanov D, Micelli A, Murzi M, Solinas M, Cerillo AG, Glauber M. Sutureless Aortic Valve Prosthesis Sizing: Estimation and Prediction Using

Multidetector-Row Computed Tomography. *Innovations* (Phila). 2015 Jul-Aug;10(4):230-5; discussion 235.

[14] Leon MB, Smith CR, Mack MJ, Makkar RR, Svensson LG, Kodali SK, Thourani VH, Tuzcu EM, Miller DC, Herrmann HC, Doshi D, Cohen DJ, Pichard AD, Kapadia S, Dewey T, Babaliaros V, Szeto WY, Williams MR, Kereiakes D, Zajarias A, Greason KL, Whisenant BK, Hodson RW, Moses JW, Trento A, Brown DL, Fearon WF, Pibarot P, Hahn RT, Jaber WA, Anderson WN, Alu MC, Webb JG; PARTNER 2 Investigators. Transcatheter or Surgical Aortic-Valve Replacement in Intermediate-Risk Patients. *N Engl J Med.* 2016 Apr 28;374(17):1609-20.

[15] Martuza B, Pepper JR, Stanbridge RD, Jones C, Rao C, Darzi A, Athanasiou T. Minimal access aortic valve replacement: is it worth it? *Ann Thorac Surg* 2008;85:1121-31.

[16] Fischlein T, Pfeiffer S, Pollari F, Sirch J, Vogt F, Santarpino G. Sutureless Valve Implantation via Mini J-Sternotomy: A Single Center Experience with 2 Years Mean Follow-up. *Thorac Cardiovasc Surg*. 2015 Sep;63(6):467-71.

[17] Glauber M, Gilmanov D, Farneti PA, Kallushi E, Miceli A, Chiaramonti F, Murzi M, Solinas M. Right anterior minithoracotomy for aortic valve replacement: 10-year experience of a single center. *J Thorac Cardiovasc Surg*. 2015 Sep;150(3):548-56.

[18] Semsroth S, Matteucci-Gothe R, Heinz A, et al. Comparison of Anterolateral Minithoracotomy Versus Partial Upper Hemisternotomy in Aortic Valve Replacement. *Ann Thorac Surg*. 2015 Sep;100(3):868-73.

[19] Laborde F, Fischlein T, Hakim-Meibodi K, Misfeld M, Carrel T, Zembala M, Madonna F, Meuris B, Haverich A, Shrestha M; Cavalier Trial Investigators. Clinical and haemodynamic outcomes in 658 patients receiving the Perceval sutureless aortic valve: early results from a prospective European multicentre study (the Cavalier Trial)†. *Eur J Cardiothorac Surg*. 2016 Mar;49(3):978-86.

[20] Vogt F, Pfeiffer S, Dell'Aquila AM, Fischlein T, Santarpino G. Sutureless aortic valve replacement with Perceval bioprosthesis: are there predicting factors for postoperative pacemaker implantation? *Interact Cardiovasc Thorac Surg*. 2016 Mar;22(3):253-8.

[21] Barnhart GR, Accola KD, Grossi EA, Woo YJ, Mumtaz MA, Sabik JF, Slachman FN, Patel HJ, Borger MA, Garrett HE Jr, Rodriguez E, McCarthy PM, Ryan WH, Duhay FG, Mack MJ, Chitwood WR Jr; TRANSFORM Trial Investigators. TRANSFORM (Multicenter Experience With Rapid Deployment Edwards INTUITY Valve System for Aortic Valve Replacement) US clinical trial: Performance of a rapid deployment aortic valve. *J Thorac Cardiovasc Surg*. 2017 Feb;153(2):241-251.

[22] Accola KD, Chitwood WR Jr, Mumtaz MA, Barnhart GR. Step-by-Step Aortic Valve Replacement With a New Rapid Deployment Valve. *Ann Thorac Surg*. 2018; 105(3):966-971.

[23] Borger MA, Dohmen P, Misfeld M, Mohr FW. Current trends in aortic valve replacement: development of the rapid deployment EDWARDS INTUITY valve system. *Expert Rev Med Devices*. 2013;10(4):461-470.

[24] Borger MA, Moustafine V, Conradi L, et al. A randomized multicenter trial of minimally invasive rapid deployment versus conventional full sternotomy aortic valve replacement. *Ann Thorac Surg*. 2015;99(1):17-25.

[25] Kocher AA, Laufer G, Haverich A, et al. One-year outcomes of the Surgical Treatment of Aortic Stenosis With a Next Generation Surgical Aortic Valve (TRITON) trial: a

prospective multicenter study of rapid-deployment aortic valve replacement with the EDWARDS INTUITY Valve System. *Thorac Cardiovasc Surg*. 2013 Jan;145(1):110-5; discussion 115-6.

[26] Barnhart GR, Accola KD, Grossi EA, et al. TRANSFORM (Multicenter Experience With Rapid Deployment Edwards INTUITY Valve System for Aortic Valve Replacement) US clinical trial: Performance of a rapid deployment aortic valve. *J Thorac Cardiovasc Surg*. 2017;153(2):241-251.e2.

[27] Capelli C, Corsini C, Biscarini D, et al. *Pledget-Armed Sutures Affect the Haemodynamic Performance of Biologic Aortic Valve Substitutes: A Preliminary Experimental and Computational Study. Cardiovasc Eng Technol*. 2017;8(1):17-29.

[28] Theron A, Gariboldi V, Grisoli D, et al. Rapid Deployment of Aortic Bioprosthesis in Elderly Patients With Small Aortic Annulus. *Ann Thorac Surg*. 2016;101(4):1434-1441.

[29] Takagi H, Umemoto T; ALICE (All-Literature Investigation of Cardiovascular Evidence) Group. Prosthesis-Patient Mismatch After Transcatheter Aortic Valve Implantation. *Ann Thorac Surg*. 2016;101(3):872-880.

[30] Romano MA, Koeckert M, Mumtaz MA, et al. Permanent Pacemaker Implantation After Rapid Deployment Aortic Valve Replacement. *Ann Thorac Surg*. 2018;106 (3):685-690.

[31] Mogilansky C, Balan R, Deutsch C, Czesla M, Massoudy P. New postoperative conduction abnormalities after the implantation of a rapid-deployment aortic valve prosthesis. *Interact Cardiovasc Thorac Surg*. 2019;28(4):581-586.

[32] Phan K, Tsai YC, Niranjan N, et al. Sutureless aortic valve replacement: a systematic review and meta-analysis. *Ann Cardiothorac Surg*. 2015;4(2):100-111.

[33] Grant JK, Braghiroli J, Panakos A, De Marchena E. Balloon aortic valvuloplasty: Treatment of rapid deployment aortic valve replacement complicated by a paravalvular leak. *J Card Surg*. 2019;34(8):738-741.

[34] Moore M, Barnhart GR, Chitwood WR Jr, et al. The economic value of INTUITY in aortic valve replacement. *J Med Econ*. 2016;19(10):1011-1017.

In: Perspectives in Aortic Valve Disease
Editor: Giovanni Concistrè
ISBN: 978-1-53618-769-4

Chapter 19

Aortic Valve Repair

Stefano Mastrobuoni*, MD, Laurent De Kerchove, MD and Gebrine El Khoury, MD
Cardiovascular and Thoracic Surgery Department, Saint-Luc's Hospital, Catholic University of Louvain, Brussels, Belgium

Abstract

Aortic valve (AV) sparing and repair procedures are advantageous alternatives to valve replacement in patients with aortic aneurysm with or without aortic regurgitation but also for patient with isolated AV regurgitation without severe leaflet disease. A successful repair strategy proceeds first from a clear understanding of the anatomy and function of the AV and the potential mechanisms of valve dysfunction. The fundamental starting point is the understanding that the AV is a functional unit composed of the valve cusps and the functional aortic annulus. Lesion on any or more of these components can induce aortic regurgitation as well as a gradient across the valve. A functional classification of aortic regurgitation identifies 3 main mechanisms of AV regurgitation although more than 1 type of lesion can coexist in any given patient. The goal of AV repair is to improve the surface of coaptation by restoring the functional relation between the leaflets and the FAA, while preserving the mobility of AV cusps. We present our preferred surgical techniques for valve sparing-root replacement (VSRR) in the context of tricuspid (TAV) and bicuspid (BAV) aortic valve. Further we will discuss our current approach to isolated aortic valve regurgitation.

Keywords: aortic valve, repair techniques, sparing techniques

Introduction

During the past 25 years, important advances in the field of aortic valve (AV) repair have transformed it from an infrequent and anecdotal technique to a feasible and advantageous

* Corresponding Author's Email: stm919@mail.harvard.edu.

alternative to valve replacement in patients with ascending aorta aneurysm or aortic regurgitation (AR). These advances included first a deeper understanding of the anatomy of the AV and the mechanisms of AR; the development of surgical techniques aimed to restore on the one hand the geometry of the aortic root while sparing the AV and on the other hand to improve the leaflet coaptation while ensuring cusp mobility; and the development of a common language that can be used by all clinicians to describe the lesions, discuss repair techniques, and compare immediate and long-term results after repair.

Aortic regurgitation and aortic root aneurism concern mainly adolescent and young adults with connective tissue disorders or other abnormal congenital valve diseases like bicuspid aortic valve (BAV). In these patients, aortic valve sparing and repair procedures represent a particularly interesting alternative to replacement because of the limitations of currently available aortic valve substitutes. Although xenografts don't need long-term anticoagulation therapy, the high structural failure rate in young patients expose them to multiple re-replacements and increased morbidity and mortality . Mechanical valves have an excellent freedom from reoperation, but a freedom from major bleeding and thromboembolic events of around 90% at 10-year in young patients. Nonetheless recent studies showed very similar long-term survival after AV replacement regardless of the type of prosthesis implanted. AV replacement with the pulmonary autograft (the Ross operation) is ideal for young patients with AV stenosis because of its durability, excellent survival, and low risk of thromboembolic complications. However, the presence of aortic insufficiency and aortic root dilatation are considered as important predictors of late pulmonary autograft failure .

This chapter attempts to describe the principles of correction of AV regurgitation by focusing on functional anatomy and surgical techniques.

Anatomy of the Aortic Valve

For the purpose of AV repair the AV should be considered as a functional unit composed of two structures: 1- the functional aortic annulus (FAA) made by the Sino-Tubular junction (STJ) and the Ventriculo-Aortic junction (VAJ) (Figure 1), 2- the valve cusps. The integrity of these 2 components (the FAA and the cusps) is the basis for good valve function, and dysfunction of one of them is frequently associated with dysfunction of the other as well. Thus, a first fundamental principle in AV repair is that both lesions of the cusps and the FAA should be addressed at the time of valve repair. Further, similarly to the annuloplasty during mitral valve repair, dilatation of the VAJ should be addressed during AV repair even in the absence of ascending or aortic root aneurysm.

The VAJ is the anatomical line of transition between the endocardium and the endothelium and is a complex and non-planar structure (Figure 2). The aortic root inserts on fibrous tissues in approximately one half of its circumference and on muscular tissues on the other half. The fibrous portion, beneath the non-coronary cusp and half of the left coronary cusp, consists in the aorto-mitral valve continuity and the two trigones. The muscular portion, beneath the other half of left coronary cups and right coronary cusp, consists in the left ventricular and interventricular myocardium. Beneath the right/non coronary commissure stands the membranous septum and, below it, the bundle of Hiss. The basal ring is the virtual plane passing through the nadir of the three cusps and is a surgical landmark. A clear comprehension of the relationship between the VAJ and the basal ring is of paramount important for AV annuloplasty.

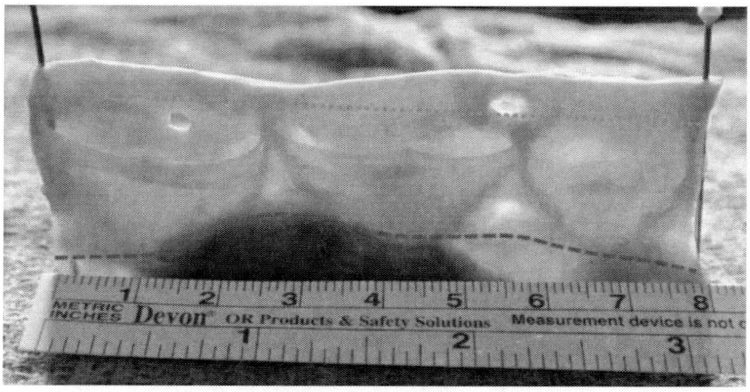

Figure 1. Anatomical specimen of the aortic root showing the position of the Ventriculo-aortic junction (VAJ) (red line) and the Sino-tubular Junction (STJ) (blue line), in between, the three sinuses of Valsalva and inter-leaflets triangles.

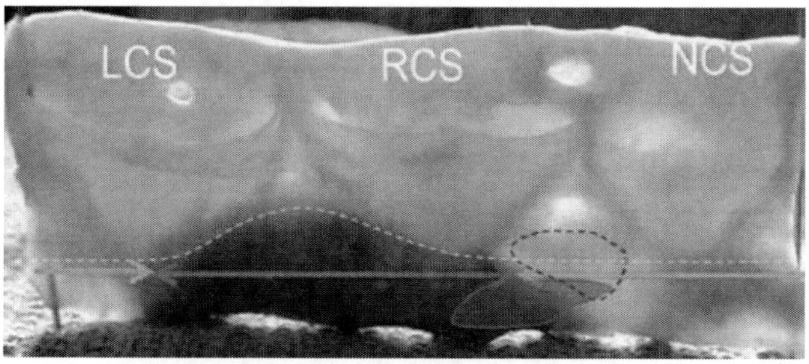

Figure 2. Anatomical specimen of a tricuspid aortic valve showing the fibrous (green arrowed line) and the muscular portion (red arrowed line) of the VAJ (yellow dotted line). The membranous septum (black dotted area) and the conduction bundles (red shadowed area) are also indicated. LCS: left coronary sinus; RCS: right coronary sinus; NCS: non-coronary sinus. (Reprinted with permission).

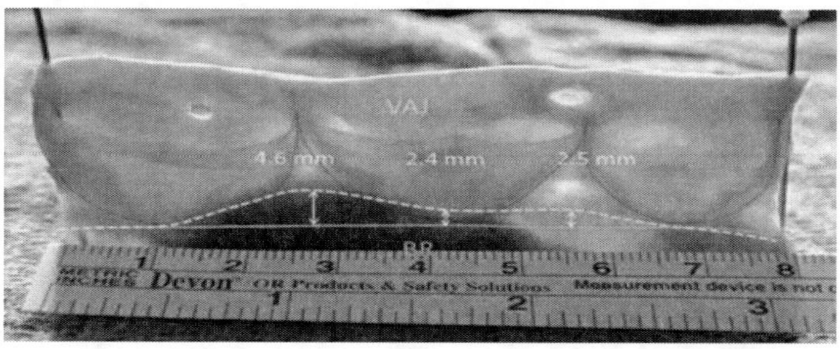

Figure 3. Anatomical specimen of a tricuspid aortic valve showing the relation between the VAJ (yellow line) and the basal ring (green line). At the level of the non-coronary and the left-coronary sinuses the VAJ reaches the BR, but at the level of the right-coronary sinus the VAJ lays few millimeters above the BR due to the presence of the muscular tissue of the inter-ventricular septum and the right outflow tract. The picture shows also the mean distance observed between these two lines. (Reprinted with permission).

On its fibrous portion the VAJ is at the level of the basal ring while on its muscular portion and at the level of the membranous septum the VAJ is a few millimeters higher than the basal ring (Figure 3).

The diameter of the aorta at the level of the basal ring has a mean of 23±2mm in women and 26±3mm in men without aortic root or valve disease and it is closely related to the body surface area . In the context of chronic AR, oftentimes the VAJ and the basal ring are dilated, particularly in patients with bicuspid AV (mean diameter of 27-28mm in TAV and 28-30mm in BAV).

The distance between the lower point of the cusp insertion in the aortic wall and the middle point on the free margin is the cusp height (also called geometric height) (Figure 4).

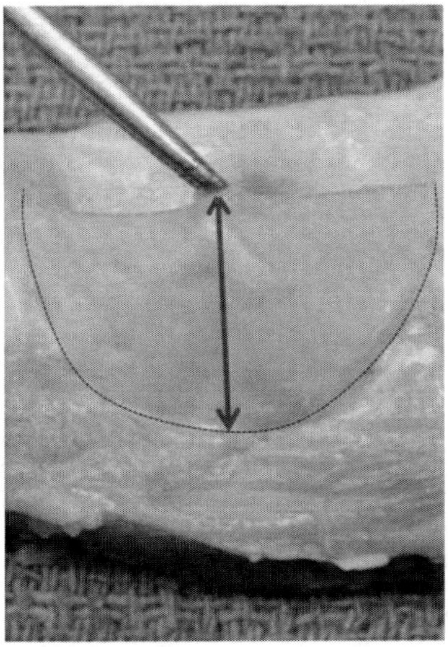

Figure 4. Anatomical specimen of a tricuspid aortic valve showing the geometric height (red arrowed line): from the lowest point of the base of insertion of the cusp (black line) to the middle point on the free margin (green dotted line).

The mean cusp height is 20mm in Tricuspid Aortic Valve (TAV) and 24mm in Bicuspid Aortic Valve (BAV) (at the non-fused cusp) . A cusp height of 15mm or less in adult may be considered as a sign of cusp retraction which in turn may reduce the cusps coaptation hence causing regurgitation across the valve. Only part of each cusp joins the others during valve closure. Indeed, on each cusp the coaptation surface area (mean of 1.25 cm^2) corresponds approximately to 40% of the total cusp surface. Therefore, the effective height is the distance between the lower point of the cusp "belly" and the tip of coaptation in the center of the valve (Figure 5). In competent AV, the effective height measures 9 to 10mm8. Moreover, the effective height normally reaches approximately the mid-height of the commissures. Nonetheless the length of coaptation varies along the cusp. The coaptation surface is indeed bigger close to the commissures and smaller in the center of the valve.

The free margin of the cusp is on average 34mm long and is usually elongated in root or ascending aorta dilatation involving the STJ as a compensatory mechanism11. Cusp prolapse is nothing less than an elongated free margin.

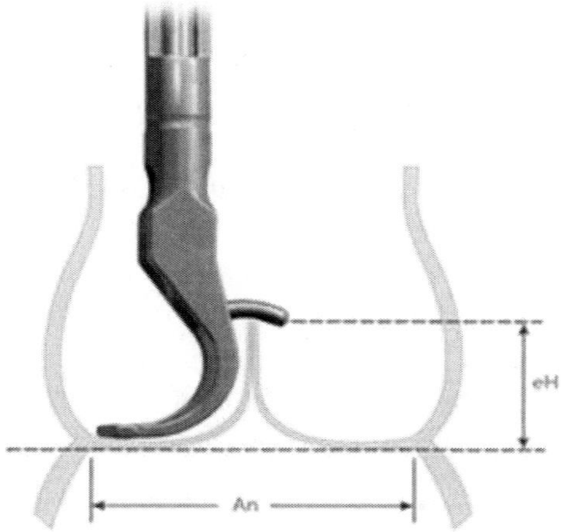

Figure 5. Diagram illustrating the use of the caliper in a tricuspid aortic valve to measure the effective height of the cusp. The effective height corresponds to the height of the caliper hook when the convex part sits perfectly on the cusp while the hook touches the free margin. eH: effective height, An: annulus diameter.

FUNCTIONAL CLASSIFICATION OF AORTIC REGURGITATION

We have developed and implemented since many years a classification of the aortic regurgitation that encompasses all the different causes of AR (Figure 6). This classification aims to provide a common ground for surgeons, cardiologists, and cardiac echo specialists. We further intended to point out the technique of choice for a specified mechanism.

AI Class	Type I Normal cusp motion with FAA dilatation or cusp perforation				Type II Cusp Prolapse	Type III Cusp Restriction
	Ia	Ib	Ic	Id		
Mechanism	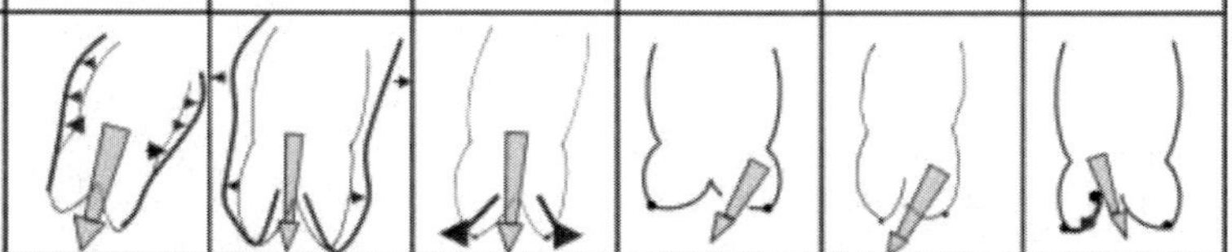					
Repair Techniques (Primary)	STJ remodeling *Ascending aortic graft*	Aortic Valve sparing: *Reimplantation or Remodeling with SCA*	SCA	Patch Repair *Autologous or bovine pericardium*	Prolapse Repair *Plication Triangular resection Free margin Resuspension Patch*	Leaflet Repair *Shaving Decalcificatio Patch*
(Secondary)	SCA		STJ Annuloplasty	SCA	SCA	SCA

Figure 6. Repair-oriented functional classification of Aortic Insufficiency with description of disease mechanism and repair techniques used. FAA: Functional Aortic Annulus; STJ: sino-tubular junction; SCA: sub-commissural annuloplasty. Reprinted with permission.

Briefly, similar to the classic Carpentier's classification of mitral valve regurgitation, in the classification that we proposed, type 1 disease is caused by lesions of the FAA in the setting of normal cusp motion, type 2 disease is caused by excessive cusp motion due to cusp prolapse, and type 3 disease is caused by restrictive cusp disease. Nonetheless multiple lesions can simultaneously contribute to AR, therefore correction of all contributing lesions is critical for successful repair. Moreover, as in mitral valve regurgitation, severe chronic AR can lead to dilatation of the ventricular-aortic junction. Therefore, also in patients with type 2 lesions (without aortic dilatation) annuloplasty of the VAJ should be considered particularly if the VAJ is already enlarged. It is a matter of debate which is the cutoff for dilatation.

General Principles of AV Repair

The goal of AV repair is to restore an effective surface of coaptation by reestablishing the functional relation between the leaflets and the FAA all the while preserving mobility of the AV cusps. The mobility of the valve cusps depends on both the length of the free margin and the length of the base of implantation. If increased cusp mobility may occur because of excess free margin length (as in cusp prolapse) or over-reductive annuloplasty, a reduced mobility may occur for dilatation of the VAJ (as frequently observed in bicuspid AV), overcorrection of prolapse, and in cases of severe dilation of the STJ.

As aortic regurgitation can be isolated or associated with aortic root aneurysm, we will discuss in the next sections the specific techniques of valve sparing – aortic root replacement (VSRR) and of isolated cusp repair. Nevertheless, cusp repair is oftentimes required during VSRR while aortic annuloplasty is required in isolated AR to stabilize the repair and ensure durability. Further, the reimplantation of the valve during VSRR can elicit a cusp prolapse that needs to be address for the good result of the operation. We will further discuss the specific case of AV repair in cases of bicuspid AV.

Aortic Valve Repair in Tricuspid AV

Valve-Sparing Aortic Root Replacement with the Reimplantation Technique

The aortic valve sparing – aortic root replacement (VSRR) with the Reimplantation of the aortic valve into a cylindrical Dacron graft has been introduced over two decades ago by Dr. David and coll. as alternative option to composite replacement of the aortic valve and root with a prosthesis (Bentall operation) in patients with aortic root aneurysm with or without significant aortic insufficiency. VSRR-reimplantation is our technique of choice in cases of root aneurysm with normal valve.

Compared to valve replacement with a prosthesis, VSRR allows a significant reduction of prosthesis-related complications. However, the technical complexity of this procedure and the concern for the durability of the re-implanted aortic valve have initially limited the wide diffusion of this operation. Nowadays long-term results of this operation confirm the excellent clinical results in terms of valve-related complications and survival, and the stability of valve function over time with a low risk of recurrent aortic regurgitation or reoperation on the valve . Although severe calcifications or fibrosis determining valve stenosis or reduced cusp mobility represent a contraindication to valve-sparing procedure, other cusp lesions such as fenestration or prolapse should not deter to the use of this technique but they must be addressed during the procedure in order to obtain a lasting result . Cusp plication to correct prolapse has been applied in up to 60% of the patients with a tricuspid aortic valve undergoing VSRR in our Institution15. Further, cusp prolapse can become evident after valve reimplantation therefore a careful reassessment of the valve should be carried out before termination of the procedure. Nonetheless, cusp prolapse can be easily corrected (as we will see later on) and should not therefore preclude VSSR.

We have already and extensively described the technique of VSRR with reimplantation that we have implemented and detailed videos are also available . Briefly, the procedure is systematically carried out through a number of steps and allows no shortcut. The ascending aorta is opened 1 cm above the sino-tubular junction and three traction stitches of 4-0 polypropylene are placed at the tip of each commissure. These stitches are extremely useful to assess valve coaptation through all the steps and help expose the aortic root during external dissection. A careful and thorough examination of the valve, aortic wall, coronary ostia and VAJ is performed at this point and the decision to valve repair is eventually confirmed.

The first step of VSSR is the external dissection of the aortic root aimed to reach the level of VAJ, given the constraints of the surrounding heart structures (Figure 7).

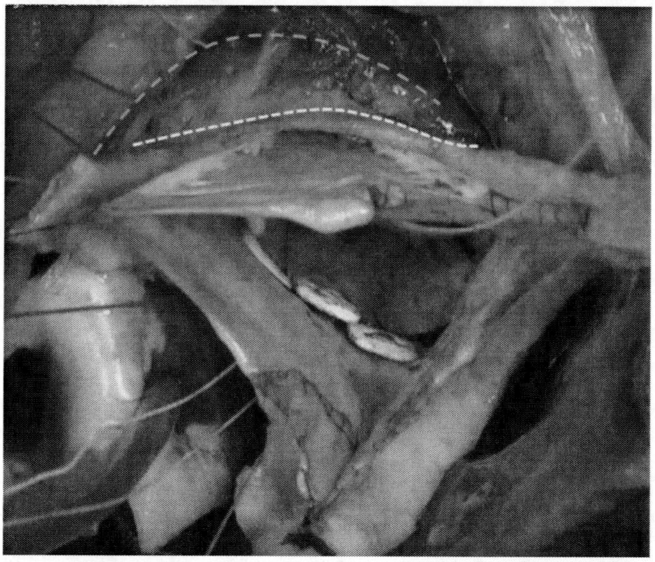

Figure 7. Intraoperative picture of VSRR in tricuspid AV showing the limits of external root dissection in the area of the right ventricular outflow tract. The dissection should go beyond the VAJ (yellow line) and reach the basal ring (green line) in order to have a horizontal suture line in this area. The pledgeted stitches of the proximal suture have been already placed in the area of the left cusp.

The vascular graft should indeed necessarily sit at the level of the VAJ in order to both realize a complete circumferential annuloplasty and avoid valve distortion during the reimplantation. It is easier to start the root dissection along the Non-Coronary (NC) sinus because there is not the constraint of the coronary arteries or other heart structures here. The sinus of Valsalva is then resected leaving few millimeters of aortic rim towards the base of the cusp. Before the external dissection of the right and left sinuses, the coronary buttons are isolated leaving a generous patch of aortic wall. Importantly, along the non-fibrous portions of the annulus the external dissection of the aortic root should go as deep as the real level of the VAJ, avoiding injuries to both the aortic root and the right ventricular outflow tract. The external dissection is properly completed if the valve is completely free from the surrounding structures and fully mobile at this point. After completion of the external dissection, the stitches for the proximal suture line are passed horizontally through the VAJ. We usually use ten to twelve 2-0 Tycron sutures with pledget that are distributed along the circumference of the VAJ. The pledgets have to lay inside the left ventricular outflow tract (Figure 8).

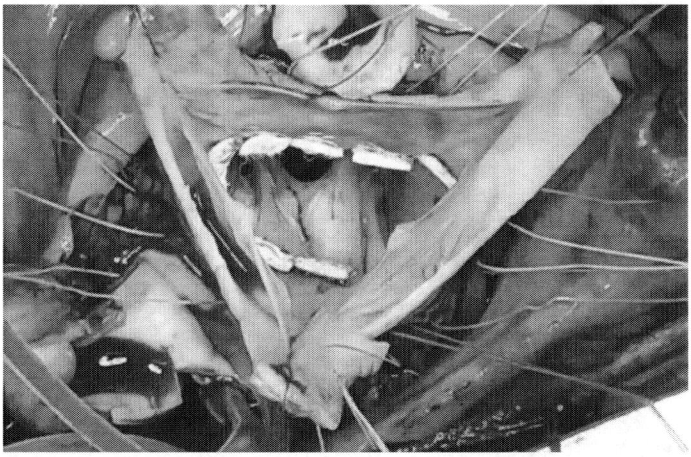

Figure 8. Intra-operative picture showing the proximal suture line in VSRR-Reimplantation. Twelve pledget stitches make a circumferential annuloplasty of the VAJ.

As we have seen before, attention must be paid to avoid the atrio-ventricular node and the conduction tissue at the level of the R/NC inter-commissural triangle. The complete annuloplasty realised by these pledget stitches prevent later dilatation and recurrence of aortic regurgitation and is therefore a key-point for the success of valve repair10.

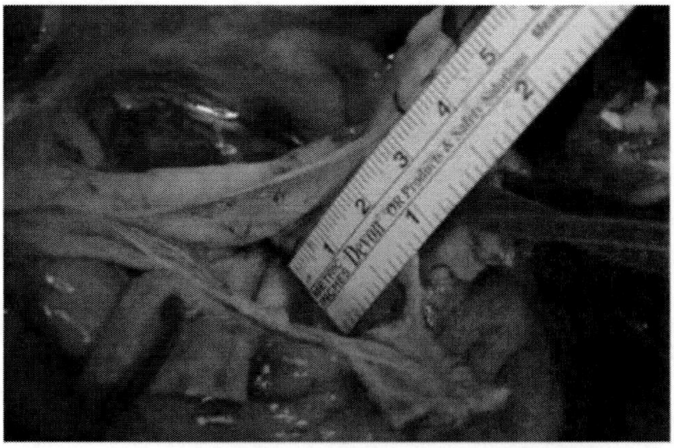

Figure 9. The height of the commissure between the left- and non-coronary cusps is the reference for the choice of graft size. The height is measured from the base of inter-leaflets triangle corresponding to the VAJ (thick purple line) to the tip of the commissure (thin purple line).

The next step is the selection of the vascular graft that replaces the aortic root and where the aortic valve will be re-implanted. The choice of a straight graft rather than a graft with neo-sinuses is still matter of debate. Nonetheless we routinely use a graft with built-in neo-aortic sinuses (GelweaveValsalva™ graft, Vascutek Ltd, a Terumo company, Renfrewshire, Scotland) because we believe that this particular type of graft eases the procedure and may have a clinical benefit on valve function. Our current graft-sizing technique has been previously described. The size of the graft should be equal to the height of NC/LC commissure measured from the base of inter-leaflets triangle to the top of the commissure (Figure 9).

The stitches of the proximal suture line are then passed through the base of the prosthesis. Finally, the graft is parachuted down and the stitches are tied to ensure appropriate seating around the aortic annulus. It is important to avoid excessive tension on these stitches that may otherwise tear the muscular tissue of the VAJ. Further, it should be recalled that this suture line aims to fix the base of the prosthesis but it is the distal suture that ensure hemostasis. During this step it is also extremely important to ensure that the stitches of the proximal suture line have not caught the valve. The aortic valve can be now reimplanted into the graft. The commissures are reimplanted first using 4-0 polypropylene sutures. To prevent valve distortion, it is of paramount importance that the three commissures must be reattached at the same level or eventually higher than the neo-sinotubular junction of the Valsalva graft. A running suture starting from the commissure and aimed to fix the rest of the valve to the graft is then performed in small regular steps. During this step, it is important to avoid a dead space between the valve and the prosthesis that may cause bleeding. After valve reimplantation, it is critical to re-examine the cusps for any residual prolapse, symmetry, and the height of coaptation. A sealing test can also carried out to assess the competency of the valve. The last step of the procedure will be the reimplantation of the coronary ostia. The left ostium, due to its posterior position, is sutured first to the graft. We usually sew the coronary ostia with a running suture of 5-0 polypropylene and a free autologous pericardial strip can also be used on the coronary side to improve hemostasis. After the ostia are re-implanted, cardioplegia can be given directly into the graft in order to distend the new aortic root, check for hemostasis and also assess valve competence by indirect signs such as root pressure and left ventricular dilatation. A further assessment of the valve is performed after cardioplegia. Cusp repair should eventually be carried out at this moment.

Cusp Prolapse Repair in Tricuspid AV

Aortic regurgitation can be the result of isolated cusp disease. Grossly, cusp dysfunction can be described as type-2 (cusp prolapse) or type-3 (cusp restriction) lesion according to our classification (Figure 6). Type-2 dysfunction is the more common mechanism of isolated regurgitation. In general, cusp prolapse is the result of an excess of length of the free margin. Although cusp prolapse can exist isolated, it is commonly associated with dilatation of one or more components of the FAA.

In the normal AV, the free cusps' margins usually run parallel at the same level and join each other in the center of the aortic root about 9-10mm above the nadir of the sinuses of Valsalva (normal effective height). Cusp prolapse is then defined as one of these 2 situations: 1- when one (or more) of the free margins is lower compared to the others because of the excessive tissue and a transverse band can be present in the middle of the cusp body (Figure 10) (usually the transverse band can also be seen on echo imaging); 2- when the free margins are the same level but their coaptation is lower than the normal reference (9 -10 mm of effective height). In the latter situation the normal parallel configuration of the free margins is respected but the entire coaptation is too low representing a risk of recurrent AI. Both type of prolapse can occur after VSSR but the second type occurs when the commissures are not re-implanted high enough inside the graft or in case of severe free margin elongation as observed in large root aneurysms.

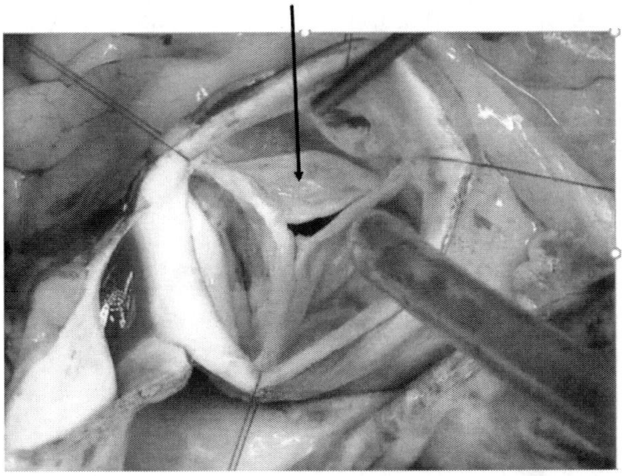

Figure 10. Intra-operative picture illustrating a prolapse of the right coronary cusp (black arrow). Compared to the left and non-coronary cusps, its free margin is lower and a transverse band is evident in the body of the cusp.

Moreover, cusp prolapse may occur after VSRR if a too small graft has been chosen. Consider indeed the exemplary case of a root aneurysm (>50mm) without significant preoperative regurgitation. Reimplantation of this valve into a smaller graft (e.g., 28mm) can be very likely associated to a relative excess of tissue and consequently cusp prolapse (Figure 11).

For tricuspid AV, prolapse of the RC or NC cusps is significantly more common than prolapse of the LC cusp. In young patients prolapse is often associated with root dilatation and connective tissue disorder.

Surgery for isolated AI starts with a transverse aortotomy 1cm above the sino-tubular junction. The incision is extended circumferentially so that only the posterior 1-2cm of aortic wall directly above the left coronary ostium is left intact. A traction suture is placed at the apex of each of the 3 commissures to assess the valve mobility and the height of coaptation in the arrested heart. Normally the cusps close at the level of the mid-height of Valsalva sinuses with an effective height of 9-10mm. Effective height can be quantified also intra-operatively by using a dedicated caliper . A cusp prolapse can be identified if the free margin is below the reference point and lower than the other cusps. Once cusp prolapse is confirmed, the choice of repair technique depends on the quality and quantity of cusp tissue. Central leaflet plication and free margin resuspension are usually indicated in case of cusp of good quality with flexible tissue. Triangular resection and pericardial patch repair are instead indicated in cases of poor tissue quality with thickening, fibrosis or calcification.

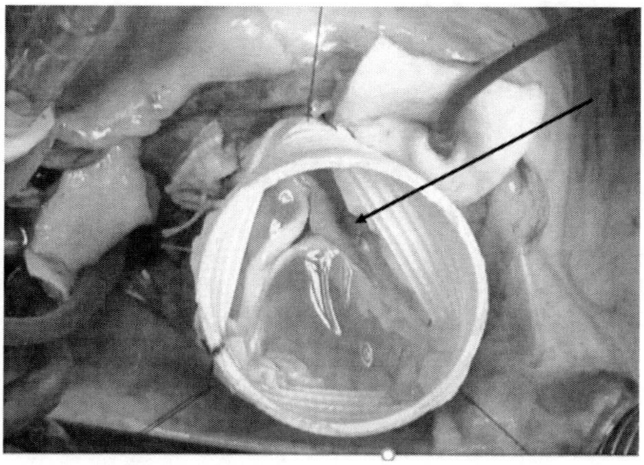

Figure 11. Intra-operative picture showing prolapse of the RCC after valve sparing-reimplantation. Injecting saline solution with pressure into the aortic root allows closure of the valve and can unveil cusp prolapse.

Central Leaflet Plication and Triangular Resection

The central plication is the most used technique in our experience to correct cusp prolapse. Videos of this and other techniques of cusp repair are also available on line . A 5-0 or 6-0 polypropylene suture, depending on the thickness of the cusp tissue, is used for plication passing the stitch from the aortic to ventricular side of the leaflet and back to the aorta in order to have a fold of excess tissue on the aortic side of the cusp (Figure 12). If the excess of tissue is substantial, the plication can be extended onto the body of the leaflet by a running suture (Figure 13) and eventually a triangular resection of the leaflet can also be performed.

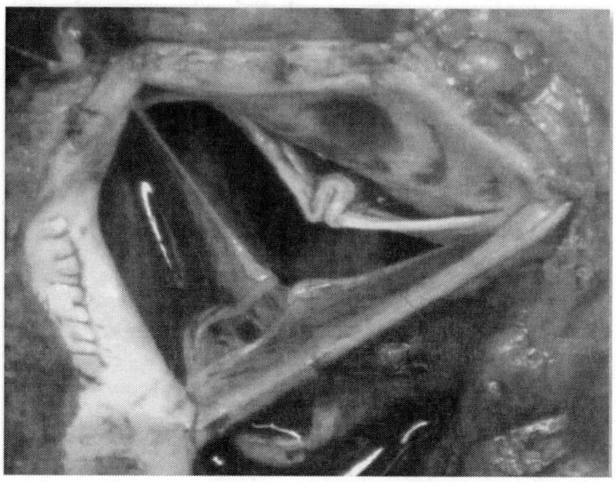

Figure 12. Intra-operative pictures showing the result of central plication to treat RCC prolapse. The reference stitch passes through the middle point of both the LCC and NCC. After alignment of the RCC, the excess of tissue on the RCC becomes evident.

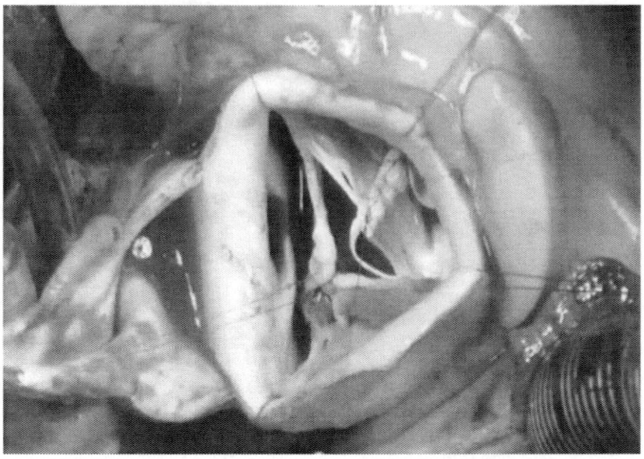

Figure 13. Intra-operative pictures showing the result of central plication and triangular resection to treat RCC prolapse. The locked running suture starts from the belly of the cusp, where the fold of the plication begins, to the free margin. The plication stitch and the running suture stitch are then tied together.

Free Margin Resuspension

For resuspension of the prolapsing free margin, we use two 7-0 polytetrafluoroethylene (PTFE) sutures that will shorten the free margin by pulling up the cusp (Figure 14).

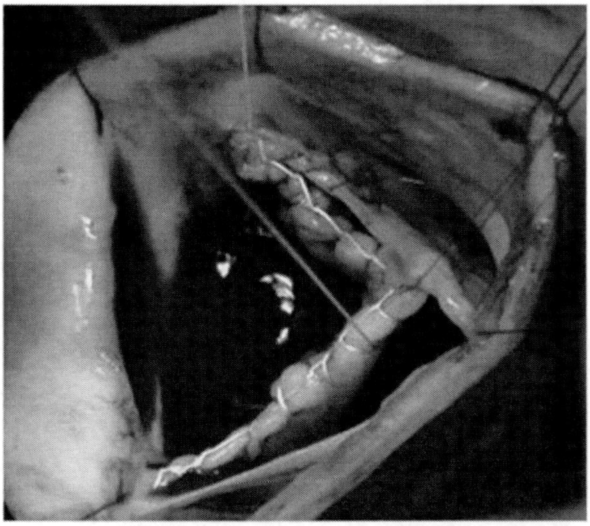

Figure 14. Intraoperative picture showing the result of free-margin resuspension to treat prolapse of left coronary cusp (LCC). Two running sutures of PTFE are passed over and over the free margin from one commissure to the other. These stitches are then pulled gently to shorten the excessive length of the LCC free margin.

Each PTFE suture is first secured to the apex of the commissure and then run over the full length of the free margin to reach the opposite commissure. The length of the free margin is therefore reduced by gently pulling the PTFE sutures until the free margin reaches the reference point. This 2-steps technique allows symmetric and homogenous shortening of the free margin.

In general, the free margin plication is a more adaptable and versatile technique and is our preferred approach for prolapse repair. There are, however, a few situations in which resuspension is particularly useful. This technique is indicated in the setting of a fragile free margin with multiple small fenestrations. In either case, these cusp repair techniques can restore leaflet coaptation and provide a durable solution to cusp prolapse.

Cusp Fenestration Repair

Small fenestrations in the area of the commissures in an otherwise normal cusp do not usually need to be repaired. When the fenestration is large or when it is ruptured with a lack of continuity in the free margin, then the fenestration must be repaired with patch material. The decision for the type of patch material is principally at the surgeon's discretion as no strong evidence exists on the superiority of one material over another and different types of patches have been used. We currently use either bovine pericardial patch or autologous pericardium. Non-treated autologous pericardium is preferred in cases of simpler repairs, like small fenestration or perforation, while treated autologous or bovine pericardium are employed in more complex repairs such as commissure reconstruction.

The patch is trimmed in the form of the defect but 2 mm bigger the size, so as to prevent restriction of cusp surface following the suture. The patch is usually sutured on the aortic surface of the cusp with a continuous 6-0 polypropylene sutures. One edge of the patch is used as new free margin in case of ruptured fenestration or is used to reinforce the free margin when the fenestration is not ruptured. Large fenestrations are frequently present on both sides of the commissure and one patch fixed to the commissure and distributed between the two cusps (Figure 15) or two separate patches can be used to treat the lesion. Small fenestration close to the free margin can be repaired with free margin resuspension by PTFE as seen above.

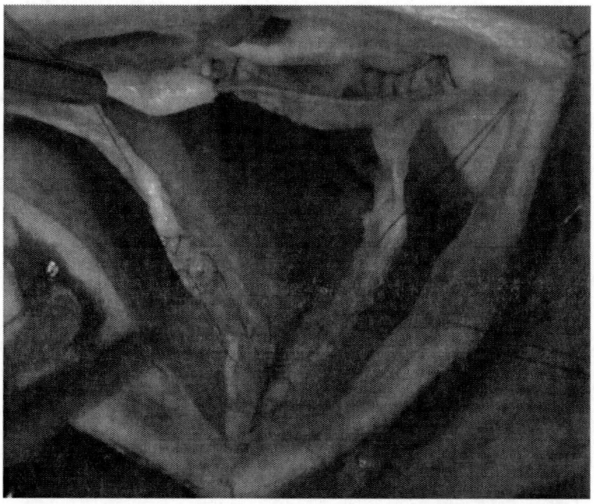

Figure 15. Intraoperative picture showing the result of repair of a commissural fenestration at the level of the LCC/NCC with a single heterologous patch.

Cusp Perforation

Perforation is defined as tissue defect at the belly of the cusp with preservation of the free margin and it might represent the only cause of AI. The perforation can be the result of an endocarditis, resection of a fibroelastoma or iatrogenic. Very small perforation (up to 2-3mm) can be closed directly with 6-0 polypropylene sutures. Large perforations of one or more cusps will need a patch repair (Figure 16).

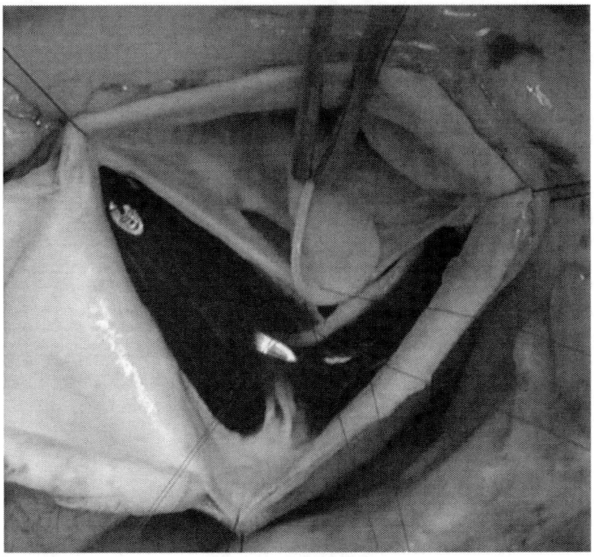

Figure 16. Intraoperative picture showing a large perforation, due to infective endocarditis, of the RCC. A heterologous pericardial patch has been trimmed to close the defect. The patch has a diameter 1mm larger than the defect in order to avoid cusp tension following the suture.

Aortic Valve Repair in Bicuspid AV

Bicuspid aortic valve (BAV) is the most common congenital cardiac anomaly in the adult population and is also associated with a peculiar aortopathy. For the purpose of valve repair, it is noteworthy that BAV is almost constantly associated with dilatation of the VAJ, which should be therefore addressed during BAV repair.

Anatomical Considerations

Bicuspid aortic valves may be divided into 2 general types . Type 0 BAVs have 2 very symmetric aortic sinuses, 2 commissures facing at 180°, and a symmetric base of implantation of the 2 cusps. This configuration is nonetheless present in a minority of cases (±7%). The mechanism of aortic regurgitation in this setting is usually related to cusp prolapse or dilatation of the aortic root.

Type 1 BAVs, which are significantly more common, present 2 cusps fused together along a median raphe (Figure 17).

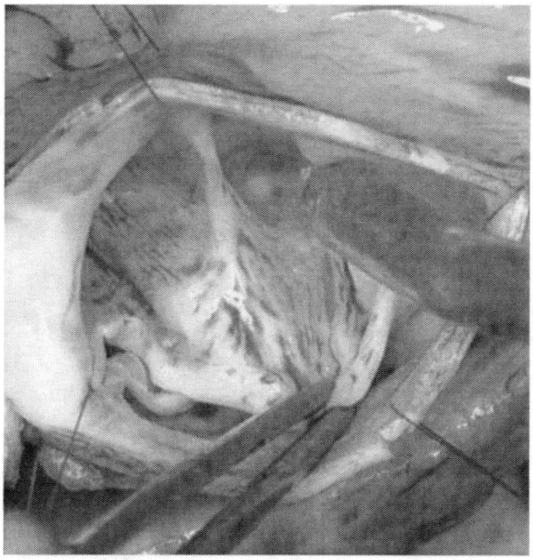

Figure 17. Intra-operative picture illustrating a Type-I BAV with incomplete fusion of the LCC and RCC, a small raphe and a pseudo-commissure.

In most of the cases the fusion involves the LC and RC cusps, and much less frequently the other possible combinations. The conjoined cusp is usually larger than the non-conjoined cusp (usually the non-coronary cusp) resulting therefore in a more or less asymmetric valve apparatus. The conjoined cusp accounts for a proportion of valve circumference that varies between 180° and 240°. Depending on the degree of cusp fusion, the raphe can be more or less developed and can forms a ''pseudo-commissure'' on the aortic wall which is nonetheless lower than the true commissures. Commissural orientation is defined as the angle limited by the lines passing through the 2 commissure and the central axis of the valve. The angle is measured on the non-conjoined cusp (Figure 18). We have extensively described the relation between commissure orientation in type 1 BAVs, length of fusion and height of the commissure . We have also proposed a new surgical-oriented classification22 grouping type 1 BAVs in 1) very symmetric BAVs with a 160-180° commissural orientation resembling type 0 valves, 2) quite asymmetric BAVs with 140-160° orientation, 3) very asymmetric BAVs and tricuspid-like with a commissure orientation angle <140°. The second group of BAVs is also the most numerous. Techniques for BAV repair can differ importantly between these 3 groups. Respect or improvement of the 180° symmetry seems to be advisable and associated with better valve durability. Further, we'll see that restoring BAV symmetry during repair can in most of the cases allow to avoid use of patch that is associated to worse outcomes.

Two mechanisms of AI are commonly observed in type 1 valves. One is prolapse of the conjoined cusp ("prolapsing" Type 1) wherein the raphe is generally thin and pliable and the conjoined cusp well-developed with a near to normal geometric height (Figure 19).

The other is restriction of the conjoined cusp ("restrictive" Type 1) wherein, despite the larger base of insertion of the conjoined cusp, the raphe is thickened and rigid and the cusp is therefore restrictive with a smaller surface and small geometric height (Figure 20). Generally, prolapsing Type 1 BAVs tend to have a commissural orientation in the 160°-180° range while restrictive type 1 BAVs tend to be more asymmetric (commissural orientation of 120-160°).

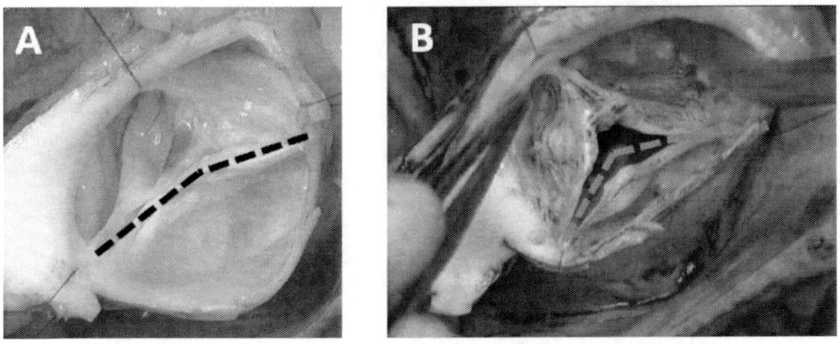

Figure 18. A. Intraoperative picture of a symmetric type-I BAV with LCC/RCC almost complete fusion, a small raphe and commissural orientation of almost 180°. B. Intraoperative picture of an asymmetric type-I BAV with LCC/RCC quite incomplete fusion, a well-developed raphe and commissural orientation of 140°.

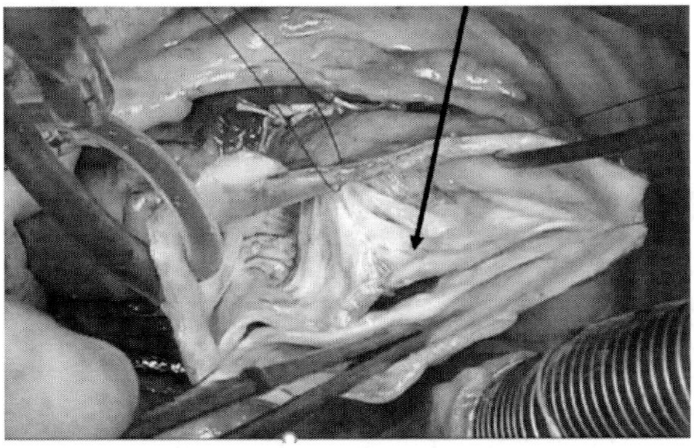

Figure 19. Intra-operative picture illustrating a symmetric type I bicuspid aortic valve with RCC/LCC fusion and prolapse of the conjoined cusp. The free margin of the conjoined cusp (black arrow) is indeed lower than the free margin of the non-conjoined cusp.

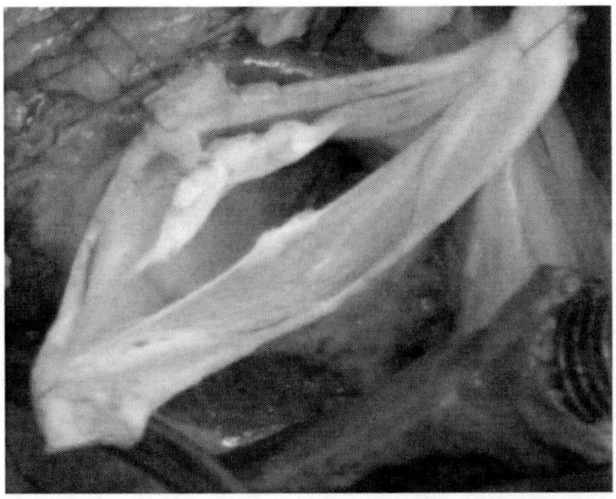

Figure 20. Intra-operative picture illustrating a symmetric type I bicuspid aortic valve with incomplete fusion of the RCC and LCC and a restrictive raphe causing aortic regurgitation.

Surgical Techniques for BAV Repair

Various surgical techniques can be employed to repair regurgitant BAV. A thorough analysis of the valve should find out any abnormality that needs to be addressed during the repair. Valve assessment should go through cusp anatomy, quantity and quality of cusp tissue, commissure orientation, dilatation of VAJ and/or aorta, and quality of aortic wall tissue. Surgical strategies should include: cusp repair, annuloplasty and root management.

Cusp Repair in BAV

In type 0 valves, the degree of prolapse should be assessed as usual by comparing the prolapsing cusp with the non-prolapsing cusp. Whenever both cusps are prolapsing, the objective of repair is to restore the height of coaptation at the mid-height of the Valsalva sinuses which usually corresponds to an effective height of 10mm. This can be achieved by a central plication of the prolapsing cusp. Thickened, fibrotic areas of the cusp (typically the central aspect of the free margin) can be thinned gently with a blade to ease the plication and make the coaptation surface more pliable and regular.

In type 1 valves, cusp repair consists essentially in the management of the fused cusp, and particularly the raphe. In prolapsing BAVs, raphe repair consists generally in closing first the unfused portion close to the free margin, then the effective height is sorted out and the residual prolapse is corrected by central plication (Figure 21).

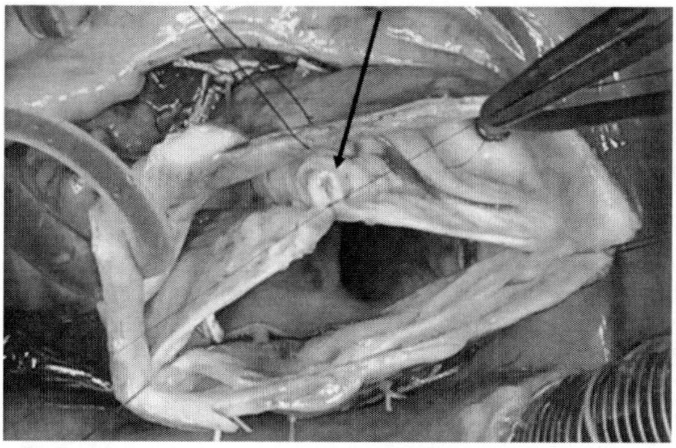

Figure 21. Intra-operative picture illustrating central plication of the conjoined cusp to treat cusp prolapse in BAV.

In restrictive Type 1, the fibrosis of the raphe is removed with a blade or scissors sparing as much as possible the leaflet tissue. After raphe resection, the quantity of remaining cusp tissue must be assessed. If the quantity of tissue is adequate and the edges of the leaflet can be re-approached without excessive tension and keeping cusp mobility, then the gap can be repaired directly with a running or interrupted 6-0 polypropylene suture. In case of lack of adequate tissue an autologous or heterologous pericardial patch should be used to fill the defect. In the past these were the most challenging cases and were associated with the worst outcome due to patch degeneration over time. Nowadays, we the implementation of a reductive annuloplasty of the VAJ, particularly in the anterior muscular area towards the RVOT, which corresponds to the conjoined cusp in the common RC-LC configuration, allows to reapproximate the edges of the leaflet and to correct the gap without using the patch or with very small ones. In general, if the valve has a commissure orientation >140° (2nd BAV group), a triangular patch may be needed to fill the defect but the valve configuration will be kept bicuspid. If the commissural orientation is even tighter (close to 120°) and the valve very asymmetric, it is convenient to create a new commissure using one patch (the "butterfly technique") and transform the valve into a tricuspid valve (Figure 22).

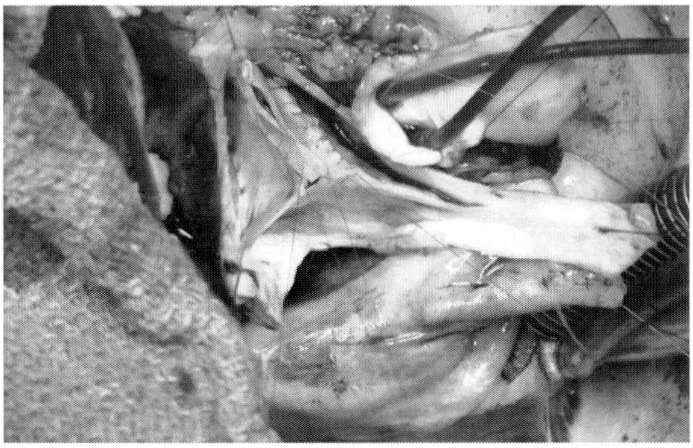

Figure 22. Intra-operative picture illustrating a type I restrictive BAV with a commissural orientation of 120°. After resection of the raphe, commissural orientation is respected and a neo-commissure is created with a single patch (butterfly technique).

The new commissure should arrive to the height of the sino-tubular junction. Once the valve is repaired, again the geometric height is measured a central plication is eventually employed if it is still too low.

When root replacement is indicated and patch repair is also needed, we advise to perform the repair before root replacement because it is much easier to work on the valve inside the native root (or eventually once the sinuses are resected) than inside the vascular graft. Nonetheless cusp plication and direct closure of the raphe are generally performed once the valve is reimplanted into the graft because the reimplantation technique itself impacts the height of coaptation. However, we also advise to put the stitches for the proximal suture line before patch or any cusp repair is performed because there is an easier access to the VAJ.

Annuloplasty and Aorta Management

In the absence of BAV regurgitation, aneurysm of the ascending aorta will be treated by classical supracoronary ascending aorta replacement.

Aortic root aneurism without regurgitation is treated with valve sparing root replacement with the reimplantation technique. The technique of reimplantation in BAV is roughly the same than in TAV. The external root dissection is performed deeply to reach the level of the basal ring all along the circumference of the valve. It is noteworthy that at the level of the anterior commissure (in the usual situation of a LC/RC fusion) the stitches for the proximal suture should be few millimeters higher than the basal ring in order to avoid injuring the membranous septum and the conduction bundle. In the rare case of a right-non (RC-NC) leaflet fusion, the nadir of the conjoined cusp is precisely et the level of the membranous septum. To avoid injury to the conduction bundle and the risk of a complete AV block, the annuloplasty stitches can be omitted at this level. The Valsalva graft sizing is based on the height of the posterior commissure (LC-NC commissure). The proximal suture line stitches are passed through the proximal end of the graft respecting the curve for the membranous septum (Figure 23).

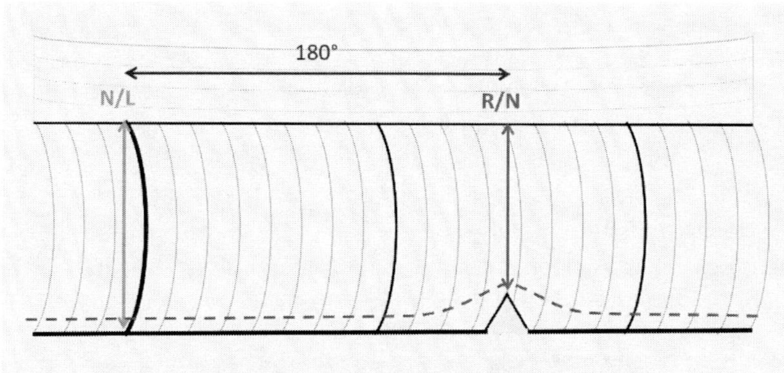

Figure 23. Diagram illustrating that during VSRR in BAVs, the vascular graft is evenly divided in order to respect, or restore, valve symmetry; the stitches for the proximal suture line (red dotted line) should be few millimeters higher at the level of the anterior commissure (purple line) (corresponding to the RCC/NCC commissure) in order to avoid the membranous septum and the conduction tissue. The height of the posterior commissure (corresponding to the LCC/NCC commissure) gives the size of the graft; the diameter of the graft is equal to the height of the neo-sinus (green line).

In absence of regurgitation the valve is reimplanted respecting the native commissure orientation. The commissures must be implanted as high as possible inside the graft, ideally at the level of the neo-STJ. In type 1 BAV, the pseudo-commissure (raphe) is reimplanted in the graft at grossly the same height as it was in the native root. Then, the distal suture line is performed. Once the valve is reimplanted, valve coaptation is assessed by measuring the effective height. Importantly, even if the valve was not leaking, the reduction of the STJ and root size can induce a prolapse of both cusps. Again, we aim to obtain an effective height of 9-10mm and central free margin plication is added as needed. Importantly effective height must be measured first at the non-conjoined cusp and adjusted accordingly. Then the effective height is measured on the non-conjoined cusp and corrected to have both free margins at the same height.

In case of BAV with significant regurgitation and without root aneurysm (>50mm), the management of the annuloplasty and aorta will be different in order to obtain a durable normal valve function. As most of these patients will present with dilated VAJ, annuloplasty must be performed at the time of surgery whenever the VAJ is greater than 26mm. Circumferential prosthetic annuloplasty is more stable over time than non-circumferential techniques like the Cabrol technique, also known as sub-commissural annuloplasty (SCA). We have shown that the SCA reduces indeed the inter-commissural triangle width and enhances coaptation. However, SCA does not really reaches the level of the VAJ and it loses its effect over time with a high risk of recurrent regurgitation. During the last decade, we have therefore limited the use of SCA in favor of circumferential annuloplasty. Currently, we use two techniques of annuloplasty, one is the valve sparing root replacement with the reimplantation technique and the other is the external ring annuloplasty.

The circumferential ring annuloplasty will be used only in case of BAV regurgitation with strictly normal root dimension (<40mm). The technique consists in fixing an external flexible prosthetic band around the VAJ, whether a strip of Dacron graft or the Simplicity® band (Medtronic Inc.). In these cases, we still need to reach the level of the VAJ therefore deep external root dissection is performed. However, the ease and depth of external root dissection is somewhat limited and a bit more difficult compared to the same dissection during the reimplantation technique because the coronary ostia and the sinuses are not removed. Moreover, below each coronary artery, a tunnel is created with right-angle forceps in order to pass the band below the vessel. The surrounding tissue around the coronaries must be left intact to decrease the risk of injury. Once the dissection is completed, 9-10 pledged stitches are placed along the basal ring. Most care must be taken to avoid injury to the coronary arteries. A band of 10mm is usually used and the stitches are distributed homogenously along its length. Finally, one of the stitches is passed through each extremity of the band in order to close the circumference. The annuloplasty stitches are tied with a 23 or 25 Hegar dilator inserted through the VAJ in order to correctly reduce its size (Figure 24).

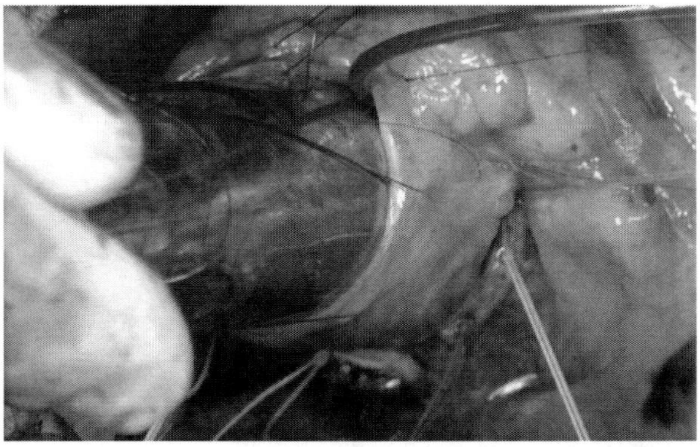

Figure 24. Intra-operative picture showing external annuloplasty with a band. A Hegar dilator is inserted through the valve to avoid excessive annular reduction.

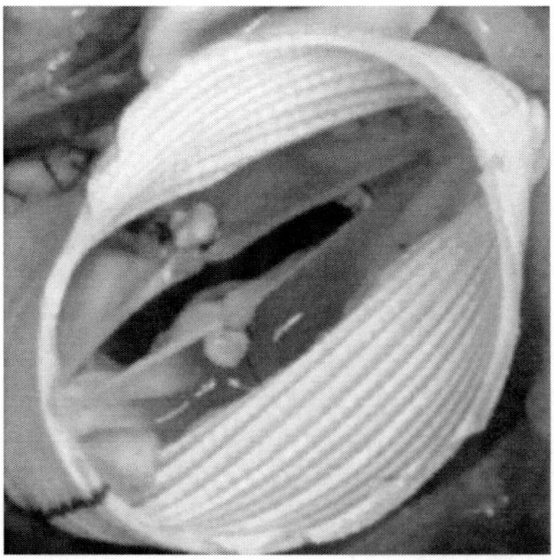

Figure 25. Intra-operative picture showing a BAV reimplanted into a vascular graft during VSRR with a commissure orientation of 180°. The selective circumferential annuloplasty and commissure reimplantation allow restoring valve symmetry.

The reimplantation technique is used whenever the root size is greater than 40mm or anytime one of the goals of repair is to improve the valve symmetry regardless of the root dimensions. Effectively, in case of regurgitation, we believe that it is easier and favorable for repair durability to re-implant the valve in a symmetric configuration (commissure orientation of 180°) (Figure 25). Arguably the symmetric configuration allows a laminar blood flow across the valve which in turn might enhance repair durability compared to a turbulent flow across an asymmetric valve. Furthermore, as we have already seen, the circumferential annuloplasty of VSRR allows an easier management of the raphe, especially in cases of restrictive type 1 BAV. VSRR allows indeed direct re-approximation of the leaflet after raphe resection and improve cusp mobility.

Valve symmetry nonetheless involves 3 levels: the VAJ, the commissures and the sinuses. Therefore, we perform a "symmetric annuloplasty" at the VAJ level that consists in distributing the proximal suture line stitches evenly onto the graft between the conjoined and non-conjoined cusps. although the portion of VAJ corresponding to the conjoined cusp accounts generally for more than 180° of root circumference (Figure 23). To complete valve symmetry, the two commissures are reimplanted at 180° inside the graft up.

In our experience, we have employed VSRR-reimplantation plus cusp repair for the vast majority (80%) of patients with BAV disease amenable to repair. During this procedure, the valve is kept symmetric in cases of Type 0 morphology, and is made symmetric in Type 1 morphologies unless the valve was very asymmetric with <140° commissures orientation. In this case indeed, the valve may be best transformed into a tricuspid valve by commissural reconstruction as already described.

RESULTS OF AORTIC VALVE REPAIR

Repair of the aortic valve should supposedly allow patients requiring surgery for aortic dilatation or valve regurgitation to avoid the risks of prosthesis-related complications, whether xenograft or mechanical prosthesis, mainly structural valve deterioration and reintervention, infective endocarditis, anticoagulation-related bleeding or thromboembolic events, and ultimately mortality. Valve replacement with the pulmonary autograft, the Ross operation, provides excellent results but in face of the technical complexity it should be reserved mainly for patients with AV stenosis. Nonetheless, results of AV repair should be first divided by indication for surgery, that means the mechanism of AR in our classification (Figure 6). Therefore, in the next paragraphs we'll discuss the results of AV sparing/repair in cases of aortic dilatation (Type I), cusp prolapse (type II) or cusp restriction (type III). However, we should not forget that more mechanisms of AR can coexist in any given patient and oftentimes the available series report the results of different techniques implemented together (e.g., valve sparing root replacement plus cusp repair) for one indication or the results of one technique (e.g., cusp repair) for different indications (root aneurysm or isolated AR).

Outcomes of Valve-Sparing Root Replacement with the Reimplantation Technique

Experience with the David operation is well entered into its third decade, therefore long-term results of this procedure are available from dr. David himself and other groups. Traditionally, the first concern relative to this procedure regarded the durability of the valve function after reimplantation into a vascular graft. David and colleagues reported a cumulative risk of developing moderate and severe AR of 10% at 20 years . These authors found that preoperative moderate or severe AR, BAV and aortic dissection were associated with increased risk of postoperative AI in univariable analysis. In our experience we observed a significant impact of time since surgery on valve function and a risk of grade 3+ and 4+ AR of 6% at 10 years10. We also found that severe preoperative AR and residual AR at the end of the procedure are associated to a higher progression of postoperative AR . Nonetheless freedom from AV reoperation was 95% at 15 years in Toronto14 and 90% at 10 years in our experience10. Further, a meta-analysis of 31 studies on VSRR comprising more than four thousand patients estimated in 0.23% patient-year the linearized rate of major bleeding events, 0.41% patient-year the rate of thromboembolism and 0.23% patient-year the occurrence of infective endocarditis . Finally, 10-year survival is in the range of 80-90% in dr. David's and in our series and higher than survival after valve replacement. Recently Klotz et al. showed that long-term survival was comparable to that of the matched general population in Germany. Predictors of late survival were, as expected, age and type A aortic dissection at time of surgery.

Surely, patient selection is a key point to get improved results. Compared to David's experience, in our series we had a higher prevalence of BAV patients and a higher percentage of cusp and patch repair. We believe indeed that many valves can be spared even if they require cusp repair and that a slightly higher risk of reoperation is the trade-off to avoid a prosthesis. It is nonetheless a matter of experience to rule out regurgitant aortic valves that are too diseased for a repair with an acceptable outcome. The key factors that predict repair success or late failure are: the quality and quantity of cusp tissue to begin with, mobility of the cusps, coaptation and residual AR at the end of repair. Limited calcifications or fibrosis do not contraindicate this procedure but extensive fibrosis that limit cusp mobility or that require resection and patch repair are associated to suboptimal results. Moreover, low coaptation into the root, low effective height and a short length of coaptation are risk factors for late failure, despite satisfactory cusp mobility.

Outcomes of Isolated Aortic Valve Repair

Sharma and coll. from the Mayo clinic reported their long-term results of AV repair for isolated cusp disease. They observed a freedom from at least moderate AR of 58% and a freedom from reoperation of 72% at 15 years following surgery. Significant predictors of late reoperation were severe AR before surgery and more than mild AR at discharge after the intervention. It is noteworthy that over 80% of patients in this series had an annuloplasty by means of the Cabrol sub-commissural stitches (SCA). A large analysis from the Cleveland Clinic, pooling a certain number of different techniques for AV repair, found a freedom from reoperation of 90% at 10 years after surgery and that annular support was associated with best valve durability. We have demonstrated improved results of AV repair with complete circumferential annuloplasty by means of valve sparing – reimplantation compared to the sub-commissural annuloplasty if the VAJ is dilated (>28mm) regardless of the root diameter10 . Schäfers and coll. and Lansac and coll. have also shown that results of isolated valve repair, particularly in BAV, are improved if the repair is associated to annuloplasty, whether by suture annuloplasty or external ring . With suture annuloplasty dr. Schäfers observed a freedom from reoperation of 92.6% and freedom from significant AR (>2) of 79.5%. With the external ring, dr. Lansac reported a freedom from reoperation and freedom from AR>3 of 97.5% and 82.2% respectively at 7-year follow-up. Padial and coll. already in the '90s demonstrated that patients with severe AR have a significantly larger aortic annulus than patients with moderate or mild AR. Therefore, it is well agreed that the annuloplasty is a necessary adjunctive technique also in isolated AV repair, particularly if the VAJ is bigger than 26-28mm.

In our current approach, we favor valve sparing-reimplantation when the VAJ is dilated (>28mm), in BAV whenever we aim to imrpove valve symmetry or when, despite the normal diameter, the aortic root presents a thin and diseased wall. Whenever the VAJ is dilated over 26mm but there is no root dilatation nor wall disease, and the valve is tricuspid, we prefer to employ an external annuloplasty with a suture band.

REFERENCES

[1] Antunes MJ. Aortic valve repair: still a dream? *Eur J Cardio-Thorac Surg* 11 (1997):266-267.

[2] Chan V, Malas, T, Lapierre H, et al. Reoperation of left heart bioprostheses according to age at implantation. *Circulation* 2011;124(suppl I):S75-80.

[3] Bouhout I, Stevens LM, Mazine A, et al. Long-term outcome after elective isolated mechanical aortic valve replacement in young adults. *J Thorac Cardiovasc Surg* 2014;148:1341-6.

[4] Chiang YP, Chikwe J, Moskowitz AJ, Itagaki S, Adams DH, Egorova NN. Survival and long-term outcomes following bioprosthetic vs mechanical aortic valve replacement in patients aged 50 to 69 years. *JAMA* 2014;312(13):1323-1329.

[5] Glaser N, Jackson V, Holzmann MJ, Franco-Cereceda A, Sartipy U. Aortic valve replacement with mechanical vs. biological prostheses in patients aged 50-69 years. *Eur Heart J* (2016)37:2658-2667.

[6] Goldstone AB, Chiu P, Baiocchi M, et al. Mechanical or biologic prostheses for aortic-valve and mitral-valve replacement. *N Eng J Med* 2017;377:1847-57.

[7] Mastrobuoni S, de Kerchove L, Solari S, et al. The Ross procedure in young adults: over 2à years of experience in our Institution. *Eur J Cardio-Thorac Surg* 2016 Feb;49(2):507-12.

[8] Bierbach BO, Aicher D, Issa OA, et al. Aortic root and cusp configuration determine aortic valve function. *Eur J Cardiothorac Surg* 2010 Oct; 38(400-6).

[9] Navarra E, El Khoury G, Glienur D, et al. Effect of annulus dimension and annuloplasty on bicuspid aortic valve repair. *Eur J Cardiothorac Surg* 2013 Aug;44(2):316-22;

[10] de Kerchove L, Mastrobuoni S, Boodhwani M, et al. The role of annular dimension in tricuspid aortic valve repair. *Eur J Cardiothorac Surg* 2016 Feb;49(2):428-37.

[11] Tamer S, Mastrobuoni S, van Dyck M, et al. Free margin length and geometric height in aortic root dilatation and leaflet prolapse: implications for aortic valve surgery. *Eur J Cardiothorac Surg* 2020 Jan 1;57(1):124-132.

[12] Boodhwani M, de Kerchove L, Glineur D, et al. Repair-oriented classification of aortic insufficiency: impact on surgical techniques and clinical outcomes. *J Thorac Cardiovasc Surg* 2009 Feb;137(2):286-94.

[13] David TE, Feindel CM. An aortic valve-sparing operation for patients with aortic incompetence and aneurysm of the ascending aorta. *J Thorac Cardiovasc Surg.* 1992 Apr;103(4):617-621.

[14] David TE, Feindel CM, David CM, Manlhiot C. A quarter of a century of experience with aortic valve-sparing operations. *J Thorac Cardiovasc Surg* 2014 Sep; 148(3):872-9.

[15] Mastrobuoni S, de Kerchove L, Navarra E, et al. Long-term experience with valve-sparing reimplantation technique for the treatment of aortic aneurysm and aortic regurgitation. *J Thorac Cardiovasc Surg* 2019 Jul;158(1):14-23.

[16] de Kerchove L, Boodhwani M, Glineur D, et al. Effects of preoperative aortic insufficiency on outcome after aortic valve-sparing surgery. *Circulation* 2009;120(suppl 1):S120-S126.

[17] Mastrobuoni S, Tamer S, de Kerchove L, El Khoury G. Valve sparing: aortic root replacement with the reimplantation technique. *Multimed Man Cardiothorac Surg* 2015 Jul 1;2015. pii: mmv012. doi: 10.1093/mmcts/mmv012.

[18] de Kerchove L, Boodhwani M, Glineur D, Noirhomme P, El Khoury G. A new simple and objective method for graft sizing in valve-sparing root replacement using the reimplantation technique. *Ann Thorac Surg* 2011;92:749-751.

[19] Schafers HJ, Bierbach B, Aicher D. A new approach to the assessment of aortic cusp geometry. *J Thoracic Cardiovasc Surg* 2006 Aug; 132(2):436-8.

[20] Tamer S, de Kerchove L, Glineur D, El Khoury G. Video-atlas of aortic valve repair. *Ann Cardiothorac Surg* 2013;2(1):124-126.

[21] Sievers HH, Schmidtke C. A classification system for the bicuspid aortic valve from 304 surgical specimen. *J Thorac Cardiovasc Surg* 2007;133:1226-33.

[22] de Kerchove L, Mastrobuoni S, Froede L, et al. Variability of repairable bicuspid aortic valve phenotypes: towards an anatomical and repair-oriented classification. *Eur J Cardiothorac Surg* 2019 Feb 20:ezz033. doi: 10.1093/ejcts/ezz033. Online ahead of print.

[23] Boodhwani M, de Kerchove L, Glineur D, et al. Repair of regurgitant bicuspid aortic valves: a systematic approach. *J Thorac Cardiovasc Surg* 2010;140:276-84.

[24] 24. David TE, David CM, Ouzounian M, Feindel CM, Lafreniere-Roula M. A progress on reimplantation of the aortic valve. 100th annual meeting of the American Association for Thoracic Surgery 2020.

[25] Mastrobuoni S, de Kerchove L, Vancraeynest D, et al. Long-term progression of aortic regurgitation following valve sparing-reimplantation. The Heart Valve Society annual meeting 2020. Abu Dabi, Feb 15-16 2020.

[26] Arabkhani B, Mookhoek A, Di Centa I, Lansac E, Bekkers JA, De Lind Van Wijingaarden R, et al. Reported outcome after valve-sparing aortic root replacement for

aortic root aneurysm: a systematic review and meta-analysis. *Ann Thorac Surg* 2015 Sep;100(3):1126-31

[27] Klotz S, Stock S, Sievers HH, Diwoky M, Petersen M, Stierle U, et al. Survival and reoperation pattern after 20 years of experience with aortic valve-sparing root replacement in patients with tricuspid and bicuspid valves. *J Thoracic Cardiovasc Surg* 2018 Apr;155(4):1403-11.

[28] Sharma V, Suri RM, Dearani JA, et al. Expanding relevance of aortic valve repair – is earlier operation indicated? *J Thorac Cardiovasc Surg* 2014;147:100-8.

[29] Zeeshan A, Idrees JJ, Johnston DR, et al. Durability of aortic valve cusp repair with and withput annular support. *Ann Thorac Surg* 2018 Mar;105(3):739-48.

[30] de Kerchove L, Boodhwani M, Glineur D, et al. Valve sparing-root replacement with the reimplantation technique to increase the durability of bicuspid aortic valve repair. *J Thorac Cardiovasc Surg* 2011 Dec; 142(6):1430-8.

[31] Schneider U, Hofmann C, Aicher D, Takahashi H, Miura Y, Schäfers HJ. Suture annuloplasty significantly improves the durability of bicuspid aortic valve repair. *Ann Thorac Surg* 2017;103:504-10.

[32] Lansac E, Di Centa I, Sleilaty G, et al. Long-term results of external ring annuloplasty for aortic valve repair. *Eur J Cardiothorac Surg* 2016;50:350-60.

[33] Padial LR, Olivier A, Sagie A, Weyman AE, King ME, Levine RA. Two-dimensional echocardiographic assessment of the progression of aortic root size in 127 patients with chronic aortic regurgitation: role of the supraaortic ridge and relation to the progression of the lesion. A*m Heart J* 1997, Nov;134(5 pt 1): 814-21.

In: Perspectives in Aortic Valve Disease
Editor: Giovanni Concistrè
ISBN: 978-1-53618-769-4

Chapter 20

AORTIC VALVE SPARING: REMODELING AND REIMPLANTATION

Ruggero De Paulis**, Raffaele Scaffa and Ilaria Chirichilli
Cardiac Surgery Department, European Hospital, Rome, Italy

ABSTRACT

"Aortic valve sparing" (AVS) surgery, introduced in the 90s by Yacoub with the remodeling and by David with reimplantation technique, has gained increasing attention and more evident scientific relevance in the last decades. In recent years the number of AVS interventions has significantly increased through a better knowledge of anatomy and pathophysiology of the aortic root. The sharing and appreciation of positive clinical results along with progressive modifications of the original techniques, has helped in the worldwide spread of this surgery.

The concept that the aortic valve regurgitation can occur in patients with normal aortic cusps is not new but, paradoxically, for many years, we have been replacing intact aortic valves while somehow preserving enlarged aortic roots. Today, the leaflets integrity in the context of aortic root pathology is evaluated only after the root has been excised and normal root anatomy has been re-established. The complex interaction between the aortic valve leaflets and the skeleton of the aortic root - annulus and sino-tubular (ST) junction - is the basis for a normally functioning aortic valve. Annular and/or ST junction dilatation are the key elements in determining aortic valve regurgitation; consequent stress on the leaflets leads to intrinsic cusp defects. It is therefore important to understand how re-establishing the normal relationship of all aortic root components is the foundation for a good AVS procedure. Based on these premises echocardiography and diagnostic radiology (computed tomography and magnetic resonance imaging) are fundamental for both the selection of the AVS surgery candidates and for the clinical follow-up and the research studies.

Today is possible to perform both the remodeling and the reimplantation procedure while achieving an anatomical root reconstruction with excellent long-term results. Especially in young patients, AVS operations have become an established alternative to Bentall procedure with the important advantage of avoiding the use of valve prostheses

* Corresponding Author's Email: rdepaulis58@gmail.com.

and their inherent incidence of complications in terms of structural valve deterioration, thromboembolism, endocarditis and hemorrhage.

Keywords: aortic root, aortic valve, aortic operation, aortic regurgitation, aortic aneurysm

INTRODUCTION

"Nothing in nature is without reason; if you understand the reason you don't need experience" ("Nessuno effetto in natura è sanza ragione; intendi la ragione e non ti bisogna sperienza"), said Leonardo da Vinci, who, besides his many attributes as an artist, architect, anatomist, and military engineer, was also a leading hydrodynamic expert of his time. Although the whole thrust of Leonardo's argument is towards experimentation ("experience"), he gave great importance to acutely observing the different forms of each anatomical portion to understand its function. Undoubtedly, Leonardo understood almost everything necessary to know how to properly approach and surgically treat both aortic valve and aortic root pathology. The surgeon's ideal to pursue the most physiologic result by the discipline of surgery in which he excels truly stands in line with the medieval genius attempts to find nature's truths through his art [1].

Aortic valve sparing (AVS) procedures - remodeling and reimplantation, respectively introduced by Yacoub and David - were first described nearly 40 years ago [2, 3]. However, they have gained popularity only in the last two decades because of an in-depth knowledge of the "functional anatomy" of the aortic root and a collective evidence of satisfactory long-term results. Basically, after excision of the Valsalva's sinuses of the native aortic root (Figure 1), the scalloped aortic valve is sutured to a triple-tongue-shaped Dacron graft (remodeling) or entirely incorporated into a straight Dacron graft (reimplantation). The "remodeling" has always been considered physiologically superior to the "reimplantation" procedure for its ability to obtain a lifelike reconstruction of the Valsalva's sinuses. On the other hand, the "reimplantation" has always been considered more radical for its stabilization and support of the aortic annulus to prevent further annular dilatation.

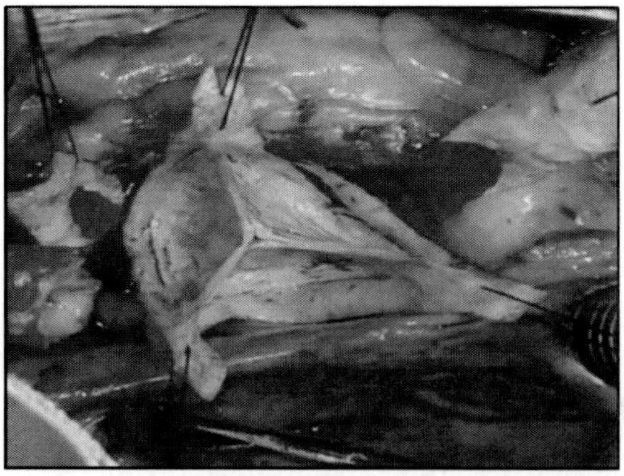

Figure 1. Aortic root preparation for a valve sparing procedure procedure in TAV (TAV: Tricuspid Aortic Valve).

During the 90's, there was an endless "philosophical" discussion about the peculiarity of the two different types of surgery but without a significant diffusion in the clinical usage of any of the two procedures. From 2000 on, it has been a progressive and worldwide diffusion of the AVS procedures with several modifications to overcome the apparent limitations of both original approaches. In fact, until 2000, AVS-focused publications did not exceed 20 articles; in the following years, almost 300 publications have progressively appeared. The most significant world literature of the past 2 years has been selected and commented by us in a recent review [4].

Despite all these years of surgical experience acquired amongst "aortic surgical teams" confusion still exists on the weaknesses and strengths of both remodeling and reimplantation procedures. It seems obvious that preoperative anatomical conditions combined with the many "customizations" of the techniques may differ significantly in the surgical scenario making it complicated an objective comparison between the two procedures.

However, in the last years, the differences between these two procedures have narrowed and nowadays both can guarantee an optimal anatomical and physiological root reconstruction with increased long-term valve durability. In the 21st century, avoidance of a valve replacement is slowly becoming mandatory in the young patient population, in which anticoagulation therapy and its related morbidity are undesirable.

THE RATIONAL

A strategy is a generalized approach to problems; a technique is something you say or do in a particular way. In team games (especially in basketball and soccer) an "assist" is the end of an action with which a player puts his teammate in a position to score (the pass that precedes a shot or goal). As a consequence of such philosophy, once the appropriate surgical strategy has been chosen ("the action and the assist"), the "goal" could be a simple and reproducible construction technique ("more science than art").

A correct approach to "spare" an aortic valve includes: 1) a wide knowledge of anatomy and physiology of the aortic root, 2) a systematic imaging assessment (echocardiography and computed tomography), 3) a knowledge of the two major procedures along with an intraoperative evaluation of aortic valve configuration. These skills facilitate patient selection and patient-tailored surgical planning.

Surgical Anatomy and Physiology of the Aortic Root

To identify an appropriate surgical strategy and technique, a deep understanding of the aortic anatomy and physiology is strongly recommended. Just like the mitral valve, also the human aortic valve and the root have been identified as a 3-dimensional complex of different elements, constituting a functionally dynamic structure. Although this aortic region has been anatomically well described, there is still controversy on the best nomenclature of its distinct elements, particularly the aortic annulus, which has several definitions.

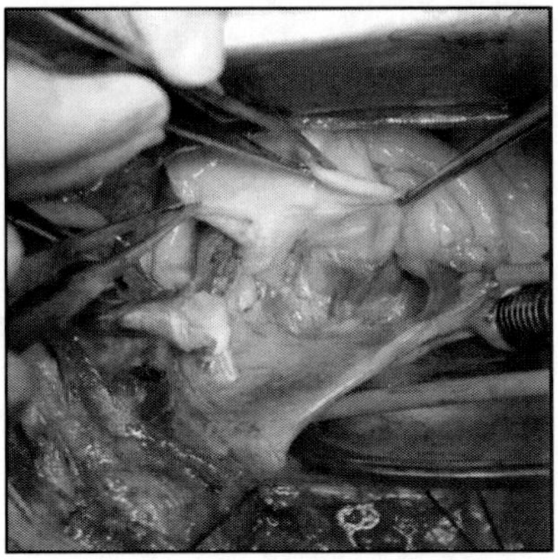

Figure 2. Dissection of the aortic root in preparation for aortic valve reimplantation. At the level of the Non-Coronary sinus the dissection reaches the level of the VBR despite the presence of muscular fibers as part of VAJ (VBR: Virtual Basal Ring; VAJ: Ventriculo-Aortic Junction).

The aorto-ventricular junction (AVJ) represents a real anatomical region with a specific histologic entity where ventricular structures (including the muscular septum, mitro-aortic curtain, and membranous septum) join the arterial system. Diagrammatically, the AVJ is characterized by a relatively circular line created by joining the base of inter-leaflet triangles with the lower third of Valsalva's sinuses, slightly above the nadir of the aortic leaflets crossing in several points the semilunar line of attachment of the aortic leaflets (this landmark is evident only at the level of the muscular portion of the aortic root). Histologically, the AVJ has a variable thickness along the circumference of the aortic root (range 1 to 4.6 mm; maximum at the level of the right coronary sinus). Differently, the virtual basal ring (VBR) it is no more than a virtual circular line positioned inside the left ventricle outflow tract, simply created by connecting the nadirs of each leaflet, without a real anatomic counterpart and it is the echocardiographic parameter considered to provide a measurement of the diameter of the aortic annulus. Noteworthy, the relationship between VAJ and VBR helps in a better understanding: the two anatomical landmarks, VAJ and VBR are further away at the level of the right coronary sinus and closer at the level of the non-coronary sinus. In the basal part of the non-coronary aortic sinus, the VAJ is entirely constituted by arterial wall, comprised in a portion of the mitro-aortic curtain, and precisely at this level VBR and VAJ coincide [5] (Figure 2).

The basal attachments of the aortic leaflets describe three semilunar lines with a distinctive crown-like formation and represent the hemodynamic boundary line between the left ventricle and the arterial system. The distal limit of the aortic root is marked by a supravalvular crest, called the sino-tubular (ST) junction. Inside the aortic lumen, the ST junction appears as a marginally elevated ridge of thickened aortic wall, while on the outside is usually less identifiable. The ST junction, with its specific relationship with the other components of the aortic root, plays a fundamental role in the function of the aortic valve. The aortic root as a whole naturally follows the curvature of the ascending aorta and it has been noted that there is the presence of a tilt angle of 5.5°–11° between the lines passing through the VBR and ST junction planes [6, 7]. In few simple words, the aortic annulus (VAJ or VBR), along with the ST junction and the three commissural posts connecting these two rings, represent the skeleton of the root (see below) that regulates the proper geometry of the aortic valve and root complex. The sinuses of Valsalva are defined as three-dimensional spaces of the aortic root surrounding the aortic leaflets that promote and regulate their opening and closing movements during the cardiac cycle. The role played by the sinuses of Valsalva in regulating movements of the aortic valve leaflets is well known. The anatomic features partially explain the complexity of valve hemodynamics: several studies shed light on the refined interactions between the aortic valve and its structures (VAJ, VBR, leaflets attachments, commissures and inter-leaflets triangles), the sinuses of Valsalva, and the ST junction ("from shape to function") [8-12].

The functional geometry of the normal trileaflet aortic valve, where the total length of the free margins equals the circumference and exceeds that of the inter-commissural distances, is an arrangement that allows wrinkle-free coaptation of the three cusps during diastole, as well as full opening during systole. In this way the aortic valve averts the systolic pressure load completely, and on the other hand, when diastole occurs, it is "ready" to receive the diastolic pressure load with its cusps smooth, fully extended, and in a linear approximation [13]. During the systole, the aortic root is more cylindrical due to annular contraction and commissures expansion (via the transmission of ventricular pressure through the inter-leaflet triangle); during the diastole, a "recoil" occurs to restore a static balance. However, the aortic root deformation during the cardiac cycle is also characterized by an overall systolic increase in its diameter in order to maintain the leaflets flat through the whole sequence of leaflet opening. The total area of the leaflets when compared to the aortic root is approximately 40% greater, with the largest area measured in the non-coronary leaflet and the smallest to the left coronary leaflet in most cases. This observation is fundamental in understanding the importance of aortic valve coaptation and the importance of the right proportion between overall root area and cusp surface. During diastole, cusp coaptation is indeed guaranteed by a long contact between the bellies of the three leaflets explaining the importance of a good proportion between cusp area and root dimension. An increase in root dimension will invariably lead to a reduction of cusp tissue available for coaptation [6].

Finally, the anatomic relationships of the external side of aortic root with the contiguous cardiac structures have fundamental relevance for surgical dissection of the root needed to reach and expose the aortic annulus. On the external surface of aortic root the limit of the surgical dissection corresponds to the roof of left atrium on the side of the non - and left coronary sinus, while it corresponds to myocardium coming from the interventricular septum and continuing laterally to the right ventricular outflow tract on the side of right coronary sinus. It is important to point out the presence of a cleavage plane between the muscular component of the left ventricle and the infundibulum of the right ventricle. This is the anatomical plane that permits externally to reach the level of the virtual basal ring despite the presence of muscular fibers as part of the VAJ [6, 7].

With these more or less virtual lines in mind El Khoury and colleagues introduced the concept of the functional aortic annulus (FAA) followed by a description of a functional classification of aortic regurgitation (AR). The FAA is comprised of (I) the ST junction, (II) the semilunar attachments of the aortic leaflets and, (III) the VBR. All the structures intersected by these lines are crucial for the anatomic and functional integrity of the aortic valve; in this way the FAA could be considered the real "skeleton" of the aortic root. The type I classification of AR represents the "pure" AR secondary to abnormalities of the aortic wall then largely due to lesions of the FAA; in this case the AR can be due to dilatation of ST junction and ascending aorta (type Ia) or dilatation of Valsalva's sinuses, ST junction and ascending aorta (type Ib) or dilatation of aortic annulus, (type Ic) that practically corresponds to the "annulo-aortic ectasia." Substantially, in these alterations the aortic valve presents various degrees of AR with relatively undamaged leaflets (highly depending on the duration of the disease). Type II AR is due to intrinsic leaflet disease like leaflet prolapse as a result of excessive cusp tissue or commissural disruption. Finally, type III AR is due to leaflet restriction as the result of calcification, thickening, and fibrosis of the aortic valve leaflets [14].

The use of a standardized functional classification is important because it will assist in the interpretation of trans-esophageal echocardiography (TEE) studies with specific reference to anatomical lesions and description of the pathology, but also in identifying optimal candidates for surgical repair. Important lessons in this regard may be learned from a parallel with the development of mitral valve repair. The Carpentier classification of mitral valve regurgitation has been instrumental in the diffusion and evolution of techniques for the mitral valve repair. Recently for bicuspid aortic valve (BAV) a new classification of phenotypes based on the commissural orientation further codified some anatomical characteristics suggesting specific surgical approaches [15]. This classification needs further validation with regards to surgical techniques and long-term outcomes but, once again, underline the importance of classification in a proper standardization of surgical techniques.

The Role of Imaging

Currently available imaging provides detailed information of the abnormalities in each component of the aortic root and these informations includes the size and shape of the annulus and ST junction as well as cusp anatomy and function. For adult male the mean diameter of aortic annulus with normal aortic valve was 23.1 ± 2.0 mm (approximately 10% smaller in women) and is closely related to body size (from 20.7 mm for 1.51 m2 to 25.2 mm for 2.61 m2 of body surface area); however regurgitant aortic valves present on average larger annulus especially in case of BAV (mean diameter 27 mm for tricuspid and 31 mm for BAV) [16].

Echocardiography has historically been used as the main form of aortic root imaging. However, computed tomographic (CT) scan has become an integral part of preoperative workup of patients undergoing AVS operations. CT imaging can be valuable in evaluating aortic diameters at the standard levels (annulus, sinuses, ST junction, tubular aorta); the precise diameters should be obtained from parasagittal multi-planar reconstruction along the centerline. Accurate measurements of aortic annulus are particularly important for managing patients with aortic root aneurysms; the ability to generate arbitrary oriented (orthonormal) images to augment the axial images is critical in assessing the size of the aortic annulus and root since they are typically located oblique to standard axial slices. Despite it having been considered a circular area, in vivo CT scan studies have accurately described the annulus elliptical shape with a minor and major diameter [17]. In a recent CT scan study we showed an elliptic annular shape in tricuspid aortic valve (TAV), a circular shape in type 0 BAV and an intermediate behavior in type 1 BAV, suggesting a possible gradual spectrum of ellipticity. In the postoperative phase after a reimplantation procedure these differences were eliminated, suggesting an active role of the annuloplasty on the geometry of the aortic annulus [18]. The continuation of this research, according to the classification for BAV as proposed by de Kerchove et al. [15], showed a linear correlation between the commissural orientation and the shape of the aortic annulus. As the commissural orientation decreases towards an asymmetric phenotype, the aortic annulus approaches a more elliptical shape [19]. Valve configuration determines long-term results after BAV repair: orientation of the commissures (>160°) as a naturally symmetrical BAV has superior results than an orientation of the commissures close to 120° [20]. Bisecting and off-center cuts represent well identifiable lines, mainly used for accurate CT measurements of the sinuses of Valsalva; measuring the annulus diameters using the bisecting cut has been proven to be more accurate while off-center cuts result in diameters significantly larger than those measured with the bisecting cut [21].

For many surgeons the direct measurement of the aortic annulus during surgery using an Hegar probe is probably the most reliable, accurate and valid method compared to the various diagnostic methods. However, sometimes, subtle dilatations are more difficult to recognize. In such cases it is always important to consider the relationship with cusp size.

The TEE and the modern 3-D TEE allow for accurate morphologic and functional evaluation of the aortic valve and aortic root complex with a good prediction of valve reparability [22, 23]. The echocardiography assessment should focus on the geometry and/or size of the components of the aortic root that influence the mechanism of opening and closing of aortic valve. Key aspects to consider include measurements of the annulus, ST junction and sinuses of Valsalva, evaluation for leaflet prolapse as well as visualization of jet origin and direction. Schematically the jet of AR is central in type I AR (mainly due to dilatation of various components of the skeleton of the root), is eccentric with a direction away from the prolapsing cusp in type II AR, while in type III is eccentric but with a jet direction towards the more restricted cusp. The number of cusps, their thickness, the appearance of the free margins must be examined in multiple views. However, the final decision is mainly based on intraoperatively evaluation of tissue quantity and quality and the presence of leaflet calcifications. Generally, smooth and large leaflets with redundant tissue are considered as more repairable than small, fibrous or thickened leaflets. In an echocardiographic representation (mid-esophageal 120° view) of the aortic root the diameter of the ST junction, in a normal healthy heart, is approximately 75% of the maximal sinus diameter, and is larger than aortic annulus at the level of the VBR with a ratio of 1.3 [24]. A mismatch in this ratio between the ST junction and the VBR (mostly 1.6 or more) is a frequent cause of secondary AR with normal aortic cusps. Cusp geometry can also be evaluated by means of echocardiography. Each cusp has a typical height between the central free margins and the aortic insertion lines. This distance is called "effective height" and is an important quantitative parameter of cusp configuration (Figure 3). The normal value of the effective height is 9 to 10 mm and it can be determined by echocardiography as well as intraoperatively with a caliper. Another important parameter to be evaluated is the "coaptation length" that is the amount of leaflet tissue that is actually in contact during systole (Figure 3).

This length should be measured between the two cusps in BAV and between each of the three cusps in TAV (Figure 4). Both effective height and coaptation length are two important parameters in the postoperative evaluation of the results. After surgery the effective height of all the leaflets should be should be 9 mm or more and the coaptation length at least 4 mm or more. A shorter effective height and/or coaptation length have been proven a risk factor for early and late residual aortic regurgitation [25, 26].

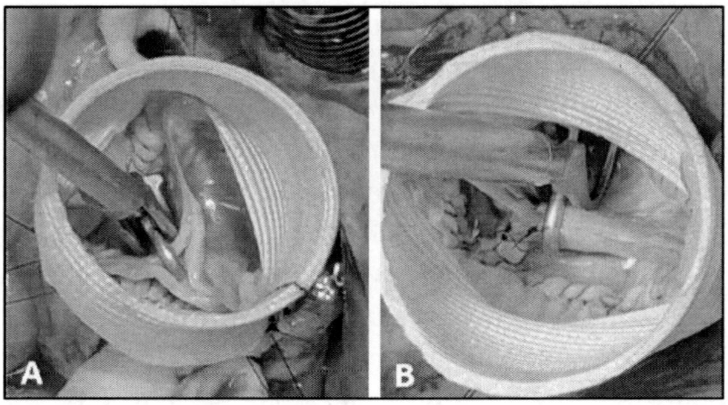

Figure 3. Schematic representation of an aortic valve reimplantation with Valsalva graft showing the eH, (the height difference between the central free margin and the aortic insertion lines), and the cL (the amount of leaflet tissue used for coaptation) (eH: effective Height; cL: coaptation Length).

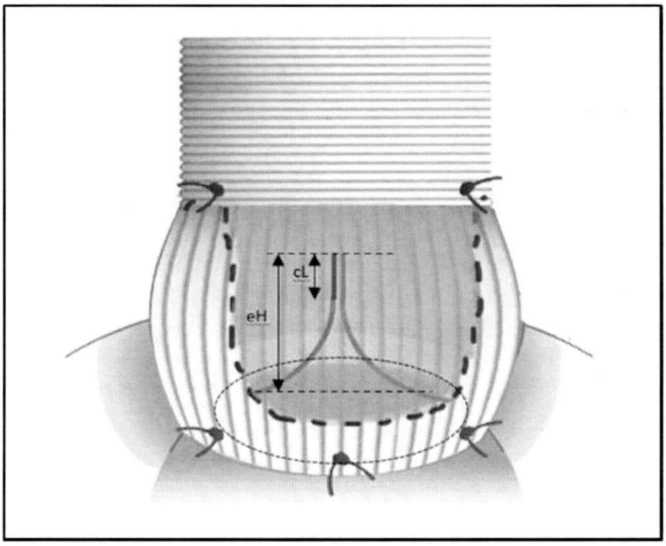

Figure 4. Use of caliper in TAV (A) and BAV (B) in order to measure the effective height (eH) of each cusp. When eH is <9 mm leaflet plication is needed. (TAV: Tricuspid Aortic Valve; BAV: Bicuspid Aortic Valve).

The History of Remodeling

The original remodeling technique was first reported in an abstract in 1983 but fully reported with the first results in 1993 [2]. Briefly, the aneurysmal tissue of the sinuses of Valsalva along with the ascending aortic wall is excised right at the annular attachment of the cusps; the end-portion of a straight Dacron graft is tailored in the form of three tongues (by excising three "triangles" to match the inter-leaflet triangles) and trimmed to match the shape of the sinuses. Then, each Dacron "tongue" is properly fixed to the aortic annulus starting at the nadir (deepest point) and suturing upwards until each commissure is fixed at the top of the triangular part of the excised Dacron. In this way the remodeling technique reshape the ST junction and at the same time creates 3 pseudo-sinuses of Valsalva with a very anatomical reconstruction of the root [10, 11]. The intrinsic characteristics of the remodeling technique have made it appealing because it is quick, require only a single suture line, and it does not need an extensive dissection and accurate mobilization of the aortic root. However, the long external sutures between the Dacron tongues and the valve remnants have always been a concern for the increased risk of bleeding and for the possibility of altering the proper geometry of the aortic valve by tissue distortion. The technical key to success in the method of remodeling is the careful prevention of bleeding by an accurate and precise suture line; to prevent postoperative bleeding small variations of the original technique have been proposed. In one of these techniques, a scalloped Dacron tube is placed inside the aortic root ("inclusion technique) without the resection of the Valsalva sinuses [27]. Other subsequent modifications were focused on creating custom made individualized reconstruction of three Dacron "patches" for the sinuses of Valsalva (Robicsek-Thubrikar graft) [28, 29]; however these techniques haven't had a worldwide diffusion.

As we have seen, the importance of a root reconstruction relies on the re-establishment of the right proportion between all root components. Unfortunately, the remodeling technique failed to address the aortic annulus. A properly reduced and supported aortic annulus is important in obtaining and maintaining a normal effective height, ensuring large leaflet coaptation and preventing cusp stress Postoperative echocardiography years after the operation have indeed shown that the lack of annular stabilization facilitates, in some patients, the development of AR over the time with an incidence of reoperation varying between 10% and 20% at 10 years [30-32]. For this reason, in the subsequent years the most important modification of the remodeling technique was aimed to adding a annuloplasty or annular stabilization to the classical remodeling technique [33-36].

The History of Reimplantation

In the classic reimplantation technique David proposed the "sparing" of the aortic valve within a cylindrical Dacron graft placed over the entire aortic root structure, reducing both the annulus and the ST junction diameters [3].

The Valsalva sinuses are resected a few millimeters above the aortic annulus and a series of sutures are placed under the annulus at the same horizontal level passing for the nadirs of each cusp without modifying the valve geometry (Figure 5). These sutures are passed through the base of a straight Dacron prosthesis and tied to secure annulus inclusion and reduction. Finally, the valve are reimplanted working from above, inside the conduit by polypropylene running suture in the same manner as the sub-coronary method used to implant a stentless bioprosthesis; in this way it is possible to obtain a complete support of the aortic wall with a very much reduced risk of bleeding due to the internal sutures. A straight Dacron re-establishes a proper proportion between the annulus and the ST junction and therefore a good geometrical condition for the aortic valve. These features are the starting point on the way to obtaining a satisfactory and effective leaflet coaptation. The drawback of the classic procedure is the elimination of the Valsalva sinuses that are important in regulating leaflets motion [10, 11].

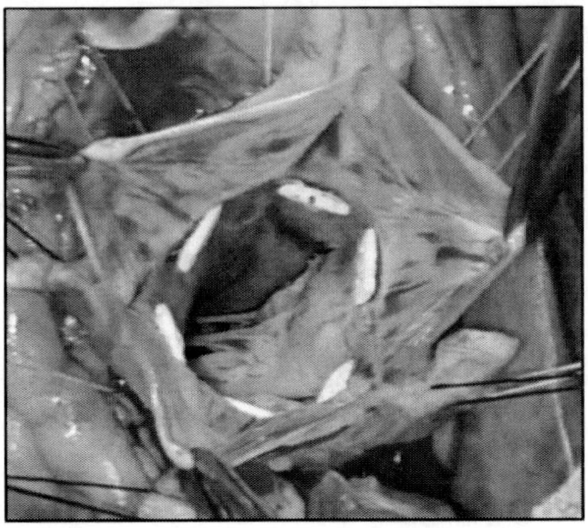

Figure 5. A series of pledgeted U-stitches are passed inside out the left ventricular outflow tract along the line of the virtual basal ring. Normally in tricuspid aortic valve 6 stitches are sufficient to complete annular stabilization and to secure the proximal part of the graft (3 at the nadirs of the cusps and 3 at the base on inter-leaflets triangles).

Although the valve can function well in the absence of sinuses, the presence of recirculating vortices inside the sinuses is a guarantee for a smooth opening and closing of the aortic valve during the cardiac cycle. The reduced leaflet stress is thought to be an important issue for the aortic valve longevity. Since the appearance of the classical reimplantation, many surgeons, including dr. David, proposed a series of technical variations in order to overcome the absence of sinuses of Valsalva. The "David II" and "David III" were already known as variations of the Yacoub's remodeling procedure (II is exactly similar to remodeling and the III is a remodeling with the addition of an external strip in the fibrous portion of basal ring), and therefore variation of the reimplantation technique were labeled as "David IV" (2001) and "David V" (2003). Both of them were progressive attempts to create pseudo-sinuses by the use of a larger straight graft opportunely plicated. The "David IV" is reimplantation with a graft size 4-mm bigger than usual with hand-made plications at the ST junction; the "David V" uses an even larger graft size (6-8 mm bigger), which is "necked down" both at the bottom and at the top ends to create graft pseudo-sinuses [37, 38]. Beginning in 2002, the Stanford group further simplified the David V procedure by using 2 separate grafts: a very large graft is used proximally to create large pseudo-sinuses of Valsalva and facilitate suturing inside the graft and a smaller graft is used to reduce the ST junction and replace the ascending portion of the aorta [39]. Other authors have described innumerable individual modifications of the reimplantation. All these modifications focused in the proximal part of Dacron conduit and tried to create a larger space" into which the leaflets could open without contact of the cylindrical conduit. In 1995 Cochran by scalloping the base of a cylindrical conduit increased the circumference of the cylinder. When this new increased circumference was sewn to the "fixed" anatomic anulus, the cylindrical shape of the conduit was somehow modified and the conduit would bulge outward at three locations creating pseudosinuses. [40]. In the following years there was a general trend to use a larger graft size than previously recommended [41]. Similarly, Takamoto et al. used a larger graft, and narrowed the distal part of the graft by three longitudinal running sutures at three sites reducing the original diameter and creating a neo-ST junction [42]. Other more complex and less convincing techniques have also been described [43]. The Florida Sleeve technique was introduced to simplify the procedural complexity; this technique involves protecting the aortic root with a Dacron "sleeve" while leaving native tissue in place and does not require coronary artery reimplantation decreasing the risk of surgical bleeding [44].

For all types of reimplantation an adequate mobilization of the base of the aortic root to place the bottom row of sutures in the sub-annular plane is mandatory and may require skeletonization of the aortic annulus and the central fibrous body of the heart. This aspect once again highlights the importance of a deep knowledge of the aortic root, the base of the heart and the surrounding structures.

The Similarity of the Two Procedures after All Modifications... from Remodeling to Reimplantation (the "Ring")

When the aortic root disease is treated by an AVS procedure, achieving a precise relationship among all the components of the aortic root and to restore near normal anatomy and function is imperative and the materials used could contribute greatly. To overcome the drawback of the remodeling technique, and to address the issue of annular dilatation several types of annuloplasty have been devised. It was demonstrated that sub-commissural annuloplasty (SCA) also known as Cabrol stitches are not appropriate in a large annulus (>28-30 mm) because the annuloplasty effect disappears with time and is associated with a high risk of AR recurrence both for BAVs and TAVs [45]. Furthermore, altering the shape of the interleaflet triangle with the SCA alter the physiologic function of this important component of the root. Ideal aortic annuloplasty should ensure good valve function, stability of annular diameter reduction and ease to implant without interference with coronary arteries, conduction system and leaflets mobility. The imperfect coincidence between the VAJ and external limit of aortic root dissection is particularly relevant when considering an internal or external annular fixation. The "internal" approach includes the use of strip of Dacron [33] or a rigid Dacron-covered titanium ring [34]. Although the subvalvular plane (particularly in the right coronary sinus) is easier to reach with internal rings, sub-aortic placement may interfere with cusps mobility and increase potential risks of hemolytic or thromboembolic events. For the "external" approach Lansac and coll. [35] has proposed a flexible ring positioned around the annulus fixed by a series of subvalvular sutures (in a manner similar to that used for reimplantation technique). Since 2009 Schäfers added, whenever the basal ring exceeds 26-27 mm a simple circular suture by braided polyester or PTFE [36]. This annulopasty consists of a suture placed from outside the aortic wall, under the coronaries, at the level of the VBR in a circumferential fashion and tighten around a Hegar dilator of an appropriate size (frequently 23 to 25 mm). This type of annuloplasty requires limited root dissection, shorter time to be performed and is associated with equal outcomes in term of stability of the results and freedom from reoperation. At this time, there is no evidence of the superiority of one technique of implant over another; moreover, the optimal material for an annuloplasty ring is still uncertain. In a recent porcine model study on the external approach for annuloplasty, Dacron ring was similar to native aortic annulus than suture annuloplasty, offering a more a physiological support [46]. Choice of material and future improvements of dedicated material for the annuloplasty procedures remain a challenge for future studies.

The Similarity of the Two Procedures after All Modifications... from Reimplantation to Remodeling (the "Space")

Traditionally the reimplantation procedures have been executed using a standard cylindrical straight tubular grafts, and, as previously described, numerous technical modifications have been added to reconstruct the anatomy of Valsalva's sinuses. At the end of the 90s, I imagined to modify a standard Dacron graft in order to create the shape of Valsalva sinuses without major modifications in the original technique as described by T. David in 1991. On February 14, 2000 our group have introduced into the clinical practice a new pre-formed Dacron conduit designed specifically for aortic root replacement. This graft is called the "Valsalva" graft (manufactured by Terumo Aortic, Renfrewshire, Scotland, UK) for its ability, when pressurized, to create the pseudo-sinuses of Valsalva. The main characteristic of the graft is a portion, called the skirt, with longitudinally directed pleats (at 90 degree with respect to the rest of the graft) that expand horizontally and, after aortic valve reimplantation, reproduce the sinuses of Valsalva. The peculiar design of the graft allows for proper root reconstruction by re-establishing the main FAA characteristics: two fixed rings (annulus and ST junction) joined by three pillars (the commissures) dividing three independent bulging sinuses [47]. The role of the Valsalva graft in AVS procedures is to combine the peculiar advantages of remodeling and reimplantation simplifying and standardizing the various steps of the operations. The theoretic arguments favoring polyester fabric pseudosinuses include slower aortic cusp closing velocities, which reduce the diastolic stresses on the cusps and thus potentially enhance valve durability [12]. The presence of pseudo-sinuses in the Valsalva graft guarantees proper and physiological aortic leaflet motion both during the opening and closing phase [8, 9, 48]. However, it is well known that the dynamics of aortic leaflet is altered not only in the absence of sinuses but also when the aortic wall is stiff (age, hypertension, atherosclerosis). Any Dacron graft is intrinsically stiffer than the natural living aortic wall and for this reason it appears even more important to guarantee a natural size and shape of neo-sinuses in order to best compensate for the loss of wall elasticity [49]. The Valsalva graft with its peculiar characteristics of longitudinally directed pleats of the graft allows a proper anatomical reconstruction in the size and shape of the sinuses (Figures 6-9). Although there is evidence that the Valsalva graft maintain certain distensibility at the level of the sinuses both in the short-term [9] and at medium-term [50] it is evident that the elastic component will remain markedly reduced when compared to natural aortic wall. More recently the Cornell International Consortium for Aortic Surgery (CICAS) evaluated the flow dynamics in the aortic root after AVS procedures with Valsalva graft or straight graft, by exploiting the capability of 4D Flow imaging to measure in vivo blood velocity fields and 3D geometric flow patterns. These studies clearly demonstrated that the recreation of the sinuses of Valsalva is associated with significantly lower wall shear stress and organized vortical flows at the level of the sinus that are not evident using the straight tube graft. Various and still unexplored knowledge can be obtained from the qualitative and quantitative analysis of these complex datasets, that could shed more light on the various surgical techniques and grafts adopted in AVS surgery [51-53].

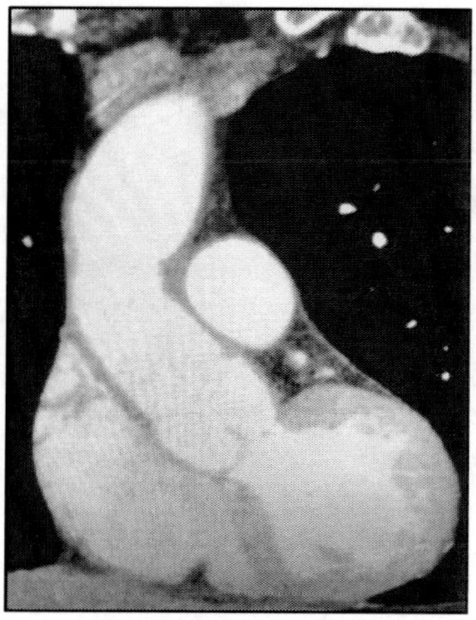

Figure 6. Postoperative sagittal CT scan view: Valsalva graft used in reimplantation procedure restores a near normal anatomy achieving a precise relationship among all the components of the aortic root. (CT: computed tomography).

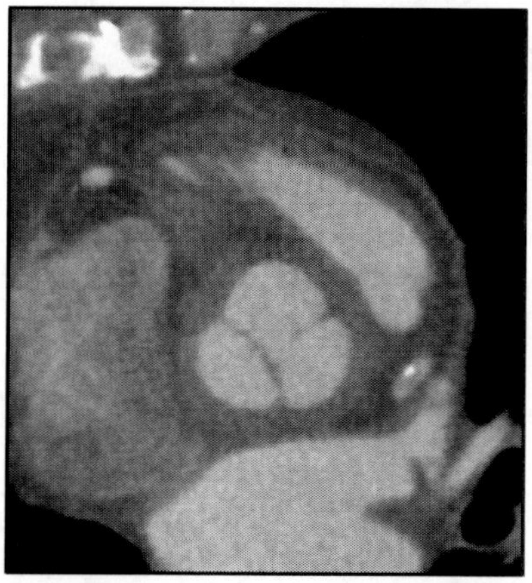

Figure 7. Postoperative sagittal cine MRI view (MRI: Magnetic Resonance Imaging).

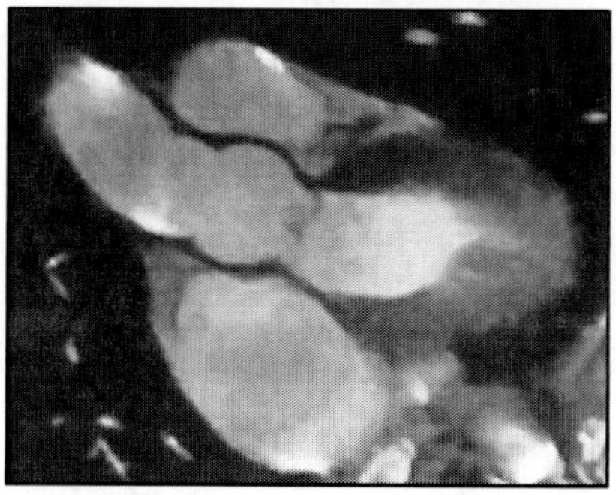

Figure 8. Postoperative cross sectional CT scan of a patient after a reimplantation procedure using the Valsalva graft shows the trilobate aspect of the root with 3 independent sinuses. (CT: computed tomography).

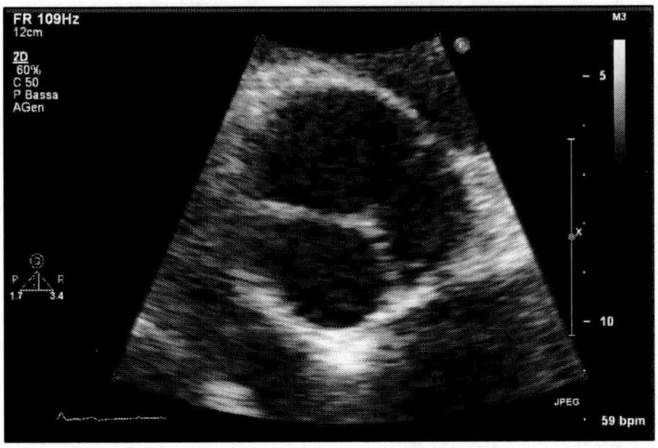

Figure 9. Postoperative short-axis TEE after a reimplantation procedure using the Valsalva graft in a patient with a TAV (TEE: Transesophageal Echocardiography; TAV: Tricuspid Aortic Valve).

These findings need confirmation in larger studies but are expected to have important implications in predicting the aortic valve durability.

Moreover, from a surgical point of view, the use of this designed graft with a sinus-like root portion can facilitate the suture of the coronary buttons during ostia reimplantation reducing the stress in the circumferential direction after the aorta has been pressurized [54]. The advantages are particularly evident in the redo cases and calcified and rigid coronary ostia. The initial hypothesis that the reduction of the stress on the coronary anastomoses may decrease the incidence of postoperative complications such as bleeding and late pseudo-aneurysm formation has been confirmed in our experience in nearly two decades of aortic root surgery including AVS and Bentall procedures [55-57].

As regarding the use of other types of preformed anatomical grafts, a new vascular graft (Cardioroot; Intervascular SAS, La Ciotat, France) has been also used for AVS operations in a prospective, multicenter study with excellent results at 1-year follow-up [58]. Considering the possibility of leaflet contact with the walls of a straight tube graft and the experimental data on suboptimal leaflet function, one would expect a much higher rate of failure following the original David procedure. In fact, despite re-creation of neosinuses in the aortic root is certainly superior from an anatomical and functional point of view, the clinical superiority of a graft with sinuses versus a cylindrical graft remains unproven. The long-term results of reimplantation using the Valsalva graft show freedom from reoperation of 90.1% ± 4.3% at 13 years [54]. In centers with longest experience, midterm and long-term outcomes with straight grafts for AVS operations are also excellent with freedom from reoperation on the aortic valve at 18 years higher than 90% [59, 60]. It is evident that no Dacron conduit can compensate for a suboptimal surgical performance or for patients selection both in the remodeling or reimplantation. The complexity of AVS procedures requires enough experience and several technical points, other than the choice of a graft, can significantly affect the final result. As an example, the technique used to reimplant the valve inside the Dacron conduit and/or the way the valve is geometrically repositioned inside the conduit, are far more important for the long-term success of the operation. The use of a straight graft or a pre-formed graft with sinuses, such as the Valsalva graft, is only a single factor and certainly not the most important.

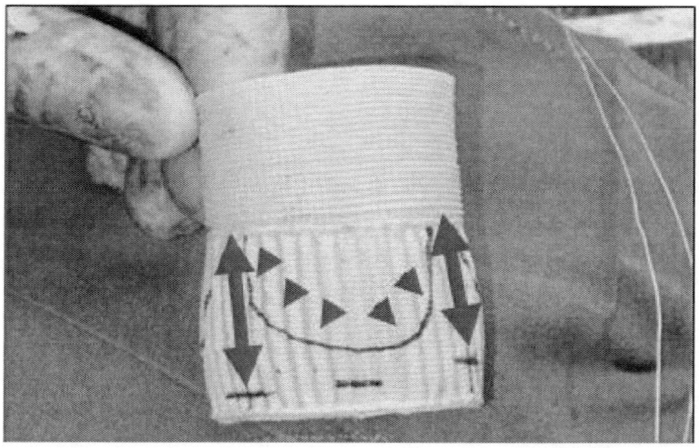

Figure 10. The level where to position the annular sutures inside the skirt is probably the most important individual point for the correct use of a Valsalva graft. The length of the commissural posts (CP) are measured and compared with the skirt of the graft from the ST junction down toward the base of the skirt. This point is marked (green arrows) to indicate the proper level where the annular sutures need to be placed along the whole circumference. This will ensure that once the commissural posts are stretched they will easily reach the ST junction where they will be anchored. Another curved line (red arrows) in the shape of the sinuses can also be used as a suturing path to simplify the fixing of valve remnants to the Dacron. (ST: sino-tubular).

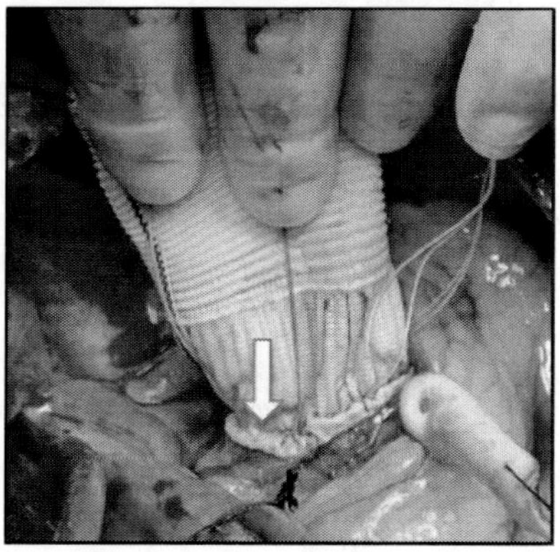

Figure 11. Once the graft is securely anchored to the annulus, the excess skirt (white arrows) will lie naturally at the base of the root and it does not need to be excised.

Nevertheless, when using the Valsalva graft some specific points need to be respected. For reimplanting the valve inside the Valsalva conduit we followed the key steps first described by David, but we introduced some details necessary to adapt the graft to each "patient's aortic valve" [61, 62]. Correct matching between native and synthetic aortic root components relies predominantly on the selection of the correct size of the graft used to replace the aortic root. We suggest the intraoperative measurement of the aortic annulus (using a Hegar dilator) at the sole criterion determining the choice of prosthetic tube graft. By adding 5 mm to the measure of the annulus, the proper conduit size is chosen [63]. As a rule of the thumb in most of the cases a 30 mm graft is required. With an annulus of 27 mm or greater, a 32 mm Valsalva graft is invariably chosen. Next, the skirt of the Valsalva graft (i.e., the section corresponding to the sinus portion of the root) is matched with the length of the commissures. When the height of commissures matches the height of the "skirt" the whole skirt is utilized and it is secured to the annulus to provide the annuloplasty effect. When the height of the commissures is shorter than the height of the "skirt," the excess of skirt is left out and the annular sutures are passed at the corresponding level inside the skirt (Figure 10, 11).

In this way we guarantee that, once the aortic valve is retrieved from inside the graft, the top of the commissures will be right at the level of the new ST junction. Once the top of the commissure are fixed at the new ST junction the aortic valve remnants can be safely sutured to the Dacron wall without risk of modifying the valve geometry (Figure 12, 13). Finally, the aortic leaflets are tested for symmetry and coaptation before proceeding to cusp plication where needed. It is very important to underline the fact that by stretching the commissural post and fixing them at the level of the new ST junction we reproduce the skeleton of the root by connecting two rings (annuls and ST junction) by means of three straight and rigid pillars (the commissural posts). Sinuses will bulge only between the commissural posts ensuring the formation of three independent pockets just like in the natural aortic root.

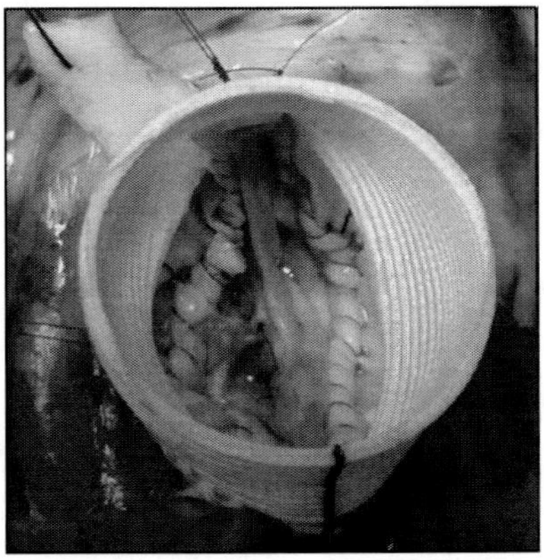

Figure 12. The aortic valve remnants are sutured to the skirt of the Valsalva graft by polypropylene running suture in the same manner as the subcoronary method used to implant a stentless valve. Note that the commissures are fixed right above the new ST junction (ie, the line connecting the skirt of the graft with the cylindrical straight portion). In this way it is possible to reconstruct the "skeleton" of the aortic valve: the commissural posts are now stretched between 2 fixed rings (annulus and ST junction). (ST: sino-tubular).

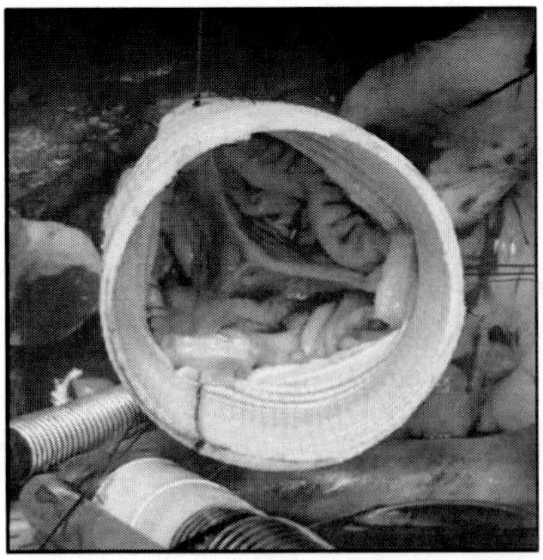

Figure 13. Same as in Figure 12. Reimplantation procedure for a BAV (BAV: Bicuspid Aortic Valve).

Indications and Choice of the Strategy (Remodeling vs. Reimplantation)

AVS operations were developed to preserve the aortic valve in patients with aortic root aneurysm with or without AR and in patients with ascending aortic aneurysm and AR secondary to dilatation of the ST junction (in both instances we are in fact in the presence of abnormality of the FAA with the aortic cusps reasonably normal). Over the years, the encouraging results have allowed to expand the indication to patients with more damaged valve leaflets (e.g., BAV and TAV with long-standing AR). The main etiologies of disease of FAA are classically heritable disorders of connective tissue, BAV with its related aortopathy, and arterial hypertension. All of them lead to abnormalities of the aortic wall and the "surgical strategy" focus on the need of replacing the whole aortic wall of the root irrespective of the type of disease in question. In this respect, the two AVS procedures are not competitive to each other. Usually the surgeon gets acquainted with one of the two procedure and invariably use it in all presenting cases. However, if we want to give direction based on the specific characteristics of the two procedures we should select the reimplantation method when the aortic annulus diameter is very large, and the remodeling method when the annular diameter is smaller. The cut-off value varies, but it seems reasonable to consider it around 27-28 mm in many cases, because long-term results after surgery worsened when this cut-off value was exceeded [64]. Usually the size of the annulus is measured by direct intubation by an Hegar dilatator or similar. Classically, young adults with aortic root aneurysms associated with genetic syndromes are ideal candidates for reimplantation; others patients with ascending aortic aneurysm and AR secondary to dilated ST junction and a normal aortic annulus can be treated with remodeling. Through the years several modifications, some repetitive and others innovative, have been proposed to the original reimplantation or the remodeling procedures. Today all changes led to perform a remodeling with the addition of annular support or a reimplantation with the creation of neo-sinuses (practically eliminating the Achilles heels of both procedures).

It is commonly known that each surgical procedure follows a learning curve and, often, AVS procedures have been criticized for complexity and for being time-consuming. Recently, the group of Hannover (Germany) analyzed whether the surgeon's level of expertise affects the outcomes after the reimplantation procedure. The study shows a significant correlation between the surgeon's experience and both cardiopulmonary bypass time and aortic cross-clamp time and a trend towards statistical significance comparing the surgeon's skills and the perioperative mortality and complications. Noteworthy, despite there was no association between residual postoperative AR grade and the surgeon's experience, there was a significant association between aortic valve-related reoperation and the surgeon's level of experience [65]. Because experience is important and the learning curve could take time, it seems reasonable to be acquainted with one of the two procedures, absorbing all "tips and tricks." To the same extent, it is advisable to avoid switching from one procedure to the other before having achieved good and stable results with the procedure of your choice.

Additional Leaflets Repair (Further Scientific Contribution)

In AVS surgery the newest and more important evolution has been the development and standardization of a technique of leaflets repair that, in addition to the graft implantation, could corrects residual AR due to "intrinsic" or "iatrogenic" abnormalities of the leaflets. In many cases alteration of the geometry of the FAA (annular dilatation and/or loss of ST junction) is the initial cause of AR that, over the time, begets cusp prolapse and leaflet degenerative changes. In our personal experience the presence of a dilated annulus (specially in a long-standing disease process) increases the probability of facing, at time of surgery, an intrinsically damaged cusps. This surgical finding has been confirmed by a study using a finite element computer-assisted stress analysis. Dilatation of ST junction was found to slightly affect leaflet coaptation with less damage on the leaflet free margins; on the other hand, annular dilatation, whether alone or combined with ST junction dilatation, was responsible for a significantly reduced coaptation and a significant damage on the leaflet structure. Data from this study indicated that the stress on the free margin and on the 'belly' of the aortic leaflet increased by 14% in case of isolated dilatation of the ST junction, while increase by 67% in case of isolated annular dilatation [66]. In the clinical practice it is indeed important, especially in young individuals with large annuli, to advise surgery at an earlier stage in order to increase the chance of finding cusps with a relatively normal structure and function.

Moreover, when performing an AVS procedure we invariably modify the leaflet configuration. By removing a dilated root and replacing it with a Dacron prosthesis of nominal normal size (average of 30 mm for an adult) we invariably reduce the root diameter and cause some form of leaflet sagging. It has to be further emphasized that, independently on the preferred procedure, remodeling or reimplantation, we might cause small distortion in the valve geometry when the valve is sutured to the Dacron graft. In fact, when suturing the Dacron to the valve remnants, attention must be paid not to distort the orientation, height and distance of the commissures. The distortion may indeed induce leaflet prolapse that will need to be addressed to avoid any early residual AR. It is indeed of paramount importance to normalize not only valve geometry but also cusp configuration. Cusp configurations are relatively difficult to standardize intraoperatively, even though these dimensions have a mathematic relationship with sinus dimensions [67]. Schäfers et al. have designed a caliper that facilitates easy and reproducible measurement of cusp height difference, called "effective height" (Figure 3). The height difference of the cusp (free edge to insertion) can be measured in millimeters and for normal tricuspid aortic valves this effective height varies from 8 to 10 millimeters [26]. In order to standardize the assessment of leaflet prolapse and cusp configuration, the use of this caliper is recommended (using an effective height of 9-10 mm as a reference) (Figure 4). If one cusp is found to be prolapsing (having an "effective height" inferior to the other two cusps), the simple shortening of the leaflet's free margin, by central plication can eliminate the tissue redundancy and normalize cusp geometry. Employing a fine polytetrafluoroethylene (PTFE) suture along the leaflet the free margin in order to reduce its length is an alternative method; however, it is more difficult, less reproducible, and slightly less accurate to perform.

At the beginning of the era of the popularity of AVS surgery additional cups intervention after both remodeling and reimplantation have been considered a risk factor, with a significant increase in the annual progression rate of AR [64]. In 2010 an Italian multicenter experience of reimplantation procedure with Valsalva graft highlighted that additional aortic leaflet repair was necessary for 9% (25 of 278 patients). At 10-years of follow-up the freedom from aortic valve reoperation rate was 91% with an incidence of reoperation significantly greater among patients who had undergone some form of leaflet plasty [56].

It seemed logical that if we started with a normally functioning TAV or BAV and the surgical procedure was only aimed at eliminating the root pathology and dilatation, the results would have been more predictable and probably better in the long-term period. On the other hand, when starting with a severely regurgitant aortic valve the need for valve plasty would necessarily add another level of uncertainty. As is often the case in surgery, every surgical additional step carries its own additional risk of failure. In this specific case the AVS procedure combined to cusp repair would carry the correspondent risk of failure usually associated with both procedures if considered separately. Nonetheless, leaflet plasty is necessary if we want to spare preoperatively regurgitant valve or correcting for intra-operative alteration of leaflet geometry resulting in suboptimal coaptation and/or induced prolapse.

With growing experience and continuing reasoning we came to the conclusion that the combined aortic valve repair and AVS surgery are intimately linked and they always need to be invariably part of the same procedure. Even when the valve looks normal after being re-implanted in a Dacron conduit, and even if the valve is not leaking at all after the procedure, it is very unlikely that all the leaflet are in fact exactly at the same level (i.e., that all have the same effective height). A not leaking valve after an AVS procedure indicates that the coaptation length (the apposition of the leaflets) is sufficient to make the valve competent but fails to indicate that the amount of coaptation is evenly distributed between the leaflets (i.e., that all leaflets have the same effective height). In fact when we perform an AVS procedure, even in a normally functioning valve (bicuspid or tricuspid), we invariably reduce the whole root diameter. It is common practice going from a root diameter of about 5.0/5.5 cm to a root diameter of 30-32 mm (the two most commonly utilized sizes of Dacron conduit). The direct and immediate effect of dramatically reducing the whole root diameter is a relative apparent excess of tissue in the leaflet free margin that would consequently tend to prolapse. This effect is much easily understandable when referring to a BAV configuration for its similarity with a suspended bridge. If in a suspended bridge we move closer to the four poles that hold the suspensions, we immediately see that the suspension will sag down. To lift the bridge to the same level we will need to shorten the suspensions. It is evident that the induced prolapse needs to be corrected almost invariably in both leaflets. Although this same process takes also place for TAV, it is more difficult to immediately appreciate it because the tricuspid geometry would better mask the induced leaflet prolapse. Even though all three leaflets might potentially be prolapsing, usually one of the three (for some reason more frequently the right one) would more often be affected. Furthermore, it must be stressed that, along with the reduced root diameter, other surgical factors might be related to the modification of a leaflet prolapse like a slightly different commissural orientation or a different tension on each reimplanted commissure.

In simple term, when we perform an AVS procedure we invariably modify the leaflet configuration resulting in some for of leaflet sagging and prolapsing. Although in most cases this can be barely recognized by the naked eye, it is evident if we individually measure the effective height with the help of a caliper. If we want to achieve a so-called "perfect anatomical reconstruction" we need to focus not only on the root anatomy and on a proper sinus reconstruction but also on a perfect length of the leaflet free margin that is invariably affected by the reconstruction of the root anatomy.

After 20 years of experience we can now acknowledge that AVS surgery associated with aortic cusp repair has further expanded its effectiveness in patients with complex aortic valve anatomy, avoiding aortic valve replacement and its inherent pitfalls. We can certainly state that the road to a continuously improved reconstruction of a dilated aortic root is unraveling and becoming clearer.

CONCLUSION

Surgical treatment of the pathology of aortic root has the aim of avoiding aortic dissection and/or rupture while restoring normal aortic valve function. However, for a long time, little attention had been paid to the fact that, in many circumstances, the aortic valve was intrinsically "healthy." Since the seminal article by H. Bentall in 1967 [68], the aortic valve has been replaced along with the root with a valve conduit. The results are indeed satisfactory albeit with a certain incidence of valve related complications.

In the current era, with the increasing age of patients who undergo aortic root surgery, and data supporting the use of a biological aortic valve in the younger population, the need for a composite biological valved conduit have significantly increased. Parallel to the increased use of biological valve in the context of a Bentall operation, AVS operation have also been performed in a growing number of patients. AVS operations, both the Yacoub "remodeling" and the David "reimplantation" have evolved and improved. The growing acceptance and applicability of these procedures are founded on a better standardization of the technique, a lower risk of surgical bleeding, and larger amount of data on favorable long-term results. Both procedures of remodeling and reimplantation can now provide excellent root reconstruction and adequate clinical results in terms of valve durability. The AVS technique offers several advantages over the Bentall procedure, such as no need for oral anticoagulation and lifestyle adjustments [69]. Nevertheless, the age criterion in patient selection has been debated. As experience and familiarity with these techniques increases, AVS procedures can also be considered excellent alternative to composite conduits with biological valve, whenever in the presence of good anatomical condition, even in elderly patients [70].

Today the strategies and techniques for AVS operations, previously viewed as difficult and unclear, have now been thoroughly analyzed and shared with the scientific community. Clinical results are piling up, clearly demonstrating a very long durability of the procedure with limited incidence of complications and without limitation in any form of physical activity. A refined multimodal imaging enables us to evaluate the results of an anatomical reconstruction along with the physiological function of the spared and repaired aortic valve. The road to avoid the use of valve prostheses is becoming wider.

REFERENCES

[1] Morea M, De Paulis R. 'Il buso' (the orifice). How much did Leonardo know of the aortic valve? *J Cardiovasc Med* 2007; 8(6):399-403.

[2] Sarsam MA, Yacoub M. Remodeling of the aortic valve annulus. *J Thorac Cardiovasc Surg* 1993; 105:435-438.

[3] David TE, Feindel CM. An aortic valve-sparing operation for patients with aortic incompetence and aneurysm of the ascending aorta. *J Thorac Cardiovasc Surg* 1992; 103:617-621.

[4] De Paulis R, Scaffa R, Chirichilli I. Valve sparing root replacement: un update. *Curr Opin Cardiol* 2020; 35(2):95-100.

[5] de Kerchove L, El Koury G. Anatomy and pathophysiology of the ventriculo-aortic junction: implication in aortic valve repair surgery. *Ann Cardiothorac Surg* 2013; 2:57-64.

[6] De Paulis R, Salica A. Surgical anatomy of the aortic valve and root-implications for valve repair. *Ann Cardiothorac Surg* 2019; 8(3):313-321.

[7] de Kerchove L, Jashari R, Boodhwani M, Duy KT, Lengelé B, Gianello P, Mosala Nezhad Z, Astarci P, Noirhomme P, El Khoury G. Surgical anatomy of the aortic root: Implication for valve-sparing reimplantation and aortic valve annuloplasty. *J Thorac Cardiovasc Surg* 2015; 149(2):425-33.

[8] De Paulis R, De Matteis GM, Nardi P, Scaffa R, Buratta MM, Chiariello L. Opening and closing characteristics of the aortic valve after valve-sparing procedures using a new aortic root conduit. *Ann Thorac Surg* 2001; 72(2):487-94.

[9] De Paulis R, De Matteis GM, Nardi P, Scaffa R, Bassano C, Chiariello L. Analysis of valve motion after the reimplantation type of valve-sparing procedure (David I) with a new aortic root conduit. *Ann Thorac Surg* 2002; 74(1):53-7.

[10] Leyh RG, Schmidtke C, Sievers HH, Yacoub MH. Opening and closing characteristics of the aortic valve after different types of valve-preserving surgery. *Circulation* 1999; 100(21):2153-60.

[11] Furukawa K, Ohteki H, Cao ZL, Narita Y, Okazaki Y, Ohtsubo S, Itoh T. Evaluation of native valve-sparing aortic root reconstruction with direct imaging - reimplantation or remodeling? *Ann Thorac Surg* 2004; 77(5):1636-41.

[12] Grande-Allen KJ, Cochran RP, Reinhall PG, Kunzelman KS. Re-creation of sinuses is important for sparing the aortic valve: a finite element study. *J Thorac Cardiovasc Surg* 2000; 119(4):753-63.

[13] Robicsek F, Thubrikar MJ, Cook JW, Fowler B. The congenitally bicuspid aortic valve: how does it function? Why does it fail? *Ann Thorac Surg* 2004; 77(1):177-85.

[14] El Khoury G, Glineur D, Rubay J, Verhelst R, d'Acoz Yd, Poncelet A, Astarci P, Noirhomme P, van Dyck M. Functional classification of aortic root/valve abnormalities and their correlation with etiologies and surgical procedures. *Curr Opin Cardiol* 2005; 20:115-21.

[15] de Kerchove L, Mastrobuoni S, Froede L, Tamer S, Boodhwani M, van Dyck M, El Khoury G, Schäfers HJ. Variability of repairable bicuspid aortic valve phenotypes: towards an anatomical and repair-oriented classification. *Eur J Cardiothorac Surg* 2019; 56:351-359.

[16] Capps SB, Elkins RC, Fronk DM. Body surface area as a predictor of aortic and pulmonary valve diameter. *J Thorac Cardiovasc Surg* 2000; 119: 975-82.

[17] Blanke P, Russe M, Leipsic J, Reinöhl J, Ebersberger U, Suranyi P, Siepe M, Pache G, Langer M, Schoepfet UJ. Conformational pulsatile changes of the aortic annulus: impact on prosthesis sizing by computed tomography for transcatheter aortic valve replacement. *JACC Cardiovasc Interv* 2012; 5:984-94.

[18] Chirichilli I, Irace F, Weltert L, Tsuda K, Scaffa R, Salica A, Galea N, De Paulis R. Morphological modification of the aortic annulus in tricuspid and bicuspid valves after aortic valve reimplantation: an electrocardiography-gated computed tomography study. *Eur J Cardiothorac Surg* 2019; 56(4):778-784.

[19] Chirichilli I, Irace FG, Weltert LP, Salica A, Guerrieri Wolf L, Fusca S. Ricci A, De Paulis R. A direct correlation between commissural orientation and annular shape in bicuspid aortic valves: a new anatomical and computed tomography classification. *Interact Cardiovasc Thorac Surg* 2020; 30(5):666-670.

[20] Aicher D, Kunihara T, Issa OA, Brittner B, Gräber S, Schäfers HJ. Valve configuration determines long-term results after repair of the bicuspid aortic valve. *Circulation* 2011; 123(2):178-85.

[21] Mori S, Anderson RH, Tahara N, Izawa Y, Toba T, Fujiwara S, Shimoyama S, Watanabe Y, Nishii T, Kono AK, Takahashi S, Hirata K. The differences between bisecting and off-center cuts of the aortic root: the three-dimensional anatomy of the aortic root reconstructed from the living heart. *Echocardiography* 2017; 34:453-61.

[22] Berrebi A, Monin JL, Lansac E. Systematic echocardiographic assessment of aortic regurgitation-what should the surgeon know for aortic valve repair? *Ann Cardiothorac Surg* 2019; 8:331-341.

[23] Hagendorff A, Evangelista A, Fehske W, Schäfers HJ. Improvement in the assessment of aortic valve and aortic aneurysm repair by 3-dimensional echocardiography. *JACC Cardiovasc Imaging* 2019; 11:2225-2244.

[24] Tamás E, Nylander E. Echocardiographic description of the anatomic relations within the normal aortic root. *J Heart Valve Dis* 2007; 16:240-6.

[25] Bierbach BO, Aicher D, Issa OA, Bomberg H, Gräber S, Glombitza P, Schäfers HJ. Aortic root and cusp configuration determine aortic valve function. *Eur J Cardiothorac Surg* 2010; 38:400-406.

[26] Schäfers HJ, Bierbach B, Aicher D. A new approach to the assessment of aortic cusp geometry. *J Thorac Cardiovasc Surg* 2006; 132:436-8.

[27] Hvass U. A new technique for sparing the aortic valve in patients with aneurysm of the ascending aorta and root. *J Thorac Cardiovasc Surg* 2000; 119:1048-9.

[28] Zehr KJ, Thubrikar MJ, Gong GG, Headrick JR, Robicsek F. Clinical introduction of a novel prosthesis for valve-preserving aortic root reconstruction for annuloaortic ectasia. *J Thorac Cardiovasc Surg* 2000; 120(4):692-8.

[29] Urbanski, PP. Valve-sparing aortic root repair with patch technique. *Ann Thorac Surg 2005*; 80: 839-844.

[30] Luciani GB, Casali G, Tomezzoli A, Mazzucco A. Recurrence of aortic insufficiency after aortic root remodeling with valve preservation. *Ann Thorac Surg* 1999; 67(6):1849-52.

[31] Leyh RG, Fischer S, Kallenbach K, Kofidis T, Pethig K, Harringer W, Haverich A. High failure rate after valve-sparing aortic root replacement using the "remodeling technique" in acute type A aortic dissection. *Circulation* 2002; 106(12 Suppl 1):I229-I233.

[32] Yacoub MH, Gehle P, Chandrasekaran V, Birks EJ, Child A, Radley-Smith R. Late results of a valve-preserving operation in patients with aneurysms of the ascending aorta and root. *J Thorac Cardiovasc Surg* 1998; 115(5):1080-90.

[33] Fattouch K, Castrovinci S, Murana G, Nasso G, Guccione F, Dioguardi P, Salardino M, Bianco G, Speziale G. Functional annulus remodelling using a prosthetic ring in tricuspid aortic valve repair: mid-term results. *Interact Cardiovasc Thorac Surg* 2014; 18(1):49-54; discussion 54-5.

[34] Rankin JS, Mazzitelli D, Fischlein T, Choi YH, Pirk J, Pfeiffer S, Wei LM, Badhwar V. Geometric Ring Annuloplasty for Aortic Valve Repair During Aortic Aneurysm Surgery: Two-Year Clinical Trial Results. *Innovations* (Phila) 2018; 13(4):248-253.

[35] Youssefi P, Di Centa I, Khelil N, Debauchez M, Lansac E. Valve sparing root replacement: remodeling root repair with aortic ring annuloplasty. *Ann Cardiothorac Surg* 2019; 8(3):411-414.

[36] Schneider U, Aicher D, Miura Y, Schäfers HJ. Suture Annuloplasty in Aortic Valve Repair. *Ann Thorac Surg* 2016; 101(2):783-5.

[37] Miller DC. Valve-sparing aortic root replacement in patients with the Marfan syndrome. *J Thorac Cardiovasc Surg* 2003; 125(4):773-8.

[38] Harky A, Antoniou A, Howard C, Rimmer L, Ahmad MU, Bashir M. Valve sparing aortic root surgery: from revolution to evolution? *J Vis Surg* 2019; 5:14. doi: 10.21037/jovs.2019.01.11.

[39] Demers P, Miller DC. Simple modification of "T. David-V" valve-sparing aortic root replacement to create graft pseudosinuses. *Ann Thorac Surg* 2004; 78:1479-81.

[40] Cochran RP, Kunzelman KS, Eddy AC, Hofer BO, Verrier ED. Modified conduit preparation creates a pseudosinus in an aortic valve-sparing procedure for aneurysm of the ascending aorta. *J Thorac Cardiovasc Surg* 1995; 109(6):1049-57; discussion 1057-8.

[41] Gleason TG. New graft formulation and modification of the David reimplantation technique. *J Thorac Cardiovasc Surg* 2005; 130(2):601-3.

[42] Takamoto S, Nawata K, Morota T. A simple modification of 'David-V' aortic root reimplantation. *Eur J Cardiothorac Surg* 2006; 30(3):560-2.

[43] Rama A, Rubin S, Bonnet N, Gandjbakhch I. New technique of aortic root reconstruction with aortic valve annuloplasty in ascending aortic aneurysm. *Ann Thorac Surg*. 2007; 83(5):1908-10.

[44] Hess PJ Jr, Klodell CT, Beaver TM, Martin TD. The Florida sleeve: a new technique for aortic root remodeling with preservation of the aortic valve and sinuses. *Ann Thorac Surg* 2005; 80(2):748-750.

[45] de Kerchove L, Vismara R, Mangini A, Fiore GB, Price J, Noirhomme P, Antona C, El Khoury G. *In vitro* comparison of three techniques for ventriculo-aortic junction annuloplasty. *Eur J Cardiothorac Surg* 2012;41(5):1117-1124.

[46] Benhassen LL, Ropcke DM, Sharghbin M, Lading T, Skov JK, Tjørnild MJ, Poulsen KB, Bechsgaard T, Skov SN, Nielsen SL, Hasenkam JM. Comparison of Dacron ring and suture annuloplasty for aortic valve repair-a porcine study. *Ann Cardiothorac Surg* 2019; 8(3):342-350.

[47] De Paulis R, De Matteis GM, Nardi P, Scaffa R, Colella DF, Chiarello L. A new aortic Dacron conduit for surgical treatment of aortic root pathology. *Ital Heart J* 2000; 1(7):457-63.

[48] Matsumori M, Tanaka H, Kawanishi Y, Onishi T, Nakagiri K, Yamashita T, Okada K, Okita Y. Comparison of distensibility of the aortic root and cusp motion after aortic

root replacement with two reimplantation techniques: Valsalva graft versus tube graft. *Interact Cardiovasc Thorac Surg* 2007; 6(2):177-81.

[49] Robicsek F, Thubrikar M. Are we implanting half-valves? The role of sinus wall compliance in aortic valve function. *Ann Thorac Surg* 1999; 67(2):597.

[50] Monti L, Mauri G, Balzarini L, Tarelli G, Brambilla G, Vitali E, Ornaghi D, Citterio E, Settepani F. Compliance of the Valsalva graft's pseudosinuses at midterm follow-up with cardiovascular magnetic resonance. *Ann Thorac Surg* 2011; 91(1):92-6.

[51] Galea N, Piatti F, Sturla F, Weinsaft JW, Lau C, Chirichilli I, Carbone I, Votta E, Catalano C, De Paulis R, Girardi LN, Redaelli A, Gaudino M; Cornell International Consortium for Aortic Surgery (CICAS). Novel insights by 4D Flow imaging on aortic flow physiology after valve-sparing root replacement with or without neosinuses. *Interact Cardiovasc Thorac Surg* 2018; 26(6):957-964.

[52] Galea N, Piatti F, Lau C, Sturla F, Weltert L, Carbone I, De Paulis R, Gaudino M, Girardi LN; Cornell International Consortium for Aortic Surgery (CICAS). 4D flow characterization of aortic blood flow after valve sparing root reimplantation procedure. *J Vis Surg* 2018; 4:95.

[53] Gaudino M, Piatti F, Lau C, Sturla F, Weinsaft JW, Weltert L, Votta E, Galea N, Chirichilli I, Di Franco A, Francone M, Catalano C, Redaelli A, Girardi LN, De Paulis R. Aortic flow after valve sparing root replacement with or without neosinuses reconstruction. *J Thorac Cardiovasc Surg* 2019; 157(2):455-465.

[54] Weltert L, De Paulis R, Scaffa R, Maselli D, Bellisario A, D'Alessandro S. Re-creation of a sinuslike graft expansion in Bentall procedure reduces stress at the coronary button anastomoses: A finite element study. *J Thorac Cardiovasc Surg* 2009; 137(5):1082-7.

[55] De Paulis R, Chirichilli I, Scaffa R, Weltert L, Maselli D, Salica A, Guerrieri Wolf L, Bellisario A, Chiariello L. Long-term results of the valve reimplantation technique using a graft with sinuses. *J Thorac Cardiovasc Surg* 2016; 151:112-9.

[56] De Paulis R, Scaffa R, Nardella S, Maselli D, Weltert L, Bertoldo F, Pacini D, Settepani F, Tarelli G, Gallotti R, Di Bartolomeo R, Chiariello L. Use of the Valsalva graft and long-term follow-up. *J Thorac Cardiovasc Surg* 2010; 140(6 Suppl):S23-7; discussion S45-51.

[57] Chirichilli I, Irace FG, D'Aleo S, Folino G, Weltert LP, Scaffa R, Nardella S, De Paulis R. Long-term follow-up of Bentall procedure using the Perimount bioprosthesis and the Valsalva graft. *Interact Cardiovasc Thorac Surg* 2020; 30(5):679-684.

[58] Tasca G, Lindner J, Barandon L, Santavy P, Antona C, Burkert J, Gamba A. Aortic root surgery with the CARDIOROOT vascular graft: results of a prospective multicenter postmarket surveillance study. *J Cardiothorac Surg* 2019; 14:94.

[59] Shrestha ML, Beckmann E, Abd Alhadi F, Krueger H, Meyer-Bockenkamp F, Bertele S, Koigeldiyev N, Kaufeld T, Fleissner F, Korte W, Schmitto J, Cebotari S, Harringer W, Haverich A, Martens A. Elective David I Procedure Has Excellent Long-Term Results: 20-Year Single-Center Experience. *Ann Thorac Surg* 2018; 105:731-8.

[60] David TE, Feindel CM, David CM, Manlhiot C. A quarter of a century of experience with aortic valve-sparing operations. *J Thorac Cardiovasc Surg* 2014; 148:872-9; discussion 879-80.

[61] De Paulis R, Scaffa R, Salica A, Weltert L, Guerrieri Wolf L, Folino G. Aortic valve sparing techniques: pearls and pitfalls. *J Vis Surg* 2019; 5:74. doi: 10.21037/jovs.2019.09.02.

[62] De Paulis R, Scaffa R, Weltert L, Salica A. Mimicking mother nature: The Valsalva graft. *J Thorac Cardiovasc Surg* 2020; 159(5):1758-176.

[63] De Paulis R, Scaffa R, Forlani S, Chiariello L. The Valsalva graft in aortic valve repair and replacement. *Multimed Man Cardiothorac Surg* 2005; 2005(1129):mmcts.2004. 000992. doi:10.1510/mmcts.2004.000992.

[64] Hanke T, Charitos EI, Stierle U, Robinson D, Gorski A, Sievers HH, Misfeld M. Factors associated with the development of aortic valve regurgitation over time after two different techniques of valve-sparing aortic root surgery. *J Thorac Cardiovasc Surg* 2009; 137:314-9.

[65] Beckmann E, Martens A, Krueger H, Kaufeld T, Korte W, Stettinger A, Haverich A, Shrestha ML. Aortic valve-sparing root replacement (David): learning curve and impact on outcome. *Interact Cardiovasc Thorac Surg*. 2020; 30(5):754-761.

[66] Weltert L, de Tullio MD, Afferrante L, Salica A, Scaffa R, Maselli D, Verzicco R, De Paulis R. Annular dilatation and loss of sino-tubular junction in aneurysmatic aorta: implications on leaflet quality at the time of surgery. A finite element study. *Interact Cardiovasc Thorac Surg* 2013; 17(1):8-12.

[67] Kunzelman KS, Grande KJ, David TE, Cochran RP, Verrier ED. Aortic root and valve relationships. Impact on surgical repair. *J Thorac Cardiovasc Surg* 1994; 107:162-70.

[68] Bentall H, De Bono A. A technique for complete replacement of the ascending aorta. *Thorax* 1968; 23(4):338-9.

[69] De Paulis R, Scaffa R, Salica A, Weltert L, Chirichilli I. Biological solutions to aortic root replacement: valve-sparing versus bioprosthetic conduit. *J Vis Surg* 2018; 4:94. doi: 10.21037/jovs.2018.04.12.

[70] Settepani F, Szeto WY, Bergonzini M, Barbone A, Citterio E, Berwick D, Gallotti R, Bavaria JE. Reimplantation valve-sparing aortic root replacement for aortic root aneurysm in the elderly: are we pushing the limits? *J Card Surg* 2010; 25(1):56-61.

In: Perspectives in Aortic Valve Disease
Editor: Giovanni Concistrè ISBN: 978-1-53618-769-4

Chapter 21

TRANSCATHETER THERAPY: DEVICES AND TECHNIQUES

Francesco Maisano[1,*] and Giulio Russo[1,2,3]
[1]University Heart Center, University Hospital, Zurich, Switzerland
[2]Fondazione Policlinico Universitario A. Gemelli, IRCSS, Roma, Italia
[3]Università Cattolica del Sacro Cuore, Roma, Italia

ABSTRACT

Transcatheter aortic valve implantation (TAVI) has established as the first treatment option for symptomatic severe aortic stenosis in inoperable patients and in those at high or intermediate surgical risk. Last August 2019, the Food and Drug Administration approved the use of TAVI for the treatment of symptomatic severe aortic stenosis also in patients at low surgical risk. This approval paved the way to application of TAVR in patients at all levels of surgical risk. Moreover, some trials are underway to further investigate possible future indications for TAVI (e.g., asymptomatic severe aortic stenosis). In spite of this, some technical issues (e.g., durability, pacemaker implantation rate, antiplatelet regimen…) as well as clinical indications (e.g., asymptomatic severe aortic stenosis, younger patients, aortic regurgitation…) still remain open and unsolved and more data are needed to better understand how far the TAVI can go. In this perspective, TAVI as compared to surgery has gained a central role although it has still many challenges to overcome.

In this chapter, a detailed overview of main available TAVI prostheses and techniques are provided with a special focus on some challenging situations.

Keywords: aortic valve stenosis, aortic valve replacement, transcatheter aortic valve implantation

[*] Corresponding Author Email: francesco.maisano@usz.ch.

INTRODUCTION

TAVI was initially intended for the high or prohibitive surgical risk patient. Although no clear definition of "high" or "prohibitive/inoperable" risk existed, a risk of 15-50% or >50% of surgical mortality or permanent disability, respectively, were arbitrarily defined to select patients unsuitable for cardiac surgery and for which the percutaneous approach was the only feasible one (Table 1). This led to a renewed interest in cardiac surgical risk algorithms and put the "Heart Team" in a central role in the patient assessment. At the same time several operative risk scores were developed [1-4] although the two most used are the European System for Cardiac Operative Risk Evaluation (EuroSCORE) and that of the Society of Thoracic Surgeons (STS). The EuroSCORE II has been found to be a better predictor of mortality than the original logistic EuroSCORE but nonetheless still lacks discriminatory power and is outperformed in TAVI patients by the STS-PROM score [5]. A EuroSCORE II of >10% or an STS >8 are considered to indicate high risk with respect to TAVI, while an STS score <4 defines low risk patients. Despite their known limitations, the enrolment of "high surgical risk" patients into TAVI trials, [6, 7] was based upon the logistic EuroSCORE I and the STS operative risk scores.

Table 1. Risk classification in cardiac sugery patients

	Low Risk	Intermediate Risk	High Risk	Prohibitive Risk
STS	<4%	4-8%	>8%	Predicted risk of death or major morbidity with surgery >50% at 1-year
Frailty	None	1 Index	>2 Indices	
Major organ system compromise (not to be improved after intervention)	None	1 organ system	1-2 organ systems	>3 organ systems
Procedure-related impediment	None	Possible impediment	Possible impediment	Severe Impediment

Current European guidelines recommend TAVI in patients who are not suitable for surgical aortic valve replacement (SAVR) as assessed by heart team [8]. Some clinical (e.g., age >75, frailty, prior cardiac surgery…) and anatomical (porcelain aorta, expected patient-prosthesis mismatch, valve and aortic root morphology…) features may help to choose between the two approaches although no clear indications are proposed and choice is mainly based upon local heart team assessment and experience.

Last August 2019, the U.S. Food and Drug Administration (FDA) approved the TAVI use for the treatment of symptomatic severe aortic stenosis in patients at low surgical risk formalizing the application of TAVR in patients at all levels of surgical risk. FDA decision was based upon the results from the PARTNER 3 and Evolut Low Risk clinical trials (Figure 1).

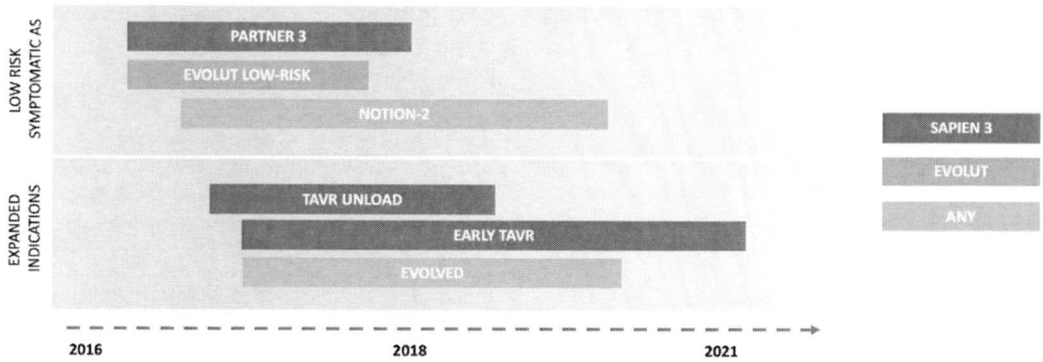

Figure 1. FDA decision based upon results from PARTNER 3 and Evolut Low Risk clinical rials.

The PARTNER 3 trial was randomized clinical trial comparing TAVI with the Edwards Sapien 3 system and SAVR in symptomatic aortic stenosis patients with STS score <4% [9]. The primary endpoint (a composite of all-cause death, stroke, or rehospitalization) at 1 year was lower in the TAVI group as compared to the SAVR group (8.5% vs. 15.1%; P = 0.001 for superiority). These data demonstrated the superiority of Sapien 3 balloon expandable prosthesis over surgery supporting the use of TAVI also in low risk category. Similar results came from the Evolut Low Risk clinical trial, which compared the Medtronic Corevalve self-expandable technology (Corevalve, Evolut R and Evolut Pro) to SAVR in low risk patients (STS score <3) [10]. Such data pave the way for a larger TAVI use, although long term data are still lacking and several issues remain still open.

TAVI DEVICES

Valves Prostheses

Currently there are several percutaneous prosthetic aortic valve systems with CE mark approval and they are classified according to their deployment mechanism (Figure 2):

- *Balloon-expandable*: the SAPIEN family valves (Edwards Lifesciences, Irvine, CA, USA) are those with widest experience and available data. More recently, the Meril Myval (Meril Lifesciences, Pvt. Ltd., India) has gained the CE mark.
- *Self-expandable*: the most studied and most implanted model is represented by the Corevalve family valves (Medtronic Inc, MN, USA). However, several devices belong to this category and each has its own peculiar features.
- *Mechanically-expandable*: the LOTUS (Boston Scientific Corporation, MA, USA) is the only example for this group.

The latest generation devices addressed some of first-generation devices issues such as paravalvular leak (PVL) regurgitation, mispositioning, atrio-ventricular block and the potential for vascular access complications. In this perspective the newest devices have different design and smaller diameter sheath and more precise device deployment mechanisms. However, still some open issues remain in this field and pacemaker implantation, prostheses durability, coronary obstruction risk and best antiplatelet/ anticoagulant will some of the future challenge for transcatheter aortic valve implantation (TAVI) devices.

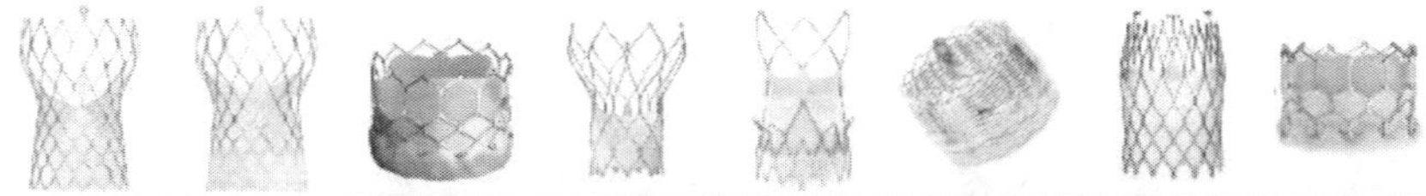

	Evolut R (Medtronic)	Evolut Pro (Medtronic)	Sapien 3 (Edwards)	Portico (Abbott)	Acurate Neo (Boston Scientific)	Lotus (Boston Scientific)	Allegra (NVT)	Myval (Meril)
Deployment	Self-expanding	Self-expanding	Balloon-expanding	Self-expanding	Self-expanding	Mechanical	Self-expanding	Balloon-expanding
Frame	Nitinol	Nitinol	Cobalt-chromium	Nitinol	Nitinol	Nitinol	Nitinol	Nickel-Cobalt
Leaflets	Porcine	Porcine	Bovine	Bovine	Porcine	Bovine	Bovine	Bovine
Delivery routes and sheath size	TF/Tao/TS 14 Fr	TF/Tao/TS 16 Fr	TF/TA/Tao 14/16 Fr	TF/TA 18/19 Fr	TF/TA/TS 18/19 Fr	TF 18 Fr	TF 18 Fr	TF 14/Fr

Figure 2. TAVI portfolio.

Sapien (Edwards Lifesciences, Irvine, CA, USA)

The very first model was pioneered by Cribier-Edwards in 2002. Currently, three models are available: SAPIEN XT, SAPIEN 3 and the brand-new SAPIEN 3 Ultra (Table 1).

They use the bovine pericardial tissue as for the Edwards surgical valves, and have dedicated outer skirt to reduce PVL risk and a row of large cells struts to allow easier coronary access. As compared to most of the self-expandable models, the SAPIEN family has the lowest profile. They can be implanted through either the transfemoral or the transapical route. In order to use smaller sheaths introducers, the balloon and the prostheses are assembled in the descending aorta for the XT and 3 models, whereas the newest Ultra valve is crimped on the balloon and has a lower crossing profile. During deployment SAPIEN XT frame foreshortens homogenously while the SAPIEN 3 has more foreshortening in the lower two-thirds compared to the upper one-third of the frame. Moreover the SAPIEN 3 needs to less oversizing than the XT in most cases unless the size falls in between two different size according to company size chart, in which case oversizing by 10-20% may be advisable.

Medtronic CoreValve (Medtronic Inc, MN, USA)

The CoreValve system is the most studied self-expandable model and following its first platform, three new system have been launched: the EVOLUT R, EVOLUT PRO and EVOLUT PRO+. It is a self-expanding valve made of single layer porcine pericardium in a trileaflet configuration with a scalloped skirt in a nitinol frame. The EVOLUT PRO models have an external pericardial wrap to improve the annulus sealing and to reduce the PVL risk. Of note, its supra-annular position allows it to maintain a circular configuration at the level of the valve leaflets achieving larger effective orifice area and optimizing coaptation in non circular anatomy.

Unlike the SAPIEN models, the EnVeo Pro delivery system does not require any sheath introducer allowing lower access site dimensions. Once mounted, the needs to be checked fluoroscopically in the anteroposterior projection and rotated to ensure that the paddles and their attachments are equidistant. Due to its supra-annular design, hemodynamic instability may occure during its deployment. The valve is resheatable, repositionable and retrievable and has been mainly used for transfemoral approaches although it is suitable for all approaches but the transapical.

Portico (St. Jude Medical, CA, USA)

It is a self-expanding nitinol valve platform with bovine pericardium valve at annular level. The stent large cells facilitate its accommodation in calcific native valve and coronary reaccess. Due to lower radial force, the aortic valve pre-dilation is highly recommended. Its new Flexnav transfemoral delivery system increases flexibility and trackability decreasing the risk for vascular complications. Alongside this, a different delivery system allows also the transapical approach. Similarly to CoreValve system, it is re-sheathable, re-positionable, and retrievable until 80% of the device is deployed in the aortic annulus. The valve can then be assessed for stability and function prior to final release.

Acurate Neo (Boston Scientific Corporation, MA, USA)

This self-expanding valve platform is the transfemoral version of the transapical device. It is made of porcine leaflets with upper and lower crowns and stabilization arches. Like the CoreValve it has a supra-annular design. A distinguishing feature is the top-down deployment to increase hemodynamic stability and precise implantation. Consequently, during the deployment sequence, the upper crown expands first, followed by the arches and finally the lower crown: the upper crowns are responsible for supra-annular anchoring of the prosthesis and capping of the native leaflets, stabilization arches contribute to axial self-alignment, and the pericardial skirt acts as a seal to prevent PVL.

Lotus (Boston Scientific Corporation, MA, USA)

It consists of three bovine pericardial leaflets attached to a braided nitinol frame with a radiopaque marker used for accurate placement. The valve is designed to expand radially as the valve shortens during deployment. Rapid pacing is not required during the implantation and it is fully repositionable during deployment and retrievable prior to release. This together with very controlled deployment mechanism and an adaptive seal limits PVL and malpositioning. The valve functions early in deployment, providing hemodynamic stability for the patient.

Allegra (New Valve Technology, Switzerland)

It is a self-expanding device made of a nitinol stent frame and a bovine pericardium (annular skirt and leaflets). The delivery system has a 18 Fr cartridge and 15 Fr catheter shaft. Valve deployment is in three steps: first, the central part of the valve is released, while both ends of the device are still captured. During the second step, the bottom of the valve is released allowing the operator to assess valve position, patency of the coronaries, hemodynamic functions, and paravalvular regurgitation. The process can be re-started till this step, and the valve can thus be retrieved. In the final step, after the operator confirms the position of the prosthesis, the safety locker is released for final deployment of the Allegra valve.

Myval (Meril Lifesciences, Pvt. Ltd., India)

The latest technology to get the CE mark approval is Myval. It is a balloon-expandable valve, made of bovine pericardium tissue in a nitinol-cobalt alloy frame. Similarly to other prostheses technology, the lower closed cell part of the valve frame is covered externally with a protective sealing cuff in order to reduce PVL. The crimped valve is inserted through a 22Fr or 24Fr (based on prostheses size) expandable sheath.

TECHNIQUES

Transfemoral Approach

Access Site Management

Transfemoral artery is the most used approach accounting for more 90-95% of all TAVI used accesses. Often it is performed under local anesthesia with or without sedation, while deep/general anesthesia and intubation is reserved for non-femoral approaches or complex femoral procedures.

Currently half of all transcatheter procedures are performed under general anesthesia worldwide. Alongside the arterial access for TAVI, a second arterial access is needed in order to have continuous invasive pressure monitoring, to perform angiography and, in case vascular complication, for bail-out procedures. Currently, several vascular accesses sites settings have been proposed (figure 3).

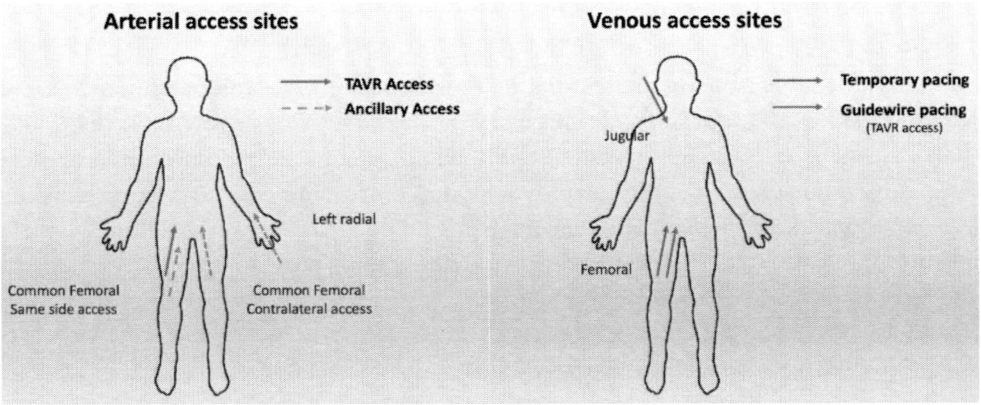

Figure 3. Vascular accesses sites for TAVI procedure.

The contralateral femoral artery and the radial artery are the most common used ones. Recently, a less invasive technique (LITE) based on the use of radial artery as ancillary access and retrograde guidewire pacing has been described by Burzotta et al. [11]. Moreover, data coming from a multicenter study accounting almost 5000 patients undergoing TAVI demonstrated a lower rate of vascular and bleeding complications in those using radial artery as secondary access as compared to femoral [12].

Due to the use of large bore sheaths, femoral puncture should always be guided by ultrasound, fluoro or both (Figure 4).

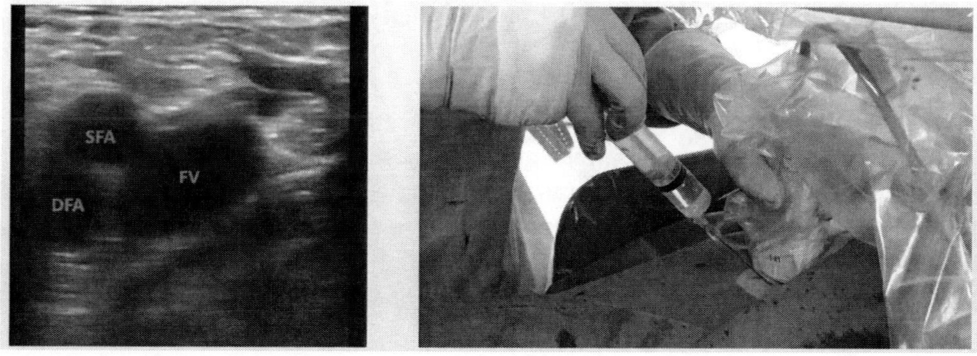

Figure 4. Echo-guided femoral puncture.

Once the artery access has been gained, preclosure devices such as Proglide (Abbott Vascular, Redwood City, CA) or Prostar (Abbott Vascular Inc, Santa Clara, CA) are implanted.

Although these percutaneous devices originally were not designed for TAVI, now they have CE approval and are able to close arteriotomies up to 24Fr in diameter.

Vascular outcomes with the use of preclosure devices as compared to surgical repair have been investigated showing a slight advantage for percutaneous devices provided that operators gain experience and know how to manage possible vascular or bleeding complications, [13, 14]. Manual compression as well as the use of additional devices such as Femostop II or Angioseal together with protamine administration are often used to achieve hemostasis.

Temporary Pacemaker Implantation

Temporary pacing is required for pre-dilation, post-dilation, or prosthesis deployment under rapid pacing to prevent device ejection by systolic contraction. In addition, it serves as protection against the potential development of bradyarrhythmia following TAVI. The right internal jugular vein or femoral vein is used typically. Alternatively, the use of guidewire for pacing in order to reduce vascular access sites and related complications has also been described [11, 15]. However, in those with higher risk for bradyarrhythmia (e.g., pre-existing atrio-ventricular block, right bundle branch block…) temporary venous pacing is advisable. During the procedure, pacing rates must be high enough to cause a fall in systolic BP and this typically occurs >160-220bpm. At the end of the procedure, temporary pacing might be removed in case of no ECG changes, especially if a balloon-expandable valve has been implanted. On the contrary, if some ECG changes occur (P-R segment prolonging, any atrioventricular or bundle branch block) temporary pacing should left in place and ECG assessed in the following hours/days.

Valve Implantation

After vascular and temporary pacing management, aortic valve crossing is the next step for the prostheses implantation. A standard straight-tipped wire through an Amplatz catheter in the LAO projection is commonly used to cross the native valve. Alternative catheters such as an internal mammary or Judkins right can be used (horizontal aorta) and hydrophilic wires can also be used in particularly challenging cases.

A pigtail catheter is placed in the non-coronary sinus of Valsalva and aortic root angiography is used to determine the position of equipment relative to the coronary cusps.

Balloon valvuloplasty prior to prostheses implantation serves the purpose to prepare the aortic landing zone for TAVI, especially in severely calcific aortic valves. Importantly, the size of the balloon should not exceed the minimum aortic annulus diameter as measured from the CT scan. Massive aortic regurgitation may follow balloon pre-dilatation, consequently, TAVI device should be ready for implantation before valvuloplasty. Although some devices strongly suggest pre-dilatation, it is not required for all of them and the operator experience plays a key role to assess clinical and anatomical characteristics to identify those cases in which valvuloplasty should be performed or not.

Following this, device positioning should be assessed carefully. In order to do so, the aortic annular plane (the nadirs of the non, right and left coronary cusp leaflets) should be perpendicular to the valve device and co-axially aligned. Modern computed tomography analysis softwares allow to calculate the "three cusps view" and the correct annular alignment, which can also be found with the "following the right cusp" rule [16]. More recently, the "cusp overlap" view has been proposed by Tang et al, in order to reduce the rate of permanent pacemaker implantation rate [17]. Correct implantation depth is a critical feature of a successful implant. Accurate placement of the prosthesis requires visualization of both the aortic annulus plane and that of the device delivery catheter overlap perpendicularly. Before final deployment, self-expandable devices allow to recapture and re-implant the device in order to obtain the correct position. Too deep implantation has been associated to higher PVL risk and higher permanent pacemaker implantation. In some cases, post dilatation can be required in order to reduce PVL and better expand the prostheses against the annulus.

ALTERNATIVE APPROACHES

Subclavian/Transaxillary

This the most frequent non-femoral access point used, according to the TVT registry data [18]. Higher incidence of stroke was observed in comparison to transfemoral route although reported vascular complications were not significantly higher.

It is more frequently performed via a surgical cut-down when in the subclavian portion. If transaxillary it can also be performed percutaneously with pre-closure sutures most frequently into the proximal third of the axillary artery. A left-sided approach is selected in >95% of cases due to a more favorable alignment of the prosthesis with the native valve, while the angulation at the subclavian-aortic junction may vary according to the aortic arch anatomy. The presence of a LIMA graft should always be considered and may represent a relative contra-indication. Of note, dissection and/or bleeding can be challenging to control even with open surgical access. For this reason, it is advisable to choose and to learn only one alternative access site on order to master it and the related complication.

Transaortic

A right anterior mini-thoracotomy is used for patients with a right sided ascending aorta or patent coronary bypass grafts and a mini-J sternotomy for middle or left-sided ascending aortas and a deep anatomical location or pre-existing lung disease. Using a purse-string suture, needle puncture and access with a hemostatic sheath is obtained. The puncture is made with a minimum of 6cm for CoreValve and 8cm for SAPIEN platforms. The valve is then deployed in the same way as via the transfemoral approach [19-21].

Transcarotid

Although only seldom used and limited by the risk for stroke, it has been demonstrated to be feasible [22]. It is performed under local anesthesia and with cerebral oximetry monitoring. Satisfactory vessel size and vessel quality are critical determinants for efficacy and safety as well as anatomically complete Circle of Willis. The short distance and provision of a direct coaxial approach to the aortic valve is an advantage.

Transapical

This is performed via a left anterolateral intercostal incision followed by needle puncture of the apex through a pledgeted purse-string suture. A dedicated hemostatic sheath is applied and the valve deployed in a similar fashion to the transfemoral approach thereafter. The advantages of this route are the short distance to the aortic valve and antegrade delivery allowing for more precise control. On the other side the risk for hemorrhage, tamponade and left ventricular pseudoaneurysm may be increased. There are many complexities that are not immediately apparent with this 'front door' access concept. In essence it is still a form of thoracotomy and can be associated with delayed recovery and hemodynamic instability especially in those with pre-existing left ventricular impairment.

Transcaval

This percutaneous route has been used in those who lack conventional access options. It is technically challenging and there is a significant 'learning curve'. The procedure consists of femoral vein access and puncture across the inferior vena cava into the abdominal aorta using a coronary guidewire to apply electrocautery energy and create a caval-aortic fistula. The remaining steps up to deployment are conducted in the conventional way and then the fistula is closed with a percutaneous device such as an Amplatz PDA occluder [23].

Additional Techniques in Complex Clinical Scenarios

Low Coronaries: When and How to Protect Them

One of the most important differences between TAVI and SAVR is that while the latter literally replaces the patient native valve, the former implants a prosthesis pushing the native leaflets and annulus outwards. For this reason, coronary occlusion by the native leaflet may represent a life-threatening complication although it is rare and is quite unpredictable.

In a large multicenter registry including 6688 patients, the overall incidence of coronary occlusion was 0.66%. Of note, elder patients, balloon-expandable valve and higher logistic EuroSCORE were associated to a higher risk for coronary occlusion. Left coronary artery was the most affected one (88.6%) with mean height 10.6±2.1 mm and alongside this, coronary occlusion occurred more frequently in those with small sinus of Valsalva diameters (mean diameter= 28.1±3.8 mm) [24].

Same data came from a review including 18 publications describing 24 case of coronary obstruction following TAVI procedure [25]. Most of them were women (83%) and received a balloon-expandable prosthesis. As for the registry, in most cases, left main coronary artery was involved with a mean height of 10.3±1.6 mm.

An even more risky category is represented by those patients undergoing TAVI in a previously failed implanted bioprosthesis. The largest experience is described in the VIVID registry where the reported rate of coronary obstruction was 2.3% in 1612 patients undergoing valve-in-valve (VIV) TAVI [26]. The virtual transcatheter valve to coronary ostium distance as well as prior stentless or stented bioprosthesis with externally mounted leaflets identified a subset of patients at higher risk for coronary obstruction. Few data exist about TAVI-in-TAVI and, similarly to the VIV TAVI, the incidence of coronary obstruction in higher than in native valve TAVI accounting for 2% of cases [27]. Interestingly, most coronary obstruction occur after valve deployment. However, more than one fifth of cases can be observed during the following 24 hours or even after two months [25, 26, 28]. Although left coronary artery is the most common involved, unlike immediate coronary obstruction, delayed obstruction occurs more frequently with self-expanding valves. The continuing stent expansion of these valves may explain this complication, while valve endothelization and neo-sinus thrombus formation may be the reason for very delayed (>7 days) coronary occlusion.

Bail-out percutaneous coronary intervention (PCI) with or without stent implantation has been the preferred strategy for the management of coronary occlusion although in many cases hemodynamic and electrical instability occur very soon and patient quickly crashes. Moreover, due to technical challenges the rate of success for PCI itself is 70-80% and in some cases (high-risk) surgery is required. For these reasons, over the years a careful patient selection and the use of preventive coronary protection before starting TAVI has improved the outcomes.

In order to avoid coronary occlusion, a preventive cannulation and coronary wiring is highly recommended. In most cases, placement (without deployment) of coronary stent downstream to the ostium is also advisable. Beside coronary arteries height and sino-tubular junction dimensions, an injection during pre-dilation valvuloplasty and careful assessment of leaflet calcification may help to detect those cases at higher risk for coronary occlusion. In some cases, single stent implantation might be not enough and a second stent inside the previous one is required (sandwich technique) [29], or multiple stents are implanted from to the ostium inside the aorta through the TAVI stent frame (tunnel technique) [30]. However, the most common technique is the so-called "chimney technique, with the stent placed between the degenerated leaflet and the aortic wall.

More recently, a new interesting technique (Bioprosthetic or native Aortic Scallop Intentional Laceration to prevent Coronary Artery obstruction, BASILICA) based on iatrogenic intentional leaflet laceration has been described, [32, 33]. It can be applied to either one or two leaflets. The leaflet is crossed with a 0.014" wire, which is snared in the left ventricle. The wire is then electrified with radiofrequency energy to lacerate the leaflet and it is finally retrieved. In this way both acute and delayed obstructions are avoided and no additional stents are implanted in the coronary ostia. However, the technique in complex and after leaflet laceration acute massive aortic regurgitation may occur leading to hemodynamic collapse. A prospective study is underway (NCT03381989) to evaluate the efficacy and the safety of this technique.

TAVI in the Setting of Acutely Decompansated Aortic Stenosis

Mortality and re-hospitalization rates of severe aortic stenosis in patients not suitable for surgery treated with medical therapy (including balloon aortic valvuloplasty, BAV) can reach up to 50% and 44% in one year, respectively [34]. Surely, prognosis of untreated patients with hemodynamic instability due to decompensated aortic stenosis is even poorer. In these cases, medical therapy solutions might be limited and due to high operative risk (hemodynamic instability, advanced age, left ventricular dysfunction, comorbidities) they are usually deemed not suitable for urgent surgery (Figure 5).

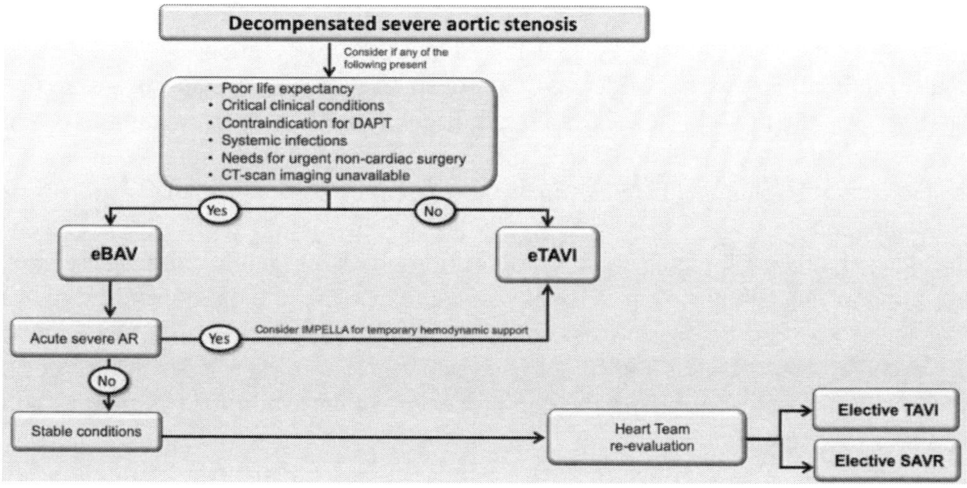

Figure 5. Strategy in decompensated severe aortic valve stenosis.

The Role of Emergent BAV

An alternative life-saving therapeutic option is the BAV. Cribier first described its efficacy in 10 patients with cardiogenic shock refractory to intensive medical therapy [35]. However, subsequent data suggested that BAV have high in-hospital mortality (up to 70%) and a high incidence of aortic valve restenosis, [36, 37]. Moreover, in some cases the procedure might be complicated by acute aortic regurgitation leading to urgent aortic valve replacement (AVR) or to death [38].

An alternative strategy to manage acute decompensated aortic stenosis is represented by emergent BAV (eBAV) followed by TAVI under stable clinical conditions. The role of eBAV as a bridge-to-TAVI/surgery has already demonstrated its superiority to eBAV alone with a mortality rate of 22% in those undergoing eBAV followed by TAVI (76%) or surgery (24%)

as compared to 55% in the eBAV alone group (median follow up 378 days and 183 days, respectively) [39].

A direct comparison between emergent TAVI (eTAVI) and eBAV followed by elective TAVI strategy, has been conducted by Bongiovanni et al. [40] in a multicentre retrospective cohort. The analysis revealed a high 30-day mortality rate in both eBAV (33%) and eTAVI (23.8%) group although no significant differences were found between the two groups as far as immediate (<72 h) and 30-day mortality are concerned. Of note, patients undergoing eTAVI showed a significant higher rate of major vascular complications and stroke as compared to eBAV group (p=0.01 for both). Overall, at the Kaplan-Meier analysis a trend towards lower mortality in the eTAVI group could be observed (OR= 0.55 and p=0.172).

Alternatively, one potential role for the eBAV is the bridge-to-decision strategy, especially in those patients with many comorbidities [41]. In a single-centre retrospective study, 202 patients underwent bridge-to-decision eBAV because of either severe clinical instability (103 patients) or when initial heart team evaluation was not conclusive and required further clinical or instrumental evaluation (99 patients). A total of 9 (4.5%) in-hospital deaths occurred with 8 patients belonging to those with hemodynamic instability (cardiogenic shock/acute pulmonary edema/New York Heart Association class IV). Of the 193 patients with bridge-to-decision BAV who survived and received a second heart team evaluation (around one month after BAV) 73% were judged suitable for definitive treatment (26% underwent AVR and 47% TAVI). Although those patients with hemodynamic instability were at highest risk of death, the in-hospital mortality rate in this group was only 8% and 76% of them were successfully stabilized and addressed for definitive treatment suggesting that bridge-to-decision BAV may represent a valuable solution in those cases where patients are not immediately suitable for percutaneous or surgical treatment or need further evaluation.

In spite of this, one of the main complications of BAV might be acute severe aortic regurgitation, which is reported in 1-5% of cases, and in some of them it may lead to death for cardiogenic shock. For this reason, it is advisable to perform eBAV with TAVI bioprosthesis available and ready to be assembled. In such situations, left ventricular assistance devices placement (e.g., Impella) may help to keep proper organ perfusion for few minutes allowing only eTAVI valve preparation.

Moreover, eBAV as a bridge to TAVI strategy exposes patients to multiple procedures and the associated complications (e.g., contrast-induced nephropathy, vascular and bleeding complications) and should, therefore, be limited to those cases where comorbidities may affect patient prognosis.

The Role of Emergent TAVI

The role of eTAVI alone has also been considered as a possible therapeutic strategy for patients with decompensated severe aortic stenosis. Although TAVI has been approved for the management of severe aortic stenosis in elective high surgical risk and in inoperable patients, current European guidelines only mention BAV as a bridge to AVR or TAVI in hemodynamically unstable patients or in patients with symptomatic severe aortic stenosis who require urgent major non-cardiac surgery [42] (recommendation class IIb, level of evidence C). Previous version of the same guidelines considered hemodynamic instability a relative contraindication for TAVI while the expert consensus paper on TAVI did not mention the role of urgent/emergent TAVI [43].

However, in carefully selected high-risk patients, TAVI has already been demonstrated to be superior to BAV, surgery and medical therapy with regards to one-year mortality and functional class improvement [44].

Currently, the role of eTAVI as a standalone therapy on patients with cardiogenic shock has been investigated in one single-centre retrospective study [45]. Among a total of 771 elective TAVI, Frerker analysed 27 patients (3.5%) treated with eTAVI due to acutely decompensated aortic stenosis and cardiogenic shock. All patients had symptomatic severe aortic stenosis, high operative risk score (mean Logistic EuroSCORE 60±21) and half of them required mechanical ventilation. All procedures guided by transoesophageal echocardiography and by angiography. Procedure success was achieved in 24 (89%) patients and only 3 deaths occurred, either intraprocedural or post-procedural (within 72 hours). Self-expandable (CoreValve) and balloon expandable (SAPIEN) bioprosthesis were equally used in the eTAVI group and the choice was based on anatomical conditions. As expected, mid- and long-term outcomes were significantly worse in emergently treated patients as compared to electively ones with a 30-days survival of 66.7% vs 92.3% and one-year survival of 59.3% vs 82.7%, respectively. However, it is noteworthy that among the 9 deaths occurred within 30 days of eTAVI, the predominant cause of death was pneumonia or sepsis, while only 3 patients died from cardiovascular causes. These data suggest that eTAVI in acutely decompensated aortic stenosis is feasible and has an acceptable one-month and one-year survival rate. Moreover, the cumulative survival curves indicate that once eTAVI patients survived for 30 days, no significant differences were noted in long-term survival as compared to electively treated patients. Similarly, in another single-centre study of 27 patients undergoing urgent TAVI for acute heart failure 30-day mortality was 3.7% [46]. The overall mortality rate of the urgent TAVI was not significantly different from that in the elective TAVI. However, unlike the previous study, none of the patients had cardiogenic shock and none of them was treated with inotropic drugs before the procedure. Only 15% of them had severe left ventricular dysfunction and 1 out of 4 patients had computed tomography available at time of urgent procedure.

According to the more recent STS/ACC TVT registry [47], urgent/emergent TAVI due to decompensated aortic stenosis is not rare as it occurs in 1 case out of 10 elective TAVI. More than one third of patients undergoing urgent/emergent TAVI had STS PROM score higher than 15% and around 40% of them showed a low LVEF (<45%). Cardiopulmonary bypass was used in 3.5% of cases while most of the procedures were performed under general sedation. Femoral access was the preferred route for both elective and urgent procedures (79% and 75% of cases respectively), followed by transapical access and, much more rarely, by transaortic, axillary, subclavian and transiliac access. Balloon-expandable was used in three cases out of four. Device success was achieved in more than 90% of cases in both groups. However, compared to elective procedures patients undergoing urgent/emergent TAVI had a higher rate of 30-day mortality (4.3% vs 8.7%, adjusted HR 1.28, 95% CI 1.10-1.48, p<0.001), of 1-year mortality (17.5% vs 29.1% adjusted HR 1.20, 95% CI 1.10-1.31, p=0.001) and showed also a higher incidence of acute kidney injury/new dialysis.

All these data suggest that eTAVI is feasible and may have some advantages as compared to eBAV. Surely, it requires a careful selection of patients: according to the large STS/ACC TVT registry those undergoing urgent/emergent TAVI and with oxygen-dependent lung disease or high baseline creatinine have worse outcome. One more issue to be considered is that often patients undergoing urgent/emergent TAVI may not have performed computed tomography scan, which is commonly used for the study of the aorta and aortic valve anatomy. Most of the urgent/emergent procedures described in the studies were angiography/trans-esophageal echocardiography guided. The lack of complete imaging assessment may help to explain why all the three studies demonstrated a higher post-procedural kidney injury, probably due to higher use of contrast agent. Moreover, in some cases implantation of a second bioprosthesis was necessary. Consequently, a highly experienced heart team and a hybrid operating room are mandatory in order to achieve acceptable short- and mid-term outcomes.

Conflict of Interest

Giulio Russo: nothing to disclose.

Francesco Maisano: Grant and/or Research Support from: Abbott; Medtronic; Edwards Lifesciences; Biotronik; Boston Scientific Corporation, NVT, Terumo.

Consulting fees, Honoraria from: Abbott; Medtronic; Edwards Lifesciences; Perifect; Xeltis; Transseptal solutions; Cardiovalve. Magenta.

Royalty Income/IP Rights from: Edwards Lifesciences (FMR surgical annuloplasty).

Shareholder (incl. stock options): Cardiovalve, Magenta, Transseptalsolutions, 4Tech, Perifect, Coregard.

References

[1] Nilsson J, Algotsson L, Hoglund P, Luhrs C, Brandt J. Comparison of 19 pre-operative risk stratification models in open-heart surgery. *European heart journal* 2006;27:867-74.

[2] Jin R, Grunkemeier GL, Starr A. Validation and refinement of mortality risk models for heart valve surgery. *The Annals of thoracic surgery* 2005;80:471-9.

[3] Brown ML, Schaff HV, Sarano ME, et al. Is the European System for Cardiac Operative Risk Evaluation model valid for estimating the operative risk of patients considered for percutaneous aortic valve replacement?. *The Journal of thoracic and cardiovascular surgery* 2008;136:566-71.

[4] Kuduvalli M, Grayson AD, Au J, Grotte G, Bridgewater B, Fabri BM. A multi-centre additive and logistic risk model for in-hospital mortality following aortic valve replacement. *Eur J Cardiothorac Surg* 2007;31:607-13.

[5] Osnabrugge RL, Speir AM, Head SJ, et al. Performance of EuroSCORE II in a large US database: implications for transcatheter aortic valve implantation. *Eur J Cardiothorac Surg* 2014;46:400-8; discussion 8.

[6] Leon MB, Smith CR, Mack M, et al. Transcatheter aortic-valve implantation for aortic stenosis in patients who cannot undergo surgery. *N Engl J Med* 2010;363:1597-607.

[7] Smith CR, Leon MB, Mack MJ, et al. Transcatheter versus surgical aortic-valve replacement in high-risk patients. *N Engl J Med* 2011;364:2187-98.

[8] Baumgartner H, Falk V, Bax JJ, De Bonis M, Hamm C, Holm PJ, Iung B, Lancellotti P, Lansac E, Rodriguez Muñoz D, Rosenhek R, Sjögren J, Tornos Mas P, Vahanian A, Walther T, Wendler O, Windecker S, Zamorano JL; ESC Scientific Document Group 2017 ESC/EACTS Guidelines for the management of valvular heart disease. *Eur Heart J.* 2017;38(36):2739-2791.

[9] Mack MJ, Leon MB, Thourani VH, Makkar R, Kodali SK, Russo M, Kapadia SR, Malaisrie SC, Cohen DJ, Pibarot P, Leipsic J, Hahn RT, Blanke P, Williams MR, McCabe JM, Brown DL, Babaliaros V, Goldman S, Szeto WY, Genereux P, Pershad A, Pocock SJ, Alu MC, Webb JG, Smith CR, Investigators P. Transcatheter Aortic-Valve Replacement with a Balloon-Expandable Valve in Low-Risk Patients. *N Engl J Med.* 2019;380:1695-705.

[10] Popma JJ, Deeb GM, Yakubov SJ, Mumtaz M, Gada H, O'Hair D, Bajwa T, Heiser JC, Merhi W, Kleiman NS, Askew J, Sorajja P, Rovin J, Chetcuti SJ, Adams DH, Teirstein PS, Zorn GL, 3rd, Forrest JK, Tchetche D, Resar J, Walton A, Piazza N, Ramlawi B, Robinson N, Petrossian G, Gleason TG, Oh JK, Boulware MJ, Qiao H, Mugglin AS, Reardon MJ, Evolut Low Risk Trial I. Transcatheter Aortic-Valve Replacement with a Self-Expanding Valve in Low-Risk Patients. *N Engl J Med.* 2019;380:1706-15.

[11] Burzotta F, Aurigemma C, Romagnoli E, Shoeib O, Russo G, Zambrano A, Verdirosi D, Leone AM, Bruno P, Trani C. A less-invasive totally-endovascular (LITE) technique for trans-femoral transcatheter aortic valve replacement. *Catheter Cardiovasc Interv.* 2020 Jan 11. doi: 10.1002/ccd.28697. [Epub ahead of print].

[12] Junquera L, Urena M, Latib A, Muñoz-Garcia A, Nombela-Franco L, Faurie B, Veiga-Fernandez G, Alperi A, Serra V, Regueiro A, Fischer Q, Himbert D, Mangieri A, Colombo A, Muñoz-García E, Vera-Urquiza R, Jiménez-Quevedo P, de la Torre JM, Pascual I, Garcia Del Blanco B, Sabaté M, Mohammadi S, Freitas-Ferraz AB, Guimarães L, Couture T, Côté M, Rodés-Cabau J. Comparison of Transfemoral Versus Transradial Secondary Access in Transcatheter Aortic Valve Replacement. *Circ Cardiovasc Interv.* 2020 Mar;13(3):e008609. doi: 10.1161/CIRCINTERVENTIONS.119.008609.

[13] Haulon S, Hassen Khodja R, Proudfoot CW, Samuels E. A systematic literature review of the efficacy and safety of the Prostar XL device for the closure of large femoral arterial access sites in patients undergoing percutaneous endovascular aortic procedures. *Eur J Vasc Endovasc Surg* 2011;41:201-13.

[14] Hernandez-Enriquez M, Andrea R, Brugaletta S, et al. Puncture Versus Surgical Cutdown Complications of Transfemoral Aortic Valve Implantation (from the Spanish TAVI Registry). *Am J Cardiol* 2016;118:578-84.

[15] Faurie B, Abdellaoui M, Wautot F, Staat P, Champagnac D, Wintzer-Wehekind J, Vanzetto G, Bertrand B, Monségu J. Rapid pacing using the left ventricular guidewire: Reviving an old technique to simplify BAV and TAVI procedures. *Catheter Cardiovasc Interv.* 2016;88(6):988-993.

[16] Kasel AM, Cassese S, Leber AW, von Scheidt W, Kastrati A. Fluoroscopy-guided aortic root imaging for TAVR: "follow the right cusp" rule. *JACC Cardiovasc Imaging.* 2013;6(2):274-5.

[17] Tang GHL, Zaid S, Michev I, Ahmad H, Kaple R, Undemir C, Cohen M, Lansman SL. "Cusp-Overlap" View Simplifies Fluoroscopy-Guided Implantation of Self-Expanding Valve in Transcatheter Aortic Valve Replacement. *JACC Cardiovasc Interv.* 2018;11(16):1663-1665.

[18] Dahle TG, Kaneko T, McCabe JM. Outcomes Following Subclavian and Axillary Artery Access for Transcatheter Aortic Valve Replacement: Society of the Thoracic Surgeons/American College of Cardiology TVT Registry Report. *JACC Cardiovasc Interv.* 2019;12(7):662-669.

[19] Bapat V, Attia R. Transaortic Transcatheter Aortic Valve Implantation: Step-by-Step Guide. *Semin Thorac Cardiovasc Surg* 2012;24:206-11.

[20] Bapat V, Khawaja MZ, Attia R, et al. Transaortic Transcatheter Aortic valve implantation using Edwards Sapien valve: a novel approach. *Catheter Cardiovasc Interv* 2012;79:733-40.

[21] Reardon MJ, Adams DH, Coselli JS, et al. Self-expanding transcatheter aortic valve replacement using alternative access sites in symptomatic patients with severe aortic stenosis deemed extreme risk of surgery. *J Thorac Cardiovasc Surg* 2014;148:2869-76 e1-7.

[22] Azmoun A, Amabile N, Ramadan R, Ghostine S, Caussin C, Fradi S, Raoux F, Brenot P, Nottin R, Deleuze P. Transcatheter aortic valve implantation through carotid artery access under local anaesthesia. *Eur J Cardiothorac Surg.* 2014;46(4):693-8; discussion 698.

[23] Greenbaum AB, O'Neill WW, Paone G, et al. Caval-aortic access to allow transcatheter aortic valve replacement in otherwise ineligible patients: initial human experience. *J Am Coll Cardiol* 2014;63:2795-804.

[24] Ribeiro HB, Webb JG, Makkar RR, Cohen MG, Kapadia SR, Kodali S, Tamburino C, Barbanti M, Chakravarty T, Jilaihawi H, Paradis JM, de Brito FS Jr, Cánovas SJ, Cheema AN, de Jaegere PP, del Valle R, Chiam PT, Moreno R, Pradas G, Ruel M, Salgado-Fernández J, Sarmento-Leite R, Toeg HD, Velianou JL, Zajarias A, Babaliaros V, Cura F, Dager AE, Manoharan G, Lerakis S, Pichard AD, Radhakrishnan S, Perin MA, Dumont E, Larose E, Pasian SG, Nombela-Franco L, Urena M, Tuzcu EM, Leon MB, Amat-Santos IJ, Leipsic J, Rodés-Cabau J. Predictive factors, management, and clinical outcomes of coronary obstruction following transcatheter aortic valve

implantation: insights from a large multicenter registry. *J Am Coll Cardiol.* 2013;62(17):1552-62.

[25] Ribeiro HB, Nombela-Franco L, Urena M, Mok M, Pasian S, Doyle D, DeLarochellière R, Côté M, Laflamme L, DeLarochellière H, Allende R, Dumont E, Rodés-Cabau J. Coronary obstruction following transcatheter aortic valve implantation: a systematic review. *JACC Cardiovasc Interv.* 2013;6(5):452-61.

[26] Ribeiro HB, Rodés-Cabau J, Blanke P, Leipsic J, Kwan Park J, Bapat V, Makkar R, Simonato M, Barbanti M, Schofer J, Bleiziffer S, Latib A, Hildick-Smith D, Presbitero P, Windecker S, Napodano M, Cerillo AG, Abdel-Wahab M, Tchetche D, Fiorina C, Sinning JM, Cohen MG, Guerrero ME, Whisenant B, Nietlispach F, Palma JH, Nombela-Franco L, de Weger A, Kass M, Sandoli de Brito F Jr, Lemos PA, Kornowski R, Webb J, Dvir D. Incidence, predictors, and clinical outcomes of coronary obstruction following transcatheter aortic valve replacement for degenerative bioprosthetic surgical valves: insights from the VIVID registry. *Eur Heart J.* 2018;39(8):687-695.

[27] Barbanti M, Webb JG, Tamburino C, Van Mieghem NM, Makkar RR, Piazza N, Latib A, Sinning JM, Won-Keun K, Bleiziffer S, Bedogni F, Kapadia S, Tchetche D, Rodés-Cabau J, Fiorina C, Nombela-Franco L, De Marco F, de Jaegere PP, Chakravarty T, Vaquerizo B, Colombo A, Svensson L, Lange R, Nickenig G, Möllmann H, Walther T, Della Rosa F, Elhmidi Y, Dvir D, Brambilla N, Immè S, Sgroi C, Gulino S, Todaro D, Pilato G, Petronio AS, Tamburino C. Outcomes of Redo Transcatheter Aortic Valve Replacement for the Treatment of Postprocedural and Late Occurrence of Paravalvular Regurgitation and Transcatheter Valve Failure. *Circ Cardiovasc Interv.* 2016 Sep;9(9). pii: e003930.

[28] Jabbour RJ, Tanaka A, Finkelstein A, Mack M, Tamburino C, Van Mieghem N, de Backer O, Testa L, Gatto P, Purita P, Rahhab Z, Veulemans V, Stundl A, Barbanti M, Nerla R, Sinning JM, Dvir D, Tarantini G, Szerlip M, Scholtz W, Scholtz S, Tchetche D, Castriota F, Butter C, Søndergaard L, Abdel-Wahab M, Sievert H, Alfieri O, Webb J, Rodés-Cabau J, Colombo A, Latib A. Delayed Coronary Obstruction After Transcatheter Aortic Valve Replacement. *J Am Coll Cardiol.* 2018;71(14):1513-1524.

[29] Ielasi A, Latib A, Montorfano M, Colombo A. [Sandwich stenting to treat an ostial left main narrowing following transcatheter aortic valve implantation]. *Rev Esp Cardiol.* 2011;64(12):1220-2.

[30] Fiorina C, Curello S, Maffeo D, Lorusso R, Chizzola G, Ettori F. Management of acute left main obstruction after transcatheter aortic valve replacement: the "tunnel technique." *Cardiovasc Revasc Med.* 2012 Mar-Apr;13(2):142.e5-9.

[31] Romano V, Buzzatti N, Latib A, Colombo A, Montorfano M. Chimney technique for coronary obstruction after aortic valve in valve: pros and cons. *Eur Heart J Cardiovasc Imaging.* 2018;19(10):1194.

[32] Komatsu I, Mackensen GB, Aldea GS, Reisman M, Dvir D. Bioprosthetic or native aortic scallop intentional laceration to prevent iatrogenic coronary artery obstruction. Part 1: how to evaluate patients for BASILICA. *EuroIntervention.* 2019 May 20;15(1):47-54.

[33] Komatsu I, Mackensen GB, Aldea GS, Reisman M, Dvir D. Bioprosthetic or native aortic scallop intentional laceration to prevent iatrogenic coronary artery obstruction. Part 2: how to perform BASILICA. *EuroIntervention.* 2019 May 20;15(1):55-66.

[34] Leon MB1, Smith CR, Mack M, Miller DC, Moses JW, Svensson LG, Tuzcu EM, Webb JG, Fontana GP, Makkar RR, Brown DL, Block PC, Guyton RA, Pichard AD, Bavaria JE, Herrmann HC, Douglas PS, Petersen JL, Akin JJ, Anderson WN, Wang D, Pocock S; PARTNER Trial Investigators. Transcatheter aortic-valve implantation for aortic stenosis in patients who cannot undergo surgery. *N Engl J Med.* 2010;363:1597-607.

[35] Cribier A, Remadi F, Koning R, Rath P, Stix G, Letac B. Emergency balloon valvuloplasty as initial treatment of patients with aortic stenosis and cardiogenic shock. *N Engl J Med.* 1992;326:646.

[36] Buchwald AB, Meyer T, Scholz K, Schorn B, Unterberg C. Efficacy of balloon valvuloplasty in patients with critical aortic stenosis and cardiogenic shock--the role of shock duration. *Clin Cardiol.* 2001;24:214-8.

[37] Moreno PR, Jang IK, Newell JB, Block PC, Palacios IF. The role of percutaneous aortic balloon valvuloplasty in patients with cardiogenic shock and critical aortic stenosis. *J Am Coll Cardiol.* 1994;23:1071-5.

[38] Otto CM, Mickel MC, Kennedy JW, Alderman EL, Bashore TM, Block PC, Brinker JA, Diver D, Ferguson J, Holmes DR Jr, Lambrew CT, McKay CR, Palacios IF, Powers ER, Rahimtoola SH, Weiner BH, Davis KB. Three-year outcome after balloon aortic valvuloplasty. Insights into prognosis of valvular aortic stenosis. *Circulation.* 1994;89:642-50.

[39] Ben-Dor I, Maluenda G, Dvir D, Barbash IM, Okubagzi P, Torguson R, Lindsay J, Satler LF, Pichard AD, Waksman R. Balloon aortic valvuloplasty for severe aortic stenosis as a bridge to transcatheter/surgical aortic valve replacement. *Catheter Cardiovasc Interv.* 2013;82:632-7.

[40] Bongiovanni D, Kühl C, Bleiziffer S, Stecher L, Poch F, Greif M, Mehilli J, Massberg S, Frey N, Lange R, Laugwitz KL, Schymik G, Frank D, Kupatt C. Emergency treatment of decompensated aortic stenosis. *Heart.* 2018;104:23-29.

[41] Saia F, Moretti C, Dall'Ara G, Ciuca C, Taglieri N, Berardini A, Gallo P, Cannizzo M, Chiarabelli M, Ramponi N, Taffani L, Bacchi-Reggiani ML, Marrozzini C, Rapezzi C, Marzocchi A. Balloon aortic valvuloplasty as a bridge-to-decision in high risk patients with aortic stenosis: a new paradigm for the heart team decision making. *J Geriatr Cardiol.* 2016;13:475-82.

[42] Baumgartner H, Falk V, Bax JJ, De Bonis M, Hamm C, Holm PJ, Iung B, Lancellotti P, Lansac E, Rodriguez Muñoz D, Rosenhek R, Sjögren J, Tornos Mas P, Vahanian A, Walther T, Wendler O, Windecker S, Zamorano JL; ESC Scientific Document Group. 2017 ESC/EACTS Guidelines for the management of valvular heart disease. *Eur Heart J.* 2017;38:2739-2791.

[43] Otto CM, Kumbhani DJ, Alexander KP, Calhoon JH, Desai MY, Kaul S, Lee JC, Ruiz CE, Vassileva CM. 2017 ACC Expert Consensus Decision Pathway for Transcatheter

Aortic Valve Replacement in the Management of Adults With Aortic Stenosis: A Report of the American College of Cardiology Task Force on Clinical Expert Consensus Documents. *J Am Coll Cardiol.* 2017;69:1313-1346.

[44] Dvir D, Sagie A, Porat E, Assali A, Shapira Y, Vaknin-Assa H, Shafir G, Bental T, Nevzorov R, Battler A, Kornowski R. Clinical profile and outcome of patients with severe aortic stenosis at high surgical risk: single-center prospective evaluation according to treatment assignment. *Catheter Cardiovasc Interv.* 2013;81:871-81.

[45] Frerker C, Schewel J, Schlüter M, Schewel D, Ramadan H, Schmidt T, Thielsen T, Kreidel F, Schlingloff F, Bader R, Wohlmuth P, Schäfer U, Kuck KH. Emergency transcatheter aortic valve replacement in patients with cardiogenic shock due to acutely decompensated aortic stenosis. *EuroIntervention.* 2016;11:1530-6.

[46] Landes U, Orvin K, Codner P, Assali A, Vaknin-Assa H, Schwartznberg S, Levi A, Shapira Y, Sagie A, Kornowski R. Urgent Transcatheter Aortic Valve Implantation in Patients With Severe Aortic Stenosis and Acute Heart Failure: Procedural and 30-Day Outcomes. *Can J Cardiol.* 2016;32:726-31.

[47] Kolte D, Khera S, Vemulapalli S, Dai D, Heo S, Goldsweig A, Aronow HD, Elmariah S, Inglessis I, Palacios IF, Thourani VH, Sharaf BL, Gordon PC, Dawn J. Outcomes Following Urgent/Emergent Transcatheter Aortic Valve Replacement: Insights from the STS/ACC TVT Registry. *J Am Coll Cardiol Intv.* 2018;Epub ahead of print.

ABOUT THE EDITOR

Giovanni Concistrè, MD

Ospedale del Cuore "G. Pasquinucci",
Fondazione Toscana Gabriele Monasterio, Massa, Italy
Email: gioconci@libero.it

Dr. Giovanni Concistrè is currently an adult cardiac surgeon at the Ospedale del cuore "G. Pasquinucci", Massa, Italy. He received his Degree cum laude in Medicine at Perugia University, discussing the following thesis: "Clinic and echocardiografic follow-up of patients with the aortic valve replacement with a stentless bioprosthesis Toronto SPV". His interest in research developed over the years and when his father underwent surgery for coronary bypass grafting, he decided that he wanted to pursue a career in cardiac surgery. In October 2019, he got a Degree cum laude in Cardiac Surgery at Genova University, discussing the following thesis: "Left ventricular reshaping in ischemic dilated cardiomyopathy: Genoa's experience". In 2010 he worked at Department of Cardiac Surgery and Heart Transplantation of San Camillo Hospital in Rome and subsequently he became Assistentarzt at Deutsch Herz Zentrum in Munich and at Klinikum Nurnberg, Germany. From February 2013 to April 2014, he worked at Clinica S. Anna in Catanzaro, Italy. Concistrè is the author of numerous publications in scientific journals. He has always been interested in sutureless aortic bioprostheses, presenting also numerous works at international conferences. His 2nd Level Master's degree in "Innovations in Cardiac surgery: advances in minimally invasive therapeutics" was obtained at Scuola Superiore S. Anna, Pisa. Concistrè is a Reviewer for *Archives of Medical Science*, *Journal of Thoracic and Cardiovascular Surgery*, *Journal of Heart Valve Disease*, *European Journal of Cardio-Thoracic Surgery*. From May 2014, he is cardiac surgeon in Massa, Italy.

INDEX

A

M

N

O

P

R

S

T

V